# Nutrition
## for Life

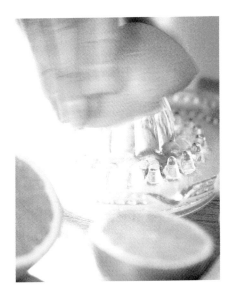

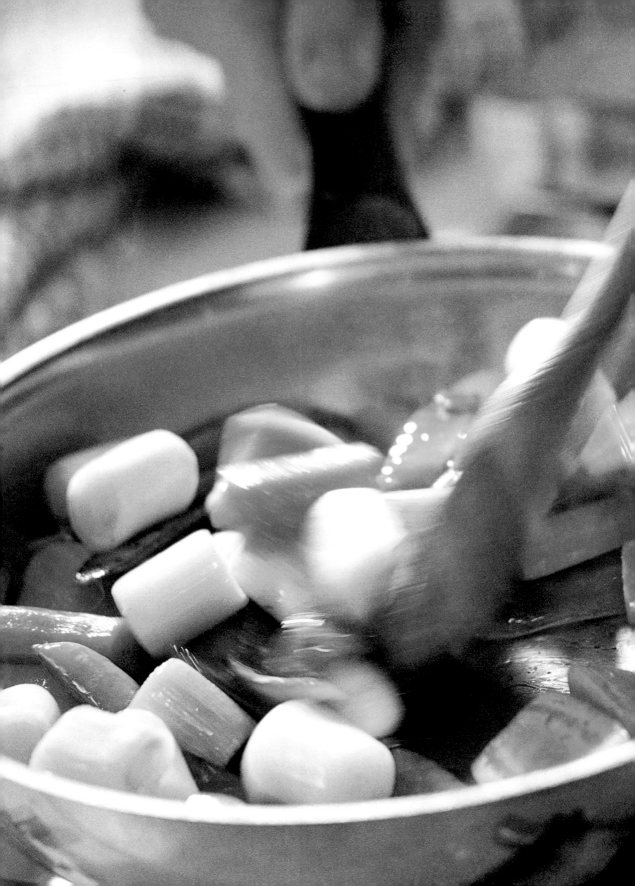

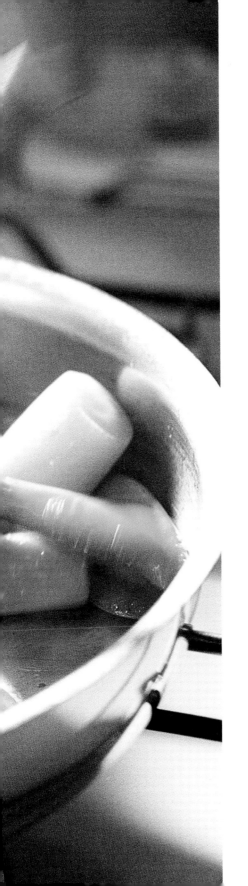

# Nutrition
## for Life

Lisa Hark PhD RD
and Dr Darwin Deen

Foreword by
Dr Ian W Campbell
President of the National Obesity Forum

LONDON, NEW YORK, MUNICH, MELBOURNE, DELHI

**Senior Editors** Irene Lyford, Liz Coghill
**Project Art Editor** Sara Kimmins
**Editor** Becky Alexander
**Editor for UK edition** Norma MacMillan
**Nutritionist for UK edition** Fiona Hunter
BSc Hons (Nutri.), Dip. Dietetics
**Designer** Isabel De Cordova
**Design Assistant** Iona Hoyle

**DTP Designer** Julian Dams
**Production Controller** Wendy Penn

**Senior Managing Editor** Jemima Dunne
**Managing Art Editor** Marianne Markham
**Category Publishers** Mary Thompson,
Corinne Roberts
**Art Director** Bryn Walls

First published in the United Kingdom in 2005 by
Dorling Kindersley
80 Strand London WC2R 0RL

Reprinted with corrections 2006

Paperback edition first published in the United Kingdom 2007

A Penguin Company

2 4 6 8 10 9 7 5 3

A CIP catalogue record for this book is available from the British Library

ISBN 978-1-4053-2835-7

All enquiries regarding any extracts or reuse of material in this book should be addressed to the publishers,
Dorling Kindersley Ltd

Publishers Note

Every effort has been made to ensure that the information in this book is accurate. The information in this book will be relevant to the majority
of people but may not be applicable in each individual case, so you are therefore advised to obtain expert medical advice for specific
information on personal health matters. Never disregard expert medical advice or delay in receiving treatment due to information obtained from
this book. The naming of any product, treatment, or organization in this book does not imply endorsement by the authors or the publisher,
nor does the omission of any such names indicate disapproval. Neither the publisher nor the authors accept any legal responsibility for any
personal injury or other damage or loss arising from any use or misuse of the information and advice in this book.

Note: Any recipes in this book are intended for people of generally good health, without specific food allergies

Colour reproduction by Colourscan, Singapore
Printed and bound by Tien Wah Press, Singapore

See our complete catalogue at
**www.dk.com**

# Contents

## Assess your health and lifestyle 10

## Food for life 32

## Elements of a healthy diet 68

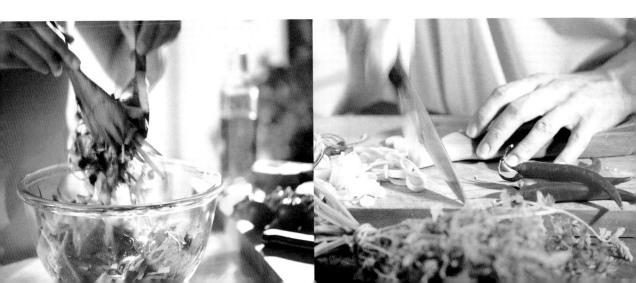

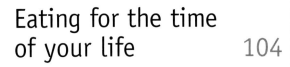

# Eating for the time of your life · 104

# The truth about weight control · 156

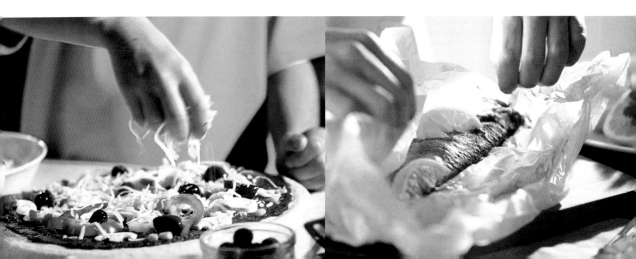

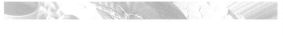

# Food as medicine 210

# The food you buy 272

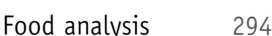

# Food analysis 294

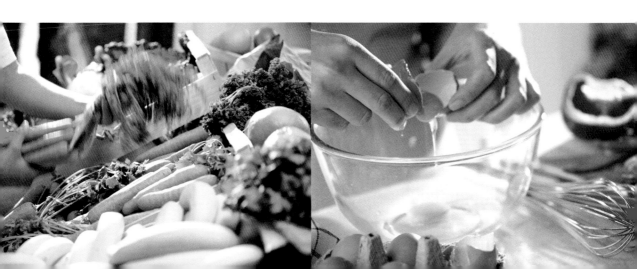

# Foreword

Recent years have seen a proliferation in our knowledge of science and improved medical care, but in the process we lost sight of one of the most fundamentally important factors influencing health: nutrition. We now recognize that what you eat can influence how you feel, your ability to concentrate, your ability to enjoy life, your resistance to infection, and your risk of developing serious diseases. The importance of a calorie-balanced diet to reduce the likelihood of overweight is clear, but so also is the need for adequate amounts of vitamins and minerals in the drive to both maintain good health and promote a better quality of life from childhood through old age.

   Much of what we regard as "modern disease" can be traced to lifestyle. Our attitudes to food, the way we prepare it, and how we eat can also positively, or adversely, influence our health. Whether our aim is to lose weight, improve management of health problems, or simply to maintain the good health we enjoy, there is so much that we as individuals can do to improve this basic foundation of good health, by improving our dietary intake.

   The difficulty for many has been knowing where to start. *Nutrition for Life* provides the practical information and advice needed. The food we eat is important both medically and socially: as we seize this opportunity for improving our health, we can also enjoy the fantastic social advantages of fun, appetizing, and nutritious food shared by the whole family. Life is for living, and nutrition is for life.

Dr Ian W Campbell
President of the National Obesity Forum

# Introduction

The publication of our book, *Nutrition for Life*, could not be more relevant today, with obesity at epidemic proportions both here, in North America, and throughout the industrialized and developing world. The World Health Organization estimates that there are now over 300 million obese adults worldwide, with more than 115 million suffering from obesity-related problems such as cardiovascular disease, cancer, and diabetes. These are overtaking more traditional health concerns such as undernutrition and infectious disease.

But what does this mean to you? Nutrition and lifestyle play a critical role at all stages of life, from infancy to old age; in *Nutrition for Life*, we show you how you can improve your health throughout your life, from many different perspectives. This is where our book is particularly relevant, since it addresses all the questions you may raise about taking care of your health and your family's health.

*Nutrition for Life* has been designed to help you to think seriously about your diet and lifestyle in an easy and enjoyable way. Whether you are single, married, have young or older children, are healthy, or suffer from a chronic medical condition, you will gain short-term and long-term health benefits from reading this book and by putting into effect the advice it contains.

LISA A HARK, PhD, RD
University of Pennsylvania
School of Medicine, Philadelphia

DARWIN DEEN, MD, MS
Albert Einstein College
of Medicine, New York

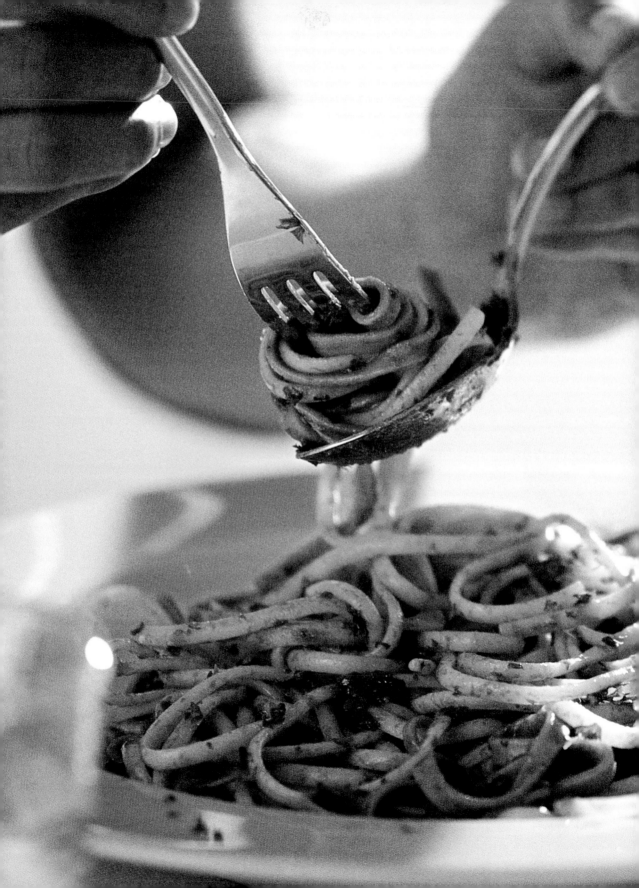

# Assess your health and lifestyle

As you think about improving your health, you will most likely start by making dietary and lifestyle changes. It is important to think about why you want to make these changes. Are they right for you, and will they help you achieve your goals? This chapter will help you identify key areas for change.

# The nutrition–energy balance

Good nutrition and regular exercise help you stay healthy and live longer.

You are what you eat. Everything that you eat and drink affects how your body functions. And, as your body's needs vary at different stages of your life and according to how you live your life, your nutritional needs vary too.

### Know your body's needs

The connection between diet and health is clear: to grow properly and function normally, you need a complete range of nutrients, including carbohydrates, proteins, fats, fibre, and water, as well as a variety of vitamins and minerals (*see Food for Life, pp.32–67*).

Many of these nutrients are not just essential for normal body functioning, but they can actually improve your state of health and protect you against a number of diseases. Eating well makes you feel well, which improves your mood and enables you to cope better with stress.

### Is your diet healthy?

If your diet lacks any nutrients or provides too much of certain factors, you will not function at an optimum level. At the same time, you may be creating future

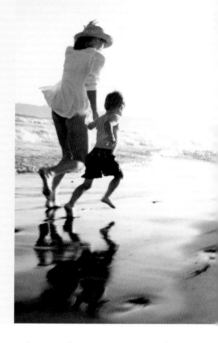

**Five-a-day** Include a minimum of five servings of fruits and vegetables each day to ensure that you have a health-giving range of vitamins and other nutrients in your diet.

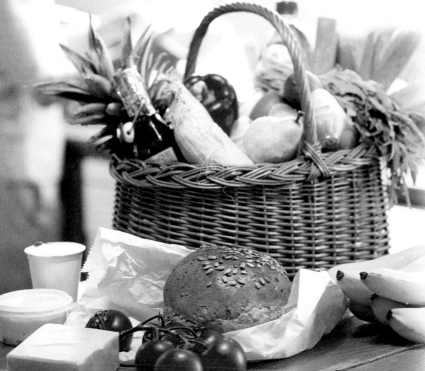

# The elements of good nutrition

To function properly, your body needs a daily intake of a full range of essential nutrients, including a variety of fruits, vegetables, pulses, whole grains, low-fat dairy products, lean meats, fish and shellfish, and healthy oils such as olive.

The foods we eat contain two main categories of nutrients: macronutrients and micronutrients. Macronutrients are needed in large quantities every day and form the foundation of any diet. They include proteins, carbohydrates, and fats, and provide energy.

Vitamins and minerals are found in small amounts in foods and make up the micronutrients. They play a critical role in maintaining the body's normal processes and functions.

Most foods contain both macro- and micronutrients in varying proportions. The key to achieving a healthy, well-balanced diet is to eat a wide variety of different foods.

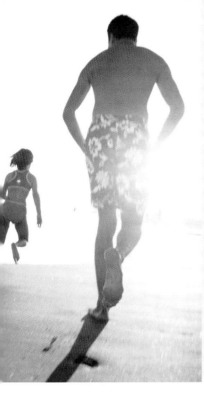

problems. For example, there is strong evidence that eating too much animal fat can lead to cardiovascular disease (*see p.214*), while skipping calcium-rich foods in your teens may lead to osteoporosis later (*see p.240*).

### The food–energy balance
To maintain a healthy weight, you need to balance the energy you take in from the food you eat with the energy you expend in the course of your daily life.

Because of our lifestyles or the type of work that we do, many of us do not get as much exercise as we need. Excess food intake is stored in the body as fat, leading to weight gain and possibly to

**Vibrant good health** A nutritious diet that meets your body's nutritional and energy needs, coupled with an active lifestyle, is the key to optimum health and well-being.

obesity. This, in turn, can lead to various medical conditions, such as diabetes, cardiovascular disease, cancer, and joint problems.

Of course the reverse is also true: if we expend more energy than we take in, we will lose weight – and this is the rationale behind many weight-loss diets (*see pp.162–197*). However, being underweight brings its own health problems and a reduced life expectancy (*see pp.208–209*).

### Is your lifestyle healthy?
In this chapter, we shall look at various aspects of diet, exercise, physical health, and weight, and invite you to review your status in those areas. If you already recognize the importance of diet and exercise, congratulations! If not, this information will help you identify any areas that are preventing you from achieving optimum health and fitness.

# Food and energy

The body gets energy, which is essential for life, from food. Our bodies expend the energy in various ways: some energy is used to maintain the critical day-to-day bodily functions that help us survive, such as breathing, heart rate, and other unconscious – also known as involuntary – activities. We also expend energy through our conscious daily activities, which can range from the sedentary – such as sitting, reading, or watching television – to participating in strenuous exercise and sport. Even activities such as thinking and sleeping require energy.

During some stages of our lives and in certain circumstances, including childhood, pregnancy and breast-feeding, athletic training, and when we are sick, or recovering from an illness,

**Energy equation** For optimum health, all of the energy we expend in activities must be balanced by the energy we obtain from food.

our bodies require extra energy to cope with the additional demands that are made. Similarly, people recovering from surgery or severe injury have extremely high energy requirements for the body's

repair mechanisms to function properly. If these extra energy requirements are not met by the food we eat, wounds may fail to heal and a full recovery will take a longer time to occur.

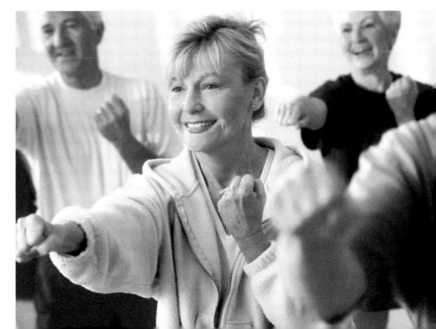

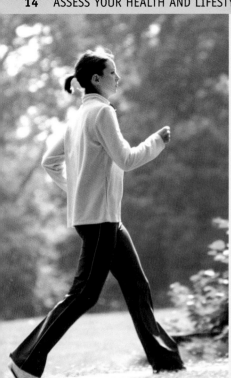

# Look at your lifestyle

## Take the first move towards optimizing your health.

Our aim in this book is to explain the link between what you eat and how you feel, whatever your lifestyle or dietary habits. We will also suggest ways of achieving optimum health and well-being for yourself and your family.

As a first step, we invite you to consider some simple questions about your diet and other lifestyle factors. We start by examining every aspect of your eating habits,

**Stepping up activity** Exercise is essential for health and well-being, so try to incorporate regular activity into your daily routine.

including how many times a day you eat, as well as what you eat and how much you eat.

Then we look at other aspects of your lifestyle. For example, how active are you? Do you take part in sport or in exercise programmes, or do you get your exercise just in walking your children to and from school each day or in your work? And finally, we consider any other factors that could have an effect on your nutritional health, such as your use of alcohol and tobacco.

## Assess your status

Once you have considered these questions, complete the quiz on page 21. Your score will identify what you are doing right as well as pinpoint any areas where changes could be made.

# The optimum number of meals a day

Do you eat three meals a day? There is no right or wrong answer to this question. Everyone's biological clock is different, and we all have different demands on our schedules. However, your body and mind need a steady supply of energy and nutrients throughout the day, so eating three balanced meals is the optimum way to achieve a healthy diet.

Studies show that people who eat less frequently than three times a day are more likely, when they do sit down to eat or have a snack, to indulge in foods that are higher in fat and calories. If you prefer to have just two meals a day, be sure that one of those is breakfast (*right*), and avoid eating big meals late at night. Children in particular need regular meals and snacks throughout the day.

**Regular meals** Eating three well-balanced meals every day gives your body a steady supply of vital nutrients.

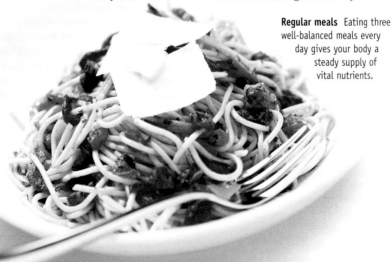

## Don't skip breakfast

Breakfast is an important meal. It breaks the long overnight fast, helping you wake up and get going; it stops you from feeling hungry later; and it helps you be more alert at school or work. If you eat before you leave home, you'll be less likely to grab a high-fat snack on the way to work.

● For a quick and healthy breakfast have a bowl of whole-grain cereal with fresh or dried fruit and milk – skimmed or semi-skimmed milk or soya milk.

● If you have more time, make an omelette or scrambled eggs. Serve with wholemeal or Granary toast.

● Make a smoothie by blending a banana or fresh berries with plain yogurt and skimmed or semi-skimmed milk or with fruit juice.

● If you must eat on the run, grab a piece of fresh fruit, such as a banana or apple, some nuts and seeds, or a low-fat yogurt.

# Snacking

Some people can get by on three meals a day, but for most of us snacking is a regular and enjoyable part of our daily routine. If you do snack, the key issues are what you snack on and why you do it. The question here is: are you really hungry or just craving food (*right*)?

If you really are hungry, then eat a healthy snack rather than wait for the next meal. This will prevent you from becoming over-hungry, and in turn will reduce the temptation to eat a nutrient-poor convenience food. Good choices for healthy snacks include fresh or dried fruit, raw vegetables, low-fat yogurt, rice cakes with peanut butter, and nuts and seeds. Stock up on healthy snacks for home, travel, and work so you always have them to hand.

Snacks are particularly important for children, who have small stomachs and so are unlikely to eat enough to meet their nutritional requirements in three meals. Regular healthy snacks are important for maintaining energy levels.

Many popular snacks, such as crisps, chocolate bars, and biscuits, contain lots of sugar, fat, and salt but have little nutritional value. So it's best to eat them once in a while rather than every day.

The key to regulating your dietary intake is to eat only when you are hungry and to stop when you are full. When you have the urge to snack, try to decide whether you really are hungry. Are you thirsty? Have a glass of water, then see if you still need food.

Think about what is triggering your urge to eat – is it boredom or maybe something you saw or smelled? Try to pinpoint exactly what it is that you are craving, and satisfy it. For example, if you really want chocolate, have just one piece – and savour it to the full.

## Hunger and cravings

When it comes to snacking, it is important to distinguish between real hunger and cravings.

**Hunger** This is a physiological response by which the body alerts the brain that nourishment is needed. If hungry, you may experience stomach discomfort or intestinal rumbling.

**Appetite** This is an instinctive physical desire to eat that occurs when you are hungry. It can be stimulated by outside influences.

**Craving** This is a psychological state affected by outside influences, such as the sight or smell of food, and by emotions, habits, moods, and imagination, rather than by hunger.

# Eating fruits and vegetables

Fruits and vegetables should form the basis of every diet. Every meal should contain them, and they should be your first choice for snacks.

Vegetarians (*see pp.100–101*) will already be reaping the benefits of these nutritious foods, but many people are not eating enough. Fruits and vegetables are fat-free, low in sodium, and provide essential nutrients, such as vitamin C, and folate, fibre, and phytochemicals. Evidence shows that eating at least five servings of fruits and vegetables a day may help prevent the development of cardiovascular disease (*see pp.214–221*) and cancer (*see pp.258–263*).

According to surveys done in the United States, the risk of cardiovascular disease is reduced in people who eat more than three servings of vegetables and fruits a day. The World Cancer Research Fund estimates that eating five or more servings every day could prevent 20 per cent of all cases of cancer. In addition, eating plenty of vegetables can help with weight control because they are high in fibre, which creates a feeling of fullness.

The British Dietetic Association, Food Standards Agency, and World Cancer Research Fund all recommend that we eat at least five servings of fruits and vegetables daily. Meeting the five-a-day target is not difficult, yet very few of us currently do so. You may be unsure what a serving actually comprises, so here are some examples:

- 1 medium-sized fruit, such as a banana, apple, or peach
- 150ml (5floz) fruit or vegetable juice
- 3 heaped tablespoons cooked peas or carrots, or a bowl of salad.

If you have a glass of fruit juice and cereal topped with a banana for breakfast, carrots as a snack, and green beans and a salad with dinner, you will easily get what you need.

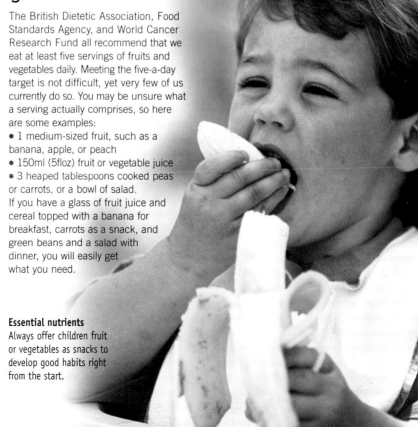

**Essential nutrients**
Always offer children fruit or vegetables as snacks to develop good habits right from the start.

# Dairy products and calcium

Milk, yogurt, cheese, and other dairy products are a prime source of the mineral calcium (*see p.62*). Calcium is the most abundant mineral in the body, but it is also the one most likely to be inadequately supplied in the normal diet. Many people in the UK do not consume enough calcium, with older adults and teenagers particularly at risk for a low intake.

## HEALTHY BONES AND TEETH

Calcium is essential for the normal growth and maintenance of bones and teeth, and calcium requirements must be met throughout life. Requirements are greatest during periods of growth, such as childhood, during pregnancy, and when breast-feeding. Calcium deficiency over the long term can lead to osteoporosis, in which the bone deteriorates and there is an increased risk of fractures (*see p.241*). You can meet your calcium needs by eating or drinking at least two to three servings of dairy products daily.

Some dairy products, such as hard cheeses and whole milk, contain a significant amount of saturated fat (*right*), a high intake of which is a risk factor for heart disease. Therefore, it's best to choose reduced- or low-fat dairy products (*see pp.82–83*) to meet your calcium requirements.

Cheese is a major source of saturated fat in the British diet, but this doesn't mean you have to give up cheese – reduced-fat versions of many popular cheeses, such as feta, Cheddar, and mozzarella, are widely available.

## Jargon buster

**Saturated fats**  Mainly of animal origin, these fats have chemical bonds "saturated" with hydrogen. A diet high in these fats is linked to raised blood cholesterol levels and cardiovascular disease.

**Unsaturated fats**  These fats, whose chemical bonds are not fully "saturated" with hydrogen, occur mainly in vegetable and fish oils. Monounsaturated fats, found in olive, rapeseed, and sesame oils, help protect against cardiovascular disease. Polyunsaturated fats, found in sunflower, groundnut, corn, and fish oils, are needed for growth, cell structure, and a healthy immune system (*see p.38*).

# Fish and shellfish are healthy choices

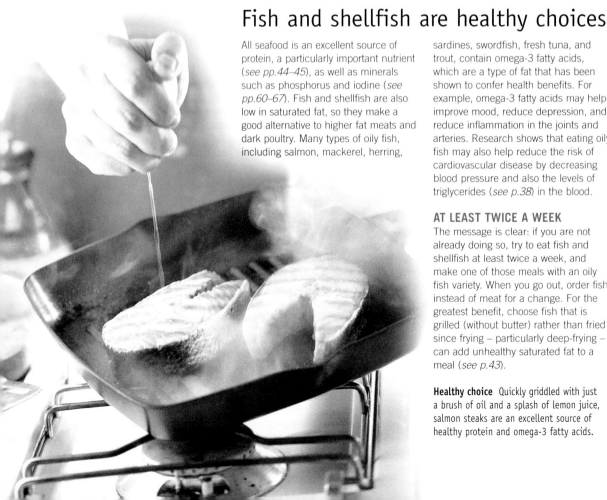

All seafood is an excellent source of protein, a particularly important nutrient (*see pp.44–45*), as well as minerals such as phosphorus and iodine (*see pp.60–67*). Fish and shellfish are also low in saturated fat, so they make a good alternative to higher fat meats and dark poultry. Many types of oily fish, including salmon, mackerel, herring, sardines, swordfish, fresh tuna, and trout, contain omega-3 fatty acids, which are a type of fat that has been shown to confer health benefits. For example, omega-3 fatty acids may help improve mood, reduce depression, and reduce inflammation in the joints and arteries. Research shows that eating oily fish may also help reduce the risk of cardiovascular disease by decreasing blood pressure and also the levels of triglycerides (*see p.38*) in the blood.

## AT LEAST TWICE A WEEK

The message is clear: if you are not already doing so, try to eat fish and shellfish at least twice a week, and make one of those meals with an oily fish variety. When you go out, order fish instead of meat for a change. For the greatest benefit, choose fish that is grilled (without butter) rather than fried since frying – particularly deep-frying – can add unhealthy saturated fat to a meal (*see p.43*).

**Healthy choice**  Quickly griddled with just a brush of oil and a splash of lemon juice, salmon steaks are an excellent source of healthy protein and omega-3 fatty acids.

# Benefits of turkey and chicken

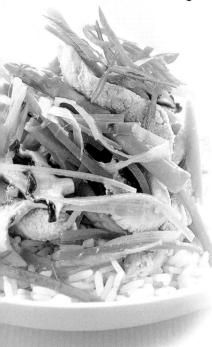

In addition to being excellent sources of protein, vitamins, and minerals, turkey and chicken are lower in both total and saturated fat than most red meat. The white meat (breast) of poultry contains less fat than the dark meat (wings and legs). However, both the fat and calorie content of turkey and chicken increase significantly if the skin is eaten.

Cooking chicken with the skin on will help to keep the meat moist, but the skin should be removed and discarded before eating. For example, a medium (150g/5oz) chicken breast, grilled and skin discarded, contains 220 calories and 3.3g fat, of which 0.9g is saturated fat. With the skin left on and eaten, the chicken breast contains 260 calories and 9.6g fat, of which 1.5g is saturated fat – almost double that when skinned.

**Oriental-style chicken** Unhealthy saturated fat is kept to a minimum in this appealing dish of lightly steamed chicken breast strips and vegetables, served with steamed rice.

# Eating red meat

Red meat – beef, lamb, veal, and pork – is a major source of protein and provides minerals including vitamin $B_{12}$, iron, and zinc. However, it can be high in saturated fat and cholesterol.

People who eat large amounts of red meat have higher rates of cardio-vascular disease than those who eat less. This is probably related to the saturated fat and cholesterol content. A high intake may also increase your risk of colon cancer. Studies have shown that people who replace red meat with chicken and fish have a lower risk of cardiovascular disease and colon cancer. Nutritionists now encourage us to eat more fish, healthy fats, and whole grains rather than red meat, saturated fat, and refined carbohydrates (see pp. 72–73).

If you really like red meat, make a point of choosing lean cuts, such as pork fillet or rump or fillet steak, and keep portion sizes modest. In addition, trim off excess fat before cooking and use low-fat cooking methods (see p.43).

# Using fats and oils

Fats are found not only in foods, but are also added during preparation, cooking, and serving. They are essential to your health, but one of the most interesting nutritional discoveries of the past decade has been that not all fats have the same effect on your health.

Saturated fats, such as butter, lard, and dripping, have been identified as having the potential to increase the risk of cardiovascular disease. This is because they raise the levels of cholesterol in the bloodstream. However, we now know that other fats, such as monounsaturated and polyunsaturated fats, found in plant-based oils and fish, are healthy and may protect against disease (see p.40).

As a first step in modifying your diet, substitute olive or rapeseed oil for animal fats in your cooking (see p.41). Bear in mind, though, that whichever oil you choose, it will provide 99 calories per tablespoon. So all fats, including oils, should be used in moderation.

**Beneficial oils** Monounsaturated fats, which are found in abundance in olive and rapeseed oils, have been shown to reduce the risk of cardiovascular disease when they are eaten as part of a healthy diet.

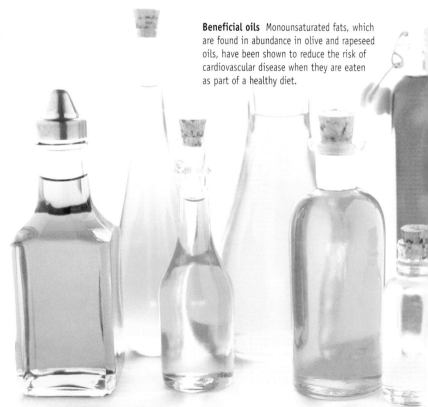

# Drinking water

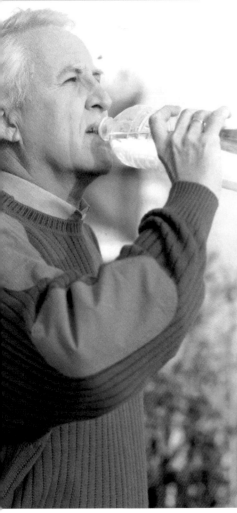

Water is an essential part of the diet. Humans are able to survive for several weeks without food, but for only a few days without water. Since the body has no means of storing water, you need a constant supply to replenish the fluid that you lose through sweating and urination. This means that you need to drink at least six to eight glasses of water every day, and more when it is hot or when playing sport or taking exercise. Do not wait until you are thirsty, since thirst may indicate that you are already lacking the water you need (see pp.96–97).

### LIMIT FIZZY DRINKS AND JUICE

In the UK, the consumption of fizzy drinks has doubled in the past 15 years – on average, we now drink over 2 litres (3½ pints) of sugary fizzy drinks, squash, and fruit juice per person every week. Although these sorts of drinks provide fluid, they also contribute a large amount of calories and sugars to the diet. The marked increase in the consumption of sugary fizzy drinks and juice is believed to be a major factor in the rising number of overweight children in Britain.

**Water of life** To help you get into the habit of drinking more water, carry a bottle with you or have one on your desk at work.

### MAKING CHANGES

You can save hundreds of calories each day by paying attention to what you drink during the day, and by trying to substitute still or sparkling water, or other low-calorie drinks, for those with a high sugar content. If you make only one dietary change after reading this book, drinking water rather than cola may be the most realistic and effective one that you can do. If you currently have a juice drink with lunch and a sugary fizzy drink with snacks, wean yourself off these gradually: substitute water for lunch for about a week, then slowly, over time, introduce more water or diet drinks. Try a glass of skimmed milk with snacks, to boost your fluid levels and also your calcium intake.

We are constantly being urged to drink six to eight glasses of water each day for better health. For many years, it was believed that caffeinated beverages did not count towards this fluid intake because they have a dehydrating effect. However, a recent study found there was no evidence to substantiate this belief, so beverages such as coffee and tea, which consist mainly of water, can count towards your daily fluid needs.

Adequate fluid intake is vital for everyone, but especially for the elderly, who are prone to dehydration because of a decline in their thirst sensation.

# Eating away from home

In the UK, the number of meals eaten away from home continues to rise. According to recent research, this trend is most likely due to the increase in the number of two-career families, who have very little time for food shopping, and preparing and cooking meals at home during the week.

It may be that you frequently have to eat away from home because of your work schedule or lifestyle. Being aware of the pitfalls will enable you to make healthy choices. For example, you could choose a grilled chicken sandwich instead of a cheese-topped burger, and order small portions or share larger ones. Instead of having chips, you can opt for a side salad, which is nutritious and much lower in fat.

Restaurant meals usually contain more fat and therefore more calories than food prepared at home. Also, portions in restaurants are often larger than those served at home. So if possible it is a good idea to share a starter when eating out,

or to eat only part of what you are served. Try to control the portion sizes by not feeling obliged to eat everything on your plate. Stop eating when you feel full.

Wherever possible, choose food that is grilled, poached, or baked, rather than fried, as the latter will be higher in calories and saturated fat content. Order sauces and salad dressings "on the side" and choose fruit or sorbet for dessert – or better still, skip it altogether.

Pizza and fast-food restaurants are frequent sources of food consumed away from home. When you are eating in these places, beware of "supersize" portions and "value meals" or "meal deals" – for example, double cheeseburger, extra large fries, and a large fizzy drink. Deals such as this are marketed together to seem like a bargain, and therefore offer a financial incentive to consume more food than you would otherwise have bought or eaten.

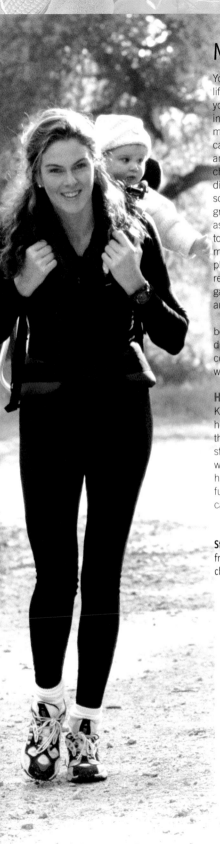

**Starting young** Walking is a healthy, cost-free activity that everyone can enjoy, so get children into the habit from an early age.

# Maintaining an active lifestyle

Your level of activity depends on your lifestyle and how you regularly spend your days. For example, if your work involves standing or moving around for most of the day, or lifting, moving, and carrying heavy objects, then you have an active lifestyle. If you have young children, you may be walking a long distance daily, taking them to and from school. Alternatively, you may expend a great deal of energy on the physical aspects of caring for babies and toddlers. Domestic and leisure pursuits may also involve you in a high level of physical activity – for example, you may regularly spend time doing housework, gardening, or carrying out home repair and maintenance work.

On the other hand, your lifestyle may be predominantly sedentary: you may drive to work, sit at a desk all day, then come home and watch television or work on a computer in the evenings.

### HEALTH BENEFITS

Keeping active will help you to stay healthy and feel good. Health is more than just the absence of disease: it is a state of physical, mental, and spiritual well-being. On a physical level, your health reflects how well your body functions in terms of allowing you to carry out your daily activities. But it is also a reflection of your state of mind. No matter how physically fit you are, if you do not feel good about yourself, then you are not healthy.

It is important to be as active as possible, incorporating activities into your life that keep you moving in an enjoyable and rewarding way. This is particularly important if you have a sedentary job, such as sitting at a computer for eight hours a day.

### INACTIVE CHILDREN

Children are born with a desire to be active; toddlers love to run around, climb, and explore, and this energy and love of exercise should be continued into later life. It is important for long-term health that parents encourage their children to be active and provide the opportunity for children to fulfill this need.

Most British children today are less active than children were in previous generations. This coincides with an increase in the number of overweight children in this country (*see p.206*). A decrease in opportunities for exercise, and an increased interest in sedentary activities for children of all ages – but especially teenagers – have led to an increase in weight problems.

Overweight children are at risk for many of the same health problems as overweight adults (*see p.206*). Statistics show that these problems may continue into adult life. Leading an active life as a family can help your child enjoy long-term good health.

## TV and weight gain

It is well documented that the more television you watch, the more likely you are to be overweight, with all the negative implications for health that this brings with it.

Excessive television watching and computer use has been linked to the increase in numbers of overweight children and adolescents in the UK. A sensible recommendation to follow is that children should be limited to no more than two hours per day of watching television and videos and using computers. To achieve this, try to limit the time your whole family spends watching television or using the computer, and find more active ways of using leisure time.

You might also try to be more active while you watch television. For example, you could buy an exercise bike or treadmill and use it while you view. If that sounds too strenuous, you could do the ironing or some light cleaning, or lift light weights while sitting on the sofa.

# Health and exercise

Recent figures indicate that 64 per cent of men and 74 per cent of women in this country do not get enough exercise. The combination of more sedentary behaviours and increased calorie intake is believed to be the major reason for the current rise in obesity in the UK.

Regular physical exercise provides many health benefits. It reduces your risk of cardiovascular disease and osteoporosis, helps with weight control, improves flexibility, reduces stress, and improves your overall quality of life. Many studies state that brisk walking for 30 minutes each day can reduce the risk of developing both cardiovascular disease and diabetes by at least 30 per cent. Even if you do not want to take up a new exercise programme, you can improve your level of physical activity by making simple modifications in your daily life. For example, take the stairs instead of the lift, park your car farther away than usual from your destination, and take a walk after dinner.

**Regular exercise** Whether you visit the gym, go swimming, or have a daily walk, regular exercise is essential for good health.

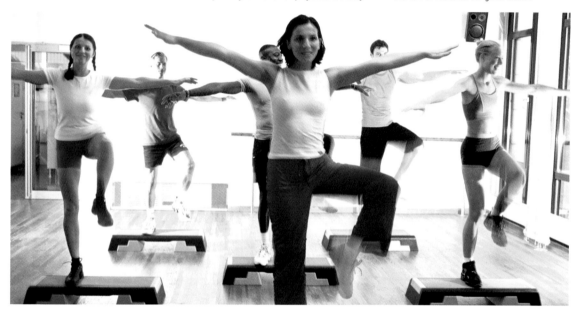

# Drinking alcohol

Alcohol has very little nutritional value, and excess consumption can lead to a number of medical problems, including certain vitamin deficiencies (*see pp.52–58*). Alcohol also adds a significant amount of empty calories to the diet, with consequent weight gain. Beer and ale are particularly high in calories, as are liqueurs.

However, moderate drinkers have lower rates of cardiovascular disease than either abstainers or excessive drinkers. Drinking alcohol in moderation may even offset some of the harmful effects of a high-fat diet. This is exemplified by the French, who tend to eat a diet that is moderately high in saturated fat, but suffer less cardiovascular disease than would be expected. This "French paradox" may be due to the antioxidants in red wine, which may protect against the harmful effects of saturated fats.

## Jargon buster

**Antioxidants** These are substances that help neutralize the damaging effect on cells and tissues of by-products known as free radicals. Sources of antioxidants available from the diet include vitamins A, C, and E and the minerals copper, selenium, and zinc.

# Smoking

Stopping smoking is the best lifestyle change you can ever make. Smoking increases your risk of cardiovascular disease, chronic lung disease, and many cancers; passive smoking – inhaling "secondhand" smoke – can cause pneumonia and asthma; and pregnant smokers put their babies at risk of prematurity, low birth weight, and even foetal death.

Within months of cutting down on the amount you smoke, your health will improve. Many smokers are concerned about gaining weight if they stop, but from a health standpoint, smoking is much more risky than carrying a few extra pounds in weight.

# Questionnaire How healthy is your lifestyle?

Circle the letter corresponding to the answer that best describes your habits. Then find your score by adding the points associated with the circled letters.

## 1 How many meals do you usually eat each day ?

a  Three meals and one snack.
b  Three meals with no snacks.
c  Two meals, skipping breakfast or lunch.
d  I usually eat only one meal a day.

## 2 What types of snacks do you eat?

a  Fruits, vegetables, nuts, and/or yogurt.
b  Salted nuts, popcorn, fruit, and/or yogurt.
c  Crisps, pretzels, popcorn, and/or other "junk" food.
d  Sweets, such as chocolate, pastries, and/or biscuits.

## 3 How many servings of fruits and vegetables do you eat each day?

a  I always eat five or more servings of fruits and vegetables a day.
b  I usually eat three or four servings.
c  I usually eat about one serving.
d  I usually eat fruits and vegetables only a few times per week.

## 4 Which dairy products, if any, do you usually eat or drink?

a  Fat-free dairy products, such as yogurt and skimmed milk.
b  Skimmed milk, low-fat yogurt, and reduced-fat cheeses.
c  Semi-skimmed milk, low-fat cream cheese, and reduced-fat ice cream.
d  Regular fat dairy products, such as whole milk and ice cream.

## 5 How often do you usually eat fish or shellfish?

a  I eat fish or shellfish at least twice a week.
b  I usually eat fish or shellfish once a week.
c  I usually eat fish or shellfish a few times a month.
d  I rarely or never eat fish or shellfish.

## 6 Which types of poultry do you eat?

a  Chicken or turkey breast with the skin removed.
b  Chicken or turkey breast with the skin on.
c  I occasionally eat breadcrumbed fried chicken or turkey breast.
d  I frequently choose the dark meat of chicken, duck, goose, etc.

## 7 How often do you eat red meat?

a  I never eat red meat.
b  Once or twice a month.
c  Several times a week.
d  I eat red meat every day.

## 8 Which fats and oils do you use?

a  I try to limit my use of any fat or oil when cooking.
b  I usually use olive or rapeseed oil.
c  I usually use butter when cooking.
d  I frequently use bacon fat, lard, or dripping when cooking.

## 9 Apart from coffee or tea, what do you usually drink during the day?

a  I usually drink water exclusively.
b  100 per cent fruit juice, water, and diet cola.
c  Sugary fizzy drinks, sports drinks, and juice drinks.
d  Sugary fizzy drinks and other sugar-sweetened drinks.

## 10 When eating out, which of the following would you usually choose?

a  Grilled, baked, or steamed main courses.
b  Pasta with seafood in marinara or tomato sauce.
c  Roast beef, steak, veal, lamb, or pasta in a cream sauce.
d  Pizza, sausages, burgers, and deep-fried foods.

## 11 How much exercise do you get?

a  I usually exercise for at least 30–60 minutes on most days.
b  I usually exercise for 30 minutes a few days a week.
c  I exercise for 30 minutes a few times a month.
d  I rarely participate in any physical activity.

## 12 How much TV do you watch?

a  I rarely watch television.
b  I watch a few hours of television every week.
c  I watch less than two hours daily.
d  I usually watch three or more hours of television every day.

## 13 How often do you drink alcohol and how much?

a  I usually have one or two units of alcohol a week.
b  I usually have one or two units of alcohol every day.
c  I rarely drink alcohol.
d  I usually have at least three units of alcohol daily.

## 14 Do you smoke? If so how many cigarettes do you smoke per day?

a  I have never smoked, or I stopped more than eight years ago.
b  I smoke fewer than five cigarettes a day.
c  I smoke five to ten cigarettes a day or up to five cigars.
d  I smoke more than ten cigarettes a day.

**Score  a** 1  **b** 2  **c** 3  **d** 4

**11–20 points**  Congratulations! Your diet is healthy and you should be proud of yourself. Keep up the good work. Read on to learn more.

**21–29 points**  You are making good choices, but are you ready for the next step? This book will give you the information you need to improve your health now and for the future. Set realistic goals that you can achieve and maintain.

**30–52 points**  Your diet may be too high in fat and too low in fruits and vegetables. You are risking your future health by selecting fatty foods and not getting enough exercise. Use the information in this book to help you understand your barriers to making changes and how you can really improve your health and the health of your family.

# Check your physical health

## Understanding your own health status helps you take control.

Once you begin to understand your health status in the context of both your lifestyle behaviours and your medical history, you will be in the best possible position to work with your doctor and dietitian to take charge of your health. Being able to understand why changes in diet and exercise will improve your health, longevity, and mental well-being will make it easier for you to achieve any changes necessary.

### Get a check-up
As part of the assessment of your current physical health, you may visit your doctor for a check-up. Many of the procedures that he or

**Family traits** To help you assess your risks of developing certain diseases, it is useful to look at your family medical history.

she carries out, such as measuring weight, height, pulse, and blood pressure, relate to your risk for developing cardiovascular disease, which is an important cause of premature death in the UK.

Some of the risks, such as your age, gender, and family history, cannot be altered (*below right*), but other risk factors can be modified by making changes to your diet and lifestyle. If you are in a high-risk category for cardiovascular disease because of non-modifiable risk factors, then it is vital that you tackle the areas where changes are possible to improve your overall health and long-term wellness.

### Look at your family
You should consider your family medical history to become aware of the medical conditions from which your parents, grandparents, and other blood relatives suffered. This will provide you with an opportunity to identify potential health issues in your own life and

to take the appropriate action to modify your risks of developing those conditions yourself.

The risks of asthma, migraines, diabetes, high blood pressure, and cardiovascular disease have all been shown to run in families or to have a genetic component.

If you are reading this book because you currently suffer from a health problem, there is much that you can do yourself to control and improve matters with diet and lifestyle changes. This is covered in detail in the chapter Food as Medicine (*see pp.210–263*). It is a good idea to discuss any changes you wish to make with your GP or a state-registered dietitian.

## Risk factors for cardiovascular disease

Many factors are known to increase your risk of developing cardiovascular disease. Some you cannot control, others you can.

### Non-modifiable high risk factors
Factors such as age, gender, and family history are predetermined, but you can reduce their impact with nutrition and exercise.
- Age: men over the age of 45 and women over the age of 55.
- Gender: cardiovascular disease is more common in men than in pre-menopausal women.
- Heredity: the risk of heart attack is greater if there is a family history of cardiovascular disease before 60.

### Modifiable high risk factors
You can change the following by adopting a healthier lifestyle:
- High cholesterol or LDL level
- Current cigarette smoking
- High blood pressure
- Diabetes
- Overweight or obesity
- Physical inactivity

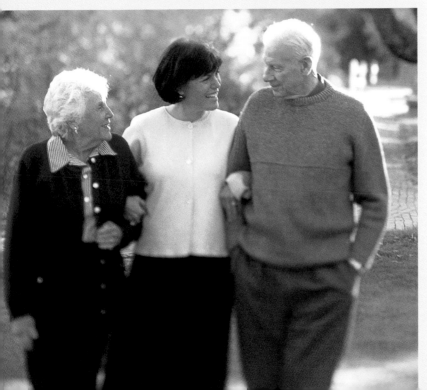

# Having a medical check-up

When you visit your doctor for a medical check-up, he or she will take a number of measurements, all of which will help assess your current state of health. These could include checking your pulse rate, listening to your heart and lungs with a stethoscope, measuring your blood pressure, and checking your weight and height.

Depending on your personal and family medical history, your GP may also take a blood sample that will be sent to the laboratory to be tested for specific conditions (*below*).

## CHECKING YOUR PULSE

Pulse is a measure of heart rate and can be felt where an artery (a blood vessel carrying blood away from the heart) runs close to the skin. In adults, the pulse rate is usually felt at the wrist.

A low resting pulse rate is a good indicator of physical fitness: the stronger your heart, the less frequently it needs to pump to provide oxygen to your tissues. Babies have a high pulse rate, but as we age the pulse rate decreases. The normal pulse rate for adults is 60–80 beats per minute. Know your figures, and how these compare to others of your age and gender.

## MEASURING BLOOD PRESSURE

This is a measure of the pressure of the blood in your arteries as your heart is pumping. The value depends on the strength of your heart muscle and the elasticity of the arterial walls, as well as the volume and viscosity of your blood.

The blood pressure of a healthy adult should ideally be no higher than 120/80mmHg. A diagnosis of high blood pressure is made if the reading is persistently above 140/90mmHg.

## LIFESTYLE CHANGES

If you are diagnosed with high blood pressure, make lifestyle changes, such as losing weight, increasing the amount of exercise you take, and limiting your use of salt and alcohol (*see p.220*). If these are not enough to normalize your blood pressure, your GP may prescribe medication, since high blood pressure is a risk factor for other cardiovascular diseases such as heart attack.

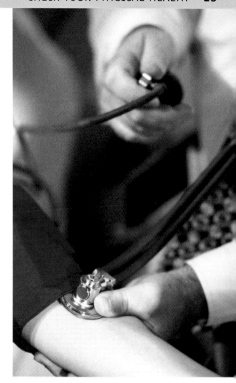

**Blood pressure**  Persistently high blood-pressure levels are associated with an increased risk of cardiovascular disease, so regular checks are essential.

# Blood tests and health

Depending on the reason for your medical check-up, the symptoms that you have described, or your family medical history, your doctor may take a blood sample that will be sent to a laboratory for testing. The tests help to assess your health and diagnose certain diseases.

**Cholesterol**  A waxy substance in the blood that is necessary for the normal functioning of the body (*see p.40*). Excess amounts of cholesterol can form deposits on the inside of blood vessels, leading to narrowing of the arteries and cardiovascular disease.

A total cholesterol level above 5mmol per litre may be hereditary and/or due to a diet that is high in saturated fat (*see p.38*). For information on how to help lower your blood-cholesterol levels, see page 217.

**Low density lipoprotein (LDL)**  Often called the "bad" cholesterol, LDL carries cholesterol from the liver to tissues. Levels greater than 3.0mmol per litre are linked with increased risk of cardiovascular disease (*see p.214*).

**High density lipoprotein (HDL)** Carries cholesterol from the tissues back to the liver. It is often referred to as the "good" cholesterol, since high levels (greater than 1.0mmol per litre for men and 1.4mmol for women) are associated with a reduced risk of cardiovascular disease (*see p.214*).

**Triglycerides**  Fatty substances in the blood that are absorbed from the diet or synthesized from excess calories. High levels of triglycerides (above 2.0mmol per litre) may be a risk factor for cardiovascular disease.

**Glucose**  The predominant sugar in the blood and may be measured at different times during the day – for example, first thing in the morning, before eating, or two hours after meals. Interpreting the results depends on when the glucose was measured. If the level of glucose in a fasting blood sample is over 6.7mmol per litre, diabetes is diagnosed (*see p.246*).

**Haemoglobin**  The protein in red blood cells that carries iron. Anaemia occurs when haemoglobin levels are lower than 13.5g per decilitre for men or 11.5g for women (*see p.66*).

**Haematocrit**  The measure of the volume percentage of red blood cells in whole blood. Levels lower than 40 per cent for men and 36 per cent for women indicate anaemia.

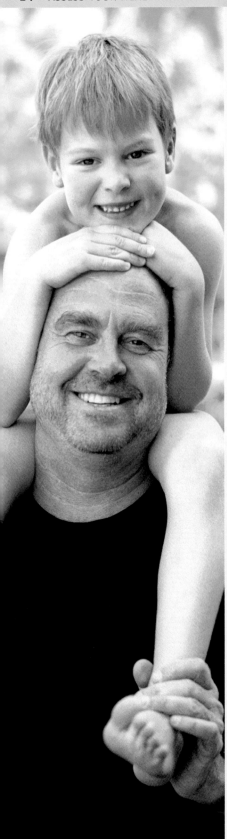

# Assess your shape and weight

## Body shape and weight provide vital clues to your health.

Most of us will wind up looking like one of our parents. Just as the colour of our hair and eyes is transmitted through our genes, so too is our height and weight distribution, though these can be influenced by diet and exercise.

### Weight distribution

Studies show that in overweight people, the distribution of excess body fat can affect their risk of developing cardiovascular disease and diabetes. Compared to "pear-shaped" individuals, who store fat around their hips and thighs, "apple-shaped" people are at an increased risk. Having a "beer belly" is no joke: a few extra centimetres around the waist may be a signal of bad things to come.

### Assessing healthy weight

Healthy weight is now defined according to body mass index (BMI), which is calculated as a ratio of weight to height (see pp.26–27). This index provides a more accurate measure of body fat than weight alone. Along with body shape, BMI assesses the risk of developing diabetes, cancer, and cardiovascular disease.

Guidelines in the UK define overweight people as those with a BMI of 25–29.9. People with a BMI of 30 and above are classified as obese and those with a BMI over 35 as extremely obese. These

definitions are based on evidence that many people with a BMI of 25 or greater begin to develop an increase in LDL, total cholesterol, and blood-sugar levels, in addition to prehypertension (see p.214) or high blood pressure.

### Risks of excess weight

The National Diet and Nutrition Survey showed that 41 per cent of men and 33 per cent of women in the UK are overweight, and that a further 22 per cent of both men and women are obese. Obesity is becoming common – in adults and children – and this is having an impact on our national health: the National Audit Office estimated for England that 30,000 deaths a year result from obesity.

If your BMI is above 25, we suggest you read the information and advice on weight control and weight reduction (see pp.156–207).

## Health risks of obesity

If your BMI is 30 or above, you are considered to be "obese", and your health may be at risk. Therefore, it is advisable to see your doctor and make every effort to lose weight.

Statistics show that being obese greatly increases your chance of diabetes and of cardiovascular diseases such as hyperlipidaemia, high blood pressure, and stroke.

Being obese also increases your chance of gall-bladder disease, sleep apnoea, osteoarthritis, and respiratory problems. You are also more at risk of certain types of cancers, including breast, colon, prostate, and endometrial.

If you need to have surgery of any kind, you may be required to lose weight first to minimize risk; this could lead to a lengthy delay.

**Family likeness** Body shape and weight are associated with various health risks, but although our basic body type is inherited, this can be modified by diet and exercise.

# Where is your fat located?

Men and women store fat in different areas of the body. In men, it is deposited mostly in the upper arms, shoulders, and abdomen; in women, it is mainly deposited in the breasts, hips, buttocks, and thighs. For both sexes, measuring your waist gives a good indication of whether you are carrying excess weight:
• In your underwear, find the mid-point between the uppermost part of your hip bone and your lowest rib.
• Mark this point and measure round your waist with a tape measure, keeping the tape parallel to the floor and snug, but not tight. Make sure you breathe normally as you take the measurement.

A waist circumference above 94cm (37in) in men and 80cm (32in) for women indicates that you are carrying excess weight around your middle, which increases your risk of developing high blood pressure, raised cholesterol levels, diabetes, and cardiovascular disease. Men with a waist measurement of 102cm (40in) and women of 88cm (35in) puts you at high risk.

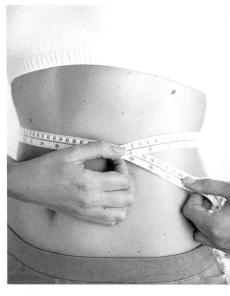

## Are you an apple or a pear?

People who tend to gain weight mainly in the abdominal region (a paunch or "beer belly") are said to have an apple shape. If you tend to gain weight mostly on your hips, buttocks, and thighs, you are said to have a pear shape. The location of your body fat affects your health. If you are apple shaped, you are at increased risk for the health problems associated with obesity, including cardiovascular diseases, such as high blood pressure, and diabetes (*opposite*). You cannot do anything to change being an apple or a pear – it is an inherited characteristic. However, you can limit its extent by controlling your weight and keeping fit.

**Identify your body shape** Measuring your waist is a simple way of checking whether you are an apple or a pear and if you are at increased risk of certain diseases.

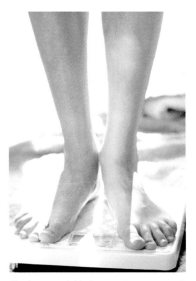

**Check your weight** An accurate measurement of your weight is an essential part of your assessment. Weigh yourself once a week – in the same clothes, in your underwear, or naked – at the same time of day, ideally in the morning before breakfast.

# How to weigh yourself

There are several dos and don'ts to be aware of if you want to get the most accurate measurement of your weight from your bathroom scales, especially if you are trying to lose weight.
• For accuracy, make sure that the bathroom scales you use are from a reputable company. Don't buy the cheapest that you can find because they may not be very accurate.
• Each time you weigh yourself, do it wearing the same clothes, in your underwear, or naked.
• Make sure that you use the same scales in the same place each time you weigh yourself. If possible, get yourself bathroom scales that only you can use. Because different scales vary in their accuracy and how they are calibrated, it is likely that you will get slightly different results if you change the scales that you use. For example, you might find that you are heavier on different scales just because they are not very accurate.

Beware of using the scales in the gym – they may seem accurate, but hundreds of people use them and they are prone to wear and tear.
• Always weigh yourself at the same time of day, ideally with an empty bladder and bowels and nothing in your stomach. First thing in the morning after you visit the toilet and before you have breakfast is the best time of day.
• Don't weigh yourself more than once a week. We all have normal fluctuations in body weight – especially for women during their menstrual cycle – and you may be disheartened if you weigh more than on the previous day.
• If you are trying to lose weight through an exercise regime, you should be aware that muscle weighs more than fat tissue. There may be a point in your regime when you look slimmer and more toned but you stay the same weight or even weigh more because you are more muscular. Don't get discouraged.

# Are you a healthy weight for your height?

Body mass index (BMI) is based on a ratio of your weight to your height. Use the chart below to find out whether or not your weight is within the normal range for your height.

If you find that you are overweight, it is advisable that you consult your GP, nurse, or a state-registered dietitian to discuss how to begin a weight-control programme (see also pp.156–207).

While BMI is a more useful indicator of body fat than the gender-specific height–weight tables that were used previously, it does have limitations. For example, it may overestimate body fat in very muscular people because muscle weighs more than fat. It may underestimate the amount of body fat in some underweight people who have lost lean tissue, such as older adults. Also, people who are tall but have a small frame might have excess fat around their waist, yet show a normal BMI. If you are puzzled or concerned by your BMI result, talk to your GP, who will explain the implications to you and give you advice on modifying your diet and lifestyle. If you have not had your height measured for many years, arrange to have it measured again because height can change with age.

There are other devices for measuring the proportion of fat in the body, and your doctor may employ one of these to double-check your findings. In the most widely used device, a harmless electric current passes through the body and identifies areas of muscle and fat.

**Using the BMI table** Find your height in the left-hand column of the body mass index (BMI) table (below), then move across that row until you find the column that corresponds with your weight (as given at the top of the chart). The number shown where your height and weight converge is your BMI score.

The colour coding in the key below will indicate whether you are underweight, in the healthy weight range, overweight, or obese. For example, if your height is 1.68m (66in) and your weight is 64kg (140lb), your BMI is 23. This means that your weight is in the healthy range. If your height is 1.68m (66in) and your weight is 70kg (155lb), your BMI is 25, which means that you are classified as being overweight.

For a more detailed interpretation of BMI scores, and advice on nutritional or lifestyle changes that may be beneficial to your health, see opposite.

## Key

**Underweight:** BMI 18.5 or below
**Healthy weight:** BMI 19.0–24.9
**Overweight:** BMI 25–29.9
**Obese:** BMI above 30

## BODY MASS INDEX (BMI) TABLE

| Height \ Weight | 45kg/ 100lb | 48kg/ 105lb | 50kg/ 110lb | 52kg/ 115lb | 55kg/ 120lb | 57kg/ 125lb | 59kg/ 130lb | 61kg/ 135lb | 64kg/ 140lb | 66kg/ 145lb | 68kg/ 150lb | 70kg/ 155lb | 73kg/ 160lb | 75kg/ 165lb | 77kg/ 170lb |
|---|---|---|---|---|---|---|---|---|---|---|---|---|---|---|---|
| 1.53m (60in) | 20 | 21 | 21 | 22 | 23 | 24 | 25 | 26 | 27 | 28 | 29 | 30 | 31 | 32 | 33 |
| 1.55m (61in) | 19 | 20 | 21 | 22 | 23 | 24 | 25 | 26 | 26 | 27 | 28 | 29 | 30 | 31 | 32 |
| 1.58m (62in) | 18 | 19 | 21 | 22 | 22 | 23 | 24 | 25 | 26 | 27 | 27 | 28 | 29 | 30 | 31 |
| 1.60m (63in) | 18 | 19 | 20 | 21 | 21 | 22 | 23 | 24 | 25 | 26 | 27 | 27 | 28 | 29 | 30 |
| 1.63m (64in) | 17 | 18 | 20 | 21 | 21 | 21 | 22 | 23 | 24 | 25 | 26 | 27 | 27 | 28 | 29 |
| 1.65m (65in) | 17 | 17 | 19 | 20 | 20 | 21 | 22 | 22 | 23 | 24 | 25 | 26 | 27 | 27 | 28 |
| 1.68m (66in) | 16 | 17 | 19 | 19 | 19 | 20 | 21 | 22 | 23 | 23 | 24 | 25 | 26 | 27 | 27 |
| 1.71m (67in) | 16 | 16 | 18 | 19 | 19 | 20 | 20 | 21 | 22 | 23 | 23 | 24 | 25 | 26 | 27 |
| 1.73m (68in) | 15 | 16 | 17 | 18 | 18 | 19 | 20 | 21 | 21 | 22 | 23 | 24 | 24 | 25 | 26 |
| 1.76m (69in) | 15 | 16 | 17 | 18 | 18 | 18 | 19 | 20 | 21 | 21 | 22 | 23 | 24 | 24 | 25 |
| 1.78m (70in) | 14 | 15 | 17 | 17 | 17 | 18 | 19 | 19 | 20 | 21 | 22 | 22 | 23 | 24 | 24 |
| 1.81m (71in) | 14 | 15 | 16 | 17 | 17 | 17 | 18 | 19 | 20 | 20 | 21 | 22 | 22 | 23 | 24 |
| 1.83m (72in) | 14 | 14 | 16 | 16 | 16 | 17 | 18 | 18 | 19 | 20 | 20 | 21 | 22 | 22 | 23 |
| 1.86m (73in) | 13 | 14 | 15 | 16 | 16 | 16 | 17 | 18 | 18 | 19 | 20 | 20 | 21 | 22 | 22 |
| 1.88m (74in) | 13 | 13 | 15 | 15 | 15 | 16 | 17 | 17 | 18 | 19 | 19 | 20 | 21 | 21 | 22 |
| 1.91m (75in) | 12 | 13 | 14 | 14 | 15 | 16 | 16 | 17 | 17 | 18 | 19 | 19 | 20 | 21 | 21 |
| 1.93m (76in) | 12 | 13 | 13 | 14 | 15 | 15 | 16 | 16 | 17 | 18 | 18 | 19 | 19 | 20 | 21 |

# What does my result mean?

Once you have found out what your BMI (Body Mass Index) is, check below to see whether it indicates that you are underweight, a normal, healthy weight, overweight, or obese and what you should then do about your weight.

**BMI 18.5 or below: Underweight** You need to eat more food to provide your body with the fuel it needs. You may need to eat more at each meal and have more snacks during the day. Be sure to choose nutritious foods from a range of food groups (*see pp.208–209*).

**BMI 19.0–24.9: Healthy weight** You are eating the right amount to keep your weight at a healthy level, but you still need to make sure that your diet is balanced, healthy, and nutritious.

**BMI 25–29.9: Overweight** It would be beneficial to your health if you lose some weight and avoid gaining any additional weight. Follow the advice in this book about healthy eating and

regular exercise to help manage your weight long-term. Making just one or two adjustments to your diet each day, such as cutting out high-fat or high-sugar snacks, should result in a healthy, gradual weight loss.

**BMI 30–34.9: Obese (Class 1)** Your health may be at risk at your current weight. Look for healthy ways of losing the excess weight; do not be tempted to try any "crash" diets, which could place more strain on your health.

**BMI 35–39.9: Obese (Class 2)** Your health is at risk at your current weight. You should use this book to find ways of changing your eating habits. You are advised to seek advice from your GP and a state-registered dietitian.

**BMI 40 or higher: Obese (Class 3)** Being this overweight poses a serious risk to your health. You are advised to consult your GP and a state-registered dietitian for a weight-loss plan.

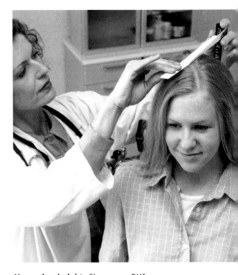

**Measuring height** Since your BMI score is based on your height and your weight, accurate measurements are essential.

| 79kg/ 175lb | 82kg/ 180lb | 84kg/ 185lb | 86kg/ 190lb | 89kg/ 195lb | 91kg/ 200lb | 93kg/ 205lb | 95kg/ 210lb | 98kg/ 215lb | 100kg/ 220lb | 102kg/ 225lb | 104kg/ 240lb | 107kg/ 235lb | 109kg/ 240lb | 111kg/ 245lb | Weight |
|---|---|---|---|---|---|---|---|---|---|---|---|---|---|---|---|
| | | | | | | BMI | | | | | | | | | Height |
| 34 | 35 | 36 | 37 | 38 | 39 | 40 | 41 | 42 | 43 | 44 | 45 | 46 | 47 | 48 | 1.53m (60in) |
| 33 | 34 | 35 | 36 | 37 | 38 | 39 | 40 | 41 | 42 | 43 | 43 | 44 | 45 | 46 | 1.55m (61in) |
| 32 | 33 | 34 | 35 | 36 | 37 | 37 | 38 | 39 | 40 | 41 | 42 | 43 | 44 | 45 | 1.58m (62in) |
| 31 | 32 | 33 | 34 | 35 | 35 | 36 | 37 | 38 | 39 | 40 | 41 | 42 | 43 | 43 | 1.60m (63in) |
| 30 | 31 | 32 | 33 | 33 | 34 | 35 | 36 | 37 | 38 | 39 | 39 | 40 | 41 | 42 | 1.63m (64in) |
| 29 | 30 | 31 | 32 | 32 | 33 | 34 | 35 | 36 | 37 | 37 | 38 | 39 | 40 | 41 | 1.65m (65in) |
| 28 | 29 | 30 | 31 | 31 | 32 | 33 | 34 | 35 | 36 | 36 | 37 | 38 | 39 | 40 | 1.68m (66in) |
| 27 | 28 | 29 | 30 | 31 | 31 | 32 | 33 | 34 | 34 | 35 | 36 | 37 | 38 | 38 | 1.71m (67in) |
| 27 | 27 | 28 | 29 | 30 | 30 | 31 | 32 | 33 | 33 | 34 | 35 | 36 | 36 | 37 | 1.73m (68in) |
| 26 | 27 | 27 | 28 | 29 | 30 | 30 | 31 | 32 | 32 | 33 | 34 | 35 | 35 | 36 | 1.76m (69in) |
| 25 | 26 | 27 | 27 | 28 | 29 | 29 | 30 | 31 | 32 | 32 | 33 | 34 | 34 | 35 | 1.78m (70in) |
| 24 | 25 | 26 | 26 | 27 | 28 | 29 | 29 | 30 | 31 | 31 | 32 | 33 | 33 | 34 | 1.81m (71in) |
| 24 | 24 | 25 | 26 | 26 | 27 | 28 | 28 | 29 | 30 | 31 | 31 | 32 | 33 | 33 | 1.83m (72in) |
| 23 | 24 | 24 | 25 | 26 | 26 | 27 | 28 | 28 | 29 | 30 | 30 | 31 | 32 | 32 | 1.86m (73in) |
| 22 | 23 | 24 | 24 | 25 | 26 | 26 | 27 | 28 | 28 | 29 | 30 | 30 | 31 | 31 | 1.88m (74in) |
| 22 | 22 | 23 | 24 | 24 | 25 | 26 | 26 | 27 | 27 | 28 | 29 | 29 | 30 | 31 | 1.91m (75in) |
| 21 | 22 | 23 | 23 | 24 | 24 | 25 | 26 | 26 | 27 | 27 | 28 | 29 | 29 | 30 | 1.93m (76in) |

# Do you need to change?

## Take charge of your health by evaluating your diet and lifestyle.

The purpose of this chapter is to help you identify any dietary and lifestyle habits that you could change to improve your health. The fact that you are now reading this book shows that you are interested in making changes.

### Putting health in context
The results of the questionnaire on page 21 have to be interpreted in the context of both your current health and your family history.

If you are aware of a medical condition that runs in your family, you may be able to reduce your risk of developing the condition by following the advice that we offer in this book.

### Minimizing risk
This is not a "diet" book in the usual sense. Our goal is to translate the best medical research available into a sensible programme that will help you to maintain and improve your health in the long-term. Evidence shows that "crash" diets do not work and that very rarely do they help people change their eating habits or lifestyle. The

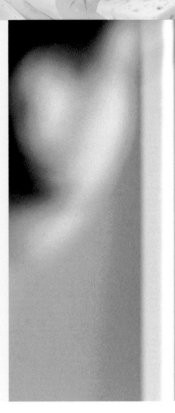

# Assess yourself

Now it is time to review your findings about your current nutritional and lifestyle status. When you understand the connection between these and your health, you will be ready to move on to making the necessary changes.

### REVIEW YOUR STATUS
In the first part of this chapter, we looked at various nutritional and lifestyle factors that have an important bearing on your health. We invited you to think about what you eat and drink and how active or inactive your lifestyle is, as well as other important factors.

Whatever your final score in the quiz, look back over your answers now and think about those questions where you scored three or four points. These pinpoint the areas where making changes will improve your long-term health. For example, you would have scored three or four points if you eat red meat more than twice a week. Make replacing red meat with other sources of protein, such as chicken, fish, or pulses, one of your goals.

This book will help you understand why your current habits are likely to create health risks and offers you advice on how to make changes.

### MINIMIZING RISKS
In the second section of the chapter we invited you to look at your current state of health and to understand it in the context of your family medical history. When you visit your doctor for a check-up, he or she will carry out various tests (for example, blood pressure) to assess your health and then will look at the results of the tests in the context of your family history. Many medical conditions have a hereditary component, but you can minimize your risk of developing the diseases by tackling the associated risk factors that can be modified by making alterations in diet, exercise, and lifestyle.

In this book, we explain in detail why these modifiable risk factors are significant, and help you find ways of making the changes that will benefit your long-term health and well-being.

### CONTROLLING YOUR WEIGHT
Finally, we looked at the issue of weight, body shape, and body mass index (BMI) and their implications for your health. Because obesity increases the risk of several other medical problems, the importance cannot be overstated. In a later chapter, The Truth about Weight Control (see pp.156–207), we look in detail at the risks associated with being overweight and provide comprehensive information and advice on how you can control and reduce your weight.

### MAKING CHANGES
Use this book to help you identify areas of your health that need improvement and to find ways of making the changes (see pp.30–31). Don't try to be perfect right from the start – or all the time. No one is. Just do as well as you can and remember that your journey to health is as important as your final destination. Each small change you make can have a long-term benefit. You need to accept the choices you make, and give yourself permission to do the best you can.

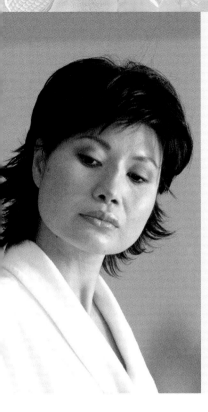

aim of this book is to help you make and benefit from these long-term changes in diet and lifestyle.

There are no guarantees in life. You may exercise regularly and eat the right foods, yet still develop a medical problem. But we know – from all of the research evidence available – that those who enjoy a nutritious diet and exercise, to maintain a healthy weight, are less likely to develop problems.

Use the knowledge you have gained throughout this chapter to determine the most important areas of nutrition, exercise, and lifestyle for you to work on – and get started right now.

**Taking stock** Take time to reflect in detail on your current health status, your diet, and your lifestyle. Consider what changes you need to make, and draw up a list.

## Checklist for change

In this chapter we have looked at various aspects of diet and lifestyle that can affect your health and well-being. Before moving on to the next section, check whether you have understood these clearly:

● Have you completed the questionnaire on page 21 and checked your score?
● Are you familiar with your family medical history (*see p.22*)?
● Have you checked your body mass index (*see pp.26–27*) and looked at how to interpret it?
● Have you identified your body shape (*see p.25*) and considered whether it places you at risk of ill health or disease?
● Are you aware of the health risks associated with being overweight and obesity (*see p.24*)?

# Case study  Lawyer with fatigue and weight gain

**Name**  Richard

**Age**  30 years

**Problem**  Richard has gained 6.75kg (15lb) in the last year. He complains of feeling tired all the time and has been drinking more and more coffee to stay alert. However, this keeps him awake at night so he is not getting enough sleep. He has sought advice from a nutritionist for his fatigue and to help him lose some weight. He also suffers from constipation, but has no other serious medical problems.

**Lifestyle**  Richard is a lawyer who eats most of his meals on the run. He skips breakfast, snacks on biscuits at work, and drinks at least four large cups of milky coffee with sugar every day. During the week, Richard has to eat out a lot with clients and colleagues at lunchtime. On other days, he

usually eats lunch in fast-food or pizza restaurants. Since he works late, he often has an Indian or Chinese take-away for dinner.

At weekends, Richard eats cereal with milk for breakfast, skips lunch, and eats out with friends in the evening, choosing starters such as pâté or deep-fried calamari, and main dishes such as steak and chips. He rarely eats any vegetables and does not take a multivitamin supplement. He usually drinks two beers on Friday and Saturday nights in the restaurant. He does not smoke and doesn't have time to exercise.

**Advice**  Richard's main complaints are most likely related to his diet and sedentary lifestyle. He does not eat fruits and vegetables, so his diet is low in fibre as well as in vitamins and minerals. He has gained weight because he takes in more calories than he burns. This is not helped by the fact that he eats out so much.

Richard's constipation and fatigue can be corrected by incorporating more fibre and water into his diet and decreasing his intake of coffee and fizzy drinks. He can increase his fibre intake by eating a bowl of bran cereal or muesli for breakfast, substituting fresh or dried fruit for the biscuit snacks, and including some vegetables in his lunch and dinner menus.

Richard's diet is high in saturated fat and calories. If he had a tuna salad sandwich rather than the fast-food burgers and fries or pizza for lunch, this would be a good start. When he eats out with clients at lunchtime or with his friends in the evening, he could skip a starter and choose lean proteins, such as grilled fish or chicken, with boiled new potatoes and a salad for his main course.

Finally, Richard needs to exercise in order to improve his health. Simply making time for a brisk walk each day would be beneficial.

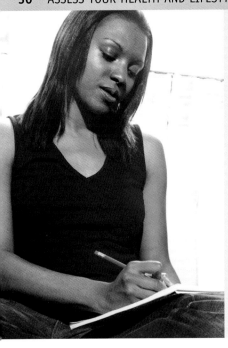

# Making changes

## Forge new habits in diet and lifestyle for optimum health.

Confidence and conviction are prime requisites for any behaviour change. Confidence reflects your attitude about your ability to make changes: if you don't believe you will succeed, the chances are you won't. Boost your confidence by believing in yourself, and enlist the aid of family and friends if necessary. Conviction, on the other hand, reflects your determination to accomplish change. If you don't believe a change is important, you are unlikely to make it; so be sure to select a change that you firmly believe will make a difference to your future health – and go for it.

### Don't give up
When it comes to changing your behaviour, your motto should be: "If at first I don't succeed, try, try, try again". Studies of people who

**Planning for change** Thinking about which behaviour change – dietary or lifestyle – will best benefit your health is a vital step. Find ways to begin making that change.

# Key stages in behaviour change

Therapists who specialize in helping people change behaviour recognize that most people pass through certain key stages as they proceed. Developed by two psychologists, the following six stages are often used to assess an individual's readiness for change.

### PRE-CONTEMPLATION
This refers to the time before you are aware that you need to change. As you are reading this book, it is likely that you have already passed this stage.

### CONTEMPLATING CHANGE
Now you are thinking about making changes but haven't done anything yet. It may be that in reading this book you are seeking expert advice on what changes are most important.

It is important to select a specific dietary behaviour to target for change. The questionnaire on page 21 should have helped you identify areas that could be improved. We suggest that you select the change you think would be easiest for you to make, and start there.

Why choose an easy goal? Simply because if you try and succeed, you will feel much better than if you try and fail; and once you have achieved the first target, you are more likely to go on to set another one. Base your initial target on your current diet. For example, if you eat fruits only a few times a week, set as your goal the intention to eat at least one piece of fruit every day.

### PREPARING FOR ACTION
This is the stage when you think about the best way of bringing about whatever changes are necessary to establish your new habit. For example, if your goal is to eat at least one piece of fruit each day, it is a good idea to decide exactly how you will achieve this goal. Try to be as specific as possible. For example, you may need to change your shopping habits – you may need to shop more often in order to have a supply of fresh fruit.

You must think about how you can have fresh or dried fruits available all the time and how to include it in your daily life, whether it is to be eaten after a meal as a dessert or as a snack – for example, in the car when travelling or taken with you to work.

If you do not do your homework and fail to prepare a realistic plan of action, your new habit will not stick, and you will soon revert to your old ways.

### INITIATING CHANGES
Now is the time to put your plans into action. Remember that small changes are easier to make than large ones, and that you must give yourself enough time for new habits and tastes to be established before moving on to the next change. For example, make sure you always take your piece of fruit in the car to work and eat it. And if you forget to eat your fruit in the car, eat it as soon as you can.

Bear in mind, too, that eating one unhealthy meal won't undermine an otherwise healthy diet. If you overeat at lunch, just have a salad and a serving of vegetables for dinner. And if you are going out to dinner in the evening, be sure to exercise during the day.

### MAINTAINING NEW HABITS
New behaviours take about six weeks to become established. Once you are confident that your first change is well established, then you can move on to the next one. This stage is about ensuring that all the effort you put into making a change doesn't go to waste. Don't worry about occasional lapses – you are aiming to improve your eating habits for the long-term and, as long as you keep trying, you are succeeding.

stopped smoking show that most of them tried and failed several times before they finally succeeded. However, changing your dietary habits will be more difficult than successfully giving up smoking. At some point after stopping smoking, you lose the desire to smoke and are then at very little risk of taking it up again. But this is not the same for your diet: you must eat and drink, day in and day out, making decisions about what to eat or drink several times a day, every day, for the rest of your life.

## How to change your diet

Throughout the book we will make suggestions for ways of improving your diet. We also include tips on how to make changes. If one way doesn't work, simply try another. If you slip up, just remember that no one needs to be perfect when it comes to how they eat – better is good enough.

If you think you might find it difficult to make a radical change in your diet or lifestyle, you can begin by selecting just one simple modification that should be easy for you to achieve, so you get off to a successful start. For example, you may choose to drink more water each day, instead of high-calorie sugary fizzy drinks. Then use more of our strategies to help you move towards your goal of achieving optimum health through improved diet and nutrition.

## Are you ready to change?

Your answers to the following questions will provide insights that may help you achieve your goals:
● What one change would bring the most significant improvement in your health?
● What other changes would you like to make?
● What would help you change?
● If you have tried to change your diet or exercise recently, did you encounter any problems?
● Are you able to deal with the occasional failure?
● Do you think you can maintain any of the changes that you have made over the past few months?

### WHAT IF I RELAPSE?

Failing is just another part of the cycle – each time you fail, you learn something that will help you the next time you try to make a change. Reviewing barriers to change, or what has impeded progress, provides useful insights. So, too, does thinking about motivations that have helped in the past and analyzing the circumstances of previous successful behaviour change or relapse. Above all, do not think of one lapse as relapse – look through the reasons why you did not succeed and start again.

## Tips for changing

The following key strategies will help when you try to change your lifestyle habits:
● Break down each change you want to make into manageable, small stages; be sure that each stage is firmly established before moving on to the next one.
● Always include your favourite foods, but look for healthier ways of preparing and cooking them. For example, brush big chips with olive oil and bake rather than fry.

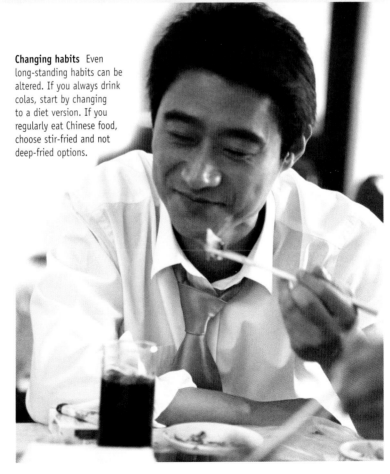

**Changing habits** Even long-standing habits can be altered. If you always drink colas, start by changing to a diet version. If you regularly eat Chinese food, choose stir-fried and not deep-fried options.

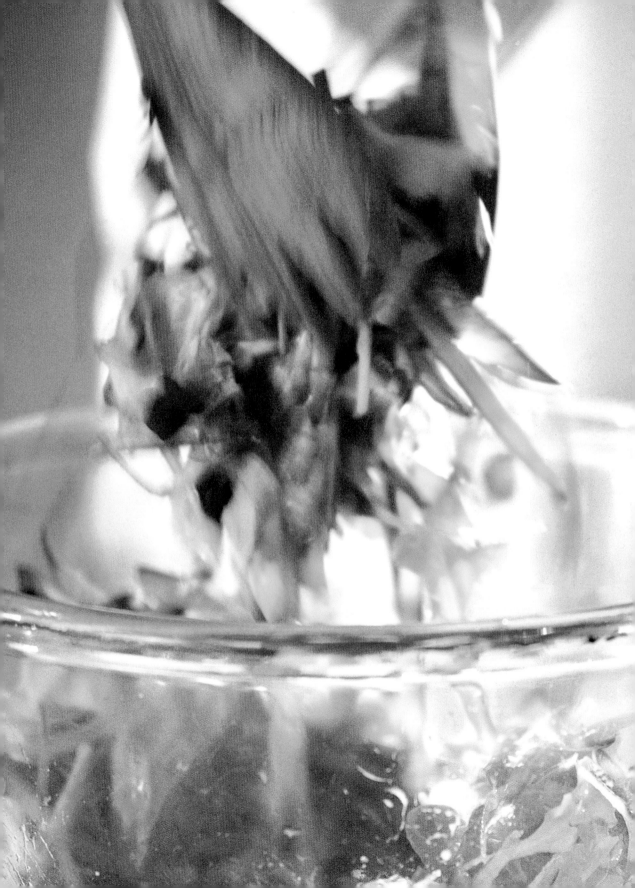

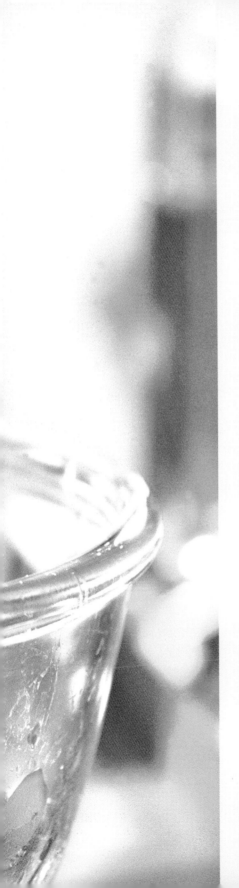

# Food
# for life

Every food we eat provides the body
with a range of nutrients, each with its
own role to play. Eating a balanced,
varied diet every day will ensure that
you have everything you need for good
health, including foods that provide
energy, fibre, protein, carbohydrates,
fats, vitamins, and minerals.

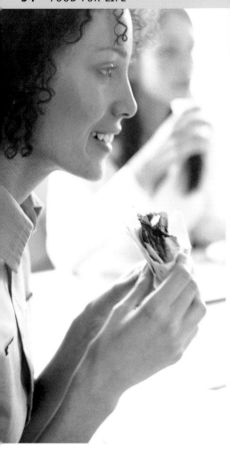

# Why we need food

## The foods we eat are the essential building blocks of life.

All foods – from apples and peas to wholemeal bread and ice cream – contain two main categories of nutrients, the macronutrients and the micronutrients.

Macronutrients are required in large amounts for healthy growth and development; they form the basis of every diet and they provide energy for all the body's everyday functions and activities. These nutrients are further categorized as being primarily fats (see pp.38–43), proteins (see pp.44–45), carbohydrates (see pp.46–47), or fibre (see pp.48–49), although most foods contain all of them in varying proportions (see p.37).

Vitamins and minerals make up the micronutrients, so called because they are found in tiny amounts in foods (see pp.50–67). Unlike macronutrients, vitamins and minerals do not provide energy and are needed in small amounts, but they play a critical role in the normal functioning of the body and digestive processes, to ensure good health.

### How we get nutrients

Take a look at what you eat in an average day: the chances are that your diet includes a wide variety of foods from all the basic food groups, and that it provides a range of essential nutrients. Your breakfast, for example, may be rich in carbohydrates and fibre

**Nutritious snack** A simple wrap, filled with lettuce, tomato, and slices of chicken breast, is a healthy snack as it contains many of the nutrients that your body needs.

# Calculating energy requirements

Your energy requirements depend on various factors, including age, gender, physical activity, muscle mass, body temperature, and whether you are still growing. Pregnancy, breast-feeding, menstruation, illness, infection, how much you eat or sleep, and hormone levels are additional factors.

Basal metabolic rate (BMR) is a measure of how much energy you need for essential functions such as breathing and heart rate. BMR is highest in the young and decreases after the age of ten. Because of their greater muscle mass, men generally have a higher BMR (and therefore require more calories) than women. Due to declining muscle mass, older adults generally have a lower BMR and require fewer calories.

Examples of the maintenance calorie requirements for different activities in adults are listed below:
- Sedentary or bedbound people: 11.5cal per 450g (1lb) of body weight per day
- People who only do light or routine activities: 13.5cal per 450g (1lb) of body weight per day
- People doing moderate activities and a regular exercise programme: 16cal per 450g (1lb) of body weight per day
- Those doing vigorous exercise, such as athletes, manual labourers, and patients recovering from injury: 18cal per 450g (1lb) of body weight per day.

## Jargon buster

**Metabolism** A collective term for all the chemical processes constantly occurring within the body, including those in which the nutrients from food are converted into substances that the body uses or excretes as waste.

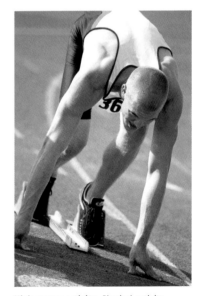

**High-energy activity** Physical activity accounts for 15–30 per cent of total energy expenditure. An athlete expends more energy than someone who sits at a desk.

from cereal or wholemeal toast; you may have a mixed salad for your lunch, and grilled fish and vegetables for dinner, providing protein and a variety of vitamins and minerals. Whatever you eat at individual meals, your diet is made up of foods from the five basic food groups (see pp.70–73).

## The energy yield of food

In addition to supplying nutrients, food provides your body with energy (right). Approximately half to two-thirds of the energy we obtain from food goes to support the body's basic, involuntary functions, which are the activities that are performed without any conscious control, such as heart rate, maintaining breathing, and body temperature. The minimum energy needed to carry out these functions is determined by your basal metabolic rate (BMR), which is your baseline rate of metabolism (opposite below), measured when the body is at rest.

You also expend energy through conscious, voluntary activities, which range from the sedentary to the strenuous. All your body's energy needs are met from the foods that you eat or from your body's energy stores.

## Nutrition and health

In the following pages of this book, we examine in detail the various elements of nutrition – proteins, fats, carbohydrates, fibre, and micronutrients (vitamins and minerals) – and how your body utilizes them. For example, you need protein for growth and repair, carbohydrates for energy, and fibre for effective digestion. We will also suggest ways of improving your general health and reducing your risks of developing certain diseases by making healthier food choices.

## Calories and energy

The energy you obtain from food is measured in calories. However, since one calorie represents a tiny amount of energy, kilocalorie units are used in nutritional analysis. 1 kilocalorie (kcal) equals 1000 calories, and this is the amount of energy required to raise the temperature of 1 kilogram of water 1° Celsius. However, the term "calorie" has come to be used as a shorthand reference to kilocalorie, and we have used this convention

(1cal represents 1kcal) in this book. Each type of nutrient generates a specific amount of energy:
- 100g (3½oz) protein: 400cal
- 100g (3½oz) carbohydrate: 400cal
- 100g (3½oz) fat: 900cal

**Kilojoules**  Energy is sometimes measured in kilojoules (kJ), and you may find this information on food labels alongside the caloric value. 1cal (1kcal) equals 4.184kJ.

# Guidelines for nutritional requirements

In addition to identifying the types of nutrients we must include in our diets on a daily basis, we also need to know how much of each is required for optimum health. Recommended daily amounts (RDAs) were originally set by the Department of Health in 1979 to specify how much of a certain nutrient was needed by different groups of the population. But RDAs were often used wrongly to assess an individual's diet.

The Department of Health replaced RDAs with DRVs (dietary reference values) in 1991, although we still use the familiar RDAs. They are benchmark intakes of energy and nutrients – they can be used for guidance, but shouldn't be seen as exact recommendations.

RDAs show the amount of energy or an individual nutrient that a group of people of a certain age range (and sometimes sex) needs for good health. Although RDAs are given as daily

intakes, people often eat quite different foods from one day to the next, and their appetite can change, so in practice the intakes of energy and nutrients need to be averaged over several days. RDAs apply to healthy people only and don't apply to children under five years of age.

## Dietary Reference Value (DRV)

DRV is a general term used to cover:
- Estimated average requirement (EAR): average amount of energy or a nutrient that is needed by a group of people.
- Reference nutrient intake (RNI): amount of a nutrient that is enough to meet the dietary needs of about 97 per cent of a group of people.
- Lower reference nutrient intake (LRNI): amount of a nutrient that is enough for a small number of people

Information given on food labels must comply with EC Nutrition Labelling Regulations, which use Nutrient and Energy Intakes for the European Community (Commission of the European Communities 1993). These are often slightly higher than UK RDAs.

in a group with the smallest needs. (Most people need more than this.)
- Safe intake (SI): recommended when there is not enough information on the physiological requirements for a nutrient.

In the Vitamin and Mineral Directories (see pp.50–67), the UK RDAs for healthy men and women are provided, followed by the RDA set by the European Community, wherever these figures are available.

# How do we process food?

Before the nutrients in food can be used, they must be broken down into components that the body can absorb. This process, which starts in the mouth and ends with the expulsion of waste products, can take between one and three days. Food is subjected to chemical changes, as digestive juices break it down into its smallest components. Proteins are broken into amino acids, fats into fatty acids and glycerol, and carbohydrates into simple sugars, such as glucose. The vitamins and minerals consist of tiny molecules that the body can absorb without breaking them down first. In the small intestine, bile produced by the liver helps digest fats, while pancreatic secretions break down carbohydrates and continue the digestion of proteins and fats. Nutrients are absorbed into the bloodstream through the intestinal walls. The food that is not digested and absorbed is passed out of the anus.

**Mouth** The process begins here as food is broken down by the mechanical action of the teeth, tongue, and jaws.

**Epiglottis** Swallowing food triggers this flap of cartilage to seal off the windpipe. At the same time the soft palate closes off the nasal cavity.

**Oesophagus** Food is propelled down this muscular tube from the throat to the stomach by rhythmic contractions known as peristalsis.

**Stomach** In the stomach, food spends up to five hours being churned to a pulp and mixed with gastric juices. These consist of acid, which kills bacteria in food, and enzymes that help break down protein into amino acids. The resulting fluid, called chyme, is squirted into the small intestine. Vitamin $B_{12}$ is released from food in the stomach.

**Gall bladder** This sac-like organ stores bile produced by the liver and releases it into the small intestine to help break down food molecules.

**Pancreas** This organ secretes digestive juice into the small intestine.

**Rectum** Stools collect here before being expelled from the anus.

**Digestive system** This is made up of the digestive tract – a long, muscular tube that extends from mouth to anus and includes the oesophagus, stomach, intestines, and rectum. Also part of this system are various organs such as the liver, pancreas, and gall bladder.

**Salivary glands** In the mouth, there are three pairs of salivary glands, which secrete saliva. The digestive enzyme amylase in saliva moistens the chewed food and helps break it down further.

**Liver** The largest internal organ, the liver produces up to 1 litre (almost 2 pints) of the digestive juice bile each day. Vitamins A, D, E, and K are stored here.

**Small intestine** Food passes from the stomach into the small intestine, a long tube consisting of the duodenum, jejunum, and ileum. Here, food mixes with more digestive juices and nutrients, including many vitamins and minerals, are absorbed into the bloodstream.

**Large intestine** The food mass moves from the small intestine into the large intestine, which is populated by bacteria that digest whatever has been left behind after small intestinal absorption. Water and nutrients released by bacteria are absorbed.

**Anus** The digestive tract opens out of the body here and stools are expelled.

# What is in the food we eat?

Foods are usually categorized as being primarily carbohydrate, protein, fat, or fibre. However, most foods contain all or most of these elements, in varying proportions, as well as traces of various vitamins and minerals.

For example, grain-based products, such as bread or pasta, are typically thought of as carbohydrate foods, but they may also contain significant amounts of protein, fat, vitamins, and minerals. Animal foods, such as meat, poultry, or fish, are rich in protein – and often in fat – and most have very low levels of carbohydrate. Even ice cream, which you may think of as just a treat or a dairy product, contains protein, carbohydrate, minerals, and vitamins, as well as fat.

Everything you eat contributes to your overall nutritional intake, but no single group of foods will provide all your nutritional needs. It is therefore important to eat a varied diet, choosing foods from all the main food groups. Combining certain foods can improve the nutrient quality of your diet. For example, eating foods rich in vitamin C with iron-rich foods can improve your absorption of the iron. Food also contains water, in various amounts. Some fruits and vegetables contain a large quantity of water, and they can provide a useful supply of liquids. The chart below shows the percentages of nutrients in the non-liquid part of various foods. See page 296 for a key to the abbreviations used for vitamins and minerals in the chart.

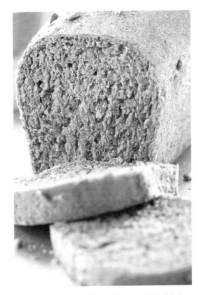

**Complete foods**  Although you might think of bread primarily as a carbohydrate source, it also contains useful amounts of protein, fat, fibre, and many vitamins and minerals.

## Macronutrients and micronutrients

Most food contains both macro- and micronutrients. When we try to plan a balanced diet, we tend to think of the macronutrient groups first: carbohydrates, proteins, and fats, and the quantities required (see p.73) for good health and weight management. These foods provide the fuel the body needs for all its key functions.

Food labels show the amount of each of these key macronutrients, to help you make the best choice for your diet (see p.277).

All foods also contain a variety of micronutrients, which are in fact vitamins and minerals. Each food contains a different selection of micronutrients, and in different quantities. Micronutrients play an important role in many processes in the body including:
• Driving metabolic processes in the body, such as enzyme reactions and manufacture of red blood cells
• Proper functioning of the heart and nervous system
• Helping to manufacture the antibodies that fight infection.

| FOOD | FAT | PROTEIN | CARBS | FIBRE | GOOD SOURCE VITAMINS/MINERALS |
|---|---|---|---|---|---|
| Wholemeal bread | 14% | 12% | 74% | 4.1% | $B_1$, Fol, Nia / Fe, K, Mg, P, Zn |
| Brown rice | 9.0% | 10% | 81% | 1.7% | $B_1$, Nia / Mg, P, Zn |
| Green beans | 0% | 9.0% | 91% | 4.0% | A, Fol, Vit K / K |
| Apple | 0% | 0% | 100% | 3.0% | K |
| Low-fat fruit yogurt | 9.0% | 17% | 74% | 0% | $B_2$ / Ca, K, P |
| Chicken breast | 27% | 73% | 0% | 0.1% | $B_2$, $B_6$, $B_{12}$, Nia / K, P, Zn |
| Fillet steak | 36% | 64% | 0% | 0% | $B_1$, $B_2$, $B_{12}$, Nia / Fe, K, P, Zn |
| Salmon | 54% | 46% | 0% | 0% | $B_1$, $B_2$, $B_{12}$, Fol, Nia, Pant / Fe, K, P, Zn |
| Lentils | 3.0% | 30% | 67% | 15.6% | $B_2$, $B_{12}$, Fol, Nia, Pant / P, K |
| Almonds | 78% | 12% | 10% | 0% | $B_2$, E / Fe, K, Mg, P, Zn |
| Eggs | 61% | 38% | 1.0% | 0% | A, $B_2$, $B_{12}$, D / Ca, P, Zn |

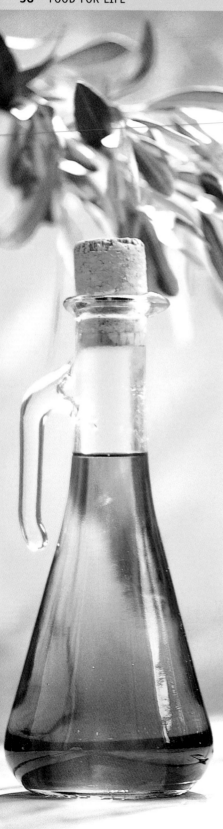

# The need for fats

## Some fats are vital for healthy body functioning.

Part of a group of compounds known as lipids, and composed of the elements carbon, oxygen, and hydrogen, fats are found mainly in plants, fish, and meats. They form a major part of all cell membranes in the body and play a vital role in the absorption of the fat-soluble vitamins A, D, E, and K (see pp.52–58) from foods.

Fat gives the body insulation, helping to maintain a constant temperature against extremes of hot and cold. It is also serves as an important source of energy.

### Lipids and lipoproteins
In addition to fats, lipids include phospholipids, triglycerides, waxes, and sterols. The most well-known sterol is cholesterol (see p.40), which circulates in the blood attached to compounds known as lipoproteins. Low-density lipoproteins (LDL), which carry cholesterol to tissues and organs, are often called "bad" cholesterol, since high levels in the blood are associated with an increased risk of cardiovascular disease (see p.216).

High-density lipoproteins (HDL), which carry cholesterol away from the tissues and back to the liver, are known as "good" cholesterol, since high levels decrease the risk of cardiovascular disease.

Fats are also referred to as good or bad according to whether their chemical bonds are "saturated" with hydrogen. Unsaturated fats are further classified into mono- and polyunsaturates, which differ in their nutritional makeup.

**Beneficial oil** Olive oil is a rich source of monounsaturated fat, which is now known to confer important health benefits.

### Avoid saturated fats
With the exception of palm and coconut oils, most saturated fats are derived from animal and dairy products. Red meat and meat products such as sausages are major sources of saturated fat in the diet, along with whole milk and its products, such as cheese, cream, and ice cream.

Excessive intake of saturated fats and trans fatty acids (below) are now believed to increase the risk of cardiovascular disease by raising the unhealthy LDL levels, so they should be restricted in the diet.

### Unsaturated fats
A diet high in monounsaturated fats, which are found in plant oils, avocados, and nuts, helps lower levels of LDL and triglycerides in the blood, without lowering healthy HDL levels.

Polyunsaturated fats consist of two major types: omega-3 fatty acids, found in fish oils (opposite), and omega-6 fatty acids, found in vegetable oils such as sunflower, rapeseed, and corn (see p.41). Your diet should include both types.

### Trans fatty acids

These occur naturally – in small amounts – in meat and dairy products, but they are also produced during the process of hydrogenation, which is used to convert liquid vegetable oils into semi-solid fats in the manufacture of some types of margarine. Trans fats are most commonly found in biscuits, cakes, pastries, meat pies, sausages, crackers, and take-away foods. Although chemically trans fats are still unsaturated fat, studies show that in the body they behave like saturated fat, causing blood cholesterol levels to rise. In fact, some studies suggest that trans fats are worse than saturated fats.

# Choosing healthier meats

Meat and meat products are one of the major sources of fat, especially saturated fat, in the diet, but – as the chart on the right shows – there is a wide variation in the amount of total fat and saturated fat in different types of meat.

Manufactured products such as sausages and salami contain the most fat, so if you are trying to lose weight or improve your diet, you could begin by replacing these with healthier choices. When shopping, choose products without visible white fat or marbling.

An easy way to reduce the fat content of chicken or turkey is to avoid eating the skin. If you cook poultry with the skin on to retain moisture, remove it and discard after cooking. Also, opt for the white meat of poultry rather than the dark meat, which contains more fat.

| FOOD TYPE | TOTAL FAT | SATURATED FAT |
| --- | --- | --- |
| Bacon (streaky) | 77% | 27% |
| Sausage | 72% | 26% |
| Minced beef | 64% | 27% |
| Chicken wing (with skin) | 58% | 16% |
| Lamb (lean) | 56% | 26% |
| Chicken thigh (with skin) | 56% | 16% |
| Ground beef (extra lean) | 50% | 21% |
| Bacon (lean back) | 45% | 16% |
| Beef (lean) | 35% | 13% |
| Pork (lean) | 29% | 10% |
| Venison | 18% | 6.0% |
| Chicken breast (no skin) | 17% | 5.0% |
| Turkey breast (no skin) | 7.0% | 2.0% |

# Eat more fish and shellfish

Seafood is a good source of protein (see pp.44–45) as well as being low in saturated fat and providing B vitamins (see pp.53–56) and many minerals. In addition, oily fish provide the heart-healthy omega-3 fatty acids. It was once advised that shellfish, in particular prawns, should be avoided in a healthy diet because of their high cholesterol content. However, recent studies show that although prawns and other shellfish do contain high levels of cholesterol, they are very low in saturated fat (as long as they are not battered and deep-fried) – it is saturated fat that is the crucial risk factor for heart disease for most people. The benefits from fish and shellfish mean they should be eaten at least twice a week.

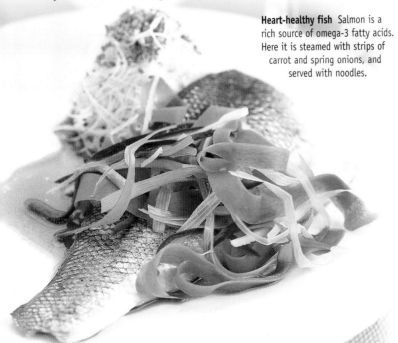

**Heart-healthy fish** Salmon is a rich source of omega-3 fatty acids. Here it is steamed with strips of carrot and spring onions, and served with noodles.

## Good sources

Most fish contain less than five per cent fat, most of it polyunsaturated. "Oily" fish contain five to 15 per cent fat; a few have more than this. This list ranks fish by their relative fat content, from oily to lean:

- Herring
- Mackerel
- Sardines
- Anchovies
- Salmon
- Tuna
- Halibut
- Cod
- Crab
- Scallops
- Prawns
- Lobster

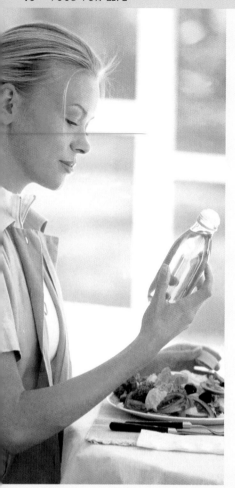

**Salad dressing** High in monounsaturated fat and low in saturates, olive oil is the perfect accompaniment to a fresh salad. Use it alone or as the basis of a vinaigrette.

# Good fats, bad fats

## Some types of fat confer important health benefits.

In recent years, countless words have been written about fat – how much we need, and which types are "good" or "bad". It's not enough to know which foods are high or low in fat; now we also need to identify the different kinds of fats contained in various foods, and to understand why some fats are good for us while other fats can pose serious health risks.

### Healthy fats

Scientific studies have shown that a diet high in monounsaturated fat reduces the levels of "bad" low-density lipoprotein (LDL) and triglycerides without decreasing levels of "good" high-density lipoprotein (HDL). This is doubly advantageous, since very low HDL levels, like high LDL levels, increase the risk of cardiovascular disease. Oils high in monounsaturated fat (*opposite above*) are also especially good for cooking because they develop fewer free radicals (*see p.58*) than polyunsaturated oils when they are heated.

The two major categories of polyunsaturated fats—omega-3 and omega-6—are known as essential fatty acids since they cannot be synthesized by the body. Omega-3 fatty acids are found in oils from cold-water fish such as tuna, herring, and sardines. They are involved in regulating blood pressure, blood clotting, and immune responses, as well as for the normal functioning of the brain, spinal cord, and the retina of the eye.

Omega-6 fatty acids are found in vegetable oils, such as sunflower and corn oil. These fatty acids are essential for growth, cell structure, and the maintenance of a healthy immune system.

### Avoid animal fats

Unlike unsaturated fats, which have an essential role to play in the diet, saturated fats are known to increase the risk of cardiovascular disease (*see pp.214–221*). These fats come mainly from animal sources, such as meat and dairy products, and from certain plant oils (*opposite above*). Due to their damaging effects on health, you should try to limit the amount of saturated fat you consume in your diet.

## What is cholesterol?

Cholesterol is a waxy substance in your blood that is a major component of every cell wall in your body. It is required for the production of some hormones, such as the sex hormones oestrogen and testosterone.

Cholesterol occurs in very high concentrations in the cells protecting the brain and nervous system. It is particularly important, therefore, that cholesterol intake is not restricted in children under the age of two years, whose brain and nervous system are still developing.

Cholesterol is also required to make bile acid and in the manufacture of vitamin D in the skin (*see p.57*). Bile acids assist with the absorption of fat from the diet.

Most of your body's cholesterol needs are met by the cholesterol your body manufactures for itself. The rest is obtained from food (high levels of cholesterol are found in egg yolks and offal such as liver and kidneys).

Excessive amounts of cholesterol in the blood can cause cardiovascular disease (*see pp.214–221*). Cholesterol forms fatty deposits in the arteries, which may lead to narrowing of the arteries, restricted blood flow, and eventually to heart attack or stroke.

An elevated blood cholesterol level (*see p.23*) may be hereditary or influenced by dietary factors – specifically by a diet that is high in cholesterol, total fat, and saturated fat. However, studies have found that dietary intake of saturated fat has a greater impact on cholesterol levels and associated health risks than the intake of dietary cholesterol alone.

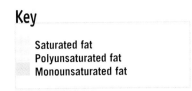

# Choosing the best oils

Advice to limit your intake of saturated fat is unequivocal, but it may not be immediately obvious which oils should be chosen for cooking, since they all contain a combination of saturated, monounsaturated, and polyunsaturated fats. The graph (*right*) ranks vegetable oils according to their monounsaturated fat content and will help you make the healthiest choices.

Whichever one you choose, remember that oil is 100 per cent fat, and one tablespoon equals 99 calories. If you are trying to control your weight, you should limit all fat intake.

When choosing oil for cooking, look for one with a high smoking point, to minimize the risk of unpleasant odours, impaired flavour, and reduced vitamin content. Some oils, such as corn and groundnut, are suitable for heating to high temperatures, but olive oil is not.

**Which oil?** It is easy to see from this graph that coconut oil is particularly high in saturated fat. It should be avoided in favour of healthier oils such as olive and rapeseed, which are high in beneficial monounsaturated and polyunsaturated fats.

## Key

■ Saturated fat
■ Polyunsaturated fat
■ Monounsaturated fat

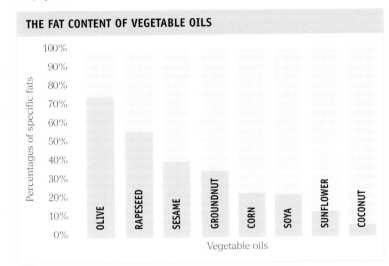

THE FAT CONTENT OF VEGETABLE OILS

---

# Questionnaire: How much fat do you add to food?

Circle the letters that accompany your answers to these questions, then check your score.

**1 How often do you fry food in either shallow or deep fat?**
a  Three or more times a week.
b  About once a week.
c  Less than twice a month.

**2 What type of fat do you generally use for cooking?**
a  Butter, lard, or beef dripping.
b  Margarine or vegetable oil.
c  Olive or rapeseed oil.

**3 What type of milk do you generally use in sauces or soups?**
a  Whole milk or cream.
b  Semi-skimmed milk.
c  Skimmed milk.

**4 Do you add butter to cooked vegetables?**
a  I always add butter.

b  I occasionally add butter.
c  I never add butter.

**5 Which method do you generally use when cooking meat, fish, or poultry?**
a  Roasting or frying.
b  Baking or sautéing.
c  Grilling or griddling.

**6 What fat do you usually have with bread?**
a  I always have butter on my bread.
b  I usually have low-fat margarine or spread.
c  I dip bread in olive oil.

**7 What fat do you use when you make gravy?**
a  Dripping from the roast meat or poultry.
b  The sediment in the roasting tin with the fat removed.
c  None; I use vegetable stock.

**8 What topping do you usually serve with desserts such as an apple crumble?**
a  Cream or crème fraîche.
b  Ice cream or Greek yogurt.
c  Low-fat yogurt.

**Score** a 1  b 2  c 3

**20–24 points** Well done! You are aware of the health benefits of low-fat cooking. Aim to continue with your healthy ways.

**13–19 points** You are making some good choices. Now look for even more ways of reducing the fat content in your cooking.

**8–12 points** You are using too much fat and your health could be at risk. Experiment with the low-fat cooking methods described on page 43 and learn how easy it is to reduce fat levels in your diet.

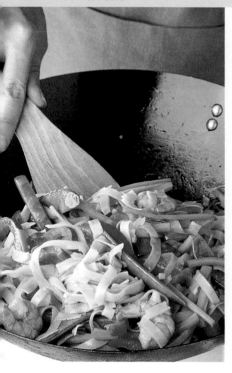

# Reducing saturated fat

## Lessen your risks of developing disease by modifying your dietary fat intake.

From the previous few pages, you will now be familiar with two key factors that should be considered in relation to fats in the diet. First, you need to know which fats should be included in your diet because of their health benefits,

and which fats should be avoided because they increase your risk of developing certain diseases.

The other important factor is the need to regulate the intake of all fats in your diet to avoid unhealthy weight gain. This is important since being overweight and obesity are associated with an increased risk of developing certain diseases, especially diabetes and cancer.

## Making healthy choices

You should aim to reduce sources of saturated fat in your diet by choosing healthy ingredients, and by preparing and cooking them in ways that do not add unhealthy fat. This means eating more fish

**Oriental technique**  Stir-frying finely cut ingredients in a wok is a quick and healthy cooking method derived from Chinese cuisine.

## Same food, less fat

Unhealthy high-fat meals are easily converted to tasty low-fat alternatives. For example, the meals shown here are similar in many respects: chicken is the main ingredient of both, and preparation and cooking times are roughly the same. However, the total fat and saturated fat contents of the meal below are almost one-fifth that of the meal above, and the total calorie content is nearly halved (*see captions*).

The reduction in the fat and calorie content was achieved by using chicken breast rather than drumsticks, which have a higher fat content (*see p.39*); by removing the skin from the chicken before cooking; by grilling or griddling with just a light brushing of oil instead of coating in crumbs and deep-frying; and by serving with a salad and boiled potatoes rather than with chips. Other healthy substitutions include:
• Lean ham instead of bacon
• Sliced turkey breast instead of corned beef or pastrami
• Chicken pie topped with filo pastry instead of shortcrust or flaky.

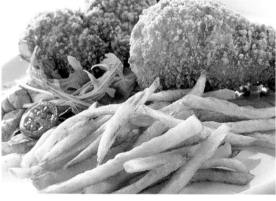

**Deep-fried chicken** This meal is loaded with 492 calories and 26g of fat, of which 5.8g is saturated. Chicken drumsticks have been coated in crumbs and, with the chips, have been deep-fried in oil, then served with minimum vegetables.

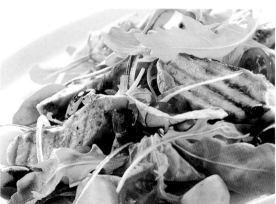

**Griddled chicken breast** Served with a fresh salad (no dressing) and boiled new potatoes, this is an appealing, healthy variation on the meal above. The result provides just 264 calories and 6g of fat (of which only 1.4g is saturated).

and shellfish, poultry, and plant proteins such as pulses instead of red meat; choosing low-fat dairy products; avoiding cream- and butter-based sauces; and using low-fat cooking methods (*below*).

## Recommended fat limits

Fat intake should be no more than 30–35 per cent of total calories each day, and saturated fat should be less than ten per cent of your total caloric intake. If we take an average of 33 per cent fat and 2000 calories per day for women and older adults and 2500 calories for men, the recommended daily limit for women and older adults is then 73g of fat, with no more than 22g of saturated fat; and for men, 92g of fat, with no more than 27g of saturated fat.

## Butter versus margarine

The controversy about whether to use butter or margarine as a spread or for cooking rests on how much saturated fat, trans fatty acids, and cholesterol each contains. With this information you can make your own decision.

Butter contains only very small amounts of trans fatty acids, but it does have high levels of cholesterol and saturated fat: 15g (½oz) of butter contains 33mg of cholesterol and over 7g saturated fat. Healthy people should keep saturated fat intake to 22–27g each day (in the UK there are no guidelines for cholesterol).

Margarine contains no cholesterol and has low levels of saturated fat; however, some magarines have high levels of trans fatty acids, which can pose the same risks to health as saturated fats. Many manufacturers in the UK have removed trans fats from their margarines.

At the moment, food labels do not mention trans fats in the Nutrition Information, although hydrogenated fat is included; however, in the future all food labels are likely to include weights of trans fats.

At the end of the day, the choice about whether to use butter or margarine is a personal one. If you don't consume much fat or large amounts of saturated fat elsewhere in your diet, you may prefer to use butter, but as with all types of fat, the amount should be limited in a healthy diet.

# Low-fat cooking

Frying – and particularly deep-frying – is a cooking method that can greatly increase fat content. It should be used rarely if you are trying to reduce fat intake in your diet.

Instead, look for methods that help keep fat levels to a minimum, such as those illustrated here. These are all simple to use and allow you to cook meat, fish, vegetables, and fruit in quick and healthy ways, retaining essential nutrients without adding unhealthy fat. Other low-fat cooking tips include:

• Add water, wine, and lemon juice if the ingredients require extra moisture.
• Choose lean cuts of meat and poultry and remove visible fat before cooking.
• Use a rack when grilling or roasting so the fat can drip through, and use a gravy separator to remove the fat from roast meat or poultry juices before making gravy.
• Reduce the amount of oil or fat needed by using non-stick pans.
• Stir-fry in stock rather than in oil.
• Microwave or steam food.
• Instead of deep-frying, brush food with a little oil and grill or roast for the same crisp effect.

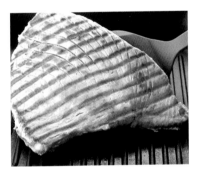

**Griddling** Very little oil is needed to prevent food from sticking, and excess fat drains into the grooves of the ridged grill pan.

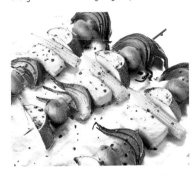

**Grilling** This method, which needs no fat, gives foods a crisp, browned exterior. Basting or marinating add flavour and keep food moist.

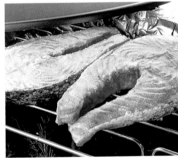

**Hot-smoking** Fish, meat, and poultry can be cooked on a rack in a covered wok over a layer of tea leaves and other interesting flavourings.

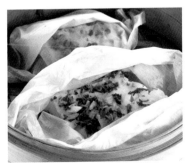

*En papillote* Seal in the flavour, nutrients, and juices by putting food in parchment or foil parcels and then baking or steaming.

# Proteins for growth

## These are a major component of every cell in our bodies.

Like fats (see pp.38–43) and carbohydrates (see pp.46–47), proteins are complex compounds that contain the elements carbon, hydrogen, and oxygen. They are also rich in the element nitrogen, which makes up about 16 per cent of their total weight. The building blocks of proteins are called amino acids (opposite).

### How we use protein

Every type of tissue in the body, including bones, skin, muscles, and organs, has its own set of proteins that help it perform its characteristic functions. Proteins help give structure to our cells and are important in cell growth, repair, and maintenance. Like carbohydrates and fats, they can also serve as an energy source. In addition, enzymes, hormones, and antibodies are all different types of proteins.

The protein that we eat has to be broken down, or digested, into amino acids and peptides (chains of amino acids) and then absorbed into the bloodstream. This pool of amino acids provides most of the elements that are needed to build new proteins in the body.

### Good sources

When we think of dietary protein, we tend to think of meat, eggs, and dairy products such as milk, cheese, and yogurt. While these foods are rich sources of this vital dietary element, protein is also found in many plant foods, such as pulses, grains, and nuts and seeds. In order to obtain the full range of essential amino acids (opposite), you should eat a variety of protein foods. Many people choose red meat (beef, pork, lamb, and veal) as their main source of protein, and eat it on a regular basis. But eating other types of protein-rich foods, such as fish, pulses, and nuts and seeds, can yield benefits for your health.

Studies have shown that people who eat less red meat and eat more fish and chicken lower their risk of developing cardiovascular disease (see pp.214–221) and colorectal cancer (see p.259). In addition, fish provides a range of key nutrients such as omega-3 fatty acids (see pp.90–91) that can improve health, and pulses and grains are a useful source of fibre and phytochemicals.

**Changing requirements** Protein needs are greatest during periods of growth, such as childhood, pregnancy, and convalescence.

## How much protein do you need?

According to the recommended daily amount (RDA) guidelines, the amount of protein needed by adult men and women is the following:
• Women aged 19–50 years need to consume 45g of protein per day.
• Men aged 19–50 years need to consume 55.5g of protein per day. The difference in the protein needs is due to the fact that, in general, men's bodies have more muscle mass than women's bodies.

How much protein you need in your daily diet is determined, in large part, by your overall energy intake, as well as by your body's need for nitrogen and essential amino acids. Physical activity and exertion increase your need for protein (see p.147). Requirements are also greater during childhood for growth and development, during pregnancy or when breast-feeding in order to nourish your baby, or when your body needs to recover from malnutrition or trauma or after an operation.

Because the body is continually breaking down protein from tissues, even adults who do not fall into the above categories need to include adequate protein in their diet every day. If you do not take in enough energy from your diet, your body will use protein from the muscle mass to meet its energy needs, and this can lead to muscle wasting over time.

### IS DEFICIENCY COMMON?

Protein deficiency is rare in developed countries, but it can occur in people who are dieting to lose weight, or in older adults who may have a poor diet. Convalescent people recovering from surgery, trauma, or illness may become protein deficient if they do not increase their intake to support their increased needs. A deficiency can also occur if the protein you eat is incomplete and fails to supply all the essential amino acids (opposite above).

### CAN YOU EAT TOO MUCH?

Since the body cannot store protein, it has to break down and dispose of any excess obtained from the diet. The liver removes nitrogen from amino acids, so that they can be burned as fuel, and the nitrogen is incorporated into urea, the substance that is excreted by the kidneys. These organs can normally cope with any extra workload, but if kidney disease occurs a decrease in protein will often be prescribed.

Excessive protein intake may also cause the body to lose calcium, which could lead to bone loss in the long-term. Foods that are high in protein (such as red meat) are often high in saturated fat, so excessive protein intake may also contribute to increased saturated fat.

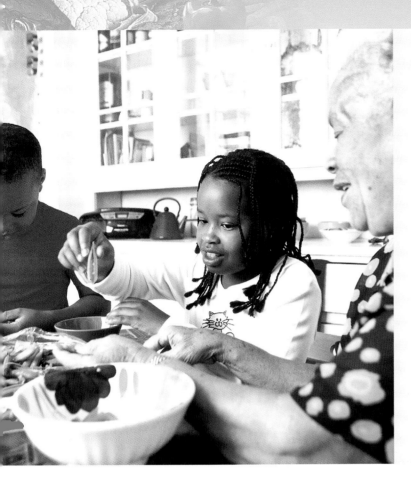

## What are amino acids?

Just as the letters of the alphabet can be combined in different ways to form an endless variety of words, amino acids can be linked together in varying sequences to form a huge variety of proteins. The unique shape of each protein determines its function in the body.

**Essential amino acids**  Our bodies require about 20 amino acids for normal functioning. Nine of these are considered essential – that is, your body cannot make them by itself and must get them from food. The essential amino acids are lysine, histidine, isoleucine, phenylalanine, leucine, methionine, tryptophan, threonine, and valine.

**Non-essential amino acids**  The remaining 11 amino acids are non-essential: although you can obtain them from food, the body can also synthesize them as needed.

# Good protein sources

Meat, poultry, fish, eggs, milk, and milk products such as cheese are excellent sources of protein, providing all of the amino acids that your body requires (*above*). However, the many nutritional advantage of these animal foods must be weighed up against their undesirable fat content (*see pp.40–43*) and lack of carbohydrates and dietary fibre.

Protein is also available from plants, in the form of pulses, nuts and seeds, and grains. With the exception of soya and soya products, plant proteins don't provide the full complement of amino acids, and so must be combined with other foods if they are the sole source of dietary protein (*see p.100*). Plant foods also contain useful amounts of dietary fibre (*see pp.48–49*) and carbohydrates (*see pp.46–47*), which are essential in a healthy, well-balanced diet.

| FOOD | SERVING SIZE | PROTEIN | CALORIES |
|---|---|---|---|
| Almonds | 100g (3½oz) | 21.1g | 612 |
| Tofu | 100g (3½oz) | 8.1g | 73 |
| Turkey breast (no skin) | 100g (3½oz) | 29.9g | 157 |
| Chicken breast (no skin) | 100g (3½oz) | 30.9g | 173 |
| Beef fillet (lean) | 100g (3½oz) | 29g | 188 |
| Pork fillet (lean) | 100g (3½oz) | 21.4g | 122 |
| Salmon | 100g (3½oz) | 20.2g | 180 |
| Eggs | 2 medium | 16g | 196 |
| Low-fat cottage cheese | 100g (3½oz) | 13.3g | 79 |
| Prawns | 80g (3oz) | 19.6g | 85 |
| Lentils, cooked | 100g (3½oz) | 7.6g | 100 |
| Low-fat fruit yogurt | 100g (3½oz) | 4.2g | 78 |
| Semi-skimmed milk | 100ml (3½floz) | 3.4g | 46 |

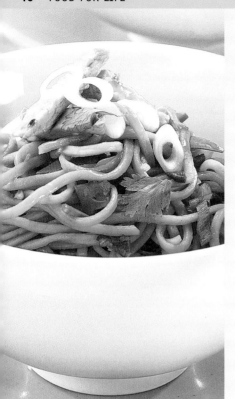

**Soba noodles** Made from buckwheat, soba noodles are high in fibre. They are quick to prepare and very versatile.

# Carbohydrates for energy

Carbohydrates form the foundation of a healthy diet, providing a readily available source of energy.

Carbohydrates are compounds composed of carbon, hydrogen, and oxygen and are generally classified as simple or complex, depending on their structure. Carbohydrates are obtained from grains, bread, rice, and pasta, as well as from fruits, vegetables, pulses, and dairy products.

## Variable complexity

All carbohydrates are composed of chains of sugar molecules. Those composed of just one or two sugar molecules are known as simple carbohydrates, and are divided into monosaccharides and disaccharides. Monosaccharides include glucose, which is present in the blood; fructose, which is found in fruits; and galactose, which is found in dairy products. Disaccharides include sucrose (table sugar) and lactose (the primary sugar present in milk).

## Choose the right carbohydrates

Some carbohydrates are really good sources of energy and nutrients, but others are a waste of calories. So which are the best carbohydrates, and how should you choose them?

The health benefits of complex carbohydrates are well established. These are found in nearly all foods of plant origin – grains, vegetables, and pulses – which also contain valuable nutrients, such as vitamins, minerals, phytochemicals, protein, and fibre, in addition to providing a good source of energy for the body. Grains, however, lose much of their nutrient content once they are refined (see p.75). To benefit from plant foods' natural goodness:
• Choose wholemeal bread and pasta and whole, unrefined grains and cereals to form the foundation of your diet.
• Limit your consumption of refined products such as cakes, biscuits, and sweets, and also of sweetened drinks.
• Eat plenty of fruits and vegetables (skin on when possible), raw or cooked for a minimum time (see p.288).

| CARBOHYDRATE SOURCE | BETTER CARBOHYDRATE SOURCE |
| --- | --- |
| White bread | Wholemeal or Granary bread |
| White rice | Brown rice |
| Croissant | Wholemeal English muffin |
| Pearl barley | Pot barley |
| Apple juice drink (sweetened) | Apple (with skin) |
| Chips | Jacket baked potato |
| Sweetcorn | Lentils |
| Fried tortilla chips | Baked tortilla chips |
| Cream crackers | Oatcakes |
| Cornflake cereal | Raisin bran cereal |
| Instant porridge | Traditional porridge |
| White pasta | Whole-grain pasta |
| Egg noodles | Soba noodles |
| Couscous | Bulgur wheat |

Complex carbohydrates, also called polysaccharides, are composed of many simple-sugar molecules that are linked together. Examples of complex carbohydrates include starch, which gives potatoes and grains their hearty character; glycogen, which the body stores as a source of energy; and dietary fibre (see pp.48–49).

## Why do we need them?

Carbohydrates provide energy for all the body's activities. As they are digested, carbohydrates are broken down into simple sugars, such as glucose. Glucose supplies energy for most of the body's activities, and in some cells and tissues such as red blood cells and the brain it is the sole source of energy.

Carbohydrates are needed for building the non-essential amino acids that the body uses to create proteins (see p.45). They also help in the processing of fat and in the building of cartilage, bone, and tissues of the nervous system.

## Choosing carbohydrates

As the major source of energy, carbohydrates must form a large part of your diet, but you should choose the best types to optimize your health. This means eating a wide variety of different types of

## Jargon buster

**Insulin resistance**  A reduced sensitivity in the tissues of the body to the action of the hormone insulin (see p.246). As a result of this sensitivity, blood glucose does not enter those tissues to be used as a source of energy, so blood glucose levels remain abnormally high. The condition is found frequently in overweight and obese people.

grains, fruits, and vegetables. As far as possible, try to eat whole grains and products made from unrefined grains in preference to refined varieties. In this way, you will benefit from the nutrients and fibre that are removed during the refining process (see p.75).

Some researchers believe that the glycaemic index (GI; below) provides a useful guide to the best carbohydrates, and that low-GI foods, which release sugar more slowly into the blood, are of particular benefit to people with diabetes (see p.246) and insulin resistance (left). However, we believe that while the concept of the glycaemic index is interesting, it should not be relied on as the sole indicator of a carbohydrate's healthfulness. Nutritional content and fibre are also important and these should be borne in mind when choosing carbohydrates.

# Understanding the glycaemic index

The glycaemic index (GI) classifies foods according to how fast they release sugar (glucose) into the bloodstream. High-GI foods release glucose quickly, causing a rapid rise in blood-glucose levels, to which the body reacts with insulin, which turns on fat storage. Low-GI foods, in contrast, release glucose steadily over several hours, so less insulin is required. Diets based on low-GI foods are therefore recommended for those with diabetes (see p.246) and insulin resistance (above), as well as for people with cardiovascular disease (see p.214) and certain digestive disorders (see p.226).

**GI value**  This figure depends on various factors, including the type of carbohydrate the food contains, how it has been processed, and the presence of fat and dietary fibre. In general, low-GI foods contain more fibre, are less processed, and do not contain as much glucose as high-GI foods. However, there is not a simple correlation between complex carbohydrates and low-GI values. For example, wholemeal bread is a healthy carbohydrate, but it has a high-GI value, whereas fructose – the type of sugar found in fruits and frequently added to soft drinks in the form of corn syrup – has a low-GI value. However, this does not mean that products sweetened with corn syrup are healthy.

**Glycaemic loading**  This is a concept developed to deal with anomalies thrown up by the glycaemic index that cast doubt on its usefulness as a nutritional tool. For example, a well-known brand of chocolate fudge cake has a relatively low GI of 41, while a 100 per cent whole-grain loaf has a GI of 69 – though common sense tells us

that the latter is healthier. To deal with such paradoxes, glycaemic load is calculated by multiplying the GI value of a food by the amount of carbohydrate in one serving. This gives a figure that reflects both the time the food takes to be broken down into glucose and also its carbohydrate content.

**Conclusion**  Our view is that while glycaemic loading is a better indicator of glycaemic response than glycaemic index alone, this is still only part of the story. Other aspects of the nutritional value of foods must also be considered, including vitamin and mineral content, phytochemicals, fibre, and protein. In terms of health benefits, the evidence is clear that eating only refined grain products can increase the risk of a variety of diseases, while eating whole grains has beneficial health effects.

# Facts about fibre

**Fibre is essential for maintaining a healthy digestive system.**

Dietary fibre, which is obtained solely from foods of plant origin, plays a vital role in the digestive process. There are two types of dietary fibre: soluble fibre, which can dissolve in water; and insoluble fibre, which does not have the ability to dissolve in water.

## Soluble fibre

The inclusion of soluble fibre in the diet slows the breakdown of complex carbohydrates, such as starch, into simple sugars, such as glucose, thereby slowing the absorption of sugar and possibly leading to reduced levels of sugar in the blood. During digestion, soluble fibre forms a gel-like mass that binds cholesterol to the stool; if eaten in sufficient quantities, soluble fibre can also help reduce the levels of cholesterol in your blood. Good sources of soluble fibre include whole grains such as oats, barley, and rye, fruits, vegetables, and pulses.

## Insoluble fibre

This type of fibre occurs naturally in brown rice, wholemeal bread, whole-grain cereals, seeds, pulses, and in the skins of vegetables and fruits. It will not dissolve in water and is not digested or absorbed by the body. Including insoluble fibre in your daily diet will help keep the gastrointestinal tract clean and promote regular bowel movements. It does this by drawing water into the stools, making them larger and softer, and easier to pass.

## The benefits of fibre

Foods that are high in dietary fibre often take longer to eat, and they increase the feeling of fullness after

## Gut flora

The bacteria in the large intestine, which are referred to as gut flora, can break down some of the chemical bonds in fibre that are resistant to the digestive enzymes. People who eat plenty of fibre have healthy colons teeming with millions of these bacteria.

Researchers have suggested that the action of gut flora on fibre creates an acidic environment in the colon that decreases the risk of developing colorectal cancer (*see p.259*), which is currently the second most common cause of cancer death in the UK.

a meal because they slow down the passage of food through the intestine. This improves the body's blood-sugar response because fibre slows the rate at which glucose is released from food. This, in turn, slows the rise of blood-sugar levels so that less insulin (*see p.246*) is released into the bloodstream. In addition, because fibre-rich foods increase the feeling of fullness, they can help with weight control.

## Fighting disease

By promoting bowel regularity and keeping the gastrointestinal tract clean, inclusion of insoluble fibre in the diet may also reduce the risk of developing conditions such as diverticular disease (*see p.234*) and constipation (*see p.229*).

Studies have also shown that a high-fibre diet helps prevent diabetes (*see p.246*) and, as a result of the activity of gut flora, reduces the risk of developing colorectal cancer (*see p.259*). This cancer is rare in countries where the traditional diet consists mainly of cereals, fruits, and vegetables.

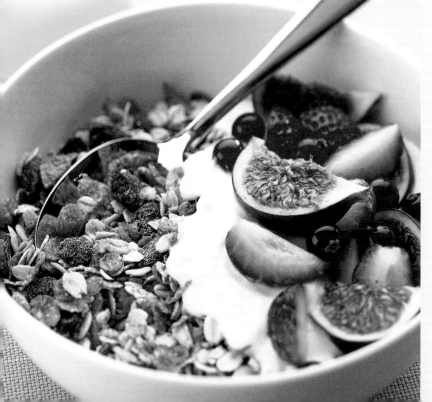

**High-fibre breakfast** Get your day off to a healthy start with a bowl of mixed-grain muesli topped with fresh fruit (skin on) and a serving of low-fat yogurt.

# How much fibre do I need?

According to the latest government guidelines, your total fibre intake should be 18g per day, depending on your age and gender (*see p.136 and p.151*). Most adults in the UK, however, get less than 12g of fibre each day. In order to ensure an adequate intake of both soluble and insoluble fibre, you should include a wide variety of fruits, vegetables, and whole grains in your daily diet.

| FOOD | SERVING SIZE | FIBRE |
|---|---|---|
| Kidney beans, cooked | 100g (3½oz) | 6.2g |
| Lentils, cooked | 100g (3½oz) | 1.9g |
| Bran flakes | 1 bowl (30g/1oz) | 3.9g |
| Peas, boiled | 80g (3oz) | 4.1g |
| Baked beans | 100g (3½oz) | 3.5g |
| Prunes, canned | 100g (3½oz) | 6.0g |
| Wholemeal bread | 1 slice | 2.0g |
| Porridge, cooked | 1 bowl (200g/7oz) | 1.8g |
| Apple (with skin) | 1 medium | 1.8g |
| Brown rice, boiled | 100g (3½oz) | 0.8g |

## Increasing fibre intake

If you plan to increase your fibre intake, do so gradually to give your system time to adjust. As you increase your intake, drink plenty of water to balance that absorbed by the fibre. The tips below can help you meet the recommended intake:
- Eat more vegetables, either raw or steamed. Cruciferous vegetables such as cabbage and broccoli are particularly high in fibre.
- Eat more fruit with skin and seeds, such as apples, pears, and berries.
- Choose high-fibre breakfast cereals, cold or hot.
- Add rolled oats or canned beans to casseroles, or use rolled oats for crumble toppings and stuffings.
- Eat whole-grain products, such as wholemeal bread, brown rice, and biscuits made from wholemeal flour rather than white flour.
- Add wheatgerm or oats to pancakes, meatballs, or burgers.
- Use cereal in place of nuts or in place of flour when making biscuits.

# Recipe  Crunchy high-fibre apricot and apple bars

### INGREDIENTS

**175g (6oz) dried apricots**

**2 apples**

**120ml (4floz) apple juice**

**225g (8oz) butter**

**75g (2½oz) soft brown sugar**

**175g (6oz) wholemeal flour**

**200g (7oz) porridge oats**

**Makes 16 bars**

**1** Preheat the oven to 180°C (350°F, gas 4). Very lightly oil a shallow baking tray measuring 31 x 21cm (12½ x 8½in).

**2** Chop the apricots, and peel, core, and finely chop the apples. Place in a pan with the apple juice and simmer for 10 minutes.

**3** Allow the mixture to cool slightly, then blend in a food processor until smooth.

**4** In a bowl, beat together the butter and sugar until creamy, then fold in the flour and oats.

**5** Spread half of the flour and oat mixture in the baking tray. Spoon over the apricot and apple mixture and spread out evenly. Spread the remaining flour and oat mixture on top and press down lightly.

**6** Bake for 30 minutes, until light golden. Cut into 16 bars while in the tray, and leave to cool before removing. Store in an airtight container.

**Each bar provides:**

Calories 231, Total fat 13g (Sat. 7.0g, Poly. 0.5g, Mono. 3.0g), Cholesterol 30mg, Protein 3.5g, Carbohydrate 27g, Fibre 2.8g, Sodium 120mg. Good source of – Vits: A; Mins: Ca, Mg, P.

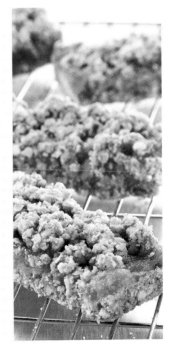

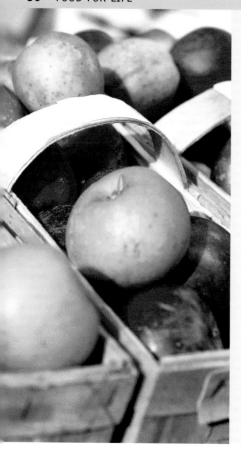

# What are vitamins?

## These are naturally occurring chemicals essential for health.

For many of us, the word "vitamin" conjures up the image of bottles of pills lining the shelves of the local chemist, or perhaps the fortified cereals that we eat for breakfast each morning. But these chemical substances occur naturally, in minute quantities, in most of the foods that we eat and, for the most part, we rely on food sources to meet our vitamin needs. However, there are a few vitamins that we obtain by other means: for example, micro-organisms in the intestine –

**Getting vitamins** Most of the foods we eat – either of plant or animal origin – contain some vitamins. Fruits such as apples and pears are useful sources of vitamin C.

commonly known as gut flora – produce vitamin K and biotin, while one form of vitamin D is made in the skin with the help of natural ultraviolet sunlight.

### Why we need vitamins

Although vitamins contain no calories, they are essential for normal growth and development, and many chemical reactions in the body. Vitamins are necessary for the body to use the calories provided by the food that we eat and help process proteins, carbohydrates, and fats. Vitamins are also involved in building cells, tissues, and organs – vitamin C, for example, helps produce healthy skin.

Vitamins are classified as fat-soluble or water-soluble, based on how they are absorbed by the body. Vitamins A, D, E, and K are fat-soluble, while the water-soluble

# How do you get vitamins?

For the most part, we rely on food sources or supplements to meet our vitamin and mineral requirements. However, there are a few exceptions to this; for example, gut flora (the micro-organisms in the intestinal tract) produce vitamin K. Vitamin D is also converted by the skin into a form that the body can use with the help of ultraviolet light in sunlight.

Because your body makes only a few vitamins itself, a balanced diet is very important – it ensures that your body receives the sufficient amount of vitamins, as well as minerals, that it requires each day.

### EAT A VARIETY OF FOODS

The key to getting enough vitamins in your diet is to eat a variety of foods. This is because while some nutrients tend to be found in substantial amounts in certain groups of foods, such as

vitamin C in fruits and vegetables, other nutrients, such as the B vitamins, are found in smaller amounts in a wide range of foods. No one food contains an adequate amount of all the vitamins that you require daily, but if you make healthy choices from a variety of foods, you are less likely to miss out on any one particular nutrient.

Most people buy the same foods each week, which can result in a limited range of vitamins. If you think this applies to you, we suggest that you read the "Good sources" boxes on the following pages, and aim to try some different foods each week. For example, eat two apricots instead of one orange, for a boost of vitamin A. Or choose salmon on your bagel instead of your usual cream cheese, to boost your intake of vitamin D. Buying vegetables and fruits in season also helps to vary your shopping choices.

## What are enriched and fortified foods?

During processing, some foods have vitamins or minerals added to them. For example, by law all white flour in the UK is fortified with calcium, iron, vitamin $B_1$ (thiamin), and niacin.

**Enriched foods** Nutrients originally present in a food that were lost during processing are replaced. For example, vitamin C is added back to fruit juices.

**Fortified foods** Nutrients are added that were never naturally a part of the food. For example, calcium is sometimes added to orange juice, and many vitamins and minerals are added to breakfast cereals to boost their nutritional value.

vitamins include vitamin C and the B-complex vitamins ($B_1$ or thiamin, $B_2$ or riboflavin, niacin, pantothenic acid, $B_6$, $B_{12}$, biotin, and folate).

Research has shown that foods rich in antioxidants are particularly beneficial for health. Antioxidants include vitamins A, C, and E, and they are found in a wide range of vegetables and fruits. Antioxidants neutralize free radicals (see p.58). A buildup of free radicals can damage body cells and tissues, resulting in disease. Studies have shown that diets rich in vegetables and fruits result in a lower incidence of some diseases, including certain cancers.

## Vitamin deficiencies

Deficiencies of vitamins are either primary or secondary. A primary deficiency occurs because you do not get enough of the vitamin in the food you eat. A secondary deficiency may be due to a lifestyle factor, such as smoking, excessive alcohol consumption, or the use of certain medications that interfere with the absorption or the body's use of the vitamin. Prolonged use of antibiotics will kill off the useful gut flora that make vitamin K (see p.58). Vitamin deficiencies may also be due to an underlying problem, such as an intestinal disorder, that prevents or limits the absorption or use of the vitamin.

Well-known vitamin deficiencies (and the diseases they cause) are $B_1$ (beriberi), niacin (pellagra), vitamin C (scurvy), and vitamin D (rickets). In Britain today, however, such deficiencies are rare due to an adequate food supply for most people, as well as food fortification programmes that add vitamins and minerals to common foods.

Scientists now have shifted their focus to discovering ways in which vitamins can promote health, prevent disease, boost the body's protection against infection, and slow down the ageing process. At the same time, public interest in vitamins has heightened. This has been prompted by headlines in the media and widespread advertising by the manufacturers of nutrient supplements.

The definitions of the amounts of vitamins (and minerals) that you should aim to receive every day – the recommended daily amounts (RDAs) – are discussed at the start of this chapter (see p.35).

## Vitamin overdosing

The likelihood of consuming too much of any vitamin from food is remote, but overdosing from vitamin supplementation often occurs (see pp.266–271). For example, many people take large amounts of vitamin C, usually in the belief that this will relieve or "cure" a cold (see p.57). However, overdosing on vitamin C can lead to diarrhoea or kidney stones. If you take vitamin supplements, you should always do so on the advice of your GP or a dietitian, and first consider whether your diet could be improved instead.

# Preserving the vitamin content of food

Many vitamins are easily destroyed by lengthy storage of food, processing, and cooking at high temperatures.
• Fruits and vegetables contain their highest level of nutrients when they are harvested at full ripeness and eaten soon thereafter, with minimum processing. The most nutritious produce consists of fresh fruits and vegetables picked at full maturity (avoid picking prematurely and allowing them to ripen off the vine) and eaten immediately.
• Frozen foods are a good choice for produce because they are generally picked at their peak freshness, quickly frozen, and stored at cold temperatures to preserve nutrients.
• Store foods properly to prevent nutrient losses. A cool, dark place is best since vitamin degradation accelerates at higher temperatures and several of the water-soluble vitamins, such as vitamin C and $B_2$, are very light-sensitive.

• Cooking contributes to vitamin losses, and many water-soluble vitamins are destroyed by heat. Therefore, it is best to keep cooking times to a minimum. Avoid boiling vegetables in large amounts of water because vitamins will leach out into the water. Instead, steam vegetables or microwave in a small amount of water in order to preserve the maximum nutrient content.

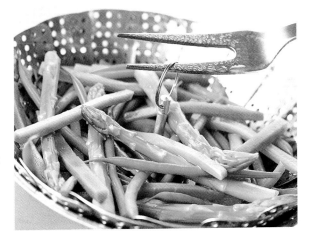

**Keeping nutrients**
Steam rather than boil vegetables to prevent vitamins, minerals, and other key nutrients from being leached out into the water.

# Vitamin directory

Here, we look at the role of each vitamin, how much we need, the symptoms and signs of a deficiency, and which foods are good sources. The recommended daily amounts (RDAs) given here are for healthy adults aged 19–50 years (*see p.35*); needs do vary at different stages of life (*see Eating for the Time of your Life, pp.104–155*).

## Vitamin A

### DAILY REQUIREMENT
**Men** 700mcg (EC 800mcg)
**Women** 600mcg (EC 800mcg)

This vitamin plays an essential role in vision, particularly night vision, normal bone growth, reproduction, and the health of skin and mucous membranes (the mucus-secreting layer that lines body regions such as the respiratory tract). Vitamin A also acts in the body as an antioxidant (*see p.58*), a protective chemical that may reduce the risk of certain cancers.

There are two sources of dietary vitamin A. Active forms, which are immediately available to the body, are obtained from animal products. These are known as retinoids and include retinal and retinol. Precursors, also known as provitamins, which must be converted to active forms by the body, are obtained from fruits and vegetables that contain yellow, orange, and dark green pigments or carotenoids. The

best known is beta-carotene. Vitamin A is measured in micrograms (mcg) as well as in Retinol Equivalents (RE): 1.0mcg RE is equivalent to 1.0mcg of retinol or 6.0mcg of beta-carotene.

In the intestine, vitamin A is protected from being chemically changed by vitamin E. Vitamin A is fat-soluble and can be stored in the body. Most of the vitamin A you eat is stored in the liver. When required by a particular part of the body, the liver releases some vitamin A, which is carried by the blood and delivered to the target cells and tissues.

### VITAMIN A DEFICIENCY
In many developing countries, a dietary deficiency of vitamin A is common, with pregnant women and infants being the most often affected. In the West, a deficiency is rare, but may occur in people who abuse alcohol or those with long-term conditions that affect their ability to absorb fats, such as cystic fibrosis or Crohn's disease (*see p.233*). This is because vitamin A is absorbed in fats. A common symptom of a severe deficiency of vitamin A is

the eye disorder xerophthalmia, in which the cornea (the transparent membrane at the front of the eye) hardens. This may progress to night blindness, corneal ulceration, and irreversible blindness.

Other signs and symptoms include growth problems in children, poor wound healing, and dry, bumpy skin rashes known as follicular hyperkeratosis. Vitamin A deficiency can also affect the health of the epidermis (skin) and the normal functioning of mucous membranes throughout the body.

## Good sources
**Vitamin A** This is found naturally in all these foods, which contain at least 0.15mcg of the vitamin, or 150mcg RE, per 50–200g (2–7oz):
- Sweet potatoes
- Carrots
- Cabbage
- Kale
- Pumpkin
- Spinach
- Peppers
- Butternut squash
- Apricots
- Orange-fleshed melon
- Mango
- Liver (beef, pork, chicken, or turkey)
- Eggs

## Vitamin A helps night vision

Night blindness – the inability to see well in dim light – is associated with a deficiency of vitamin A. This vitamin is needed for the formation of rhodopsin. This is a pigment located in the eye's retina, which is the light-sensitive tissue lining in the back of the eye.

When stimulated by light, rhodopsin splits into two proteins: opsin and retinal (a form of vitamin

A); in dim light or darkness, the reverse occurs: the retinal and opsin combine to re-form rhodopsin, a reaction that requires extra retinal.

Without adequate amounts of retinal, regeneration of rhodopsin is incomplete and night blindness occurs. Since carrots are a good source of beta-carotene, there is truth in the old saying that carrots can help you see better in the dark!

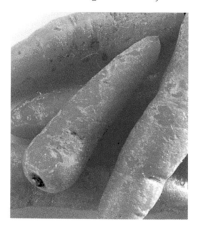

**Carrots** Rich in beta-carotene (a form of vitamin A), one medium carrot gives almost all the vitamin A you need for one day. Carrots also contain vitamins $B_1$ and $B_6$.

# Vitamin B$_1$

## DAILY REQUIREMENT
**Men** 1.0mg (EC 1.4mg)
**Women** 0.8mg (EC 1.4mg)

Also known as thiamin, vitamin B$_1$ plays an important role in helping the body convert carbohydrates and fats into energy. It is essential for normal growth and development and helps to maintain proper functioning of the heart and the nervous and digestive systems. Vitamin B$_1$ is water-soluble and cannot be stored in the body; however, once absorbed, the vitamin is concentrated in muscle tissue.

## VITAMIN B$_1$ DEFICIENCY
Primary deficiency is rare; however, deficiency sometimes occurs in people who abuse alcohol because excessive alcohol intake significantly decreases the body's ability to absorb this vitamin and interferes with its chemical reactions in the body.

In the early stages of a vitamin B$_1$ deficiency, symptoms may include poor appetite, irritability, fatigue, and weight loss. As the deficiency becomes more advanced, weakness, nerve damage that may affect the hands and feet, headache, and a rapid heart rate may also develop.

A form of vitamin B$_1$ deficiency, known as beriberi, affects babies who are breast-fed by mothers with a B$_1$ deficiency. Beriberi also affects people who abuse alcohol and those who eat a

## Good sources
**Vitamin B$_1$** This is found naturally in all these foods, which contain at least 0.1mg of the vitamin per 25–100g (1–3½oz):
- Peas
- Spinach
- Liver
- Beef
- Pork
- Wholemeal bread
- Nuts
- Bran flakes
- Soya beans

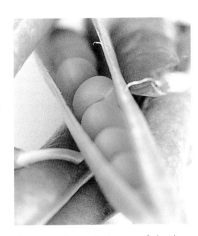

**Green peas** An excellent source of vitamin B$_1$, peas also contain significant amounts of beta-carotene (a precursor of vitamin A), niacin, folate, vitamin C, and protein.

lot of refined carbohydrates – especially polished rice, from which vitamin A is removed during processing. In its most advanced stages, beriberi will cause problems with the nervous system and the heart, leading to an abnormal heart rhythm (arrhythmia) and heart failure (see pp.216–221).

# Vitamin B$_2$

## DAILY REQUIREMENT
**Men** 1.3mg (EC 1.6mg)
**Women** 1.1mg (EC 1.6mg)

This water-soluble vitamin, also known as riboflavin, is necessary for the release of energy from carbohydrates (see p.46). Vitamin B$_2$ is needed for normal growth and development. It helps to build up glucose molecules into the complex carbohydrate glycogen, which is stored in the liver for future use; helps digest fats; is involved in changing the amino acid tryptophan into niacin; helps protect the nervous system; and also maintains mucous membranes – the mucus-secreting layer that lines body regions such as the respiratory tract.

## VITAMIN B$_2$ DEFICIENCY
A deficiency of vitamin B$_2$ can be primary – due to not getting enough of the vitamin from the diet – or

## Good sources
**Vitamin B$_2$** This is found naturally in all these foods, which contain at least 0.1mg of the vitamin per 85–300g (3–10½oz):
- Asparagus
- Okra
- Cottage cheese
- Milk
- Yogurt
- Meat
- Eggs
- Fish

secondary, which may be a result of conditions that affect absorption in the intestine, the body not being able to use the vitamin, or an increase in the excretion of the vitamin from the body.

Signs and symptoms of vitamin B$_2$ deficiency include cracked and red lips, inflammation of the lining of the mouth and tongue, mouth ulcers, cracks at the corners of the mouth, and a sore throat. A deficiency may also cause dry and scaling skin, fluid in the mucous membranes, and iron-deficiency anaemia (see p.55). The eyes may also become bloodshot, itchy, watery, and sensitive to bright light.

# Niacin

## DAILY REQUIREMENT
**Men** 17mg (EC 18mg)
**Women** 13mg (EC 18mg)

Also known as nicotinic acid or nicotinamide and abbreviated to Nia, niacin participates in at least 200 different chemical reactions involved in energy production. It is also necessary for the production and breakdown of glucose, fats, and amino acids; the development, maintenance, and function of the skin, intestine and stomach, and nervous system; and in manufacturing DNA (the substance that makes up our genes). This vitamin can also be made in the body from the amino acid tryptophan, provided that there is also sufficient vitamin B$_6$ (see p.54).

Although excessive amounts of the vitamin may be harmful to some people,

## Good sources

**Niacin** This is found naturally in all these foods, which contain at least 1.0mg niacin per 25–100g (1–3½oz):
- Peas
- Liver
- Red meat
- Poultry
- Mackerel
- Mullet
- Salmon
- Swordfish
- Kidney beans
- Peanuts
- Soya beans

doses (1–3g per day) have been used successfully in the treatment of high blood-cholesterol levels (see p.216). Niacin has also been used to treat dizziness and ringing in the ears and to prevent premenstrual headaches.

### NIACIN DEFICIENCY
Dietary deficiency of niacin is rare in Britain as this vitamin is found mainly in protein-rich foods. However, it does affect people whose diet consists primarily of maize, because maize does not contain the essential amino acid tryptophan (see p.45).

Niacin deficiency can be caused by a deficiency of vitamin $B_6$ (right) since the manufacture of niacin from tryptophan

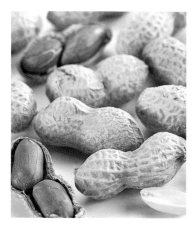

**Peanuts** Not only rich in niacin, peanuts – which are actually a legume and not a nut – are also a good source of protein and the minerals magnesium, iron, and zinc.

requires vitamin $B_6$. People who drink excessive amounts of alcohol are also at increased risk of niacin deficiency because alcohol significantly reduces the body's ability to absorb this vitamin from the intestine.

Early symptoms of niacin deficiency – which is known as pellagra – include fatigue, loss of appetite, weakness, mild diarrhoea, anxiety, irritability, and sometimes depression. The lining of the mouth and the tongue may become inflamed and sore and have a burning sensation. If the pellagra becomes advanced, symptoms may then include severe diarrhoea, skin rashes, delirium, and death if not treated.

# Pantothenic acid

### DAILY REQUIREMENT
**Men** none set in UK (EC 6.0mg)
**Women** none set in UK (EC 6.0mg)

This B-complex vitamin, also known as vitamin $B_5$ and abbreviated to Pant, helps to break down proteins and their amino acids, fats, and carbohydrates, enabling the production of energy. It is also required for the manufacture of vitamin $B_{12}$, haemoglobin (the oxygen-carrying pigment in red blood cells), and cell membranes, which enclose the contents of body cells.

## Good sources

**Pantothenic acid** This is found in all these foods, which contain at least 0.5mg of the vitamin per 100–250g (3½–8½oz):
- Sweet potatoes
- Avocado
- Mushrooms
- Yogurt
- Kidneys
- Liver
- Red meat
- Mackerel
- Mullet
- Salmon
- Trout
- Lentils
- Broad beans
- Haricot beans

### PANTOTHENIC ACID DEFICIENCY
There is no evidence that a deficiency of pantothenic acid occurs naturally, because the vitamin is made by the body. The nerve inflammation seen in people who abuse alcohol may be due to a deficiency of this vitamin; however, further evidence is needed to confirm this association.

Symptoms may include stomach pain, cramp, and fatigue, but this may mean a deficiency in all B-complex vitamins.

# Vitamin $B_6$

### DAILY REQUIREMENT
**Men** 1.4mg (EC 2.0mg)
**Women** 1.2mg (EC 2.0mg)

Also known as pyridoxine, vitamin $B_6$ is involved in the production and digestion of amino acids (see p.45). This vitamin helps the body manufacture the hormone insulin (see p.246); antibodies that fight infection; and certain chemicals that send messages between nerve cells. It is involved in the production of the chemical histamine, which is involved in allergic reactions. Vitamin $B_6$ also plays a key role in the production of haemoglobin (the oxygen-carrying molecule in red blood cells) and in the ability of oxygen to bind with the haemoglobin molecule.

A form of vitamin $B_6$ is used to treat or relieve the symptoms of a variety of disorders, including premenstrual syndrome, gestational diabetes, asthma, and depression. The vitamin may also help prevent cardiovascular disease in people who have high blood levels of the amino acid homocysteine – which may lead to cardiovascular disease (see pp.214–221).

### VITAMIN $B_6$ DEFICIENCY
This can occur in babies fed infant formula that does not contain vitamin $B_6$. It can also affect people who abuse alcohol, cigarette smokers, and women who use oral contraceptives. Certain medications can lower the level of vitamin $B_6$ in the body. For example, some of the medication used to treat or prevent the lung infection tuberculosis makes vitamin $B_6$ inactive.

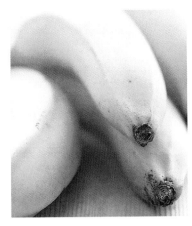

**Bananas**  A particularly good source of vitamin B$_6$, bananas also provide folate, potassium, and soluble fibre. They are best eaten ripe – when the skin is speckled brown.

Medical conditions that are thought to decrease the levels of vitamin B$_6$ in the blood are asthma, kidney disease, Hodgkin's disease, sickle-cell anaemia, and diabetes.

The symptoms of a mild vitamin B$_6$ deficiency include cracked lips, oily, flaky skin, nausea, and diarrhoea. If the deficiency becomes more severe, loss of appetite, depression, and confusion may then develop.

Because vitamin B$_6$ is required to convert the amino acid tryptophan into niacin, there may also be signs and symptoms of a deficiency of niacin (*opposite*), which include weakness, fatigue, irritability, and anxiety.

## Good sources

**Vitamin B$_6$**  This is found in these foods, which contain at least 0.5mg of vitamin B$_6$ per 100–200g (3½–7oz):

- Potatoes
- Sweet potatoes
- Bananas
- Chicken
- Turkey
- Mackerel
- Mullet
- Salmon
- Swordfish
- Trout
- Tuna

# Vitamin B$_{12}$

### DAILY REQUIREMENT
**Men**  1.5mcg (EC 1.0mcg)
**Women**  1.5mcg (EC 1.0mcg)

Also known as cyanocobalamin or cobalamin, vitamin B$_{12}$ is released from food in the stomach. In order for this vitamin to be absorbed into the blood, it has to bind with a protein called intrinsic factor, which is produced by the cells lining the stomach.

Vitamin B$_{12}$ is necessary for normal growth and development, especially in babies, young children, and teenagers and, with the vitamin folate (*see p.56*), in the production of oxygen-carrying red blood cells. It is also required for the proper functioning of the nervous system; manufacturing DNA (the substance that makes up our genes); and the processing of fats and carbohydrates.

The vitamin is found naturally only in foods of animal origin, including seafood, although many other foods are now fortified with it. Vegetarians, especially vegans (*see p.100*), are therefore at risk of a vitamin B$_{12}$ deficiency and should take a supplement.

## Anaemia and deficiencies

This is any of various disorders in which haemoglobin (the oxygen-carrying pigment in red blood cells) is deficient or abnormal, resulting in body cells and tissues not getting enough oxygen. Symptoms include constant fatigue, pale skin, and shortness of breath on exertion. Some types result from vitamin or mineral deficiencies.

**Iron-deficiency anaemia**  This is caused by low levels of iron in the body. Iron is part of haemoglobin. This type of anaemia is usually due to an insufficient intake of iron in the diet (*see p.66*) or severe blood loss.

**Megaloblastic anaemia**  This results from either low levels of vitamin B$_{12}$ (*above*) or folate (*see p.56*). These two vitamins are essential for the

## Good sources

**Vitamin B$_{12}$**  These foods naturally contain at least 0.5mcg of vitamin B$_{12}$ per 50–250g (2–8½oz):

- Dairy products
- Offal (liver, heart, kidneys)
- Eggs
- Beef
- Seafood

### VITAMIN B$_{12}$ DEFICIENCY
A deficiency may also occur in people who cannot produce intrinsic factor, placing them at risk of pernicious anaemia (*below*). Because vitamin B$_{12}$ is absorbed towards the end of the intestine (*see p.36*), people who have had their ileum surgically removed need injections of the vitamin.

Many older people lose their ability to produce sufficient gastric acid and pepsin, which is an enzyme necessary to separate vitamin B$_{12}$ from food, so that they absorb less vitamin B$_{12}$. As a result, they may need to take vitamin B$_{12}$ supplements (*see p.150*).

In addition, older people may have too many bacteria in the stomach that are normally killed by stomach acid.

formation of red blood cells, and a deficiency of either one causes the formation of abnormally large red blood cells known as macrocytes, or megaloblasts, because the red blood cells do not divide properly and cannot carry oxygen effectively.

**Pernicious anaemia**  Megaloblastic anaemia will sometimes develop because of an autoimmune reaction in which the body's immune system attacks the stomach lining. This decreases the amount of intrinsic factor made by the stomach lining, and leads to vitamin B$_{12}$ deficiency – B$_{12}$ has to bind with intrinsic factor in order for it to be absorbed into the bloodstream and used by the body. When megaloblastic anaemia is caused by an autoimmune reaction, it is known as pernicious anaemia.

These bacteria use up dietary vitamin $B_{12}$ for their own needs, leaving less available for the body to use.

Symptoms of vitamin $B_{12}$ deficiency include megaloblastic anaemia (*see p.55*), nerve damage (often felt as tingling in the hands and feet), and inflammation of the tongue and mouth. A long-term deficiency can cause irreversible nerve damage. Dementia has also been linked to a deficiency of vitamin $B_{12}$.

# Biotin

### DAILY REQUIREMENT
**Men** none set in UK (EC 150mcg)
**Women** none set in UK (EC 150mcg)

Another of the B-complex vitamins, biotin is essential for converting proteins, carbohydrates, and fats into forms that the body can use.

### BIOTIN DEFICIENCY
Pregnant women, people who abuse alcohol, and those who do not produce sufficient amounts of stomach acid, such as older people, may have low levels of biotin.

Symptoms and signs of biotin deficiency include inflammation and increased sensitivity of the skin; hair loss; muscle pain; loss of appetite; nausea; mental problems; high levels of cholesterol in the blood; and a reduction in levels of haemoglobin, the oxygen-carrying pigment in red blood cells, leading to the symptoms of anaemia (*see p.55*).

## Good sources
**Biotin** This is found in these foods, which contain at least 1.5mcg of biotin per 25–100g (1–3½oz):
- Cauliflower
- Mushrooms
- Liver
- Egg yolks
- Mackerel
- Sardines
- Kidney beans
- Peanuts
- Yeast

# Folate

### DAILY REQUIREMENT
**Men** 200mcg (EC 200mcg)
**Women** 200mcg (EC 200mcg)

Another of the B vitamins, also called folacin or folic acid and abbreviated to Fol, folate cannot be made by the body and must therefore come from food or supplements. Folate plays a vital role in making DNA (the substance that makes up our genes) and RNA (a substance needed to make proteins), in normal growth and development, and in the production of new cells. It works with vitamin $B_{12}$ to form haemoglobin for red blood cells, and helps convert the amino acid homocysteine to methionine.

A good supply of folate prior to and in early pregnancy reduces the risk of the baby developing a neural tube defect such as spina bifida (*see p.140*). If you are thinking of having a baby or are in the first trimester of a pregnancy, you should take a supplement of 400mcg (0.4mg) of folate every day.

### FOLATE DEFICIENCY
A deficiency of folate is common today since many people consume diets high in fat and processed foods and eat less than the daily recommended five servings of fruits and vegetables. A folate deficiency occurs in people with an

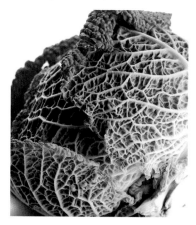

**Cabbage** This is a superfood. Rich in folate, cabbage is also a good source of beta-carotene (a precursor of vitamin A), vitamin C, fibre, and cancer-fighting phytochemicals.

## Good sources
**Folate** This is found naturally in all these foods, which contain at least 30mcg of folate per 85–200g (3–7oz):
- Sweetcorn
- Asparagus
- Brussels sprouts
- Cabbage
- Cauliflower
- Fresh green vegetables
- Peas
- Spinach
- Oranges
- Liver
- Black-eye beans
- Black beans
- Chickpeas
- Lentils
- Pinto beans
- Kidney beans

intestinal disorder such as Crohn's disease (*see p. 233*), in which they cannot absorb this and other vitamins. Folate deficiency in older people may be the result of a poor diet and normal ageing. In addition, older people produce less of the stomach acid needed for the digestion of folate. Certain medications and alcohol can affect the body's ability to take up folate.

Lack of folate causes megaloblastic anaemia (*see p.55*), with symptoms such as fatigue, shortness of breath on mild exertion, and pale skin. Other symptoms include diarrhoea, weight loss, sore mouth, and heartburn. A deficiency also results in raised levels of homocysteine (an amino acid), which may lead to cardiovascular disease.

# Vitamin C

### DAILY REQUIREMENT
**Men** 40mg (EC 60mg)
**Women** 40mg (EC 60mg)

Also known as ascorbic acid, vitamin C cannot be manufactured by the body so it must be acquired from the diet. It is the least stable of the vitamins and is easily destroyed during cooking and food processing. If consumed in high quantities, excess vitamin C is excreted

## Vitamin C and the common cold

The role of vitamin C in fighting infection has been controversial for decades. At present, research shows that vitamin C reduces histamine levels in the body, and it can be helpful in reducing the symptoms as well as the duration of a cold. However, there is no evidence to suggest that vitamin C can prevent or cure the common cold. It is advisable to try to get all your vitamin C from your diet. If you do take supplements, limit them to less than 1000mg per day because higher doses may cause problems such as diarrhoea and kidney stones.

in the urine. Vitamin C is essential for the formation of collagen, an important structural protein that strengthens bones and blood vessels and anchors teeth into the gums, in addition to being necessary for body growth, tissue repair, and wound healing. It also acts as an antioxidant (see p.58), protects against infection by enabling white blood cells to break down bacteria, is involved in the production of red blood cells and their oxygen-carrying pigment haemoglobin, and helps the body absorb iron from the intestine.

### VITAMIN C DEFICIENCY
People who do not get enough fresh citrus fruits and juices may have insufficient vitamin C intake, as may those who are following a restricted diet. Regular drinkers and smokers are at risk of vitamin C deficiency since alcohol prevents the absorption of the vitamin and cigarette smoking depletes levels. People with wounds and burns, pneumonia, tuberculosis, and rheumatic fever, as well as those recovering from surgery, may need more vitamin C to help with the healing process.

Vitamin C deficiency causes scurvy, which is a condition that leads to muscle weakness, joint pain, problems with wound healing, loose teeth, bleeding and swollen gums, easily bruised skin or little red spots on the skin, fatigue, and sometimes depression.

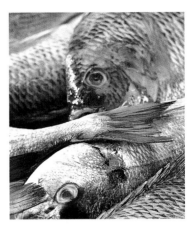

**Mackerel** A good source of vitamin D, this fish also contains niacin, vitamins $B_6$ and $B_{12}$, phosphorus, iodine, selenium, potassium, and heart-protecting omega-3 fatty acids.

## Good sources

**Vitamin C** This is found in these foods, which contain at least 10mg of the vitamin per 50–200g (2–7oz):
- Plantain
- Asparagus
- Broccoli
- Brussels sprouts
- Cabbage
- Peppers
- Tomatoes
- Blackberries
- Grapefruit
- Guava
- Kiwi fruit
- Mango
- Melon
- Oranges
- Pineapples
- Strawberries

# Vitamin D

### DAILY REQUIREMENT
**Men**  none set in UK (EC 5.0mcg)
**Women**  none set in UK (EC 5.0mcg)

This fat-soluble vitamin has an essential role in the absorption and use of calcium (see p.62) and phosphorus (see p.63), and therefore in the formation and health of bones, teeth, and cartilage (the tough, fibrous tissue that covers the ends of bones at joints). Vitamin D occurs in two forms: vitamin $D_2$, which is found in a small number of foods, and vitamin $D_3$, which is formed in the skin when exposed to sunlight. Both $D_2$ and $D_3$ are converted into a form that the body can use (active form) in the liver and kidneys.

When calcium levels in the blood are low, parathyroid hormone is released by the parathyroid glands, which are located in the neck. This hormone stimulates the kidneys to convert vitamin D into its active form, which in turn stimulates the intestine to increase the absorption of calcium and phosphorus. Vitamin D is also measured in International Units (IU), in which 40IU equals 0.001mg.

### VITAMIN D DEFICIENCY
In countries where milk and dairy foods are enriched with vitamin D, deficiency is rare. Because sunlight is so important in the manufacture of vitamin D, people most at risk are older adults, especially those who are bed-ridden or unable to get out and about easily.

Deficiency may also occur in people who cover themselves for religious or cultural reasons or for necessity, such as in cold climates, and those living in urban areas with high air pollution who get little exposure to sunshine. Other groups at risk of vitamin D deficiency include those requiring long-term use of certain anti-convulsant medications, which interfere with the conversion of vitamin D into its active form. In addition, people with chronic kidney disease are at risk of a deficiency due to the kidney's

## Good sources

**Vitamin D** This is found naturally in all these foods, which contain at least 3.0mcg of the vitamin per 50–100g (2–3½oz):
- Egg yolk
- Cod and halibut liver oils
- Mackerel
- Salmon
- Sardines
- Tuna

inability to convert vitamin D into its active form. Deficiency of the vitamin is characterized by softening of the bones, a condition called osteomalacia in adults and rickets in children. Osteomalacia may lead to pain in the legs, ribs, hips, and muscles, easily broken bones, and difficulty in climbing stairs or getting up from a sitting position. Rickets leads to deformity of the bones, especially bowing of the legs and abnormal curvature of the spine.

# Vitamin E

### DAILY REQUIREMENT
**Men** none set in UK (EC 10mg)
**Women** none set in UK (EC 10mg)

This fat-soluble vitamin is considered to be one of nature's most effective antioxidants, which protect the body against free radicals (*right*). Vitamin E also protects vitamin A from becoming chemically changed, helps make red blood cells, and prevents blood from clotting. It is stored primarily in the liver, in fat, and in muscle tissue.

### VITAMIN E DEFICIENCY
Dietary deficiency of vitamin E is very rare. The deficiency only really occurs in people with long-term conditions that prevent the absorption of fats from the intestine, such as cystic fibrosis or Crohn's disease (*see p.233*).

Signs and symptoms of vitamin E deficiency include problems with the nervous system and anaemia (*see p.55*), which is due to the shortened lifespan of red blood cells.

## Good sources
**Vitamin E** This is found in these foods, which contain at least 0.5mg of the vitamin per 25–50g (1–2oz):
● Wheat germ
● Prawns
● Almonds
● Hazelnuts
● Peanuts
● Pistachio nuts
● Soya beans
● Sunflower seeds

# Jargon buster

**Free radicals** These are chemical by-products generated during normal biochemical reactions in the body. They are highly reactive and are used by the body to kill bacteria, to fight inflammation, and to maintain smooth muscle tone. If they build up, free radicals can damage – by a process that is called oxidation – proteins, fats, DNA (the substance that makes up genes), and – if enough accumulate – body cells and tissues.

**Antioxidants** These are chemicals that occur in fruits and vegetables, and are also made naturally in the body, which can neutralize free radicals (*above*). Antioxidant sources include vitamins A, C, and E and the minerals copper, selenium, and zinc.

# Vitamin K

### DAILY REQUIREMENT
**Men** none set in UK or for EC
**Women** none set in UK or for EC

This fat-soluble vitamin is an essential component in the body's normal blood-clotting process. Most of the vitamin K that we require is produced by the gut flora, which are the micro-organisms living naturally in the intestine, but the vitamin is also obtained from food. It is stored mainly in the liver.

If you have been prescribed blood-thinning medication, consult your GP about your vitamin K intake because vitamin K may interfere with the effect of your medication.

## Antibiotics and vitamin K
If you take antibiotics for more than a few weeks, it is likely that such treatment will kill off helpful gut flora (micro-organisms in the intestine including the bacteria that make vitamin K) as well as the harmful bacteria targeted by the

## Good sources
**Vitamin K** This is found in these foods, which contain at least 0.01mg of the vitamin per 50–200g (2–7oz):
● Asparagus
● Broccoli
● Brussels sprouts
● Cabbage
● Carrots
● Cauliflower
● Celery
● Peas
● Spinach
● Apricots
● Grapes
● Pears
● Plums

### VITAMIN K DEFICIENCY
A dietary deficiency of this vitamin is rare because we get almost all that we require from the gut flora. However, a deficiency may occur in people who have any condition that affects the absorption of fats from the intestine, such as cystic fibrosis. In addition, the long-term use of antibiotic medication can lead to a deficiency of vitamin K because of the effect of the antibiotics on gut flora (*below*).

Because vitamin K deficiency reduces the ability of blood to clot, symptoms may include bleeding from the mouth, genital and urinary tracts, stomach, intestine, and skin. The skin may also bruise easily.

In newborn infants, the manufacture of vitamin K in the intestine takes about a week to become established; therefore, there is a risk of the bleeding disorder called haemorrhagic disease of the newborn. Infants now routinely receive a vitamin K injection at birth to help the blood clot if bleeding occurs.

medication. This will therefore reduce the amount of vitamin K you absorb. To restore the gut flora, you can eat yogurt with active cultures; otherwise, you should discuss taking a vitamin K supplement with your GP or a state-registered dietitian.

# Phytochemicals

## Protective chemicals found in foods of plant origin.

Phytochemicals, also known as phytonutrients, are naturally occurring protective chemicals that are found in foods of plant origin (*phyto* is derived from the Greek word for plant). Studies show that there may be as many as 100 different phytochemicals in just one serving of vegetables.

### Phytochemicals and health
Evidence has shown that people who consume a diet rich in fruits and vegetables, and therefore in phytochemicals, have a lower incidence of many disorders, including cardiovascular disease, diabetes, and certain types of cancer. Phytochemicals have an antioxidant effect (*opposite*) that protects cells from cancer and cardiovascular disease, as well as from urinary tract infections, rheumatoid arthritis, and reduced immunity. Make sure you eat at least five portions of fruits and vegetables a day to get plenty of phytochemicals.

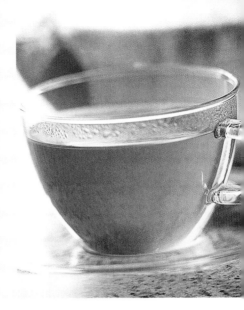

**Healthy cuppa**  A potent phytochemical called polyphenol, thought to lower the risk of stomach cancer, is found in tea.

# What are the different types of phytochemicals?

There are hundreds of phytochemicals found in foods of plant origin. The key benefits of some of the best known phytochemicals are listed below.

**Bioflavonoids**  These are helpful in the absorption of vitamin C and protect it from oxidation (damage). Citrus fruits, such as lemons, limes, grapefruit, and oranges, are particularly good sources of bioflavonoids.

**Carotenoids**  These may protect against cardiovascular disease. Carotenoids are found in orange-fleshed melon, carrots, sweet potatoes, and butternut squash.

**Glucosinolates**  Found in vegetables, these help the liver in its detoxification function. They help regulate certain white blood cells involved in immunity. They may also help reduce tumour growth, particularly in the breast, liver, colon, lung, stomach, and oesophagus.

**Organosulphides**  These give onions and leeks their pungent odour. They stimulate anti-cancer enzymes, slow the formation of blood clots, and are known to boost the immune system.

**Phytoestrogens**  These protect the body against cardiovascular disease and osteoporosis. Phytoestrogens may also slow the progression of cancer. They are found in soya products and linseeds.

**Flavonoids**  These may protect the body from inflammation, allergic reactions, and viral infections.

**Indoles**  These phytochemicals are thought to help prevent breast cancer.

**Isoflavones**  These may inhibit oestrogen-promoted cancers and lower high levels of blood cholesterol.

**Limonoids**  Found in the peel of citrus fruits, these phytochemicals appear to protect lung tissue.

**Lycopene**  Found in tomatoes, this may protect against cancers of the cervix, stomach, bladder, colon, and prostate, as well as cardiovascular disease.

**Para-coumaric acid**  This phytochemical helps prevent cancer by interfering with the development of cancer-causing nitrosamines in the stomach.

**Phenols and polyphenol**  These protect plants from chemical damage and perform the same function in humans. Found in tea, polyphenol is thought to protect against stomach cancer.

**Phytosterols**  These include stanols, which can reduce the absorption of cholesterol from the diet and therefore lower cholesterol levels in the blood. Stanols are found in soya products and fortified margarines.

**Terpenes**  These may block action of cancer-causing factors (carcinogens) and may inhibit hormone-related cancers such as ovarian cancer.

## Good sources
**Phytochemicals**  These are found in all foods of plant origin. The plant foods in the list below are thought to contain particularly beneficial phytochemicals:
- Whole grains
- Broccoli
- Brussels sprouts
- Cauliflower
- Citrus fruits
- Dark green leafy vegetables
- Garlic
- Tea
- Herbs and spices
- Onions
- Tomatoes
- Soya beans
- Wine

# What are minerals?

## These are substances originating in rocks and metal ores.

Many minerals are essential for health. We obtain them by eating plants, which take up minerals from the soil, by eating animals that have eaten plants (or eaten other animals that have eaten plants), and, to some extent, by drinking water that contains minerals.

Minerals are needed by the body in only tiny quantities and are termed macrominerals or microminerals, according to the percentage of your total body weight they constitute and how much you need in your daily diet.

Macrominerals make up more than 0.005 per cent of the body's weight and you need to be getting more than 100mg of these daily. They include calcium, magnesium,

phosphorus, potassium, sodium, and sulphur. Microminerals, which are also known as trace elements, make up less than 0.005 per cent of the body's weight and you need less than 100mg daily. Those microminerals with identified roles in health include chromium, copper, fluoride, iodine, iron, selenium, and zinc.

### Why we need minerals

Minerals work together in making and breaking down body tissues and in regulating metabolism – the chemical reactions constantly occurring in the body. Bone, for example, consists of a framework of the protein collagen in which most of the body's calcium, phosphorus, and magnesium are deposited. Minerals are stored in your bones so that in the event of a dietary deficiency such as a calcium deficiency, some of the

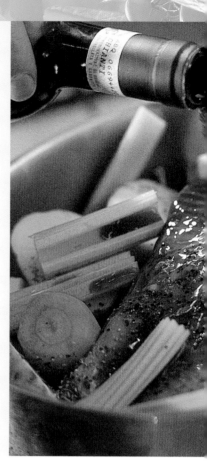

# How do you get minerals?

No single food is the best source of all of the minerals, but eating a variety of foods usually ensures that you get enough of these important nutrients. In addition, the body can store minerals for future use when intake might be low.

Animal foods are generally the best sources of minerals because they tend to contain minerals in the proportions our bodies need. Fruits and vegetables can be useful sources of some minerals such as potassium. Mineral water can also be a source of minerals (*right*), including magnesium.

Minerals are often lost when a food is processed. For example, potassium, iron, and chromium are removed from whole grains during the refining process. Refined grains described as "enriched" on the label contain minerals added back to compensate for those that were lost. Other examples of foods fortified with minerals are table salt, which

sometimes has iodine added to it, and breakfast cereals, many of which are now fortified with a range of minerals that are essential for good health.

Minerals differ from vitamins in that they are not damaged by heat or light, but some can be lost in the water used for cooking. To help preserve the mineral content of vegetables, avoid boiling them. Instead, steam them if possible or use the microwave, and keep the cooking time short. If you do boil, wait until the water is bubbling before you add the vegetables: if you put them in cold water and then bring it to the boil, more nutrients will be lost. Consider saving the water that you used for soup stock or a sauce.

Sometimes, you may need to take mineral supplements. For example, if you do not eat enough calcium-rich foods you may need a supplement to prevent osteoporosis (*see pp.268–271*).

## Minerals in water

We also get minerals from tap water and bottled mineral water, both of which have varying amounts of many minerals.

Fluoride is present naturally in many water sources. In other areas, water supplies are often fluoridated since fluoride prevents tooth decay.

Hard water contains calcium and magnesium – leaving the evidence as scaly deposits in pipes and on kitchen utensils. These minerals can be neutralized with salt crystals in order to produce softer water that leaves less scaling.

Bottled mineral water has a unique mineral content dependent on the geographical area of origin. The water collects minerals as it percolates through rocks. It may contain calcium and iron.

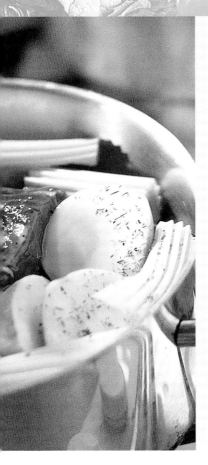

mineral can be released from the bones for the body's needs. The teeth also contain significant amounts of the minerals calcium and phosphorus.

Minerals are found in many key molecules in the body and are involved in essential chemical reactions. For example, calcium activates a digestive enzyme that helps to break down fats; copper is needed to incorporate iron into haemoglobin, the oxygen-carrying molecule that is present in red blood cells; and sulphur is a part of vitamin $B_1$. The minerals calcium, magnesium, potassium, and sodium are all very important in cell functioning, particularly in muscle contractions and in the transmission of electrical impulses along nerve fibres.

**Mineral-rich dish** Minerals are present in most foods in varying quantities. Red meat is a particularly good source of iron, needed by the body to make red blood cells.

## Mineral deficiencies

The most widespread mineral deficiencies in the UK (and the diseases they cause) are calcium (osteoporosis), iodine (enlarged thyroid gland), fluoride (tooth decay), and iron (iron-deficiency anaemia). Because the body stores and re-uses minerals, it may be years before symptoms first occur.

Causes of a mineral deficiency can be primary or secondary. Primary deficiency occurs if you do not get enough of a mineral in your diet. Secondary deficiency occurs when the dietary intake is adequate but another factor results in the body not being able to absorb or use a mineral. Poor absorption may be caused by disorders of the intestine, such as Crohn's disease, the effects of medications, or because other substances in food bind to minerals and prevent them from being absorbed. Minerals can be lost from the body as a result of alcohol abuse, excessive sweating, or medications.

# Case study Teenage girl who feels constantly cold and tired

**Name** Jennifer

**Age** 18

**Problem** Jennifer is constantly tired and in spite of doing regular exercise, she is not able to run a mile due to overwhelming fatigue. Over the last year, her fatigue has gradually become worse.

Jennifer also complains of "always being cold". She has a history of heavy menstrual periods, which usually last for seven days. Jennifer also has a history of iron-deficiency anaemia, which was initially diagnosed two years ago. Her GP prescribed iron supplements to treat this condition. Unfortunately, Jennifer found that the supplements caused

abdominal pain and constipation, so she decided to stop taking them.

**Lifestyle** Jennifer is a college student who avoids red meat, but regularly eats chicken and fish. She usually has dairy products with each meal. Her vegetable intake comes mostly from salads. She does not eat much fruit. Jennifer used to be a keen runner.

**Advice** The fatigue is almost certainly caused by iron deficiency. Therefore, Jennifer needs to obtain more iron in her diet. Because she loses iron on a monthly basis from menstrual periods, her iron stores need to be continually replenished.

Good sources of iron in the diet are red meat, poultry, fish and shellfish, nuts and seeds, green leafy vegetables, dried fruits, whole grains,

and fortified cereals. In Jennifer's case, dietary factors contributing to her ongoing iron deficiency include her avoidance of red meat and her intake of dairy products, which may reduce the absorption of iron.

She should take a multivitamin and mineral supplement that contains iron. Vitamin C-rich foods, such as citrus fruits and berries, or a vitamin C supplement, will increase the body's absorption of iron.

Because Jennifer suffers from constipation and abdominal pain when she takes iron supplements, she should add fibre to her diet and drink plenty of water. Both will help her avoid constipation. She could consult her GP or a gynaecologist about taking an oral contraceptive that can decrease the flow of her menstrual periods.

# Mineral directory

Here we look at the role of each mineral, good sources, and what happens if there is a deficiency. Macrominerals are discussed first, followed by the microminerals. The recommended daily amount (RDA) for adults aged 19–50 is given, although needs do vary at different stages of life (*see Eating for the Time of your Life, pp.104–155*).

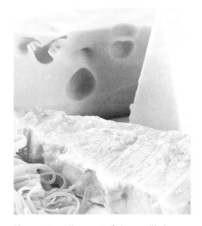

**Cheese** A small amount of cheese will give you your daily requirement of calcium. Available in many different textures and types, cheese is also a good source of protein and zinc.

## Calcium

**DAILY REQUIREMENT**
**Men** 700mg (EC 800mg)
**Women** 700mg (EC 800mg)

This is the main mineral present in bones and teeth – between them they contain about 99 per cent of the body's calcium (Ca). The remaining one per cent is used for various functions in the body such as blood clotting, nerve signals, and muscle contraction. Absorption of calcium in the intestine is regulated by vitamin D (*see p.57*). People who have problems absorbing vitamin D also have poor calcium absorption.

The body's absorption of calcium can be enhanced by lactose, which is the sugar naturally found in dairy products. Conversely, the body's ability to absorb calcium is reduced by the compounds oxalate and phytate, which are present in vegetables such as spinach, beetroot, celery, and parsley. People who are following a high-protein diet will excrete more calcium in the urine. It is for this reason that people who have kidney stones may be advised to reduce their dietary intake of protein.

Adolescents – children aged between nine and 18 years – need much more calcium in their diets than younger children or adults, in order to fuel bone development during their growth spurt.

### CALCIUM DEFICIENCY

A deficiency of this mineral is likely to remain undetected for several years because if the dietary intake of the mineral is low the bones will continue to release calcium into the blood to maintain normal blood levels.

Symptoms of calcium deficiency include bone pain, pins and needles in the hands and feet, muscle cramps and twitching, convulsions, and osteoporosis (*see p.242*), which is characterized by weakened bones that may fracture and crumble, leading to loss of height.

If you do not get enough calcium in your diet during childhood, the result will be reduced bone mass. This can increase your risk of osteoporosis later in life. The signs and symptoms of a calcium deficiency during childhood include irritability, muscle weakness, stunted growth, and muscle cramps and twitching. Untreated, a childhood deficiency of calcium may be fatal.

## Calcium and body fat

The mineral calcium has been found to help weight loss. Studies have shown that when your dietary intake of calcium is increased, there is also an increase in the breakdown of fat and a decrease in the production of fat. As a result, body fat is lost.

This relationship was discovered when studies of children and adults who consumed higher levels of calcium and dairy products were shown to have less body fat. Obese adults who were following a reduced-calorie diet high in calcium lost more weight and fat than those on a reduced-calorie diet with a low intake of calcium.

Researchers believe that each 300mg increase in calcium intake is associated with approximately 1kg (2lb) less body fat in children and 2.25–2.7kg (5–6lb) lower body weight in adults.

When calcium intake is low, levels of a hormone called calcitriol, which is involved in calcium metabolism, increase in order to help conserve calcium in the body. Calcitriol also causes fat cells to expand and increase fat stores in the body. Conversely, by maintaining your calcium levels, you can suppress the calcitriol and therefore help your body increase the breakdown of fat.

## Good sources

**Calcium** This is found naturally in all the foods listed below, which contain at least 150mg of calcium per 100g (3½oz):
- Cheese
- Milk
- Yogurt
- Spinach
- Whitebait and sardines
- White bread
- Canned salmon (eaten with bones)
- Almonds
- Tofu

# Magnesium

### DAILY REQUIREMENT
**Men** 300mg (EC 300mg)
**Women** 270mg (EC 300mg)

This mineral plays a vital role in the formation of bones and teeth and, with the minerals calcium, sodium, and potassium, is involved in transmitting nerve signals and causing muscle contractions. Magnesium (Mg) also helps the body process fat and protein and make proteins, and is necessary for the secretion of parathyroid hormone, which helps control the levels of calcium in the blood. Vitamin D increases the absorption of potassium in the intestine. Once absorbed, magnesium is stored in bone, muscles, cells, and the fluid that surrounds cells.

Because of magnesium's role in muscle contraction, it is used medically to reduce irregular heart rhythms (arrhythmias) or contractions of the uterus in pregnant women.

### MAGNESIUM DEFICIENCY
A dietary, or primary, deficiency of magnesium is rare. However, it can result from problems with the absorption of nutrients from the intestine, long-term use of diuretic medications, excessive vomiting, kidney disease, chronic alcohol abuse, hyperparathyroidism,

### Good sources
**Magnesium** This is found naturally in all the foods below, which contain at least 50mg of magnesium per 100g (3½oz):
- Whole grains
- Globe artichokes
- Spinach
- Wholemeal bread
- Bran flakes
- Lamb's kidneys
- Red meat
- Beans and pulses
- Nuts such as Brazils, almonds, cashews, and peanuts
- Sunflower seeds
- Sesame seeds
- Tofu

and liver cirrhosis. Because magnesium is also needed for the normal functioning of the parathyroid glands, which secrete parathyroid hormone, low magnesium levels may adversely decrease the levels of calcium in the blood.

A magnesium deficiency leads to low levels of calcium and potassium in the blood, as well as changes to the digestive system, nervous and muscular systems, heart and circulatory systems, and the development of blood cells.

People who develop a magnesium deficiency may have the following signs and symptoms: fatigue, weakness, poor appetite, impaired speech, irregular heart rhythms, anaemia, and tremors. Affected babies and young children may fail to thrive. The advanced signs of a deficiency include an abnormally rapid heart rate and convulsions, and it may be fatal if not treated.

# Phosphorus

### DAILY REQUIREMENT
**Men** 550mg (EC 800mg)
**Women** 550mg (EC 800mg)

Essential for bones and teeth, phosphorus (P) is also found in carbohydrates, lipids (fats and fat-like compounds), proteins, enzymes, and DNA (the substance that makes up our genes). It is also a part of ATP (adenosine triphosphate) – a

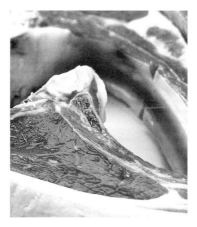

**Red meat** Not only a reliable source of protein, red meat is rich in phosphorus and other micronutrients, including B vitamins, magnesium, potassium, chromium, and iron.

### Good sources
**Phosphorus** This is found naturally in all the following foods, which contain a minimum of 150mg of phosphorus per 25g (1oz):
- Whole grains, especially oats
- Dairy products
- Red meat
- Poultry
- Seafood
- Pulses, especially lentils
- Nuts such as almonds, Brazils, peanuts, and pine nuts
- Sunflower seeds

compound that stores energy needed by all cells. The amount of phosphorus absorbed from food varies depending on your need for the mineral. Vitamin D (*see p.57*) is essential for the absorption of phosphorus.

### PHOSPHORUS DEFICIENCY
People who take excessive amounts of antacid indigestion medication for a prolonged period may develop a phosphorus deficiency. Antacids bind with dietary phosphorus and prevent its absorption into the bloodstream.

Symptoms of a deficiency of this mineral include muscle weakness and bone pain. Anaemia, impaired function of red and white blood cells, problems with the nervous system including psychological disorders, abnormal excretion of calcium in the urine, and kidney stones (*see p.238*) may also result from phosphorus deficiency.

# Potassium

### DAILY REQUIREMENT
**Men** 3500mg (none set for EC)
**Women** 3500mg (none set for EC)

Together with sodium and chloride, potassium (K) is involved in controlling the amount of water and maintaining the correct acid–alkali balance in the body.

Potassium also helps the body store blood sugar in the form of glycogen, which is the principal source of energy required by all muscles in the body, in order to work properly.

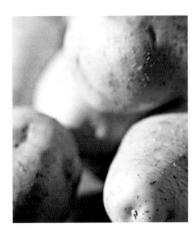

**Potatoes** Rich in potassium, potatoes are also a good source of folate, iron, and fibre. If boiled or baked rather than fried, potatoes are filling and not fattening.

Potassium is also essential for the normal functioning of muscles, nerve cells, the heart and heart valves, the kidneys, and the adrenal glands.

According to the most recent studies, regular consumption of potassium-rich foods can help to lower and control blood pressure, so it is especially important for people with heart failure (see p.221) or high blood pressure (see p.220) to eat enough of this mineral. Good sources of potassium include avocados, bananas, and potatoes (below). A high potassium intake has also been linked to decreasing the risk of stroke (see p.216), the bone

### Good sources

**Potassium** This is found naturally in all the foods listed below, which contain at least 160mg of potassium per 100g (3½oz):

- Whole grains
- Potatoes
- Asparagus
- Avocados
- Spinach
- Tomatoes
- Bananas
- Orange-fleshed melon
- Oranges
- Dairy products
- Red meat
- Broad beans

disease osteoporosis, and calcium-containing kidney stones (see p.238). In addition, you may need to eat more potassium-rich foods in warm weather as the mineral is lost from the body through sweating.

### POTASSIUM DEFICIENCY

A dietary deficiency of potassium is rare. Low levels of potassium in the blood, known as hypokalaemia, are usually caused by loss of potassium through excessive vomiting or diarrhoea, or as a result of kidney disease or a metabolic disorder in which the body chemistry is affected in some way. A potassium deficiency may also be due to taking too many laxatives or eating disorders, such as anorexia nervosa and bulimia nervosa, that may involve vomiting (see p.207).

Symptoms include fatigue, muscle weakness, constipation, cramps, and reduced kidney function. Severely low levels can lead to heart problems such as abnormal heart rhythms.

## Sodium

### DAILY REQUIREMENT
**Men**　1600mg (none set for EC)
**Women**　1600mg (none set for EC)

Best known as a component of table salt (sodium chloride), sodium (Na) is vital for controlling the amount of water in the body, maintaining the normal pH (degree of acidity or alkalinity) of blood, transmitting nerve signals, and helping muscular contraction. It is present in all foods in varying degrees, and almost all processed foods also have added salt.

Unlike all the other minerals, sodium is, on the whole, overconsumed. Dietary intake of salt is very high in the UK – far in excess of the recommended daily requirement. Symptoms of increased salt intake include nausea, vomiting, diarrhoea, and abdominal cramps.

High concentrations of sodium in the body can also result from excessive water or fluid loss. Persistently high levels of sodium in the blood can result in swelling, high blood pressure (see p.220), difficulty in breathing, and heart failure (see p.221), and may be fatal.

### SODIUM DEFICIENCY

A deficiency of this mineral is rare as our dietary intake is so high. However, the levels of sodium in the body can become too low as a result of prolonged vomiting or diarrhoea, or during periods of prolonged illness. Levels of sodium in the body can also become low as a result of dehydration or excessive or persistent sweating, which may occur during very hot weather or affect marathon runners, athletes who participate in triathlons, or people who have certain forms of kidney disease, such as acute kidney failure.

Symptoms of a deficiency of sodium include headache, nausea and vomiting, muscle cramps, drowsiness, fainting, fatigue, and possibly coma.

## Sulphur

### DAILY REQUIREMENT
**Men**　none set in UK or for EC
**Women**　none set in UK or for EC

The macromineral sulphur plays a key role in the manufacture of amino acids (see p.45) and in the conversion of carbohydrates to a form that the body can use. Sulphur (S) occurs in insulin, the hormone secreted by the pancreas that helps to regulate the levels of the sugar glucose in blood. Sulphur is also involved in manufacturing connective tissue (which surrounds body structures

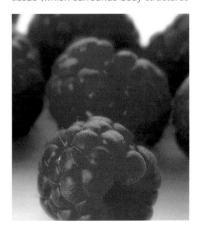

**Raspberries** An excellent source of sulphur, these fruits also contain vitamin C, calcium, magnesium, potassium, and iron, and are one of the best fruit sources of soluble fibre.

## Good sources

**Sulphur** This is found naturally in all the foods listed below, which contain at least 100mg of the mineral per 100g (3½oz):
- Bean sprouts
- Leafy green vegetables such as cabbage, kale, and turnip greens
- Raspberries
- Dairy products
- Red meat, especially offal
- Egg yolks
- Chicken
- Seafood
- Pulses
- Nuts

and holds them together), skin, hair, and nails, and in the manufacture of vitamin B$_1$ (see p.53) and biotin (see p.56) in the body.

A deficiency of sulphur has not yet been diagnosed in humans because the mineral occurs naturally in all foods.

# Chromium

### DAILY REQUIREMENT
**Men** none set in UK or for EC
**Women** none set in UK or for EC

This micromineral works with insulin, the hormone that regulates the levels of the sugar glucose in blood. Chromium (Cr) helps insulin bind to its receptors on the membrane of body cells, which

## Good sources

**Chromium** This is found naturally in these foods, which contain at least 1mg of the mineral per 50g (2oz):
- Potatoes
- Broccoli
- Green beans
- Tomatoes
- Apples
- Bananas
- Grapes
- Oranges
- Red meat, especially beef, pork, and ham
- Turkey

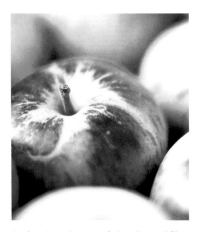

**Apples** A good source of chromium and fibre, all apples also contain quercetin, a flavonoid phytochemical that can help lower the levels of cholesterol in the blood.

then allows for the sugar glucose to move into the cell where it is used to produce energy for the cell's needs.

### CHROMIUM DEFICIENCY
A deficiency of chromium is very rare and is most likely to occur in people who have had long-term intravenous feeding. Some studies of male runners have shown that urinary chromium loss was increased by endurance exercise. This finding suggests that your need for chromium is greater if you exercise on a regular basis.

# Copper

### DAILY REQUIREMENT
**Men** 1.2mg (none set for EC)
**Women** 1.2mg (none set for EC)

Copper (Cu) plays a key role in several body functions. These include the production of pigment in skin, hair, and eyes; the development of healthy bones, teeth, and heart; the protection of body cells from chemical damage since it acts as an antioxidant (see p.58); the maintenance of the myelin sheath, which surrounds and protects nerve fibres; and the functioning of the nervous system. It is also involved in the processing of iron in the body and the formation of red blood cells.

## Good sources

**Copper** This is found naturally in all the foods listed below, which contain at least 1mg of the mineral per 50g (2oz):
- Whole grains, especially barley
- Liver
- Seafood such as crab, lobster, and oysters
- Nuts such as almonds, Brazils, and pistachios
- Sesame seeds

### COPPER DEFICIENCY
A deficiency of copper is rare, though it can occur in malnourished infants. The deficiency results in anaemia (see p.55) and its related symptoms.

Left untreated, a deficiency can lead to lung damage and excessive bleeding due to reduced production of red blood cells and damage to the connective tissues (which surround body structures and hold them together).

# Fluoride

### DAILY REQUIREMENT
**Men** none set in UK or for EC
**Women** none set in UK or for EC

This micromineral is found at varying concentrations in tap water – it is often added by water companies – and in soil; fluoride (F) is also present in very small amounts in the body. About 99 per cent of the fluoride in the body is in the teeth and bones; it helps increase tooth mineralization and bone density and reduce the risk of tooth decay. It also promotes enamel remineralization throughout life.

Fluoridation of water supplies has been endorsed by many professional health organizations as the most effective dental public health measure in existence. However, not all water companies add fluoride to their supply (see p.66).

Fluoride can be obtained from any food that is prepared in or with water that has been fluoridated. You can also obtain the mineral from fluoridated mouthwashes and toothpastes.

## Water fluoridation

By definition, water fluoridation is the adjustment of fluoride in a water supply to an optimum concentration of 0.7–1.2 parts per million, in order to prevent tooth decay in the people who use the supply. The value of fluoridation has been demonstrated beyond question. Schoolchildren living in an optimally fluoridated community were shown to be at much lower risk of tooth decay compared with those children who do not live in such an area.

There is evidence that fluoridation reduces tooth decay in children by 20–40 per cent, and helps to prevent tooth decay and loss in adults. Water fluoridation is beneficial for those living in poor communities, who are at greater risk of tooth decay and have less access to dental care and alternative fluoride resources.

### FLUORIDE DEFICIENCY

A deficiency of this mineral can lead to an increased incidence of tooth decay. If you live in an area where fluoride is not added to the drinking water supply, you would benefit from taking a fluoride supplement (*p.270*). Talk to your dentist about an appropriate supplement.

# Iodine

### DAILY REQUIREMENT
**Men** 140mcg (EC 150mcg)
**Women** 140mcg (EC 150mcg)

Although iodine (I) is found in all body cells, about 40 per cent of the body's iodine is stored in the thyroid gland. Here, it is used for making thyroid hormones, which are required for normal body metabolism and growth. Iodine occurs naturally in the sea; our dietary iodine has to come from seafood or from plants grown in soil near to the sea. However, most table salt is now fortified with iodine. Excess iodine is secreted in the urine.

### IODINE DEFICIENCY

If the body does not get enough iodine, there is a decrease in the production of the thyroid hormones. To compensate, the thyroid gland becomes enlarged, which can lead to an underactive thyroid (hypothyroidism).

A deficiency of iodine is a common worldwide cause of goitre (swelling in the neck due to an enlarged thyroid gland) and cretinism (dwarfism and learning difficulties) in those who do not get enough iodized salt or live in regions where iodine is not found.

Signs and symptoms of low iodine levels include slow metabolism and possibly weight gain. The signs and symptoms of cretinism include reduced growth of the muscles and skeleton and learning difficulties during childhood.

# Iron

### DAILY REQUIREMENT
**Men** 8.7mg (EC 14mg)
**Women** 14.8mg (EC 14mg)

This is an essential mineral in all cells of the body even though it is needed only in minute quantities. Iron (Fe) is a component of haemoglobin (the oxygen-carrying protein in red blood cells), and it plays a major role in transporting oxygen around the body. It is also part of myoglobin (a protein found in muscle cells) and is involved in the release of energy from glucose and fatty acids in the intestine.

Iron absorption requires gastric acid, which is secreted by the lining of the stomach, to convert it into a form that is best absorbed. Dietary iron from animal products – known as haem iron – is more easily absorbed by the body than the iron found in plants. However, the presence of vitamin C in the body is known to increase the absorption of iron from foods of plant origin.

A greater amount of iron is absorbed from food if the need is greater, such as during pregnancy, in adolescent girls, in people with anaemia (*see p.55*), and in those who have suffered from bleeding, such as heavy menstruation or following childbirth, surgery, or injury.

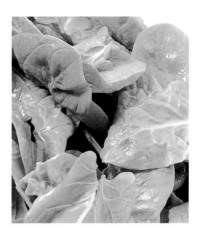

**Spinach** A useful source of iron, especially for vegetarians, spinach also contains beta-carotene (a precursor of vitamin A), vitamins C, E, and folate, calcium, and potassium.

### IRON DEFICIENCY

This deficiency is most frequently caused by a poor intake of iron. It is one of the most widespread, and also most easily remedied, nutritional problems in the world. Pregnant women and breast-feeding and new mothers, infants and children, menstruating females, especially adolescents, and older adults are at greatest risk because of changes in their metabolic rate. Babies who are not breast-fed and not given iron-fortified formula or cereal may develop iron deficiency.

Vegetarians are also at risk of this deficiency since the amount of iron that the body can absorb from plants is lower than that from meats.

## Good sources

**Iron** This is found naturally in all these foods, which contain at least 2.0mg of iron per 100g (3½oz):
- Spinach
- Dried fruit, especially prunes
- Offal (kidneys and liver)
- Red meat
- Egg yolks
- Poultry
- Sardines
- Tuna
- Prawns
- Pulses such as soya, broad, and kidney beans, and chickpeas

Iron deficiency is characterized by anaemia (*see p.55*). Signs and symptoms of iron-deficiency anaemia are common and include weakness, pale skin, fatigue and faintness, cold or numbness in the fingers and toes due to poor blood circulation, shortness of breath, greater susceptibility to infections, poor work performance, soft or brittle nails, and behavioural changes.

Young children with iron deficiency can become very tired and have low concentration. They may develop learning difficulties and behavioural problems that become permanent.

# Selenium

### DAILY REQUIREMENT

**Men** 75mcg (none set for EC)
**Women** 60mcg (none set for EC)

This micromineral is an antioxidant (*see p.58*) and part of an enzyme that protects cells from the damaging effects of free radicals (*see p.58*), which can lead to cardiovascular disease. Selenium (Se) is vital for the normal functioning of the immune system and the thyroid gland. It is found naturally in fish and shellfish, poultry, and Brazil nuts.

Selenium is also thought to have anti-cancer properties, possibly due to its antioxidant function, as well as its ability to block the action of many of the

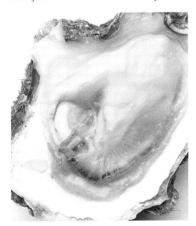

**Oysters** Shellfish such as oysters are a useful source of selenium and various other nutrients, including the B vitamins niacin and B$_{12}$, and the minerals potassium and zinc.

## Good sources

**Selenium** This is found naturally in all the foods listed below, which contain at least 10mg of the mineral per 25g (1oz):
- Brown rice
- Wheat germ
- Wholemeal bread
- Poultry
- Fish, especially tuna
- Shellfish, especially oysters
- Brazil nuts

enzymes that are involved in cell division and growth – which occur uncontrollably in cancer.

### SELENIUM DEFICIENCY

A deficiency of this mineral is rare. However, it has been seen in people who rely on intravenous nutrition, in people with intestinal problems that affect their body's ability to absorb nutrients, in severely malnourished infants and children, and in those with rheumatoid arthritis. A sign of selenium deficiency is an enlarged heart that is not able to pump blood efficiently.

# Zinc

### DAILY REQUIREMENT

**Men** 9.5mg (EC 15mg)
**Women** 7mg (EC 15mg)

Although needed in minute amounts, zinc (Zn) is essential for the breakdown of carbohydrates, fats, and proteins; in normal cell division, growth, and repair – especially during foetal growth; in the manufacture of both DNA (the substance that makes up our genes) and RNA (a substance that is involved in making proteins); in the functioning of the immune system, including wound healing; in sexual maturation, fertility, and reproduction; and in the senses of taste and smell.

Zinc is also necessary to maintain normal levels of the male sex hormone testosterone in the blood and convert this hormone into the female sex hormone oestrogen. This is why oysters have a reputation for increasing desire.

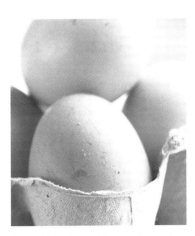

**Eggs** Rich in zinc, protein, and vitamins A, B$_{12}$, D, and E, eggs also contain, in their yolk, a substance called lecithin, which can protect against cardiovascular disease.

### ZINC DEFICIENCY

This deficiency may be primary (due to insufficient zinc in the diet) or result from decreased absorption from the intestine or increased needs because of recovery from disease. Those most at risk include people who abuse alcohol, those with HIV infection or diabetes, people on protein-restricted diets, anyone with diseases that affect absorption from the intestine, and those with liver disease.

Symptoms of zinc deficiency include poor appetite, loss of sense of taste, digestive problems, diarrhoea, vomiting, night blindness, hair loss, skin problems, poor wound healing, problems with growth in children, and delayed onset of puberty and sexual maturation.

## Good sources

**Zinc** This is found naturally in all these foods, which contain at least 1.0mg of the mineral per 25g (1oz):
- Dairy products
- Red meat
- Eggs
- Poultry
- Crab
- Lobster
- Oysters
- Brazil nuts
- Haricot beans
- Soya beans

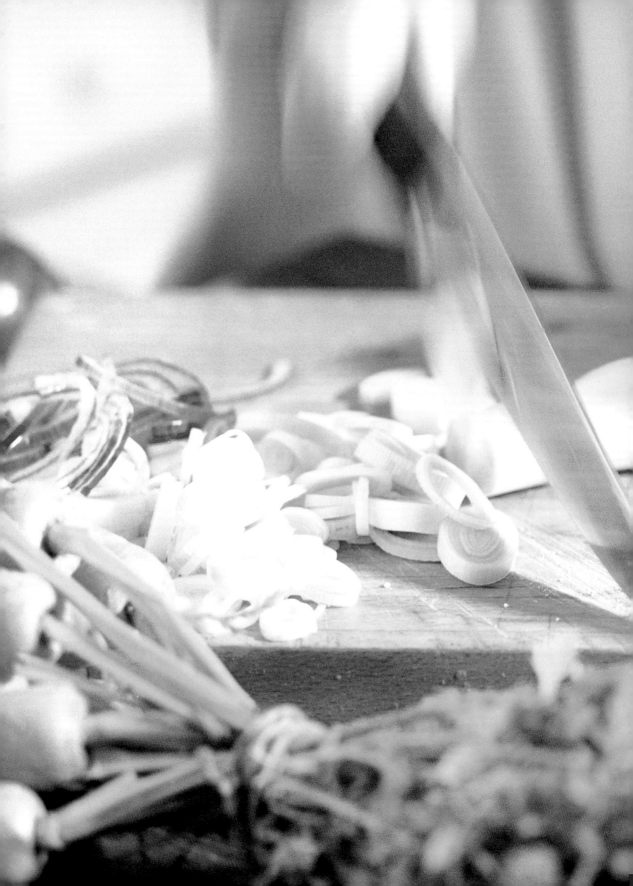

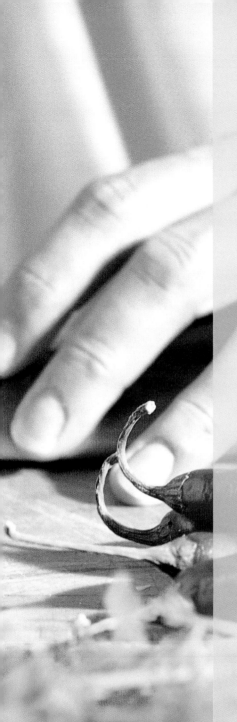

# Elements of a healthy diet

The choices you make each time you buy food have an impact on your health, vitality, and well-being, as well as your weight. Eating foods from all the food groups, and in the right quantities, as outlined in this chapter, will help you achieve the maximum benefits from your diet.

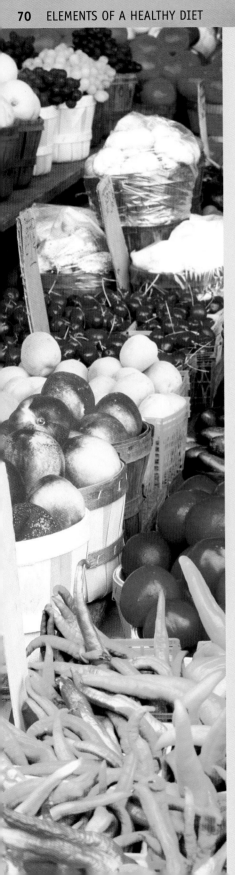

# Making the best dietary choices

## Choose your foods carefully to achieve optimum health.

In the first two chapters, we looked at why our bodies need food and how it is digested and used, and discussed the different types of nutrients that are needed in the diet – carbohydrates, proteins, fats, vitamins, and minerals.

Now we turn to the foods that supply these essential nutrients and the food groups from which they should be selected.

### The main food groups
During the 1990s, the government developed a National Food Guide – which is called The Balance of Good Health – to encourage the consumption of a nutritionally balanced diet and also to simplify meal planning.

The Balance of Good Health classifies foods into five groups. The four main groups are starchy or complex carbohydrates such as grains, pasta, rice, bread, and potatoes (see pp.74–75); vegetables (see pp.76–77) and fruits (see pp.78–79); milk and dairy products (see pp.80–83); and protein foods such as poultry, fish, meat, eggs, pulses, and nuts (see pp.84–95).

The fifth group includes foods that contain fat and sugar. Eating a lot of fatty food is a major cause of weight and health problems, and sugary foods provide calories but few useful nutrients. So the recommendations are that these foods be eaten sparingly.

**Choosing wisely** Understanding the link between good nutrition and optimum health will help you to make the best choices from the vast array of available foods.

### The need for water
Fluids are also a vital element of every diet: a man's body is about 60 per cent water and a woman's about 50 per cent, and every cell needs water to function properly. To remain healthy, you need to drink at least six to eight large glasses of fluids, preferably water, every day, and more when it is hot or when you are perspiring, such as during exercise (see pp.96–97).

### Beneficial compounds
In recent years, scientists have extended their understanding of the link between nutrition and health: it is now clear that eating particular foods contributes to good health and prevents disease. Thousands of potentially beneficial compounds in foods have now been identified, including vitamins, minerals, antioxidants, fibre, and phytochemicals. The list of foods that may help protect your health continues to grow – from many different vegetables and fruits to red wine, linseeds, and oily fish.

### Making good choices
Any food can fit into a healthy way of eating. The key is to balance your choices over time so that your overall diet is sound. You can continue to eat your favourite foods, even if they are high in fat, salt, or sugars, but try to reduce your portion sizes.

Making good choices in your diet starts with educating yourself on sound nutritional guidelines and incorporating that knowledge into your eating habits. For example, by eating a variety of nutrient-rich foods, enjoying plenty of whole grains, vegetables, and fruits, and eating regular meals with moderate portions, you can manage your weight and stay healthy.

# The four main food groups

Each of the food groups shown here provides some of the nutrients you need. No group is more important than another: you need food from all for good health.

Foods from grains, such as bread, are necessary for fibre, vitamins, minerals, and complex carbohydrates, which are an important source of energy for the body. Vegetables and fruits are needed for vitamins and minerals. Naturally low in fat, they are also a source of fibre. Dairy foods and protein foods both provide protein and a range of important vitamins and minerals. Milk and dairy products also provide calcium.

Fats, oils, and sweet foods contain calories and little else of nutritional value, so eat them sparingly.

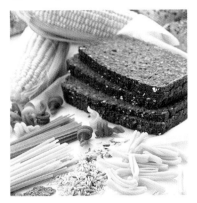

**Breads, cereals, pasta, and potatoes** The foods in this group are a valuable source of carbohydrates (*see pp.74–75*) and fibre.

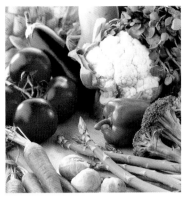

**Vegetables** A vital source of vitamins, minerals, and fibre, vegetables should form a major part of your diet (*see pp.76–77*).

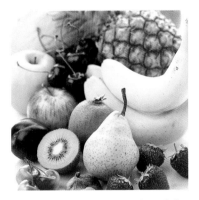

**Fruits** Packed with essential nutrients, fruits provide a good source of carbohydrates, fibre, vitamins, and phytochemicals (*see pp.78-79*).

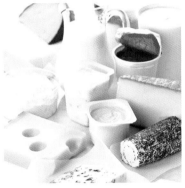

**Dairy foods** Milk and dairy products are an important source of protein, vitamins, and minerals, especially calcium (*see pp.80–83*).

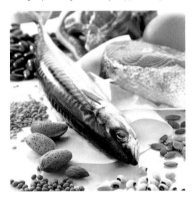

**Protein foods** This group includes meat, poultry, and fish and shellfish, as well as plant proteins such as pulses (*see pp.84–95*).

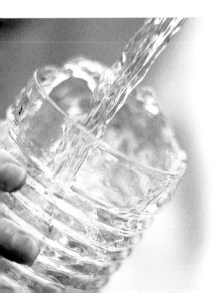

# Water

Pure water is calorie-free and the best drink to quench thirst. Your body cannot store water, so you must drink plenty of it to replenish losses and maintain healthy function of all your body cells. It is the most abundant substance in the body and is necessary for survival.

**Essential element** Although water has little nutritional content, it provides the perfect means of satisfying the body's vital need for fluid, since it contains no sugar, caffeine, or other unhealthy additives.

The quality of drinking water in the UK is regulated by the government. Their reports consistently show that it is of a very high quality. Despite this fact many people prefer to drink bottled or filtered tap water. Bottled water is convenient to carry, making it easier for you to drink your six to eight glasses a day. Sparkling, still, and flavoured waters are excellent, but watch out for "enhanced" water, which can contain unnecessary calories. Also check labels if you are controlling your sodium intake, as some brands can contain high levels of sodium.

# Dietary guidelines

## The key message is to eat a variety of foods from the basic groups.

The British government's dietary guidelines, called The Balance of Good Health, are presented in the form of a plate showing the basic food groups (*see p.71*) and the proportional amount of space they should occupy in a healthy diet.

### Balance of Good Health
Starchy carbohydrate foods – breads, cereals and grains, rice, pasta, and potatoes (*see pp.74–75*) – should take up one-third of your "plate": at least five daily servings from this group are recommended. Vegetables (*see pp.76–77*) and fruits (*see pp.78–79*) also take up one-third of the plate. The current recommendations are that you should eat at least five servings from this group every day.

Only two to three daily servings are recommended from the animal and plant protein group (*see pp.84–95*), which includes meat,

poultry, fish, pulses, eggs, and nuts. At about the same level are dairy foods (*see pp.80–83*), with a recommendation of two to three daily servings. Sweet foods and fatty foods (*see pp.98–99*), which should be eaten sparingly, occupy the smallest area on the plate.

### Suggested modifications
The latest findings on nutrition and health can help you refine the guidelines in the Balance of Good Health. For example, there is evidence that eating a lot of red meat may be harmful to your health because red meat is high in saturated fat (*see pp.86–87*). On the other hand, since it has been shown that eating oil-rich fish (*see p.39*) can help reduce the risk of developing cardiovascular disease, current recommendations suggest that the consumption of oily fish should be increased.

With regard to the carbohydrate foods, it is important to remember that whole-grain products differ significantly in nutritional value from refined products (*see p.75*).

Whole grains should form the foundation of the diet, and refined grains be eaten sparingly.

### The Mediterranean diet
Some dietary recommendations are based on studies of people living in Mediterranean countries who have lower cholesterol levels and rates of cardiovascular disease and cancer than people in northern Europe. The Mediterranean diet, low in saturated fats and high in monounsaturated fats (*see p.38*), includes more grains, vegetables, fruits, pulses, nuts, and olive oil, while protein is supplied by fish, poultry, cheese, eggs, and yogurt.

A word of caution though: a diet that is high in fat – even if it is the healthy monounsaturated fats – will also be high in calories and can lead to weight gain if you do not take enough exercise.

**Healthy lifestyle**  A diet of fresh, locally grown produce, rich in beneficial fats, and an active, outdoor lifestyle, contribute to the good health enjoyed in Mediterranean areas.

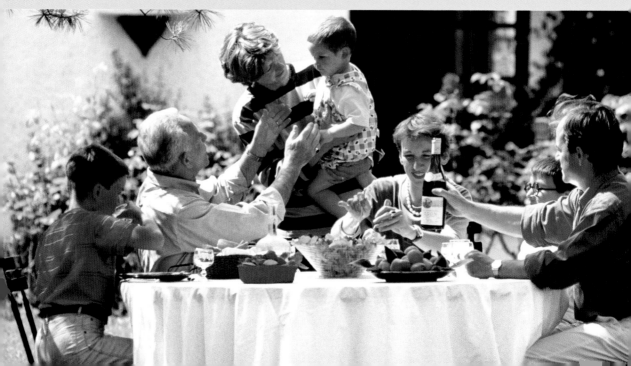

# What is a serving?

The official guidelines suggest how many servings should be eaten per day from each food group. The recommendations are expressed as ranges, to cater for different energy needs (*see p.34*). The lower number in each group applies to people with low energy requirements, such as older adults and sedentary people; the higher number in each group is appropriate for teenage boys, active men, and very active women.

## SERVINGS VERSUS PORTIONS

You may wonder whether these servings are the same size as the food portions served at home or in restaurants. They are not. Recommended servings are of a fixed, standard quantity (*right*), while portion sizes are variable. However, many people tend to eat particularly large portions of food and as a consequence have high rates of obesity.

It is a good idea to start thinking of food portions in terms of these standard serving sizes because this will help you maintain a healthy weight and eat less if you are trying to lose weight.

| FOOD GROUP | DAILY SERVINGS | WHAT IS ONE SERVING? |
|---|---|---|
| **Bread, cereal, rice, pasta, and potatoes** | 5–14 servings | • 1 slice wholemeal bread<br>• 1 egg-sized potato<br>• 3 tbsp breakfast cereal<br>• 2 heaped tbsp cooked pasta or rice |
| **Vegetables** | 2–3 servings (as part of the min 5-a-day) | • 1 medium-sized mixed salad<br>• 3–4 tbsp cooked vegetables<br>• 150ml (5floz) vegetable juice |
| **Fruit** | 2–3 servings (as part of the min 5-a-day) | • 1 medium fresh fruit (eg banana)<br>• 2 satsumas or kiwi fruit<br>• 7 strawberries<br>• 150ml (5floz) fruit juice |
| **Milk, yogurt, and cheese** | 2–3 servings | • 200ml (7floz) semi-skimmed milk<br>• 150g (5oz) low-fat yogurt<br>• 125g (4½oz) cottage cheese<br>• 40g (1½oz) hard cheese |
| **Meat, poultry, fish, pulses, nuts, seeds, and eggs** | 2–3 servings | • 85–100g (3–3½oz) cooked poultry, fish, or lean red meat<br>• 3–4 tbsp cooked dried beans<br>• 2 eggs<br>• 2 tbsp peanut butter<br>• 3 tbsp nuts or seeds |

# Five-a-day campaign

The Five-a-day Campaign encourages the consumption of at least five servings of vegetables and fruits every day. It was launched in response to evidence that diets high in these foods reduce the risk of developing certain cancers.

While the programme has helped raise public awareness of the need to eat more of these valuable foods, the recent National Diet and Nutrition Survey found that fewer than one in five adults in the UK were eating five servings of fruits and vegetables every day. In any case, the recommendation of five-a-day is only a minimum target – more is even better.

Servings each day should be chosen from a good variety of different types and colours of vegetables and fruits, in order to maximize all of their potential health benefits.

**Take five servings** One apple, a 150ml (5floz) glass of carrot juice, a handful of strawberries, and some broccoli and beans – that is all it takes to meet the five-a-day minimum target for fruit and vegetable intake.

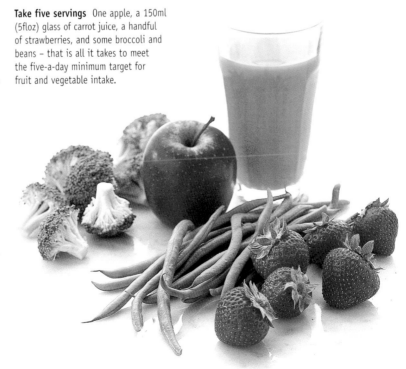

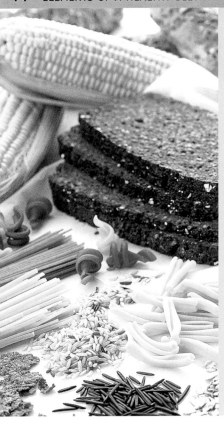

# Wholesome grains

## Choose whole rather than refined grains for optimum benefits.

Bread, rice, pasta, and potatoes are important sources of starchy carbohydrates (*see pp.46–47*), and this food group should form the basis of your diet. The guidelines are that you should eat at least five servings from this group each day.

It is important to distinguish between whole and refined grains (*opposite*), and to make a point of choosing whole grains. Studies show that certain starchy foods may have a negative effect on

**Whole-grain foods** Rich in fibre, complex carbohydrates, and many other key nutrients, whole grains reduce the risk of many diseases.

health. For example, people whose diets consist primarily of potatoes, white rice, and foods made from refined (white) flour have higher rates of diabetes and cardiovascular disease than those who primarily eat whole grains. Therefore, try to obtain most of your carbohydrates from whole-grain foods, such as wholemeal bread, brown rice, and wholemeal pasta, and limit the amount of refined grain products.

By including whole grains in your diet, you may lower your risk of cardiovascular disease because they are low in saturated fat and high in fibre, vitamins, minerals, and antioxidants. If you follow a vegetarian diet, whole grains are an important source of protein when they are combined with pulses or dairy products (*see p.100*).

## The versatility of whole grains

Grains are a dietary staple in most cultures, and a look at other cuisines can provide inspiration for your own cooking. For example, long-grain rice is used as the basis of pilafs in Indian and Middle Eastern cuisine, while short-grain rice cooked in simmering broth produces the creamy risottos of Italy. These and other grains are now widely available, and you can be as creative as you like when cooking them.

### WHICH GRAINS CAN I USE?
Grains can be eaten whole or processed into cold and hot cereals or flour for many food products, such as breads and pasta. In general, grains are a good source of vitamins, especially B vitamins, and the minerals calcium, potassium, and phosphorus. Healthy grains to use include:
**Wheat** Used to make cereals and flour, wholewheat grains or "berries" can also be cooked as a cereal or as you would rice. Whole-grain wheat is packed with

B vitamins. For cracked wheat the grains are broken into small pieces for faster cooking. Bulgur wheat is cooked and dried, then ground coarsely.
**Oats** These have more protein than most other grains. They are also high in soluble fibre, which helps eliminate cholesterol from the body. Whole oats (or groats) are the whole grain but with the hull removed. Rolled oats are whole oats that have been flattened between rollers.
**Maize** Rich in starch, maize can be eaten fresh, as sweetcorn, or hulled and dried to become hominy (in whole or broken kernels) or grits (ground hominy). When ground to a meal, it is called polenta or cornmeal.
**Barley** Whole pot barley is nuttier and chewier than pearl barley (polished barley without the hull and bran) and must be soaked before cooking. In malted barley, the grain is allowed to begin sprouting; it is the main ingredient in beer and malt whisky.

**Rye** Similar to wheat in nutritional value, rye flour is frequently used with wheat flour in bread. Rye is available in whole and cracked rye grains, which can be cooked as cereal or rice, and as rye flakes for muesli.
**Millet** This grain contains nearly as much protein as wheat. It is available in whole and cracked forms and is usually stripped of its tough, inedible hull. It is used in cakes, puddings, and soups, and as a substitute for rice.
**Quinoa** An excellent source of protein, this grain can be substituted for, or added to, nearly any other grain and is particularly good in pilafs.
**Brown rice** Retaining both the bran and the germ of the rice kernel, brown rice is a source of protein, carbohydrates, and fibre. Brown rice needs more water and longer cooking than white rice.
**Wild rice** Not really a rice but a type of grass, this has twice the protein of white rice and fewer calories. Use it in the same way as white or brown rice.

## What are whole grains?

A whole grain is a grain that has not been processed. It consists of the bran, germ, and endosperm inside an inedible outer coating (hull). The bran forms a protective inner covering and is an excellent source of fibre (*see pp.48–49*). The germ – the embryo of a new plant – is a source of protein, vitamins, and minerals; and it contains polyunsaturated fats.

The endosperm supplies most of the carbohydrates, mainly in the form of starch. When grains are processed, the hull, bran, and germ are removed, leaving a product – such as white flour – that is deficient in protein, vitamins, and fibre. While some of these nutrients may be replaced and other important nutrients added to products, whole grains are undoubtedly the better choice.

## Jargon buster

**Refined grains** These are whole grains that have been stripped of their outer coating, bran, and germ during the milling process, leaving only the endosperm to be ground into flour or other products.

Since 90 per cent of the nutritional content of each grain is contained in the germ and bran, the refined product is deficient in many nutrients that are not only essential for good health but are known to provide protection against various diseases, including cardiovascular disease (*see p.214*), diabetes (*see p.246*), and some cancers (*see p.258*).

One of the most commonly used refined grains in Britain is white flour, which is found in most commercially produced cakes and biscuits.

## What is a serving?

At least five daily servings are recommended from this food group, which includes bread, cereal, rice, pasta, and potatoes. Suggested servings include:

- 1 medium bowl cooked porridge
- 3 tbsp cold breakfast cereal
- ½ whole-grain bagel
- 1 slice wholemeal bread
- ½ English muffin
- 1 medium flour tortilla (wrap)
- 1 egg-sized potato
- 4 whole-grain crispbread
- 2 heaped tbsp cooked brown rice
- 2 heaped tbsp cooked wild rice
- 2 heaped tbsp cooked macaroni
- 2 heaped tbsp cooked noodles
- 2 heaped tbsp cooked spaghetti
- ½ large baked sweet potato
- 175g (6oz) mashed potatoes
- 2 heaped tbsp cooked barley
- 2 heaped tbsp cooked couscous
- 2 heaped tbsp cooked quinoa

## Recipe Spicy whole-grain pilaf

| INGREDIENTS |
| --- |
| 1 onion |
| 2 garlic cloves |
| 1 tsp cumin |
| 1 tsp turmeric |
| 200g (7oz) long-grain brown rice |
| 50g (2oz) wild rice |
| 3 peppers |
| 1–2 chillies |
| 2 tbsp tomato purée |

**Serves 4**

**1** Slice the onion and crush the garlic. Sauté the cumin and turmeric for 2 minutes in a little vegetable oil. Add the onion and garlic and sauté for a further 2 minutes.

**2** Add the brown and wild rices to the pan and mix with the onion and garlic. Pour in enough water or vegetable stock to cover the rice, and simmer for 20 minutes.

**3** Remove the seeds from the peppers and slice lengthways. Slice the chillies into rings. Add to the pan with the tomato purée. Stir, then simmer for a further 5 minutes until the rice and peppers are tender.

**4** Remove the pilaf to a serving dish. If you like, garnish with flaked almonds.

**Variations** Other grains can be substituted for the rice, and other vegetables and nuts or diced chicken breast added.

**Each serving provides**
Calories 276, Total fat 1.7g (Sat. 0.3g, Poly. 0.7g, Mono. 0.5g), Cholesterol 0mg, Protein 7.6g, Carbohydrate 59g, Fibre 3.0g, Sodium 39mg; Good source of – Vits: A, Fol, C, K; Mins: Ca, K, Mg, P.

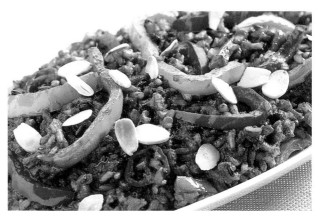

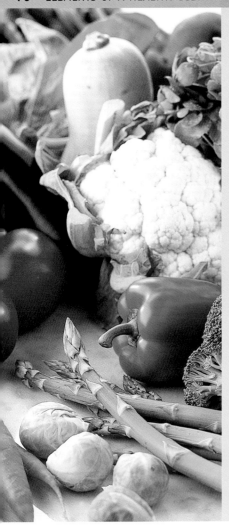

# Vegetables for health

## Improve your health by increasing your intake of vegetables.

According to the guidelines, you should eat a minimum of five servings of vegetables and fruits daily. Very few people meet this target, and miss out on one of the most potent ways of improving health and preventing disease.

### Vital nutrients

Vegetables are excellent sources of beta-carotene (see p.52), as well as vitamin C (see p.56) and some B vitamins (see pp.53–55). These help to keep your skin and eyes healthy and your bones strong, and help fight infection. They work with other vitamins and minerals to keep muscles healthy.

In addition, vegetables are an excellent source of potassium (see p.63) and of fibre, which plays an important role in the diet: studies show a reduced incidence of cardiovascular disease in those countries where a high-fibre diet is the norm.

Fibre also helps to keep the intestinal tract in good working order and may help reduce the risk of colon cancer (see p.259). In addition, a high-fibre diet is often low in fat while providing a feeling of satiety, or fullness, without adding unnecessary calories. Because of this quality, fibre can play an important role in weight control (see pp.48–49).

**Naturally healthy** Include a wide variety of vegetables in your daily diet to benefit from their potent, health-giving properties.

### What is a serving?

The recommendation is at least five servings of vegetables and fruits each day. Examples of vegetable servings include:

- 3 heaped tbsp cooked carrots, peas, or diced swede
- 1 corn-on-the-cob
- 8 Brussels sprouts
- 1 cereal bowl of salad leaves
- 1 medium or 7 cherry tomatoes
- 5cm (2in) piece of cucumber

## Increasing your vegetable intake

Vegetables are packed with vitamins and minerals and provide a great source of fibre (right), so try to eat two to three servings a day. This is not as hard as it may seem. Eat raw vegetables, such as peppers and celery, as often as possible, to benefit from their optimum nutritional content. Otherwise, you should use a cooking method that minimizes loss of nutrients (opposite above).

Always include a vegetable in your sandwich filling, and try dishes based on vegetables rather than meat. (See page 296 for a key to the abbreviations used for vitamins and minerals in the chart.)

| VEGETABLE (80g/3oz) | FIBRE | VITAMINS/MINERALS |
|---|---|---|
| Broccoli, cooked | 1.8g | Fol, C / Ca |
| Brussels sprouts, cooked | 3.4g | Fol, C / K |
| Carrots, cooked | 2.0g | Fol / K |
| Courgettes, cooked | 1.0g | K |
| Green beans, cooked | 1.9g | Fol / K |
| Mange tout, cooked | 1.9g | B₁, B₆, E |
| Peas, cooked | 4.1g | Fol / K |
| Runner beans, cooked | 1.5g | Fol, C |
| Spinach, cooked | 1.9g | Fol / Ca, Fe, K, Mg |
| Sweetcorn, cooked | 1.8g | B₁, B₆, Fol, C |

## Super vegetables

Cruciferous vegetables, such as broccoli, Brussels sprouts, cabbage, cauliflower, kale, and swede, are particularly beneficial for health. They contain phytochemicals (*see p.59*) and other compounds that may help detoxify certain cancer-causing substances before they have a chance to cause harm in the body. This family of vegetables are also rich in beta-carotene, vitamins B₁ and C, folate, calcium, iron, and potassium, as well as fibre.

Tomatoes also have important health benefits. They are rich in lycopene, a carotenoid that helps to prevent cardiovascular disease and cancers. Lycopene is a fat-soluble substance that is absorbed best when cooked in oil. Tomatoes also contain the antioxidants beta-carotene, vitamin C, and vitamin E.

Carrots are a rich source of beta-carotene, which is a precursor of vitamin A. As an antioxidant, beta-carotene helps protect against cardiovascular disease and cancer.

# Retaining the nutrients in vegetables

Vegetables are important sources of vitamins and minerals, but these delicate micronutrients are easily destroyed by heat. It is therefore best to eat at least some of your daily servings raw – for example, in salads or as snacks, such as baby carrots, celery sticks, or slices of cucumber or pepper.

When you do cook vegetables, the golden rule is to do so for the minimum amount of time and in as little liquid as possible, in order to retain their valuable nutrients. Suitable methods of cooking vegetables include steaming, stir-frying, sautéing, microwaving, and poaching (*see p.289*).

In addition to using healthy cooking methods, avoid adding saturated fat in the form of butter or cream sauces. If you think your vegetables need additional flavouring, add some fresh chopped herbs, freshly ground black pepper, or lemon.

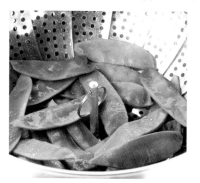

**Steaming**  Since the vegetables are not immersed in water, this method retains the maximum nutrients and fresh taste.

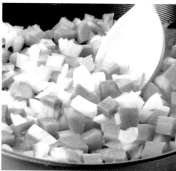

**Sautéing**  Requiring very little oil, finely diced vegetables can be quickly fried in a large shallow pan over a high heat.

# Recipe  Crunchy vegetable stir-fry

| INGREDIENTS |
| --- |
| **80g (3oz) basmati rice** |
| **1 onion** |
| **1 garlic clove** |
| **4 stalks pak choi** |
| **2 peppers (1 red and 1 yellow)** |
| **150g (5oz) mushrooms, sliced** |

**Serves 2**

**1** Steam the rice until the grains are tender.

**2** Slice the onion, crush the garlic, and shred the pak choi. De-seed the peppers and cut them into strips that are 1cm (½in) wide.

**3** Heat a little oil in a wok over high heat. Add the onion and garlic and stir-fry for 2 minutes. Add the peppers, mushrooms, and pak choi, and stir-fry for a further 4 minutes. Serve the stir-fried vegetables with the rice. If you like, accompany with ginger sauce (*right*).

**Ginger Sauce**  In a small bowl, combine 2 tbsp cold water and 1 tbsp cornflour. In a small pan, combine 5½ tbsp white rice vinegar and 2 tbsp soy sauce. Bring to the boil. Reduce the heat and add the cornflour mixture. Stir until the sauce is clear and thickened. Remove from the heat and stir in 1 tbsp finely chopped fresh ginger. Set aside until required.

**Each serving provides**

Calories 246, Total fat 1.6g (Sat. 0.1g, Poly. 0.3g, Mono. 0g), Cholesterol 0mg, Protein 8.0g, Carbohydrate 54g, Fibre 3.0g, Sodium 27mg. Good source of Vits: A, Fol, C, D; Mins: Ca, K, P.

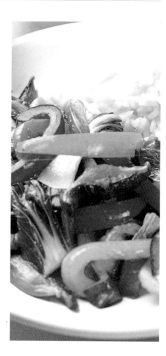

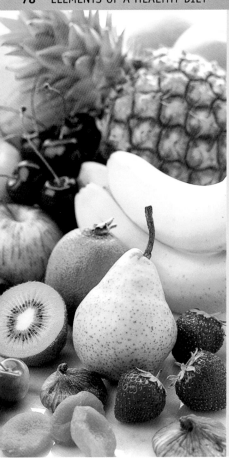

# Fruits for health

## These are easy to eat and packed with nutritional goodness.

Fruits – naturally sweet, colourful, high in vitamins and fibre, and low in calories and fat – are the ideal snack. Scientific research shows that a modest increase of one or two servings of fruit per day can dramatically reduce your susceptibility to many diseases.

### Rich in antioxidants
Vitamin C and phytochemicals, including antioxidants, abound in fruit. Antioxidants destroy harmful substances in the body, called free radicals, which can build up and cause cancer. Of particular interest

**Nature's bounty** Available in a huge array of colours, tastes, and textures, fruits are easy to eat and packed with healthy nutrients.

are two types of phytochemicals – flavonoids and polyphenols – which together have a powerful antioxidant quality. In addition, other phytochemicals in fruit have been found to be anti-allergenic, anti-carcinogenic, anti-viral, and anti-inflammatory (see p.59).

We truly do have a reason to say that an apple (or any fruit) a day keeps the doctor away.

### What is a serving?
At least five daily servings of fruit and vegetables are recommended. Suggested fruit servings include:
- 1 medium apple, pear, orange, peach, or banana
- 3 apricots or 2 plums
- ½ grapefruit
- 3 tbsp fruit salad or stewed fruit
- 1 wedge (5cm/2in) of melon
- 1 tbsp raisins
- 150ml (5floz) 100 per cent juice

## What is in fruits?

Packed with vitamins (see pp.52–58), beneficial phytochemicals (chemicals found in plants; see p.59), minerals (see pp.62–67), and fibre (see pp.48–49), fruits are an integral part of a healthy diet. They contain up to 80 per cent water and are 100 per cent cholesterol-free. Whether eaten with meals, as a snack, or on top of low-fat yogurt for dessert, eating fruits as often as possible throughout the day will help bolster the nutritive value of your diet.

The chart on the right gives several examples of the vitamin, mineral, and fibre content in commonly eaten fruits. Always bear in mind that it is better to eat fruit – preferably with the skin – rather than drink its juice, in order to receive the maximum amount of fibre and nutritional benefits. (See page 296 for a key to the abbreviations used for vitamins and minerals in the chart.)

| FRUIT | SERVING | FIBRE | VITAMINS/MINERALS |
|---|---|---|---|
| Apple, with skin | 1 medium | 1.8g | Fol, C, Vit K / Ca, K, Mg, Na |
| Apricot, dried | 4 halves | 5.0g | Vit K / Ca, Mg, P |
| Blackberries | 80g (3oz) | 2.5g | C, Vit K / Ca, Fe, Mg, P |
| Blueberries | 80g (3oz) | 2.0g | Fol, C, Vit K / Ca, K, Mg, P |
| Dates | 3 whole | 1.4g | Ca, K, Mg |
| Figs, fresh | 2 whole | 1.2g | Ca, Mg, P |
| Orange | 1 medium | 2.7g | Fol, C, Vit K / K |
| Peach | 1 medium | 1.7g | Fol, C / Ca, K, Mg, P |
| Pear, with skin | 1 medium | 3.3g | Fol, C, Vit K / Ca, K, Mg, P |
| Prunes | 3 pitted | 4.6g | Vit K / Ca, Fe, Mg, P |
| Raisins | 1 tbsp | 0.6g | Fol, C / Mg, P |
| Raspberries | 80g (3oz) | 2.0g | Fol, C, Vit K / Ca, Mg |
| Strawberries | 80g (3oz) | 1.0g | C, Vit K / Ca, Mg, P |

# How to increase your fruit intake

Fruits make ideal snacks. They are delicious and nutritious, and require little or no preparation. It is easy to take an apple, orange, or banana with you to work or when you go out for the day.

You should have no problem getting your daily minimum of five servings of fruits and vegetables in this way, once you get into the habit of having a good selection available at home and at work. In addition to eating familiar types of fruits, be adventurous and try some of the more exotic and unusual varieties available from your supermarket, such as mangoes, loquats, figs, and lychees.

**ADDING FRUIT TO YOUR MEALS**
Fruits can be incorporated easily into your main meals of the day – breakfast, lunch, and dinner – in a wide variety of interesting ways. Here are some ideas:
**Breakfast** In the morning, liven up your whole-grain cereal by topping it with a chopped apple, a sliced peach, some berries, or a handful of raisins. Or have a big bowl of fresh pineapple or melon chunks or strawberries or raspberries topped with low-fat yogurt. You can also drink a glass of 100 per cent juice – orange, apple, or grapefruit.
**Lunch** To brighten up a green salad, add some fresh fruit, such as sliced peaches and/or orange segments. Alternatively, instead of a sandwich with a meat or fish filling for your lunch, try a banana and walnut sandwich. Other ideas are to make a fresh fruit and yogurt smoothie (*see p.81*) or finish your lunch with a fruit salad.
**Dinner** Start with a slice of sweet, ripe melon, or try a sweet-savoury main dish such as grilled chicken with mango or mackerel with a gooseberry sauce. Or finish with a fruit dessert, such as a baked apple or apricots.

## Dried fruits

When fruit is dried, or dehydrated, most of the nutrients are concentrated in the remaining solids. This is why the dried versions of fruits have more nutrients – and more calories – by weight than fresh fruits.

Some light-coloured dried fruits, such as apples, apricots, peaches, pears, and sultanas, are treated with sulphur-based preservatives to prevent discoloration. People who have asthma (*see p.225*) or allergies (*see pp.252–255*) may be sensitive to sulphured foods and so should be cautious when eating treated dried fruit. If possible, buy unsulphured dried fruits.

Dried fruits are good as snacks. Soaked or cooked, they can be used to top hot or cold breakfast cereals, make compotes and stuffings, or be added to baked goods.

# Benefits of different fruits

Fruits are rich in vitamins and minerals, especially vitamin C and potassium, and in fibre. Eat a variety to reap their individual nutritional benefits.
**Apples** The skin of this refreshing fruit is an excellent source of fibre. A medium apple has about 47 calories.
**Apricots** Due to a short life span once picked, most apricots are dried or canned. A fresh apricot has about 12 calories.
**Bananas** Technically a herb and not a fruit, a medium banana (100g/3½oz) contains 95 calories and is loaded with vitamins and minerals.
**Blueberries** These delicious fruits are rich in antioxidants and help prevent urinary tract infections. There are about 50 calories in 80g (3oz) blueberries.
**Grapes** 80g (3oz) contains 48 calories, with vitamins A and C and minerals.
**Kiwi fruit** A medium kiwi fruit (60g/2½oz) has 29 calories and offers a good range of vitamins.
**Melon (orange-fleshed)** This is rich in a form of carotene (vitamin A precursor) that is known to fight cancer. A slice of melon (100g/3½oz) has 24 calories.
**Peaches** A medium peach (100g/3½oz) has about 33 calories, and offers vitamins C and D plus potassium.
**Pears** A medium pear (150g/5oz) has about 60 calories.
**Pineapple** This fruit contains a potent enzyme, bromelain, that has been used to aid digestion, reduce inflammation, and help cardiovascular disease. A large slice (80g/3oz) has 33 calories.
**Plums** A medium plum (55g/2oz) has 20 calories. Plums are a good source of vitamin C and offer potassium too.
**Raisins and sultanas** Being so rich in sugar, these dried fruits are an excellent source of energy: 1 tablespoon contains 82 calories.
**Raspberries** There are nearly 1000 varieties of raspberries. They provide 20 calories per 80g (3oz).
**Watermelon** A slice (200g/7oz) of this refreshing melon contains 62 calories plus vitamin C and some carotenoids.

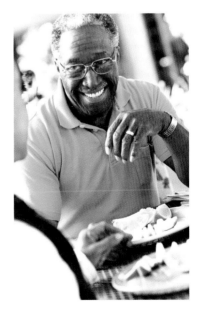

**Fruits make great snacks** Cut-up fruits, such as apples, oranges, melon, and pineapple, make a tasty, quick-to-prepare snack that is rich in fibre and beneficial nutrients such as vitamins, minerals, and phytochemicals.

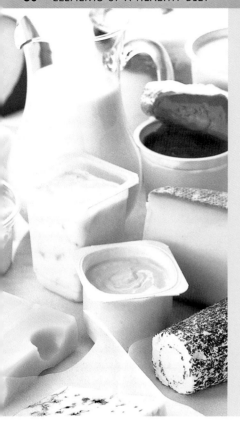

# The benefits of dairy foods

## Dairy products are nutritious – but avoid the full-fat options.

Milk and its products are excellent sources of protein, vitamins, and minerals – most particularly of calcium, which is essential for healthy bones and teeth (see p.62).

### The varieties of milk
Although cow's milk is the most common in the UK, sheep's and goat's milk are available too, as are

**Milk and milk products** These are prime sources of calcium, and there are many low- and reduced-fat options to choose from.

plant-based substitutes such as soya milk and rice milk. Cow's milk is processed in a variety of ways to create products that vary in nutritional content and storage capability. Fat content is one of the most important distinctions, varying from whole or full-fat milk (which contains 3.9 per cent fat) through semi-skimmed (1.6 per cent) to skimmed (0.1 per cent).

Since products based on whole milk are high in saturated fat and cholesterol (see p.40), it's a good idea to moderate your intake. You can reap the same health benefits, however, by choosing lower fat varieties that still contain all the important nutrients of whole milk without its saturated fat content.

## Tips on increasing your dairy intake

If you suspect that your diet does not include enough dairy products, here are some suggestions for increasing your intake each day. Try to choose low- or reduced-fat varieties so that you do not increase your intake of unhealthy saturated fats.

**Breakfast** Get your day off to a good start with any of the following:
• cereal with semi-skimmed milk
• fresh or dried fruit topped with low-fat plain or fruit yogurt
• porridge prepared with semi-skimmed milk instead of water
• a fruit smoothie made with skimmed or semi-skimmed milk or with low-fat yogurt (opposite)

**Lunch** For a healthy addition to your midday meal:
• Have a glass of chocolate-flavoured semi-skimmed milk.
• Grab a sandwich of lower fat Edam cheese on whole-grain bread.
• Enjoy low-fat cottage cheese with sliced peaches or pears on top.

• Make a mini pizza topped with reduced-fat mozzarella, tomatoes, and fresh broccoli or mixed peppers.
• Have a toasted cheese sandwich made with reduced-fat Cheddar.
• Fill a wrap with reduced-fat feta cheese, grilled peppers and onions, and tomatoes.

**Dinner** The main meal of the day provides an opportunity to add more dairy foods to your diet:
• Sprinkle grated lower fat cheese over your salad or soup.
• Make macaroni or cauliflower cheese using skimmed milk in the sauce.
• Have a baked sweet potato topped with low-fat cottage cheese and steamed broccoli florets.

**Snack** Try one of these nutritious options for a change:
• low-fat plain yogurt mixed with fresh or dried fruit
• low-fat frozen yogurt
• oatcakes or a toasted bagel half spread with reduced-fat soft cheese

## Adapting to lower fat dairy foods

If you normally eat full-fat dairy products, make a gradual transition to lower fat varieties.
• Start by mixing 50 per cent whole milk and 50 per cent semi-skimmed. Then gradually reduce the whole milk and increase the semi-skimmed content.
• When you are used to semi-skimmed milk, repeat the process with semi-skimmed and skimmed milks until you are drinking only skimmed milk.
• Use evaporated skimmed milk or fat-free fromage frais instead of cream in soups, sauces, and puddings.
• Substitute low-fat plain yogurt or fat-free Greek-style yogurt for soured cream.
• When making lasagne, substitute fat-free Quark for ricotta.

Special milks are available for people with specific dietary needs, such as lactose intolerance (*see p.232*). Milk is also available in UHT (ultra-heat-treated), dried, evaporated, and condensed forms, which are useful for cooking.

## Milk products

Cheese is milk in concentrated form, which is why cheese is such a great source of the important nutrients found in milk. It is also the reason why cheese has such a high saturated fat content. As with milk, the solution is simply to opt for reduced-fat and low-fat varieties, which contain the vital nutrients while limiting unhealthy saturated fat.

Yogurt is another milk product, made by treating milk with a bacterial culture. Yogurt is rich in protein and vitamin $B_2$, and contains living bacteria that are healthy for your digestive system.

It is available in many different types and, as with other milk products, the lower fat varieties are the healthier choice.

## The importance of calcium

It is difficult to over-emphasize the need to maintain calcium levels throughout life. Each year in the UK, over £1.7 billion are spent on treating osteoporosis (*see p.242*), a disease that may be caused by an inadequate intake of calcium. Women are most affected as they have less bone mass than men to begin with and they lose it faster as they get older, especially after the menopause. Restricting your intake of dairy products as part of a weight-loss diet is therefore not advisable for women.

Remember that your body needs an adequate supply of calcium throughout life. If you do not get enough, your body will draw it from its reserves in your bones.

## What is a serving?

Two to three daily servings are recommended from this group, which includes milk, cheese, yogurt, and other milk products. The following are examples of individual servings:

● 200ml (7floz) milk – whether it be whole or full-fat, semi-skimmed, or skimmed
● 250ml (8floz) calcium-fortified soya milk
● 40g (1½oz) hard cheese – whether it be Cheddar, feta, mozzarella, Brie, Stilton, or another
● 125g (4½oz) soft cheese such as cottage cheese, reduced-fat cream cheese, or fromage frais
● 1 small pot (150g/5oz) low-fat plain or fruit yogurt
● 200ml (7floz) low-fat chocolate milkshake
● Fruit smoothie made with 200ml (7floz) milk or 150g (5oz) yogurt

# Children's needs for calcium

Calcium is an essential nutrient for all children. The daily recommendations (RDAs) for calcium intake are: 350mg for 1- to 3-year-olds; 450mg for 4- to 6-year-olds; 550mg for 7- to 10-year-olds; 1000mg for 11- to 18-year-old boys; and 800mg for 11- to 18-year-old girls. Many children in the UK do not meet these targets, thus increasing their risk of osteoporosis when older.

Look for imaginative and appealing ways of offering lower fat dairy foods to children and adolescents. Here are some good ideas:
● Encourage them to drink more milk (rather than other drinks), eat more yogurt, and make their own milkshakes.
● Let them choose ice creams and yogurts when you go shopping, while you keep an eye on the fat content.
● Include individual cheese portions in their lunchboxes.
● Offer cheese on toast as a snack.

# Recipe  Calcium-rich fruit smoothie

| INGREDIENTS |
| --- |

**8 strawberries, hulled**

**1 orange, segmented**

**120ml (4floz) semi-skimmed milk**

**120g (4oz) low-fat plain yogurt**

**3 tbsp clear honey**

**2 tsp pure vanilla extract**

**6 ice cubes**

**Serves 2**

1 Place the strawberries, orange, milk, yogurt, honey, vanilla, and ice cubes in a food processor or blender.

2 Blend until the mixture is smooth and creamy.

**Variations** Experiment with other fruits such as raspberries, melon, peaches, and bananas.

**Each serving provides**

Calories 225, Total fat 2.0g (Sat. 1.0g, Poly. 0.1g, Mono. 0.5g), Cholesterol 6.2mg, Protein 6.0g, Carbohydrate 47g, Fibre 2.0g, Sodium 76mg. Good source of – Vits: A, Fol, C, D; Mins: Ca, K, Mg, P.

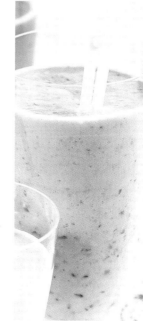

# Choosing the right milk

Most milk consumed in Britain is cow's milk. However, other milks are available as healthy alternatives.

**Cow's milk** Whole or full-fat milk has 7.8g of fat per 200ml (7floz) serving and 132 calories. Calcium content (236mg in a serving) is slightly less than that in lower fat varieties.

**Goat's milk** With slightly less lactose than cow's milk, goat's milk contains more vitamins A, $B_6$, and niacin, and calcium, potassium, copper, and selenium. Full-fat goat's milk has about the same amount of fat as cow's milk, but there are skimmed versions.

**Sheep's milk** Rich in protein, fat, and minerals, sheep's milk is not widely available. It is most often found made into cheese and yogurt.

**Soya milk** This is good for people with lactose intolerance as it does not contain any lactose or casein. A 200ml (7floz) glass contains almost 6.0g of protein, 4.8g of fat, no cholesterol, and 86 calories. Soya milk is not a good natural source of calcium or vitamin $B_{12}$, so choose a fortified variety.

**Rice milk** This is a good substitute for semi-skimmed and skimmed cow's milk for people who have allergies or who are lactose-intolerant.

**Oat milk** Lactose- and cholesterol-free, and low in fat. Choose varieties fortified with calcium and vitamin D.

**Almond milk** Lactose-free and low in saturated fat, almond milk is also very low in sugar.

**Complete food** Milk is an ideal drink for children, providing protein, carbohydrate, and micronutrients – especially calcium, which helps to build strong bones.

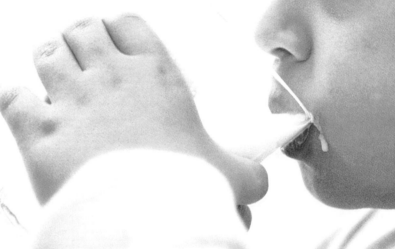

## How milk is processed

To make milk safe for human consumption and more palatable, it is processed in various ways.

**Pasteurization** By heating milk, harmful bacteria and enzymes are destroyed, without affecting taste.

**UHT** After being sterilized by this ultra-high-temperature process, milk can be stored unrefrigerated.

**Homogenization** This process breaks down the milk fat and distributes it throughout the milk.

**Evaporation** Removing 60 per cent of the water content by heating leaves a concentrated milk.

**Condensation** Up to half the water content is removed, then sugar is added to preserve the milk.

| MILK (200ml/7floz) | FAT | CALCIUM |
|---|---|---|
| Evaporated milk (whole) | 18.8g | 580mg |
| Channel Island milk | 10.2g | 260mg |
| Evaporated milk (light) | 8.2g | 520mg |
| Whole or full-fat milk | 7.8g | 236mg |
| Goat's milk | 7.4g | 200mg |
| Soya milk (calcium-enriched) | 4.8g | 178mg |
| Semi-skimmed milk | 3.4g | 240mg |
| Low-fat chocolate milk | 3.4g | 240mg |
| Soya milk (unenriched) | 3.4g | 18mg |
| Skimmed milk | 0.6g | 244mg |

# Which cheese?

Cheese is usually made from cow's, goat's, or sheep's milk. The milk is heated with the enzyme renin (rennet) to separate the curds, which are collected and pressed, then salted and left to ripen or mature – this develops the flavour and texture of the cheese. The longer a cheese is ripened, the harder the texture and the stronger the flavour. Since cheese is made from milk, they are similar in nutritive value. However, many cheeses are high in sodium and fat. Cheeses that are made from lower fat milk are not always low in fat because extra cream may be added. The more water a cheese contains, the lower its percentage of fat will be. The calorie, fat, and calcium content of some popular cheeses are shown below.

| CHEESE (28g/1oz) | CALORIES | TOTAL FAT | SATURATED FAT | CALCIUM |
|---|---|---|---|---|
| Cheddar | 116 | 9.2g | 6.1g | 207mg |
| Roquefort | 105 | 9.2g | 5.9g | 148mg |
| Parmesan | 111 | 7.3g | 4.7g | 287mg |
| Brie | 96 | 7.5g | 5.1g | 72mg |
| Goat's (soft) | 90 | 7.2g | 5.0g | 37mg |
| Camembert | 81 | 6.4g | 4.0g | 66mg |
| Mozzarella | 80 | 6.1g | 3.7g | 101mg |
| Feta | 70 | 5.7g | 3.8g | 101mg |
| Ricotta | 40 | 3.1g | 1.9g | 67mg |

# Other dairy products

There are several other dairy products widely available in supermarkets. Common products include:

**Buttermilk** Traditionally the liquid left when milk was churned into butter, today buttermilk is usually made by adding lactic acid bacteria to skimmed milk. It has a sharper taste than milk and a slightly thicker consistency.

**Crème fraîche** A French soured cream, this is wonderfully creamy but unfortunately very high in fat (40 per cent). The half fat version contains considerably less (15 per cent).

## Jargon buster

**Lactose intolerance** This is the inability to digest lactose, the sugar naturally found in animal milk. The symptoms, which develop after consuming milk products, include abdominal bloating and cramping, diarrhoea, and vomiting (*see p.232*).

**Fromage frais** This fresh curd cheese has a texture similar to yogurt but is slightly less acidic. The fat content can vary from zero to eight per cent (the higher fat version is better for cooking) and it is available plain or sweetened.

**Quark** Usually made from skimmed milk, this is a soft curd cheese with a mild, slightly sour flavour. It is virtually fat-free, although cream is added to some brands to give a smoother texture.

**Soured cream** For this rich, slightly tart cream, harmless bacteria are added to single cream to convert the sugar (lactose) into lactic acid. Soured cream has the same fat content as single cream – just under 20 per cent.

**Yogurt** Because it contains friendly bacteria, yogurt is beneficial to the digestive system – any yogurt that has to be refrigerated will be "live", which means it contains living bacteria. Yogurt may be made from whole or skimmed cow's milk as well as sheep's and goat's milk, and varies in fat content.

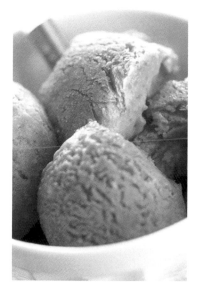

**Frozen yogurt** A refreshing alternative to ice cream, frozen yogurt is available in low-fat and fat-free varieties as well as in many flavours.

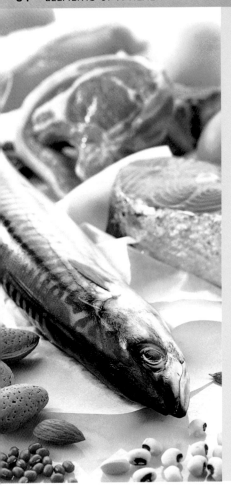

# Healthy protein sources

## Protein deficiency is rare, so the focus is now on fat content.

Protein is an essential nutrient that we must obtain from food every day, as it is not stored by the body. Deficiency is rare in the UK since protein is readily available.

For most people, protein is regarded as the basis of at least one meal a day, and this is usually more than enough to meet the recommended daily requirements.

For vegetarians, meat is not an option and so they look to plant sources for their daily protein. Here, too, there is a wide variety

**Body-building essentials** Your body needs protein for growth and repair: the healthiest sources include low-fat options such as fish, the white meat of poultry, and pulses.

to choose from, including all the different types of pulses (peas, beans, and lentils), as well as a huge variety of nuts and seeds. Unlike animal protein, most plant sources do not contain all the amino acids that make up protein, and they have to be combined to form complete protein (see p.45). One exception is soya beans, which not only contain twice as much protein as other pulses but have nearly as many amino acids as animal proteins (see p.93).

Protein is also found in milk, cheese, and bread, as well as in the foods described here.

## Choosing animal proteins

Animal sources of protein include meat, poultry, fish, and shellfish, as well as animal products such as eggs. Each of these can be further classified according to the type and amount of fat they contain.

# How much protein do you need?

Protein is essential for the repair of muscles and tissues, muscle growth, and regulation of metabolism. The amount you need depends on your body weight (right) and your health.

When you are sick or under stress, your body needs more protein as it uses energy to fight off what ails you. Your immune system depends on a constant supply of amino acids – the building blocks of protein. If you do not take in enough calories and proteins, you risk malnutrition and muscle wasting.

During pregnancy, the recommended daily amount (RDA) increases by 6g per day, and by 11g per day when breast-feeding. Children need more protein than adults for growth: about 2.2g of protein per 1kg (2¼lb) of body weight every day in the first six months of life,

and 2g per 1kg (2¼lb) for the next six months. A child's RDA then gradually decreases throughout childhood and adolescence, until age 18 when it becomes 0.75g per 1kg (2¼lb) per day.

The protein needs for athletes vary according to body weight and the type of activity (see p.147). Most athletes eat more protein than they need, believing it will help increase their muscle mass. But protein consumed in excess is either used as energy when carbohydrate and calorie intake is low or converted to fat.

Most people in the West eat far more protein than they need; deficiency is very rare. Some diets suggest eating extra protein to aid weight loss. Excess protein, however, has been linked with osteoporosis and kidney disease, and with calcium stones in the kidneys.

## How to calculate your daily protein needs

The recommended daily amount (RDA) for dietary protein is calculated on ideal body weight (the average weight for your height and gender).

Every day, adults need to eat 0.75g of protein per 1kg (2¼lb) of body weight. Therefore, a man who weighs 82kg (180lb) needs to consume about 61g of protein per day; and a woman who weighs 68kg (150lb) needs an intake of about 51g of protein each day.

However, growing children and adolescents and pregnant women require an increased amount of protein in their diet (see left).

For example, red meats, such as beef, lamb, pork, and veal, are excellent sources of high-quality protein, but they also contain high levels of saturated fats and may raise blood levels of "bad" LDL cholesterol (see p.23). Because of the link between a high intake of saturated fat and the increased risk of cardiovascular disease and other disorders, it is a good idea to reduce the amount of red meat you eat and instead choose fish and shellfish, poultry, and pulses and other plant proteins.

Poultry varies in fat content depending on the type, which parts of the bird are eaten, and whether the skin is left on, as well as on how the poultry is prepared.

## Eggs and protein
These are a good source of complete protein as well as other essential nutrients (see p.95). Although eggs do contain relatively high levels of cholesterol, it is the amount of saturated fat in a food rather than the amount of cholesterol that has the most impact on cholesterol levels in the blood.

## The benefits of eating fish
Fish is now regarded as one of the healthiest sources of animal protein (see pp.90–91). Oil-rich fish, such as salmon, mackerel, herring, tuna, trout, and sardines, are very highly recommended since they are rich in omega-3 fatty acids, which help reduce the risk of developing cardiovascular disease (see p.214). Shellfish are also a good source of protein, with the added advantage of being low in total fat.

## Plant-based proteins
Collectively known as pulses, dried peas, beans, and lentils are an important source of protein (see pp.92–94). Pulses are low in sodium and saturated fat and contain no cholesterol.

Nuts and seeds are also good sources of protein and supply a useful range of vitamins, minerals, and healthy monounsaturated and polyunsaturated fats (see p.94).

All plant proteins also have a high soluble-fibre content, which helps to reduce blood cholesterol levels (see p.217) and prevent constipation (see p.229).

## What is a serving?
Two to three servings of protein sources are recommended per day, from foods of both plant and animal origin. Suggested servings (uncooked unless otherwise indicated) include:
- 100g (3½oz) boneless meat, such as lean beef, lamb, pork, or venison, or offal such as liver
- 100g (3½oz) boneless poultry, such as chicken or turkey breast
- 100g (3½oz) boneless game, such as pheasant or quail
- 100g (3½oz) fish, such as salmon fillet, sardines, tuna steak, cod steak, or plaice fillet
- 100g (3½oz) shellfish, such as peeled prawns, lobster meat, or crab meat
- 2 medium eggs
- 100g (3½oz) tofu
- 3 heaped tbsp cooked pulses, such as soya beans, haricot beans, red kidney beans, or lentils
- 3 tbsp seeds, such as sunflower or pumpkin
- 3 tbsp nuts, such as almonds, macadamias, or walnuts

# Choosing low-fat proteins

There are two key benefits in choosing low-fat protein foods regularly instead of high-fat types:
- When you choose a lean, lower-fat animal protein (such as fish), you will get a higher concentration of protein, weight for weight, than its higher-fat counterpart such as beef steak.
- These low-fat choices are integral to a heart-healthy diet for the rest of your life. The higher fat animal proteins are associated with an increase in blood cholesterol levels and in the risk of cardiovascular diseases. They should be eaten only in limited quantities.

Low-fat protein sources include low- and reduced-fat dairy products, low-fat soya protein foods, poultry without skin, egg whites instead of whole eggs, and plenty of fish and shellfish.

| FOOD (100g/3½oz) | PROTEIN | TOTAL FAT | SATURATED FAT |
|---|---|---|---|
| Almonds | 21g | 55.8g | 4.4g |
| Salmon | 20.2g | 11g | 1.9g |
| Beef (lean) | 23g | 9.3g | 3.8g |
| Prawns (peeled) | 10.5g | 7.5g | 1.1g |
| Pork (lean) | 21.4g | 4.0g | 1.4g |
| Eggs (1 medium) | 8.1g | 7.0g | 2.0g |
| Chicken breast (no skin) | 30.1g | 4.5g | 1.3g |
| Turkey breast (no skin) | 29.9g | 3.2g | 1.0g |
| Cod fillet | 19.4g | 0.7g | 0.1g |
| Lentils, cooked | 7.6g | 0.4g | 0g |

# Red meat: good or bad?

**Protein-rich, but also high in saturated fat, red meat should be eaten sparingly.**

Red meat, which includes beef, lamb, veal, and pork, is an excellent source of protein in the diet. On the other hand, it is also a major source of unhealthy saturated fat (see pp.40–41).

The Balance of Good Health (see pp.72–73) recommends that you should eat at least two servings per day from the protein group, which includes red meat. Many people, however, eat a great deal more meat than this. Some studies show that people who eat large quantities of red meat on a daily basis have a higher incidence of cardiovascular disease than those who eat it less often.

The relationship between red meat and cardiovascular disease is believed to be due to the high saturated fat and cholesterol content of these meats. There is also evidence to suggest that a high intake of red meat may increase your risk of colon cancer. Not surprisingly, people who replace red meat with fish and chicken have been found to have lowered their risk of cardiovascular disease and colon cancer. For these reasons, it's a good idea to choose to eat lower fat sources of protein.

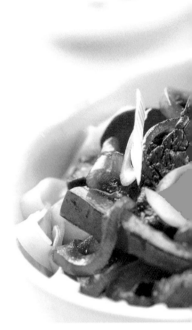

## Which meat should I choose?

Whether it is dinner in a restaurant or a barbecue at home, when you are trying to cut back on calories and fat, red meat can pose difficult decisions. If you stick with traditional favourites like beef and lamb, start by choosing cuts that have a low fat content (right) and reserve the higher fat cuts for special occasions (once or twice a month).

When buying, check any labelling on meat at the supermarket – some labels will give the fat content, particularly labels on packets of minced or ground beef. The leanest types of red meat are beef topside, rump, and fillet steak, pork leg and loin steaks, and game such as venison. Remember to trim off visible fat before cooking.

Although in general red meat is high in fat – particularly when compared to the white meat of poultry – very lean red meat (such as fillet steak) has a lower fat and calorie content than roast dark meat chicken (legs and wings) eaten with the skin.

| MEAT (100g/3½oz raw) | TOTAL FAT | SATURATED FAT |
|---|---|---|
| Sausages | 25g | 9.2g |
| Lamb | 11g | 5.0g |
| Bacon (streaky) | 23g | 8.2g |
| Bacon (lean back) | 16g | 6.0g |
| Minced beef (extra lean) | 14.3g | 5.5g |
| Lamb (lean leg) | 16.5g | 6.9g |
| Fillet steak | 16.3g | 6.4g |
| Rabbit | 5.5g | 2.1g |
| Sirloin steak | 4.5g | 2.0g |
| Pork (lean) | 4.0g | 1.4g |
| Liver (calf's) | 4.9g | 1.9g |
| Veal fillet | 2.7g | 0.9g |
| Venison | 2.2g | 0.8g |

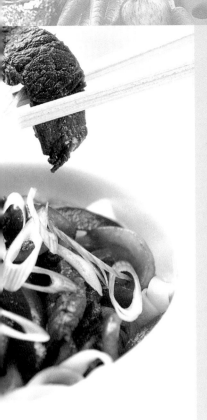

## Other types of meats

Game, such as venison, wild boar, rabbit, and, more recently, buffalo, has meat that is rich and full of flavour. Because these animals get more exercise, their meat is leaner and lower in fat than beef, lamb, and pork, and thus also lower in calories.

Offal – kidneys, liver, tongue, sweetbreads, trotters, and so on – are nutritious meats, being a good source of many of the B vitamins as well as vitamins A and D, and the minerals copper, iron, and zinc. As liver can tend to accumulate chemical residues from the animal, we suggest that you eat only the liver of young animals, such as calves and lambs.

**Beef stir-fry** Slivers of tender steak, quickly stir-fried with finely cut red peppers and spring onions, provide a quick and easy, economical, and healthy low-fat meal.

You should try to avoid eating too many preserved and processed meats, such as bacon, salami, pancetta, sausages, ham and gammon because they often contain a lot of salt as well as being high in saturated fat. Many cured meats also contain high levels of preservatives.

### What is a serving?

While two to three servings from the protein group each day are recommended, we suggest that red meat should be eaten in moderation and that you choose lean cuts. Servings include:
- 100g (3½oz) lean minced beef
- 100g (3½oz) pork loin
- 100g (3½oz) beef topside
- 100g (3½oz) fillet steak
- 100g (3½oz) sirloin steak
- 100g (3½oz) flank steak
- 100g (3½oz) venison

# Healthy ways with red meat

Rather than trying to eliminate red meat from your diet completely, the solution is to eat it less often and to select the leanest cuts possible.

You can also help minimize the fat content of meat by adopting healthy preparation and cooking methods (see p.289). For example:
- Trim off all visible fat from the meat, place it on a rack, then grill or roast it. Excess fat will drip down into the pan and can be discarded.
- Use only a light spray or brush of oil in a non-stick frying pan.
- Try stir-fried dishes where a small amount of meat, cut up into tiny strips, goes a long way mixed in with lots of vegetables.
- Cut down on portion sizes of meat and fill up instead with extra helpings of vegetables and salads.
- When eating out, order small portions or share larger ones.

## Recipe Low-fat game burgers

### INGREDIENTS

**1 onion**

**1 small carrot**

**350g (12oz) minced venison**

**50g (2oz) bulgur wheat, soaked for 30 minutes and drained**

**4 tbsp chopped flat-leaf parsley**

**1 egg white**

**black pepper**

**sunflower oil**

Makes 4

**1** Chop the onion and grate the carrot. Mix all ingredients except oil in a large bowl. Cover and refrigerate for 1 hour.

**2** Form into four burgers, each 2.5cm (1in) thick. Heat the grill. Brush each burger with oil, then grill for 5–8 minutes on each side until browned.

**Each serving provides**
Calories 180, Total fat 5.3g (Sat. 1.1g, Poly. 0.6g, Mono. 2.5g), Cholesterol 43mg, Protein 22g, Carbohydrate 12g, Fibre 1.0g, Sodium 70mg. Good source of – Vits: A, Fol, C, K; Mins: Ca, Mg, P, Se.

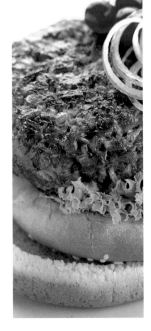

# Poultry for protein

## Lean chicken and turkey are ideal protein sources.

While chicken, turkey, and other poultry are healthier than red meat in terms of saturated fat content, there are significant differences according to which bird is chosen, which part is eaten, and how it is prepared and cooked. For example, skinned turkey breast has eight per cent fat, while skinned chicken breast contains 21 per cent fat.

The fat and calorie content of both turkey and chicken is much higher when the dark meat – from the wings and legs – and the skin are eaten (*opposite*).

To minimize the saturated fat content of poultry, grill or roast the meat and remove the skin

**Choosing chicken**  Chicken breast meat is an excellent source of low-fat protein. For a nutritious meal, stuff boneless chicken breasts with ricotta cheese and grill.

before serving or eating. There is no advantage in removing the skin before cooking: the skin helps to keep the meat moist and does not add significantly to the saturated fat content of the finished dish.

In terms of saturated fat content, ready-prepared chicken and turkey products such as burgers and sausages may not be much healthier than those made from red meat, particularly if they are breaded and deep-fried. They can also contain a lot of additives and water. If you like burgers, you could make them using minced chicken or turkey instead of beef: the result will be much lower in fat (*opposite*) and just as delicious.

### Other varieties

In addition to the popular chicken and turkey, poultry includes duck, goose, guinea fowl, and pigeon as well as game birds such as quail, pheasant, and grouse. Some are healthier than others – goose, for example, is very rich in saturated fat. Duck, too, is a fatty bird;

however, once all the skin and fat are removed (which should be done before cooking), the meat has about the same fat content as lamb. In general, the meat of game birds is quite lean.

## What is a serving?

Two to three servings daily are recommended from the protein group. Poultry makes a good choice, particularly chicken and turkey breast, which are low in saturated fat. Servings include:
- 100g (3½oz) chicken fillet or skinless boneless thigh
- 100g (3½oz) chicken nuggets
- 100g (3½oz) chicken or turkey sausage or burger
- 100g (3½oz) turkey fillet or skinless boneless leg meat
- 100g (3½oz) skinless duck breast
- 100g (3½oz) meat from a goose, without skin and bone
- 100g (3½oz) meat from a game bird, such as pheasant, quail, or pigeon, without skin and bone

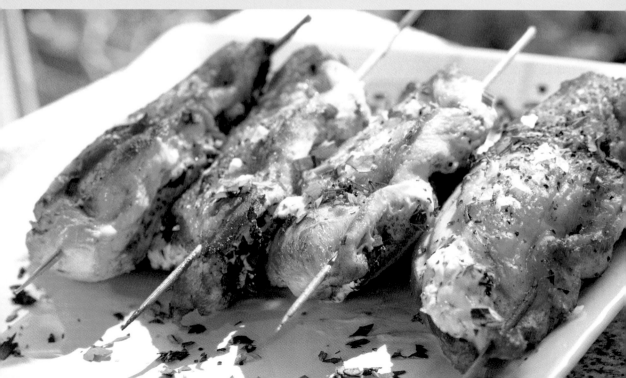

# Which poultry should I choose?

Regarding fat content, it is important to keep in mind that all poultry are not created equal. White meat from chicken and turkey has a similar calorie and saturated fat content (*right*), but duck and goose meat are much more fatty, one of the reasons they are so delicious when roasted. Ostrich and quail have the lowest content of fat and calories. All poultry has roughly an equivalent amount of protein in a standard 100g (3½oz) serving.

Of concern to many people are the growth-promoting hormones and antibiotics given to intensively reared birds to hasten their growth and immunize them against the diseases that come with being raised in close quarters. While poultry farming is closely monitored and controlled by government regulatory bodies, you may prefer to be cautious and buy organic poultry, which is not routinely given antibiotics or hormones. Free-range poultry is another option.

| POULTRY (100g/3½oz) | TOTAL FAT | SATURATED FAT |
|---|---|---|
| Duck breast (with skin) | 42.7g | 10.7g |
| Goose, roast (no skin) | 22g | 10g |
| Chicken breast (with skin) | 13.8g | 5.9g |
| Turkey roll | 9.0g | 2.7g |
| Pigeon, roast (no skin) | 7.9g | - |
| Partridge, roast (no skin) | 7.2g | 1.9g |
| Duck breast (no skin) | 6.5g | 2.0g |
| Pheasant, roast (no skin) | 3.2g | 1.4g |
| Chicken dark meat (no skin) | 2.5g | 0.8g |
| Turkey dark meat (no skin) | 2.5g | 0.8g |
| Turkey breast, roast (no skin) | 1.9g | 0.7g |
| Chicken breast (no skin) | 1.1g | 0.3g |
| Turkey breast (no skin) | 0.8g | 0.3g |

# Recipe  Low-fat turkey burgers

### INGREDIENTS

**450g (1lb) turkey breast fillet**

**1 tbsp dark soy sauce**

**1 tsp grated fresh ginger**

**1 tbsp chopped fresh coriander**

**½ tsp sea salt**

**black pepper**

**seasoned flour**

**olive oil**

**Serves 4**

1 Mince or very finely chop the turkey breast fillet.

2 In a large bowl, combine the minced turkey, soy sauce, ginger, coriander, salt, and freshly ground black pepper. Mix thoroughly, then set aside for a few minutes.

3 Shape the mixture into four burgers, each about 2.5cm (1in) thick. Dredge each burger in the seasoned flour.

4 Heat a little olive oil in a frying pan and fry the burgers for 3–4 minutes on each side until they are cooked through. Alternatively, brush each burger with olive oil and grill

or bake in a moderately hot oven until they are well cooked through, turning them once.

5 To serve, wrap each burger in a soft flour tortilla (wrap), and serve with shredded lettuce, avocado slices, and reduced-fat mayonnaise. Or serve in warm wholemeal rolls

with plain Greek-style yogurt instead of mayonnaise.

**Each serving provides**
Calories 144, Total fat 3.6g (Sat. 0.7g, Poly. 0.5g, Mono. 2.3g), Cholesterol 64mg, Protein 27g, Carbohydrate 12g, Fibre 0.3g, Sodium 569mg. Good source of – Vits: $B_6$, $B_{12}$; Mins: K, Mg, P.

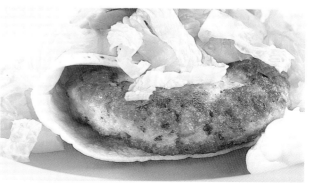

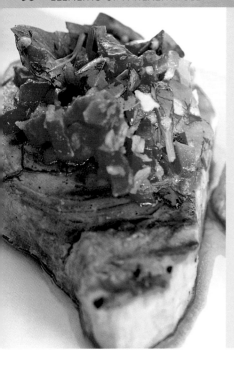

# Fish and shellfish in a healthy diet

## Eating fish twice a week reduces your risk of heart disease.

Low in both total and saturated fat content, fish and shellfish are excellent sources of protein and vitamins, so you should try to include them in your diet at least

**Griddled swordfish** Like other oily fish, swordfish are low in saturated fat but a good source of essential omega-3 fatty acids.

twice a week. Fish and shellfish are high in important nutrients, such as vitamins $B_1$, $B_6$, niacin, and D (see pp.52–57), and some are rich in omega-3 fatty acids (below).

### Benefits of fish
Ever since it was discovered that people such as Inuits, who eat a diet based on fish, have a low incidence of cardiovascular disease, the link between eating fish and reduced risk of heart attack has been a hot topic. Recent research confirms that eating fish, even a

## Choosing fish for omega-3 fatty acids

Oil-rich fish such as sardines, mackerel, and salmon contain a healthy fat called omega-3 fatty acids. This fat is believed to reduce the risk of your developing cardiovascular disease by increasing the levels of "good" cholesterol in the body and lowering the levels of "bad" cholesterol and triglycerides.

Omega-3 fatty acids have also been found to prevent blood clots by making platelets less likely to clump together and stick to artery walls. Blood vessels are also less likely to constrict, making the heart less vulnerable to life-threatening irregular heart rates. There is evidence that omega-3 fatty acids help relieve the symptoms of arthritis (see p.244), and studies show that people who regularly consume oil-rich fish are less likely to suffer from depression.

All fish and shellfish contain some omega-3 fatty acids, but the amount can vary. Generally, the fattier fish contain more than the leaner fish, but the proportion of omega-3 fatty acids can vary considerably between fish species (right). The amount of omega-3 fatty acids in farm-raised seafood can also vary depending on the diet that the fish or shellfish are fed.

| FISH (100g/3½oz) | TOTAL FAT | SATURATED FAT | OMEGA-3 |
|---|---|---|---|
| Mackerel | 16g | 3.3g | 2.2g |
| Herring | 13.2g | 3.3g | 1.83g |
| Sardine | 9.2g | 2.7g | 1.7g |
| Tuna | 4.6g | 1.2g | 1.6g |
| Anchovy | 10g | 1.6g | 1.4g |
| Salmon (canned) | 11g | 1.9g | 1.4g |
| Trout | 5.2g | 1.1g | 1.3g |
| Swordfish | 4.1g | 0.9g | 1.1g |
| Halibut | 2.2g | 0.4g | 0.9g |
| Mussel (in shell) | 0.7g | 0.1g | 0.8g |
| Oyster (in shell) | 0.2g | 0g | 0.6g |
| Crab meat | 5.5g | 0.7g | 0.4g |
| Sea bass | 2.5g | 0.4g | 0.4g |
| Cod | 0.7g | 0.1g | 0.3g |
| Haddock | 0.9g | 0.2g | 0.2g |

few times per month, can help to reduce your risk of developing cardiovascular disease.

## Shellfish is healthy

This food source has acquired a bad reputation because some shellfish contain a high level of cholesterol. However, we now know that cholesterol levels in the blood are related to the intake of saturated fat rather than to eating cholesterol-rich foods (see p.40). Since most shellfish are very low in total fat, there is no reason to exclude them from your diet, particularly if you choose them over higher fat red meat. Be sure, though, to use low-fat cooking methods, such as steaming, baking, and grilling rather than frying.

## Fish and shellfish safety

When handled properly, fish and shellfish are as safe to eat as any other source of protein. Most harmful microbes found in fish are destroyed during cooking.

Women who are pregnant or intending to become pregnant, or who are breast-feeding are advised to avoid eating any fish known to contain high levels of mercury. This is because mercury can affect the baby's developing nervous system. Shark, swordfish, and marlin contain high levels of mercury. Tuna doesn't have as high a content as these fish, but it contains more mercury than fish such as cod, haddock, plaice, and salmon. So the advice is to limit the amount of tuna eaten.

## What is a serving?

Two to three servings from the protein group are recommended daily. Twice a week, try to make these servings fish and shellfish because of their health benefits. Suggested servings include:
- 100g (3½oz) shelled mussels (20 medium)
- 100g (3½oz) peeled prawns, steamed (7 medium)
- 100g (3½oz) lobster meat
- 100g (3½oz) shelled clams
- 100g (3½oz) crab meat
- 100g (3½oz) shelled oysters
- 100g (3½oz) salmon, grilled
- 100g (3½oz) sea bass, grilled
- 100g (3½oz) tuna steak, grilled
- 100g (3½oz) sardines, grilled

# Tips for barbecuing fish

Fresh fish grilled over hot coals makes a great choice for those following a heart-healthy diet. Fish is easy to prepare and fast to cook, as well as being nutritious and delicious. Almost any kind of fish can be cooked on the barbecue. Here are some useful tips:
- Choose the freshest fish available or use thawed frozen fish.
- Do not over-cook. Fish fillets need just 4–5 minutes, depending on thickness. Fish steaks 2.5–5cm (1–2in) thick will need 6–8 minutes on each side.
- Prevent fish from sticking to the rack by marinating first, by basting with an olive oil-based mixture, or by lightly oiling the fish just before cooking.
- Always use a clean rack to avoid "off" flavours – fish will pick up the flavour of any foods previously cooked there.
- Be creative: add interesting flavouring with hickory chips, grape cuttings, or other aromatic woods on the coals.
- Use herb aromatics – soak dried sprigs of rosemary or thyme in water, squeeze dry, and sprinkle on the hot coals for a wonderful aroma.
- If the weather prevents you from cooking outdoors, griddle the fish on a well-heated ridged grill pan.

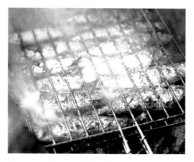

**Fresh sardines** High in beneficial omega-3 fatty acids, sardines are full of flavour and easy to barbecue with minimum preparation.

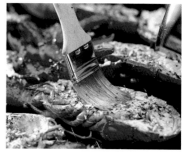

**Brushing with oil** Before barbecuing fish or shellfish, lightly brush them with olive oil to prevent them from sticking to the rack.

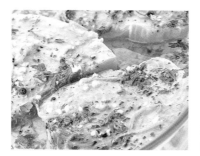

**Marinating** Lean fish steaks and shellfish will benefit from being marinated in an oil-based mixture before cooking.

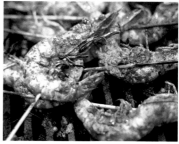

**Herb aromatics** Add flavour to barbecued seafood by sprinkling herb sprigs, such as rosemary or thyme, over the hot coals.

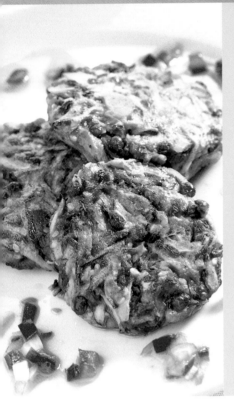

# Pulses, seeds, and nuts

## Inexpensive and versatile, these foods are nutritional gems.

Pulses, seeds, and nuts are all valuable sources of protein as well as being low in saturated fat and sodium and cholesterol-free. In addition they are good sources of fibre (see pp.48–49), complex carbohydrates (see pp.46–47), and vitamins and minerals, including

$B_1$, $B_2$, niacin, folate, calcium, potassium, iron, and phosphorus (see pp.50–67).

The term "pulse" includes a huge range of peas, beans, and lentils (below). They are important foods and have the advantage over animal proteins of being both inexpensive and versatile in how they are cooked, as well as being packed with nutrients.

Due to their high content of soluble fibre, pulses are believed to help reduce blood cholesterol levels. They also have a very low glycaemic index value (see p.47), which means that their sugars are released relatively slowly into the bloodstream and do not cause

**Healthy proteins** Lentils lend themselves to a variety of appetizing dishes. Here they are formed into burgers with almonds, grated courgettes, and sesame seeds.

## Choosing pulses

There is a myriad of pulses, in a variety of colours, shapes, flavours, and uses. They are easy to prepare and can be eaten alone, combined with many other foods, or roasted to eat as a snack. Some pulses are available precooked – canned or frozen. If you buy them dried, they need to be soaked overnight and then cooked for several hours until tender. Dried lentils do not require soaking and cook quickly.

| PULSE (100g/3½oz cooked) | CALORIES | PROTEIN |
|---|---|---|
| Aduki beans | 123 | 9.3g |
| Broad beans | 48 | 5.0g |
| Butter beans | 103 | 7.1g |
| Chickpeas | 114 | 7.7g |
| Haricot beans | 95 | 6.6g |
| Kidney beans | 103 | 8.4g |
| Lentils (brown/green) | 105 | 8.8g |
| Mung beans | 91 | 7.6g |
| Peas | 79 | 6.7g |
| Pinto beans | 137 | 8.9g |
| Soya beans | 141 | 14.0g |

## Facts about soya beans

Soya beans supply nearly as many essential amino acids as animal proteins. They contain twice as much protein as other pulses and are a good source of vitamin A, the B vitamins, and the minerals calcium, phosphorus, potassium, and iron. They also contain large amounts of isoflavones, which are phytochemicals with beneficial health effects (see p.59). Soya beans are processed into a wide variety of products, including:

**Soya milk** This has a fat content similar to semi-skimmed milk.

**Tofu** Available firm or silken, this can be used in smoothies, stir-fry dishes, soups, and burgers.

**TVP** In mince or chunk form, this has a chewy texture and nutty flavour. It can be used instead of meat in a variety of recipes.

sudden increases in blood glucose levels. This makes this group of foods particularly beneficial for anyone who has diabetes and for those at risk of developing this disease, such as people who are overweight or have a family history of diabetes (*see p.246*).

## Protein in seeds and nuts

Seeds are the embryo and food supply of new plants, whereas nuts are dried tree fruits that are contained within hard shells. Both seeds and nuts contain 10–25 per cent protein; they are both good sources of vitamins $B_1$, $B_2$, and E, the minerals calcium, phosphorus, potassium, and iron, and of fibre; and they are high in mono- and polyunsaturated fats.

Research shows that people who regularly eat nuts have a decreased risk of developing cardiovascular disease and diabetes. There are a number of possible explanations, in addition to the known benefits of unsaturated fat on cholesterol levels. For example, nuts are rich in arginine, an amino acid that boosts nitric oxide. This compound relaxes blood vessels and eases blood flow as well as making blood less likely to form clots.

## Complementary proteins

Since the protein obtained from most plants lacks one or more of the amino acids that the body needs (essential amino acids), these sources of protein must be combined with a complementary plant-derived food or soya bean product in order to form complete protein. This is not an issue when animal proteins are also included in the diet, but it is important for vegetarians who eliminate most animal products from their diets. (*see pp.100–101*).

## What is a serving?

Two to three servings daily from the protein group are recommended. Pulses, seeds, and nuts are good sources of protein, and offer an alternative to meat, poultry, eggs, fish and shellfish, and dairy foods. Here are examples of a serving.

- 3–4 tbsp cooked soya beans
- 3–4 tbsp cooked lentils
- 3–4 tbsp cooked chickpeas
- 3–4 tbsp cooked red kidney beans
- 3 tbsp sunflower seeds
- 3 tbsp sesame seeds
- 3 tbsp alfalfa seeds
- 3 tbsp pumpkin seeds
- 3 tbsp linseeds
- 3 tbsp almonds
- 3 tbsp macadamia nuts
- 3 tbsp Brazil nuts
- 3 tbsp pistachio nuts
- 3 tbsp hazelnuts
- 3 tbsp cashew nuts

# Ways of getting seeds into your diet

Seeds are ideal for snacking – they are nutritious, portable, and low in saturated fat. However, if you are trying to reduce the amount of fat in your diet, you should keep in mind that seeds are high in total fat and calories.

**Pumpkin seeds** Rich in protein, iron, zinc, and phosphorus, these seeds can be eaten raw or cooked.

**Sesame seeds** A good source of protein and calcium, sesame seeds also contain iron and niacin. Ground and mixed with sea salt, sesame seeds make a delicious condiment. You can also sprinkle the toasted seeds over stir-fries.

**Sunflower seeds** These are rich in the minerals potassium and phosphorus and also contain protein, iron, and calcium. They make a great topping for salads.

**Linseeds** A good source of fibre and omega-3 fatty acids, crushed linseeds can be added to smoothies and breads. They are often used in cereal and muesli bars.

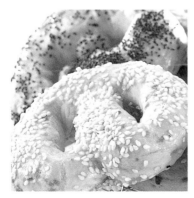

**Seeded bread** Poppy and sunflower seeds provide texture and increase the nutritional value of these individual breads.

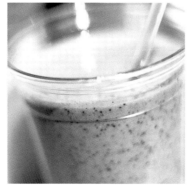

**Healthy smoothie** Crushed linseeds add fibre, omega-3 fatty acids, and a nutty flavour to a raspberry and yogurt smoothie.

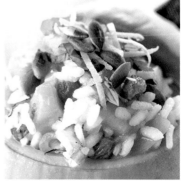

**Pumpkin risotto** Lightly toasted pumpkin seeds add texture, flavour, and a number of valuable nutrients to this savoury dish.

# Which nuts are the best?

Nuts are 10–25 per cent protein, high in mono- and polyunsaturated fats, and a good source of dietary fibre and certain vitamins and minerals. Nuts are cholesterol-free – like other plant foods – but because all nuts are high in fat, and often salted, they should be eaten in moderation.

**Almonds** High in monounsaturated fat, almonds are also a good source of protein, vitamins B$_2$ and E, calcium, iron, and zinc.

**Brazil nuts** Rich in protein, iron, calcium, and zinc, Brazil nuts also contain the highest natural source of selenium – one nut exceeds the recommended daily amount (RDA).

**Cashews** High in fat (but lower than almonds, peanuts, pecans, and walnuts), these contain essential fatty acids, fibre, protein, carbohydrate, B vitamins, and iron and zinc.

**Chestnuts** Containing less fat than most other nuts, chestnuts do have microminerals and potassium, but are not a good source of protein.

**Hazelnuts** Containing fibre, calcium, magnesium, and vitamin E, these are a good source of protein.

**Peanuts** Technically a legume, these contain more protein than most nuts (20–30 per cent), and good amounts of fibre, folate, and niacin.

**Pecan nuts** These contain vitamins A and B$_1$, fibre, and iron, calcium, copper, magnesium, potassium, and phosphorus. They are also high in mono- and polyunsaturated fats.

**Pine nuts** The small edible seeds of pine trees, pine nuts are high in protein, calcium, and magnesium.

**Pistachios** A very rich source of potassium, these contain calcium, magnesium, iron, fibre, and protein as well as vitamin A and folate.

**Walnuts** Rich in vitamins, especially folate, plus magnesium, potassium, iron, and zinc, these are also high in antioxidants and omega-3 fatty acids.

# Nuts and seeds and fat content

These foods have a high percentage of fat; however, being rich in fats does not mean that nuts and seeds are bad for our health. On the contrary, their fats are mostly mono- and polyunsaturated, which are beneficial in the prevention of cardiovascular disease and in lowering LDL cholesterol (see p.40). Some nuts, however, do contain significant amounts of saturated fats and should therefore be eaten in moderation. These include Brazil nuts, cashew nuts, macadamia nuts, and pine nuts.

Brazil nuts, pine nuts, and walnuts contain two essential fatty acids that are particularly heart-healthy: linoleic and alpha-linolenic acids. Walnuts are especially rich in alpha-linolenic acid. Seeds also contain valuable nutrients. The health benefits of nuts and seeds can be undermined if they are salted.

Because of their fat content, nuts and seeds are high in calories. If you are following a low-fat or low-calorie diet, you should be aware that you will need to watch your intake of nuts and seeds. A small percentage of people are allergic to nuts (see p.253), which is why nuts must be listed on food labels.

**Proportions of fats in nuts and seeds**
The chart below gives the breakdown of the proportions of saturated, polyunsaturated, and monounsaturated fats for some nuts and seeds. Nuts are generally high in healthy polyunsaturated and monounsaturated fats.

## Key

- Saturated fat
- Polyunsaturated fat
- Monounsaturated fat

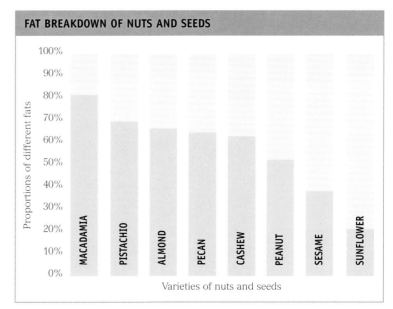

**FAT BREAKDOWN OF NUTS AND SEEDS**

Proportions of different fats: 100%, 90%, 80%, 70%, 60%, 50%, 40%, 30%, 20%, 10%, 0%

Varieties of nuts and seeds: MACADAMIA, PISTACHIO, ALMOND, PECAN, CASHEW, PEANUT, SESAME, SUNFLOWER

# Eggs and health

## An excellent source of protein and other vital nutrients.

Eggs contain all the essential amino acids in the correct proportions (*see pp.44–45*) and are therefore a good source of complete protein. They are also a significant source of vitamins $B_2$, $B_{12}$, D, E, and folate, in addition to iron (*see pp.50–67*). The iron in egg yolks, like the iron found in meat, is easily absorbed by the body.

Eggs contain other vitamins and minerals in smaller amounts, including vitamins $B_1$ and $B_6$, phosphorus, and zinc. Eggs are also one of the best sources of choline, a substance involved in the transport of fat in the body. Choline is also important for the manufacture of phospholipids, which are the major structural components of cell membranes. Most of the vitamins and minerals in eggs are found in the yolk, but the white is also a good source of protein and contains little fat and no cholesterol.

### Eggs and cholesterol

Of all the foods that are eaten in Europe today, eggs are the main source of cholesterol. Yet eggs are relatively low in calories and saturated fat – egg white does not contain any fat. Nutritionists used to advise that eating eggs should be limited, but this advice has been revised (*below*). Research also shows that there is no link between egg consumption and risk of cardiovascular disease.

**Ideal protein**  Low in saturated fat and calories, but an excellent source of complete protein, eggs provide an inexpensive and nutritious addition to your diet.

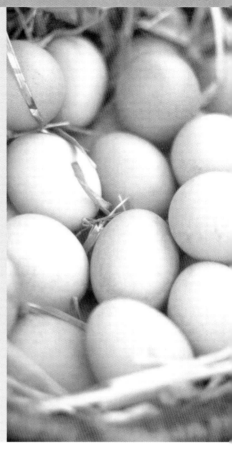

# Should I limit eggs in my diet?

Cholesterol is not found in large amounts in many foods, except in eggs and in offal such as liver and kidneys. The cholesterol in these foods does not usually make a great contribution to blood cholesterol levels. However, if you have a high level of blood cholesterol it is probably wise to limit eggs to about three a week. If you need to reduce your cholesterol levels, it is much more important to reduce the total amount of fat you eat, and to change the types of fat you eat. This is because saturated fat has more of an impact on blood cholesterol levels than eating foods high in dietary cholesterol. Eating a high-fibre diet may also help to reduce the amount of cholesterol that is absorbed into the bloodstream.

There is no limit to how many egg whites you can eat, so look at ways to use more egg whites in your cooking. When cooking eggs, avoid adding butter and cheese, which will add saturated fat.

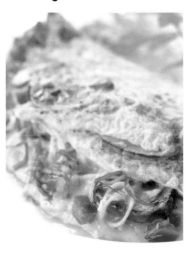

**A filled omelette**  Eggs are a useful source of many important nutrients. An omelette filled with mushrooms and tomatoes will make a quick, tasty, and nutritious lunch.

## Eggs and salmonella

Some eggs may contain salmonella bacteria, which can cause serious illness. Symptoms of salmonella poisoning include abdominal pain, vomiting, and diarrhoea.

In order to minimize your risk of this infection, always store your eggs in the refrigerator and wash your hands after handling eggs. Cook scrambled, poached, and boiled eggs until both white and yolk are firm. Home-made mayonnaise, ice cream, and mousse are made with raw eggs and so could contain salmonella. Commercial versions are based on pasteurized eggs.

Babies and toddlers, pregnant women, elderly people, and those who are already unwell should not eat raw or undercooked eggs due to the risk of salmonella poisoning.

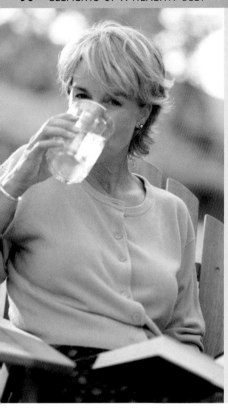

# The need for fluids

## Our bodies need fluids – and water is undoubtedly the best.

About 60 per cent of a man's body and about 50 per cent of a woman's body is made of water. Every cell in your body needs water to function properly, and if you do not drink enough you may feel tired, develop a headache, suffer from dry eyes and a dry mouth, or find it difficult to concentrate. To stay healthy, you need to drink at least six to eight glasses of water each day. When it is hot, when you are playing sport, or on any other occasions when you lose excessive fluid through perspiration, your requirement increases and you need to drink even more water or other fluids.

People who drink plenty of water gain many positive health benefits. Studies have shown that they have fewer kidney stones (see p.238), are less likely to suffer from constipation (see p.229), and are at lower risk for developing cancer of the colon or the urinary tract.

### Water power

Involved in every function of your body, water controls body temperature; gives you energy; assists in weight control; helps transport nutrients and waste products in and out of cells;

**Thirst quencher** Get into the habit of drinking water throughout the day: it is the best way of supplying your body with the fluid that it needs, without adding calories.

# Increase your water intake

Many people believe that they get enough water from coffee, tea, fruit juices, and soft drinks, but these do not fully satisfy the need for fluids. If you eat a healthy diet and exercise regularly, but do not drink enough water, you will not burn fat efficiently. This is because when the body perceives thirst, its processes slow – just as if you had skipped a meal. Whether you drink fizzy or still bottled water, filtered tap water, or just plain tap water, any increase is beneficial to your health. Aim for six to eight 225ml (8floz) glasses of water every day.

Food can also supply your body with water, especially fruits and vegetables. For example, watermelon contains more than 90 per cent water. On a warm day, eating plenty of salad leaves, tomatoes, and cucumber will boost your water intake.

## Tips for drinking more water

Most people do not drink enough water. The recommended amount is six to eight 225ml (8floz) glasses a day. Here are some ways to improve your intake every day:
• While you are studying or working at your computer, keep a bottle or large glass of water on your desk and drink from it regularly.
• Drink tap water or sparkling or still mineral water with meals instead of other carbonated drinks or alcohol.

• When you go out for the day, take a bottle of water with you in your car, briefcase, or backpack. Use an insulated sleeve to help keep it cool.
• Be sure to have a water bottle with you whenever you go to the gym, play tennis, jog or run, or play sport. Extra water is important when you are exercising.
• Buy a bottle of water instead of a sugary fizzy drink or sweetened fruit drink when you are thirsty.

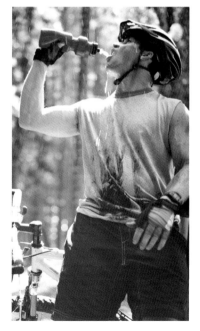

**Maintaining fluid levels** When you are being active, it is essential to replace fluids lost through perspiration by drinking lots of water – before, during, and after exercise.

helps prevent you from becoming dehydrated after sweating; and is needed for all digestive, absorptive, circulatory, and excretory functions.

Children adapt less efficiently to hot weather than adults and are more vulnerable to heat. Their bodies produce more heat but they sweat less and therefore they take longer to change their body temperature. In addition, children's thirst mechanism is not as fully developed as that of adults and they may not express the need to drink. So they must be encouraged to drink water before, during, and after exercise to prevent the risk of dehydration and heatstroke.

## What about soft drinks?
Because soft drinks are composed largely of water, sweetened fruit juice, cola, fizzy lemonade, and other popular drinks do provide the body with essential fluids.

However, they also contain large amounts of sugar, which, when consumed in excess, causes tooth decay and leads to an unhealthy increase in weight. Sweet drinks can also cause a sudden increase in blood sugar levels.

In Europe, overweight and obesity in children is increasing, and the excessive consumption of soft drinks is believed to be a major contributory factor to this problem. The UK National Diet and Nutrition Survey revealed that consumption of fizzy drinks in the UK has doubled in the past 15 years. Young adults now drink an average of six cans a week.

Studies also show that children who consume a lot of calorie-laden soft drinks eat less at their regular meals, causing them to miss out on essential nutrients. By substituting healthier drinks such as semi-skimmed milk or

water for carbonated drinks and squashes, nutritional deficiencies and obesity may be prevented in all age groups.

## Caffeine and fluids
Coffee and tea are popular drinks, not least because of the stimulating effect of the caffeine content. While caffeine also acts as a mild diuretic and increases the amounts of fluid that the body loses in urine, this effect will not cause dehydration. So coffee and tea can count as part of your daily intake of fluids.

However, some people should limit their caffeine intake (below). In addition, caffeine can interact with certain medications: it may react with some antidepressants and diminishes the effect of some tranquillizers. High consumption of caffeine may also increase the excretion of calcium in urine and the risk of osteoporosis (see p.242).

# Fruit juice

Often a good source of vitamin C, some fruit juices are fortified with calcium and other nutrients, but that does not mean they should be unlimited, especially for children. In both adults and children, drinking too much juice can contribute to overweight and obesity, tooth decay, and digestive problems, such as diarrhoea and bloating. Drinking too much juice is filling and can decrease your appetite for other more nutritious foods, including milk. Here are some useful recommendations:
• Choose 100 per cent fruit juice and not a juice drink or powdered drink mix.
• Babies should not be given juice until after the age of six months. Then until age one fruit juice should be diluted and offered only with meals.
• Fruit juice can be one of your five-a-day servings of fruit and vegetables, but regardless of how much you drink it can only count as one daily serving.
• Instead of drinking juice, eat the whole fruits so you can benefit from the fibre in fruit skins and flesh.

# Check your caffeine intake

Moderate caffeine intake is not associated with any health risk. However, The Food Standards Agency's recommendation is for pregnant women to limit their caffeine intake to about 300mg a day This is because high levels of caffeine can result in babies having a low birth weight. Note that the amount of caffeine in a drink can vary enormously according to how strong it is made. Typical content is given below.

| DRINK | SERVING SIZE | CAFFEINE |
|---|---|---|
| Coffee (drip method) | 150ml (5floz) | 115mg |
| Coffee (percolator) | 150ml (5floz) | 80mg |
| Instant coffee | 150ml (5floz) | 65mg |
| Tea | 150ml (5floz) | 40mg |
| Espresso | 30ml (1floz) | 40mg |
| Instant tea | 150ml (5floz) | 30mg |
| Soft drinks (eg cola) | 180ml (6floz) | 18mg |
| Chocolate milk drink | 225ml (8floz) | 5.0mg |
| Cocoa | 150ml (5floz) | 4.0mg |
| Decaffeinated coffee | 150ml (5floz) | 3.0mg |

# Foods to eat sparingly

If your overall diet is healthy, "once-in-a-while" foods can be enjoyed too.

The smallest section on the "plate" model for the Balance of Good Health (see p.72) is allocated to foods containing fat and sugar, such as cakes, biscuits, sweets, and crisps. The recommendation is that these foods – sometimes categorized as "junk foods" – be eaten sparingly. The reason for limiting their intake in a healthy diet is that while they provide plenty of calories, they are either deficient in nutritive value or they are high in unhealthy components such as saturated fat, trans fatty acids (see p38), and salt (see p.64) – all of which are associated with an increased risk of developing certain diseases.

## What your body needs

Following a healthy diet means choosing foods that give you the nourishment your body needs in addition to enough calories to fuel your daily activities. This does

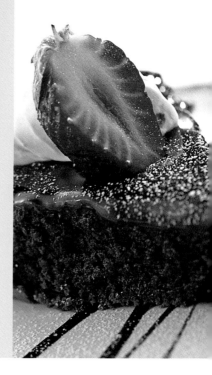

**High in sugar and fat** Although not totally devoid of nutritional value, this chocolate cake, and similar rich desserts, should be regarded as an occasional treat rather than a regular source of energy.

## Is alcohol good for you?

Several studies have suggested that moderate drinkers have a longer life expectancy than both non-drinkers and heavy drinkers. The reason why moderate drinking may confer health benefits is not completely clear, but the serious health risks posed by excessive drinking are well known.

**The health benefits of alcohol** Many studies have shown that if you drink alcohol on a daily basis, you reduce your risk of developing cardiovascular disease (see pp.214–221). The precise reason why moderate alcohol drinking is good for you is not fully understood, but it is known that alcohol raises the levels of "good" HDL cholesterol in the bloodstream.

There are other health benefits that have been attributed to moderate drinking. These benefits include:
● Lowering the risk of stroke
● Reducing levels of stress
● Increasing appetite – especially in older adults.

However, the same amount of alcohol that lowers the risk of developing cardiovascular disease may increase the risk of breast cancer (see p.259).

**The risks of excessive drinking** The risk factors associated with excessive drinking include high blood pressure, excessive weight gain and its related health risks (see p.158), increased risk of accidents, haemorrhagic strokes, and medication interactions. During pregnancy, excessive intake of alcohol is linked with premature birth, low birth weight, congenital birth defects, and poor growth in babies.

In the UK the combined cost of alcohol-related crime and disorder, health problems, lost productivity, and domestic break-up has been estimated as approaching £20 billion a year. The growing consumption of alcohol by young drinkers is also of increasing concern, because it is associated with various emotional, social, and behavioural problems.

**Alcohol and nutrition** There are seven calories in each gram of alcohol, but, since most alcoholic beverages contain insignificant amounts of vitamins and minerals, these are "empty calories". Excessive use of alcohol may lead to nutritional deficiencies since heavy drinkers tend to eat poorly and suffer from impaired digestion of food and absorption of nutrients. They also suffer loss of nutrients (especially zinc) via urinary excretion.

**Drink in moderation** The advice is that if you drink alcohol, do so in moderation – up to two to three units a day for women and three to four units for men. A half pint of beer, lager, or cider or a pub measure of spirits are about one and a half units; a glass of wine is about two units.

Alcohol should be avoided by women who are pregnant or planning to conceive and by people who are taking medication, driving cars, or operating machinery.

not mean that you have to give up delicious sweet and fatty foods altogether, but rather that you should eat them less often.

Every food group contains healthy and less healthy foods, and the healthy ones should form the basis of your diet. This means choosing whole-grain products over refined varieties; lower fat sources of protein, such as fish, chicken, and pulses, rather than meats high in saturated fat; and opting for lower-fat varieties of dairy foods. If your overall diet is healthy, you can afford to include some "once-in-a-while" foods without undue concern.

### Why we like "junk foods"
Researchers have demonstrated that the worldwide popularity of junk foods is due to their ready availability, heavy advertising, and the fact that consumers find them highly palatable. Humans are born with a taste preference for sweets and fats, so sugar and fat are added to manufactured food products to make them more palatable and flavourful.

In recent years, because of growing health concerns, many foods have been reformulated to lower their fat content. However, some of these low-fat biscuits and other foods contain added sugar to improve their taste and appeal to consumers and as a result they contain an even greater amount of calories. It is important to look at the food labels on such products to check their total nutritional content, rather than relying on the health claims that are made by the manufacturers (see p.277).

### Why we love chocolate
Universally popular, chocolate combines a sweet taste with the texture of fat to create a palatable treat whose aroma is one of the most attractive to humans. It also contains substances that help us relax and improve mood – so there is a biological reason why eating chocolate makes you feel good.

Chocolate does provide some nutrients: it is a particularly good source of magnesium and calcium. It also has antioxidant and anti-inflammatory properties.

On the down side, chocolate's high fat content can contribute to weight gain and raised cholesterol levels, with their associated health risks. It also contains caffeine, which should be limited (see p.97).

# Avoid empty calories

Eating too much of the "once-in-a-while" foods is bad for your health in a number of ways: such foods tend to be high in fat and sugar, which means that they are also high in calories and are likely to lead to overweight. Secondly, the saturated fat and trans fatty acid content of many of these products, along with their reliance on refined flour, also has a detrimental effect on health. Moreover, many of these foods provide little nutritional value – hence the term "empty calories". This means that people who eat a lot of them may be overweight, yet suffer from malnutrition.

| FOOD | SERVING | CALORIES | FAT | SATURATED FAT |
|------|---------|----------|-----|---------------|
| Cheesecake | 1 slice (120g/4oz) | 511 | 42g | 23g |
| Chocolate buttercream cake | 1 slice (65g/2¼oz) | 313 | 19g | 12g |
| Milk chocolate | 1 bar (50g) | 260 | 15g | 9g |
| Jam doughnut | 1 doughnut (75g/2½oz) | 252 | 11g | 3.2g |
| Apple pie (double crust) | 1 slice (110g/4oz) | 293 | 15g | 10g |
| Milk shake (whole milk) | 225ml (8floz) | 170 | 8g | 5g |
| Crisps | 1 small bag (28g) | 148 | 10g | 4g |
| Chocolate chip cookies | 1 cookie (25g/1oz) | 119 | 5.7g | 2.7g |
| Cola | 1 can (330ml) | 135 | 0g | 0g |
| Tortilla chips | 28g (1oz) | 129 | 6g | 2g |
| Vanilla ice cream | 1 scoop (100g) | 177 | 8.65g | 6.1g |

# Is a vegetarian diet healthier?

**A carefully planned vegetarian diet has many health benefits.**

Not all vegetarians follow the same dietary restrictions: lacto-vegetarians include dairy but no flesh, such as meat, chicken, or fish. Ovo-vegetarians include eggs in their diet, but avoid all other animal foods. Lacto- and ovo-vegetarians include both dairy and/or eggs, while vegans don't eat any animal products at all.

Because of the limitations of vegetarian diets, careful planning is needed to avoid the nutritional deficiencies that can otherwise occur. Becoming a vegetarian, however, is not difficult and there is no question that well-designed vegetarian diets are healthy for most people, including pregnant women and children.

## Benefits of vegetarianism

The diets of people who eat less animal protein and more plant-based protein tend also to contain less fat and cholesterol and more dietary fibre. This may explain why vegetarians have lower total and LDL-cholesterol levels (*see p.23*) and lower rates of cardiovascular disorders, such as high blood pressure and heart attack, obesity, diabetes, and colon cancer than those who eat meat. It is not clear, however, whether these health benefits are due solely to the diet, or are linked to factors such as regular exercise, lack of smoking, or a low alcohol intake.

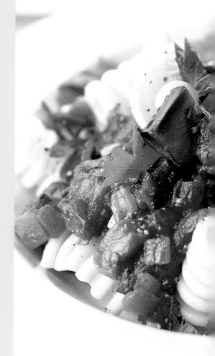

# How to combine plant proteins

Plant-based foods are described as incomplete sources of protein as (with the exception of soya beans and soya bean products) they contain insufficient amounts of one or more essential amino acids (*see p.45*). They can be combined to form good-quality protein, however, because different essential amino acids are missing from each food source.

Pulses (including soya bean products) should form the basis of your main meal. Simply add a grain and/or a seed or nut, and the meal will provide good-quality protein. Alternatively, make sure you eat something from each of these groups over each 12-hour period to ensure that all the amino acids have been included in your diet.

| MEAL IDEA | PULSE | GRAIN | SEEDS AND NUTS |
|---|---|---|---|
| **Lentil, courgette, and sesame patties** (*see p.92*) | Lentils | – | Sesame seeds |
| **Hummus with pitta bread** (*see p.127*) | Chickpeas | Wheat | Sesame seeds |
| **Spicy bean soup with corn bread** (*see p.155*) | Mixed beans | Corn | – |
| **Quinoa-stuffed peppers** (*see p.235*) | Chickpeas | Quinoa | – |
| **Vegetable and chickpea couscous** (*see p.250*) | Chickpeas | Couscous | – |
| **Tofu and vegetable stir-fry with nuts** (*see p.256*) | Soya beans (tofu) | Rice | Cashew nuts |
| **Crostini with canellini beans** (*see p.263*) | Canellini beans | Wheat | – |
| **Quick vegetable couscous with tofu** (*see p.291*) | Soya beans (tofu) | Wheat | – |

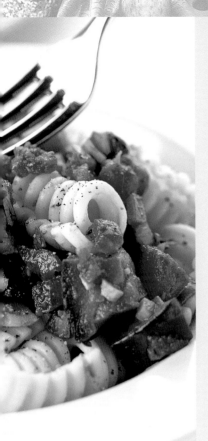

## Nutritional issues

While vegetarian diets that include cheese and eggs will be easier to balance nutritionally than those that exclude all animal products, vegetarians must still plan their diets carefully to obtain all the nutrients they need. For example, iron, which helps red blood cells to carry oxygen to the tissues, is present in both plant and animal foods, but haem iron – which is obtained from animal products – is more readily absorbed by the body than the iron that is obtained from plants (*see p.66*).

Vitamin $B_{12}$ is found only in animal foods and fortified soya products. Because this vitamin is required for the functioning of the nervous system, vegans may require a supplement in order to avoid deficiency (*see p.269*).

**Pasta with vegetables**  Making one of your daily meals a vegetarian dish is an excellent way to improve your diet.

## The macrobiotic diet

Based on ancient Eastern spiritual traditions that seek to balance the two opposing forces of Yin and Yang, this vegetarian diet claims to promote spiritual and physical well-being. By correcting what is perceived as energy imbalance, adherents of the diet claim it can prevent and cure disease.

The aim of the macrobiotic diet is to supply well-balanced meals that are composed of the essential components: grain, protein, sea vegetables, long-cooked vegetables, short-cooked (raw) vegetables, pickles, and dessert.

Strict adherence to this diet may cause health problems. Since no dairy or animal products are eaten, deficiencies in protein, vitamins $B_{12}$ and D, zinc, calcium, and iron may occur. This is very significant for people with increased nutritional needs, such as children (*see p.265, and pp.268–271*).

## Vegetarian tips

The following tips will help ensure a nutritionally sound diet, high in nutrients and low in fat:

- Choose whole grains or foods with naturally occurring vitamins.
- Select fortified or whole-grain breakfast cereals.
- Don't rely too heavily on cheese or other dairy products as they can be high in saturated fat.
- If you eat dairy products, choose low- or reduced-fat varieties.
- Eat foods containing vitamin C with meals in order to improve iron absorption.
- Have one to two servings of a good source of iron every day, for example eggs or red kidney beans.
- Strict vegans should include a good source of vitamin $B_{12}$ daily, such as a fortified cereal, fortified soya drink, or a supplement.

## Recipe  Protein-rich tofu and miso soup

### INGREDIENTS

1 litre (2 pints) vegetable stock

75g (2½oz) firm tofu, diced

4 mushrooms, finely sliced

½ carrot, cut into julienne strips

3 tbsp miso

2 spring or salad onions, finely sliced crosswise

**Serves 4**

1 Put the stock, tofu, mushrooms, and carrot in a pan. Bring to the boil and simmer for 3 minutes.

2 Dissolve miso in a little water. Remove pan from heat and stir in the miso.

Serve hot, garnished with sliced spring onions.

**Each serving provides**
Calories 126, Total fat 2.6g (Sat. 0.7g, Poly. 1.0g, Mono. 0.7g), Cholesterol 0.7mg, Protein 6.0g, Carbohydrate 21g, Fibre 0.4g, Sodium 1,933mg. Good source of – Vits: A; Mins: Ca, K, Mg.

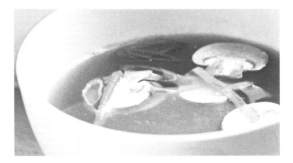

# Eating away from home

## Eating out does not have to ruin your healthy eating plan.

Whether by choice or necessity, there are many occasions when you eat away from home – and these occasions will probably present a challenge to your healthy eating programme.

But eating is not just about satisfying nutritional needs. It is also a major focus of social activities – whether it is eating in restaurants with friends, attending an office party, or meeting family at special occasions where hospitality, in the form of food and drink, is offered. There are ways to enjoy such occasions without losing sight of your long-term healthy diet goals: eating more fruits, vegetables, and whole grains; choosing lean meats and fish and shellfish; limiting your intake of refined carbohydrates, saturated fat, and salt; and being careful with portion sizes and alcohol consumption.

## Making healthy restaurant choices

There is no reason to avoid eating in restaurants, but if you want to maintain your healthy eating habits as well as preventing unwanted weight gain, you need to be very careful when ordering.

Whether you are making a quick stop at a café at lunchtime or enjoying a leisurely restaurant meal in the evening, it is possible to make healthy choices. Fast food and restaurant meals tend to be higher in calories and saturated fat than most of the meals that you prepare at home, so to enjoy a meal without sabotaging your weight-control programme, balance restaurant meals with lighter meals at home. Do not be afraid to ask questions about how a dish on the menu is prepared – it may be possible to prepare it in a different way that is healthier. And if you want to order your main dish without the rich sauce or other high-fat accompaniments, do so: the restaurant is unlikely to refuse your request.

### Party food

An inviting array of food is difficult to resist. The following tips may help you to maintain control at a celebration where food is served in a buffet style:

- Don't stand near the bowls of nuts and crisps.
- Avoid any deep-fried foods as well as mayonnaise-based dips.
- Have a small portion of fish, poultry, or meat and fill your plate with lots of vegetables and salad.
- If you fancy some bread, skip the butter or spread.
- Choose fruit or fresh fruit salad for dessert.
- Decline refills of your wineglass and ask for water instead.

## Dinner party strategies

Although you have no control over the food served when friends and family invite you to dinner, you can still limit how much you eat and drink. Fill up on salads and vegetables offered, and ask for a small portion of dessert.

You can offset any extra calories you are likely to eat by taking a walk or visiting the gym during the day: increasing your level of activity will help you burn the extra calories you are likely to take in. Exercise can also reduce your appetite and help you control how much you eat.

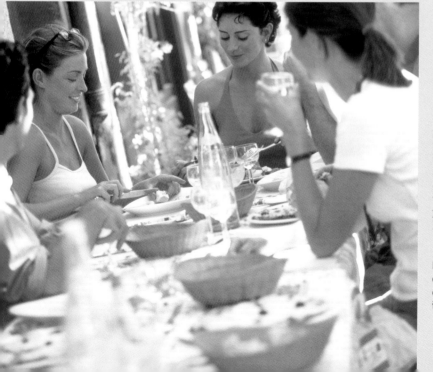

**Dining out** When eating out, don't lose sight of your long-term healthy eating plan. Order carefully, stop eating when you are full, and, if you over-indulge, eat less the next day.

# Choosing healthy restaurant options

When you eat out you need a strategy that will enable you to fully enjoy the experience without losing sight of your healthy eating habits.

## ORDERING STARTERS

When deciding on a starter, first consider whether you would eat one at home. It might be better to skip the starter, especially if you plan to have a big main dish.

● Consider ordering a starter and salad, or two starters, as your main meal, or share a starter.

● Choose low-fat, high-fibre soups such as vegetable or lentil soup. Avoid smooth, creamy soups.

● Deep-fried starters are high in fat and calories, so they are best avoided.

● If you have bread, eat it plain, or dip it in olive oil rather than spreading it with butter.

● If ordering a salad, ask for the dressing to be served separately. This way you can control the quantity.

● Choose a salad without grated cheese, fried croutons, or a special dressing such as Caesar dressing.

## THE BEST MAIN DISHES

Use eating out as an opportunity to choose main dishes you might not cook yourself. You could also try something new.

● Grilled, baked, or roast poultry breast, fish, and shellfish are the best choices, since they are low in fat.

● Opt for tomato-based pasta sauces rather than cheese- or meat-based.

● Order the smallest portion of meat, or share. If you are hungry, order extra vegetables and salad.

● Select horseradish, salsa, lemon or lime juice, or mustard instead of rich, high-fat condiments such as soured cream or mayonnaise.

## ENJOYING DESSERTS

For a healthy, refreshing dessert, have a fruit salad or fresh berries, which are packed with vitamins. You'll be able to savour the true taste of the fruit if you skip the cream.

● Avoid fruit pies and tarts as most pastry is high in fat.

● Sorbet is a good choice rather than higher fat ice cream.

## Fast food choices

The popularity of fast food is a major factor in the increasing prevalence of obesity and associated diseases. This type of food is often high in saturated fat, calories, and sodium, lacking in fibre, vitamins, and minerals, and marketed to encourage the intake of unhealthily large portions. If you do not want to eliminate fast food from your diet, balance it out with what you eat the rest of the time, and try to make healthier choices when you are in a fast food restaurant:

● Choose a small hamburger with lettuce and tomato (no cheese).

● Have salad or baked potato with your meal instead of fries.

● Eat grilled chicken sandwiches with mustard instead of deep-fried chicken sandwiches.

● Use mustard or ketchup instead of mayonnaise or "special sauce".

● Order semi-skimmed milk, water, or a small diet cola.

● Skip dessert, or try a yogurt and fruit parfait.

# Chinese meal transformation

Most of us consider Chinese food to be a healthy option. While this can be true, many of the most popular dishes are quite high in saturated fat and calories. Dishes that are battered and deep-fried, sweet and sour, or in a thick sauce are best avoided.

## CHINESE CAN BE HEALTHY

Choose dishes based on authentic, everyday Chinese cooking, which are low in fat and protein and high in fibre. The cholesterol levels in China are far lower than in the UK; this is because the diet is based mainly on grains and a wide variety of vegetables, with small amounts of protein and fat.

Stir-fried vegetables with tofu, chicken, or prawns are healthy, low-fat Chinese options. Accompany any of these with plain steamed or boiled rice for a well-balanced, healthy meal.

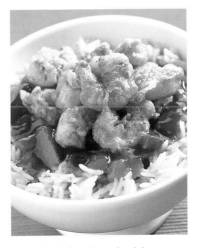

**Unhealthy choice** Battered and deep-fried prawns in sweet and sour sauce, with egg-fried rice. This meal provides 397 calories, 18g fat, and 122mg cholesterol.

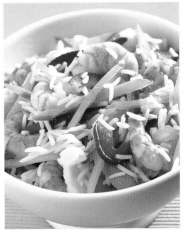

**Low-fat option** Lightly steamed prawns and vegetables, with plain steamed or boiled rice. By contrast, this meal provides only 250 calories, 1g fat, and 65mg cholesterol.

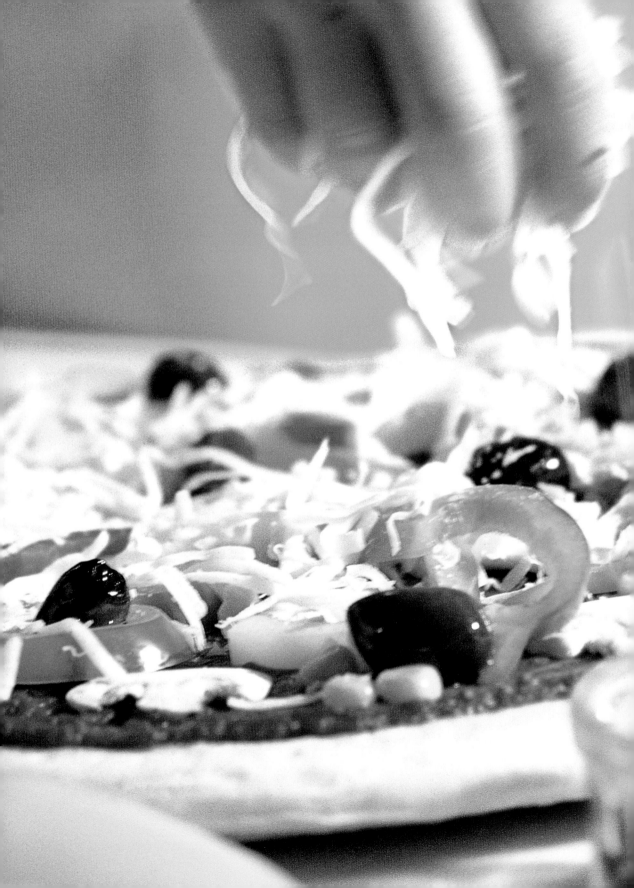

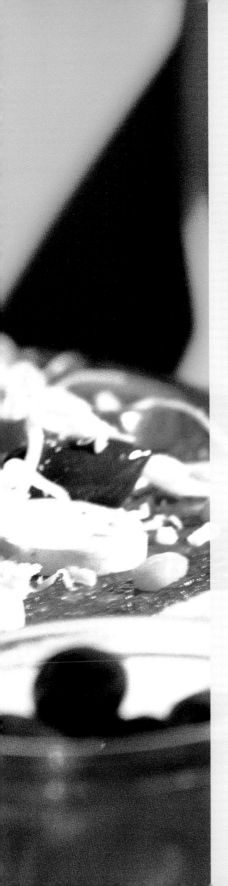

# Eating for the time of your life

Healthy eating is the foundation of a healthy body. At every stage of your life – from early childhood to old age – good nutrition can make a difference in how you feel on a day-to-day basis and in the long-term. In this chapter, you will find helpful advice on how to achieve a healthy diet for yourself, your children, and your parents.

# When our needs change

At different stages in life, we need to make sure our diet meets our body's needs.

So far in this book, we have looked at the nutritional needs of healthy adults. The focus has been on assessing your dietary habits and lifestyle and preventing disease. In this chapter, we will highlight different stages of life and show you key changes that need to be made at the different stages.

## Nutrition for children
We start with nutrition for infants, children, and adolescents. Proper nutrition has an immediate impact on your children's health, well-being, and normal growth and development, and has long-term consequences for their health as adults. Of particular importance is checking your child's growth throughout childhood to make sure he or she is getting enough calories and the right nutrients and to avoid the risk of becoming overweight or underweight.

We look at nutritional aspects of breast-feeding and bottle-feeding, when to introduce new foods during and after weaning, and the needs of preschool and school-age children, who may be fussy eaters. Adolescents' needs, including calcium for strong bones, and the need in teenage girls to replenish iron that is lost during menstrual periods, are also described.

## Nutrition for adults
In the second half of this chapter, the nutritional requirements for adults are covered. These include the specific needs of men and women. Women's extra needs for nutrients during pregnancy, after giving birth, and when breast-feeding are also covered. These topics are followed by dietary measures to lessen the symptoms and effects of the menopause. We end the chapter with nutritional tips on staying healthy and feeling good into old age.

## Nutrition for athletes
In this chapter we also address the nutritional needs of athletes – extremely active people who burn extra calories when they are performing, whether for short bursts or endurance exercises.

**Eating as a family** Make the time to eat together; encourage your children to taste new things and enjoy healthy food.

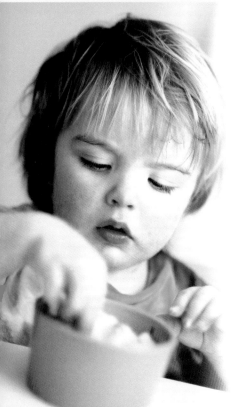

**You are what you eat** To help your child develop good eating habits that will last for life, offer him or her a variety of healthy foods at mealtimes and for snacks.

# Establishing healthy eating habits

Encouraging good eating habits in your children significantly contributes to keeping them healthy and will help them maintain the right weight throughout childhood and into adulthood.

### BE A GOOD ROLE MODEL
As a parent, you should be a good role model for your child's eating habits (see p.126). Introduce your child at a young age to a variety of healthy foods and be patient if he or she goes through a fussy eating phase (see p.127). Try to have meals together as a family as often as possible (opposite above). Since children need plenty of snacks to keep them going through the day, make sure their snacks are healthy (see p.129). In addition, if your child takes a packed lunch to school, make sure it is full of nutritious items (see p.130).

In order to prevent your children from becoming overweight, try to limit the amount of television they watch or video or computer games that they play and encourage them to be active. Also, limit junk food and sweetened fizzy and juice drinks – these are high in calories and may lead to weight gain if they are not consumed in moderation (see p.134).

### TEACH CHILDREN ABOUT FOOD
Stimulate your children's interest in food by cooking together, encouraging them to taste new foods, and planning healthy menus together (see p.131). Make sure children know the difference between healthy and junk foods and understand that what they choose to eat and drink is important for their growing body. All of this will help establish good eating habits that will stay with them for life.

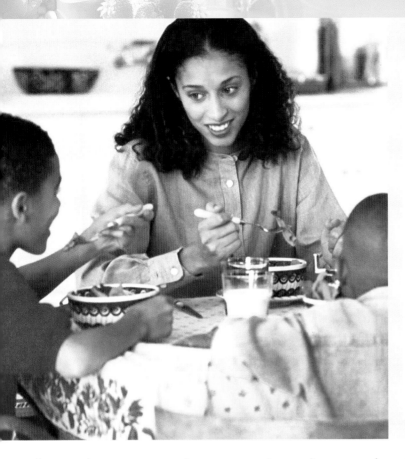

## Eating together

For many reasons it is important to eat together as a family at least once a day. In today's busy world, with children and adolescents involved in lots of extracurricular activities, it may be the only time to catch up and talk about the day. Studies of children's diets have shown that family meals are an important way in which children develop healthy eating habits.

Eating together is an opportunity for you to provide a structured, nurturing environment where healthy foods can be served and for children to learn about good table manners. It is a time to try new foods and for parents to serve as role models for good nutrition. For example, if the whole family is drinking water or semi-skimmed milk, rather than fizzy drinks, your child is less likely to choose a cola when he or she gets older.

# When do we need extra vitamins and minerals?

At certain times of life, or as a result of lifestyle factors, you may need extra vitamins (*see pp.50–59*) and minerals (*see pp.60–67*), either from your diet or by taking supplements (*see pp.268–271*).

### INFANCY TO ADOLESCENCE
The extra needs of babies, children, and adolescents are discussed on pages 114–135. Extra calcium is vital during these years to help build strong bones and protect against the bone disorder osteoporosis in later life (*see p.242*).

### ADULT NEEDS
When girls and women have menstrual periods, they lose iron in the blood. They may need to eat iron-rich foods or take a supplement, especially if their periods are heavy, to reduce the risk of iron-deficiency anaemia (*see p.55*).

During pregnancy (*see pp.138–141*), women have an increased need for vitamins $B_2$, $B_{12}$, C, and folate (which is also important for women planning to conceive). Some of these needs can be met through diet, but you could also take an ante-natal supplement (*see p.140*) to help meet increased needs for iron, folate, selenium, magnesium, iodine, and zinc during this time.

Mothers who are breast-feeding (*see pp.116–117*) need extra vitamins A, $B_1$, $B_2$, and folate to enable them to produce enough breast milk. Extra vitamins C, D, and niacin are needed to replenish vitamins passed into breast milk. You will also need extra copper, zinc, and selenium.

Men may have extra vitamin and mineral needs, depending on their activity level. For example, those involved in sport who tend to sweat a lot may need to replace sodium, potassium, and magnesium.

In addition, for the many peole who are following low-carbohydrate diets to lose weight, taking a multivitamin or a B-complex supplement is essential, since foods with carbohydrates contain important B vitamins.

### THE OVER-FIFTIES
After the age of 50 (*see pp.150–153*), you may need to focus on foods rich in vitamins $B_6$, $B_{12}$, and folate because their absorption is reduced in older age. Extra calcium is vital to keep your bones strong, especially after the menopause.

### OTHER TIMES
Strict vegetarians will not get enough vitamins $B_{12}$ and D, iron, and calcium if they do not eat fortified foods or take supplements. People who smoke may need extra vitamin C, which has the ability to neutralize the damaging free radicals (*see p.58*) that are created by inhaled smoke. Medication may interact with absorption of vitamins or minerals; if you are taking medication ask your GP about possible interactions.

# Fuel for children

**Dietary needs vary in line with a child's stage of growth and development.**

It is important to maintain a healthy diet throughout your life, but for children it is essential for their normal growth and development. Getting all the necessary nutrients from food and drinks such as milk, along with plenty of exercise, has an immediate impact on children's well-being, as well as long-term consequences for their health when they reach adulthood.

## Good habits

Establishing good eating and exercise habits early in life will help your child achieve his or her growth potential and provide the foundation for a healthy life.

Children need roughly the same basic proportions of foods from the different food groups (see p.71) as adults do, but in smaller quantities. These calories and nutrients allow a child's brain to reach its full potential. Without sufficient nutrients, a child's brain may not grow properly, which can affect intellectual development.

## Calcium for healthy bones

Although the height of a child's parents affects how tall he or she will eventually be as an adult, diet plays a key role too. Children who do not get enough vitamin D and calcium will be shorter than other children of the same age and they are also at greater risk for bone fractures compared to those who get enough of these nutrients.

**Growing children** Young children are active and curious about the world around them. Frequent snacks and meals are necessary to replenish the calories they burn.

## Energy and nutrient needs

Body composition (the relative amount of body fat, muscle, and bone), the amount of physical activity that a child does, and his or her age determine the energy (*opposite*) and nutrient needs of the child. These requirements will vary dramatically depending on the stage of his or her growth and development. For example, the more muscle an adolescent boy or girl has, the greater his or her calorie requirements will be.

## The changing body

Babies and toddlers have a high amount of body fat, which starts to decrease as they enter their primary school years. During puberty, children's body fat will increase again. Boys and girls have similar amounts of body fat until the end of adolescence, when boys lose some of the body fat. Girls, however, maintain the extra body fat deposited during adolescence throughout their adult years.

There is also a difference in the proportion of muscle that boys and girls have. Both have similar amounts until puberty, at which stage boys triple their muscle mass, but girls only double theirs. This difference helps explain the higher energy requirements of teenage boys and men compared to that of teenage girls and women.

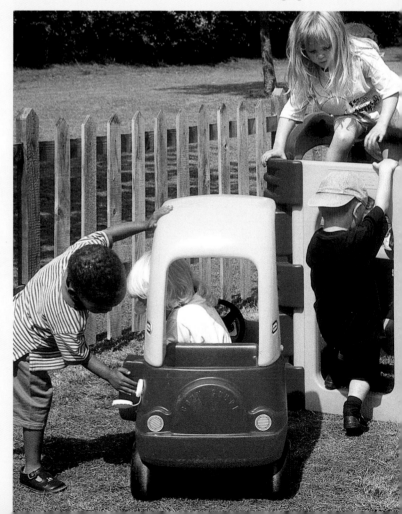

# Energy requirements

The table below shows the recommended amounts of energy in calories (*see p.35*) that boys and girls in different age groups should be getting from food each day. Although children of all ages grow rapidly, their energy needs vary. For example, the amount of energy needed – on a per kilogram (pound) basis – by an 18-year-old teenager is much lower than that of an 18-month-old toddler. Babies double their body weight over a few months, whereas older children and adolescents may double their weight over five to ten years.

Energy requirements will vary in special cases. For example, children who use up a lot of energy in sport or those who are very physically active will need more calories every day than children who are less active. In addition, children who are ill or recovering from an injury need almost double their normal amount of calories to aid the healing process and continue growing normally.

| AGE | BOYS PER DAY | GIRLS PER DAY |
| --- | --- | --- |
| 0–3 months | 545 calories | 515 calories |
| 4–6 months | 690 calories | 645 calories |
| 7–9 months | 825 calories | 765 calories |
| 10–12 months | 920 calories | 865 calories |
| 1–3 years | 1230 calories | 1165 calories |
| 4–6 years | 1715 calories | 1545 calories |
| 7–10 years | 1970 calories | 1740 calories |
| 11–14 years | 2220 calories | 1845 calories |
| 15–18 years | 2755 calories | 2110 calories |

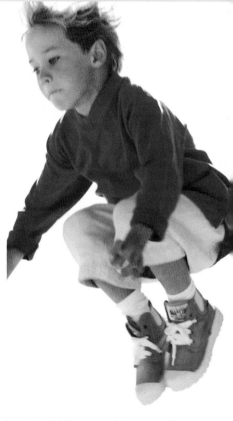

**Spring-loaded** Seven-year-olds are energetic and need 1740–1970 calories per day, ideally from nutrient-dense foods, such as lean meat, whole grains, fruits, and vegetables.

# Do children need vitamin and mineral supplements?

As long as children eat a varied diet, they should not need supplements. However, if they are fussy eaters they may get insufficient amounts of the following vitamins and minerals.

**Calcium** Most children get enough calcium as long as they drink milk and include yogurt and cheese in their diet. However, those who do not eat dairy products or do not drink milk may require a calcium supplement. Calcium needs are particularly high for adolescents because they gain more than 20 per cent of their adult height and about 50 per cent of their adult skeletal mass in this period.

**Vitamin D** If a child doesn't eat meat or oily fish, doesn't spend much time outdoors, or if their skin doesn't get exposed to daylight because they wear clothes that cover almost all of their skin when they are outdoors, you should give them vitamin drops to ensure they get enough vitamin D. A deficiency of vitamin D can cause rickets, which can lead to permanent misshaping of bones.

**Vitamin K** Most newborn babies are given an injection of vitamin K immediately after birth to prevent the bleeding disorder haemorrhagic disease of the newborn.

**Fluoride** This helps to strengthen teeth and reduce the risk of dental caries. However, as fluoride is added to some some water supplies, it is important to ask your dentist if your child needs a supplement. If so, a supplement can be given after the age of six months.

**Iron** Newborn infants usually have enough iron stores from their mother for about four months. If they are not breast-fed, they should receive iron-fortified formula. Once babies begin to eat solid foods, they should be given iron-fortified cereal to prevent the risk of iron deficiency.

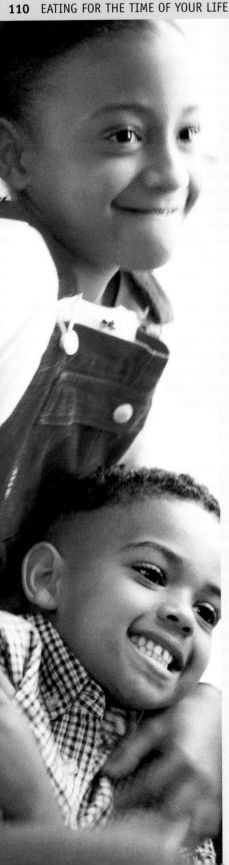

# Your child's growth

## Children's growth should be tracked to make sure they are eating enough.

Children need to be weighed and measured regularly to ensure that they are getting enough to eat for normal growth and development. This is especially important during their rapid growth spurts: the first in early childhood (first year of life) and the second, after a period of growth, in adolescence. These check-ups can help detect any disorders that may be affecting their growth or development.

### Regular health reviews
Your child should have regular health and development checks during the first year, when your doctor or health visitor will check height (length) and weight. Head circumference is also checked for children under three years, since brain growth is reflected in the growth of the skull. The results are then plotted on growth charts appropriate for your child's age and gender (opposite and see p.112) to check that he or she is growing at a steady rate. Also assessed is your child's weight for his or her height by using body mass index (BMI; see p.26). BMI charts for boys and girls aged two to 18 years are on page 113.

### Growth spurts
Babies and adolescents require an increased amount of calories and nutrients in order to ensure normal development during rapid periods of growth.

**Growing concerns** A balanced diet with the appropriate amount of food enables children to grow and develop properly. It also helps keep them healthy and happy.

From birth to the third year, your child will grow rapidly and you will see huge changes as he or she develops. During this time you may worry that your toddler is eating too little or too much. Young children need a balanced diet to grow and flourish and each child burns calories differently, so do not be tempted to put your toddler on a weight-loss diet.

During puberty, children need extra calcium in the diet, which is vital for strong bone development. Teenage boys grow very quickly: at the height of their growth spurt, they may grow more than 5cm (2in) in a year. If your child does not get enough calories during puberty, it can have long-term effects on his or her growth and sexual development.

## Plotting development

The growth charts opposite and on page 112 show the normal range of growth – weight and height for age – for 0- to 2-years-olds and 2- to 18-years-olds. These charts can help you and your GP see if your child's growth is normal.

The shaded band on each chart shows the normal range of growth. This area is made up of curves known as percentiles, based on what percentage of children of a certain age have a particular weight or height. These range from the 5th (95 per cent of children are bigger than this) to the 95th percentile (95 per cent of children are smaller than this) and show how your child compares with other children in the UK. The 50th percentile line is also shown, marking the middle of the range.

Your child's growth is considered normal if, over time, his or her measurements produce a steady upward curve within the shaded region of the chart.

# Checking your baby's growth

At the health and development checks, a doctor or health visitor will weigh your baby and measure the length from heel to crown. These figures will be plotted on growth charts: weight and height for age, with separate charts for boys and girls (*below*). The measurements can reassure breast-feeding mothers who do not know if their babies are getting enough milk.

Over time, a child's measurements should take a gradual upward curve, indicating normal growth. If growth is steady, this usually indicates that all is well, even if a child stays within a low percentile. However, if your baby's weight, height, or head circumference radically shifts or levels out in a short period of time, your doctor should investigate the cause. Most children are measured from heel to crown until 24 months, although small or ill children may be measured in this way until 36 months.

**Using the charts** Find your baby's weight or height on the left of the chart and follow the horizontal line across until it meets the vertical line from your child's age. Mark a cross here. Plotting this at regular intervals will create a curve that lets you track your child's growth and development easily.

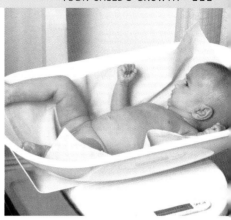

**Weighing a baby** A health visitor or doctor will weigh and measure your baby at each health check to ensure that growth is normal.

## BOYS' WEIGHT (0–2 YEARS)

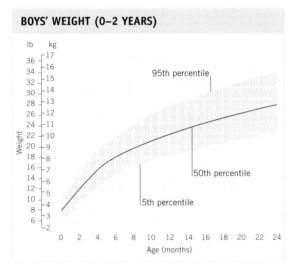

## GIRLS' WEIGHT (0–2 YEARS)

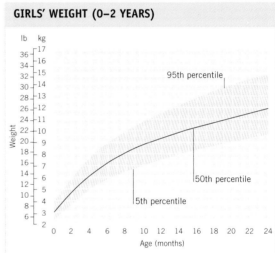

## BOYS' LENGTH (0–2 YEARS)

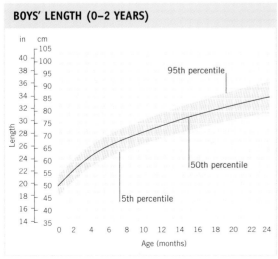

## GIRLS' LENGTH (0–2 YEARS)

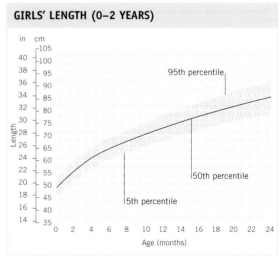

# Checking your child's growth

To monitor your child's growth, you can weigh and measure him or her yourself. This will also be done by your health visitor or doctor. The measurements can then be plotted on growth charts: weight and height for age, with separate charts for boys and girls (*below*).

Plotted over time, your child's weight and height should produce a gradual upward curve within the shaded grey band. This indicates that your child is growing normally. As long as the growth is steady, this usually means that all is well, even if a child is consistently within a low percentile, such as the 5th.

However, If your child's weight or height changes, for example from the 85th to the 45th percentile (or vice versa) in a year, this change could indicate a problem, either medical or nutritional, that requires intervention.

**Using the charts** Find your child's weight or height on the left of the chart and follow the horizontal line across until it meets the vertical line from your child's age. Mark a cross at this point. By plotting this point at regular intervals, for example every six months, you can create a curve that clearly shows how your child is growing.

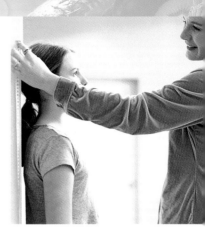

**Measuring height** When you measure your child's height, make sure she or he is barefoot and standing up straight.

## BOYS' WEIGHT (2–18 YEARS)

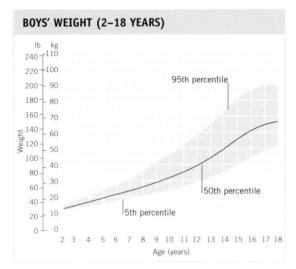

## GIRLS' WEIGHT (2–18 YEARS)

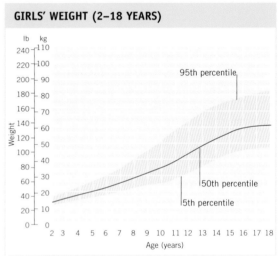

## BOYS' HEIGHT (2–18 YEARS)

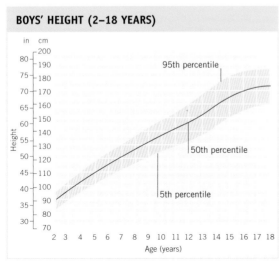

## GIRLS' HEIGHT (2–18 YEARS)

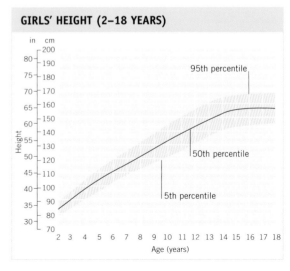

# Checking your child's weight for height

The BMI charts below show the range of body mass index (BMI) for British boys and girls aged between two and 18 years. BMI is calculated as a ratio of weight to height, and can give a more accurate reflection of your child's body fat content.

The charts have a shaded band made up of curves called percentiles. These range from the 5th percentile (95 per cent of children of a particular age have a BMI greater than this) to the 95th percentile (95 per cent of children have a BMI smaller than this). The grey band shows you how your child compares with other British children and if he or she is underweight, a healthy weight, overweight, or obese.

Regularly plotting BMI can also identify children who are at risk of becoming over- or underweight and who require nutritional or medical intervention.

The healthy weight range is within the shaded area. Most children fall into this category, which takes in a wide range of height and weight measurements. Children may be diagnosed as being underweight if their BMI for their age and gender is below the shaded area. A child with a BMI just above the shaded area is categorized as being overweight. Above the top line on the graph is the obese weight range.

**Using the charts**  To use BMI charts, you will first need to calculate your child's BMI (*right*). Then find his or her BMI number on the left of the chart and follow the horizontal line across until it meets the vertical line from your child's age. Mark a cross at this point. By plotting this every six months, you can create a curve showing your child's BMI over time. Ask your doctor or health visitor for a BMI chart to fill in.

## Working out BMI

To use the charts below, you need to work out your child's body mass index (BMI), for which you will need to know his or her height and weight in either metric or imperial measurements.

**Using metric measurements**
1. Multiply your child's height (in metres) by itself.
2. Divide your child's weight (in kilograms) by the result from step 1 to give you the BMI.

**Using imperial measurements**
1. Multiply your child's height (in inches) by itself.
2. Divide your child's weight (in pounds) by the result from step 1.
3. Multiply the result from step 2 by 703. This will tell you the BMI.

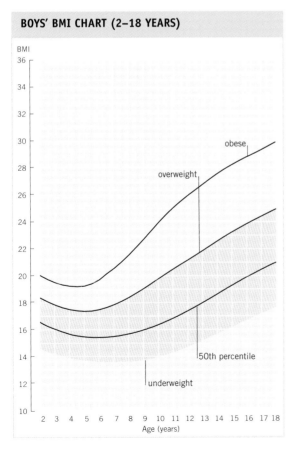

## BOYS' BMI CHART (2–18 YEARS)

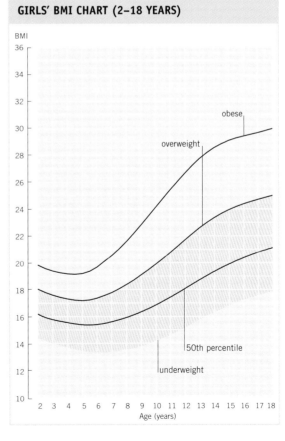

## GIRLS' BMI CHART (2–18 YEARS)

# Food in the first year

**Breast milk and infant formula are the most important sources of nutrition for babies.**

Feeding your new baby is one of the most rewarding things you do as a new parent. In the beginning, your breast-fed baby will eat every two to three hours (eight to 12 times a day) and bottle-fed babies will eat every three to four hours.

You may have heard that breast-feeding is "best for your baby". In this chapter we set out the benefits of breast-feeding, both for you and for your baby, and tell you how to do it. If you decide to use formula instead, or to introduce it while you are breast-feeding or

when you return to work, you can follow the advice given here on choosing a formula and how to prepare and store it. We also outline how formula compares with breast milk nutritionally and for convenience.

## Beginning solid foods

At about six months of age, your baby will sit up and hold his or her head up, and he or she will become much more interested in what you are eating. In the following pages, we outline why you should wait until your baby is six months old before giving any solid food and why infant rice cereal is the ideal first food (*below*). We tell you how to make the transition from giving your baby infant rice cereal to baby

foods during this critical first year, when your baby will triple his or her weight. New parents will have many questions about nutrition during this time and we make an attempt to answer most of these in this chapter.

## Food allergies

Since food allergies have become increasingly common and may be life threatening, we discuss the issues involved and provide practical information for parents with children who have a history of food allergies.

**Introducing a cup** At six to eight months, you can start offering your child diluted 100 per cent fruit juice or water in a sturdy cup with handles that she can hold herself.

## Introducing first tastes

A question often asked by new mothers is, "When can I start feeding my baby family foods?" Doctors now recommend waiting until babies are at least four, but preferably six, months old.

There are three reasons for this. First, at four months, the average baby needs at least 600ml (20floz) of breast milk or formula each day, and early introduction of solid foods may result in babies drinking less milk, thus interfering with proper nutrition during this critical period. Second, very young babies have a tongue reflex that pushes food out of the mouth. By four to six months this reflex disappears, so they can accept food from a spoon. Third, before six months, a baby's digestive system cannot properly digest the nutrients in food.

In addition, if you introduce solid foods too early, it may result in the development of food allergies (*see p.120*) or cause your baby to choke or breathe food into his or her lungs.

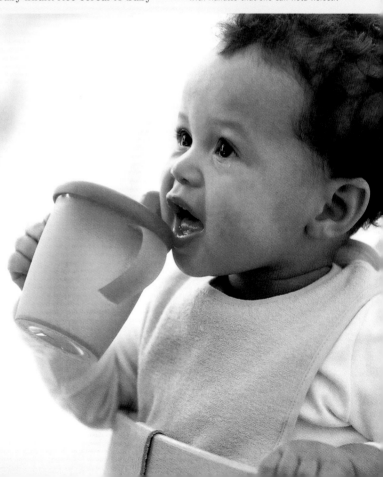

# Breast milk versus infant formula

The perfect food for your baby is breast milk; it is convenient, ready-to-serve, sterile, and tailor-made to meet all the nutritional needs of a baby until six months of age. Already at the proper temperature, breast milk does not require heating.

Giving breast milk also benefits the mother – its production burns up calories, allowing you to return more quickly to your pre-pregnancy weight. It also confers some protection against developing certain disorders, including breast and ovarian cancer. However, for one reason or another, you may decide that breast-feeding is not for you and choose to give your

baby formula instead. Most formulas are based on cow's milk or soya milk and have to be prepared with freshly boiled and cooled tap water. Your baby will still need the same amount of calories as a breast-fed baby, but since formula takes three to four hours to pass through your baby's digestive system, compared to two hours for breast milk, he or she will need fewer feedings of formula a day.

Before you decide whether you want to breast-feed or bottle-feed with infant formula, consider the points below covering nutritional and health aspects and convenience.

| BREAST MILK | INFANT FORMULA |
|---|---|
| The nutrient content of breast milk varies during each feed, and the more your baby nurses, the more milk you produce. | Infant formula always has the same nutrients, and you can estimate your baby's needs. |
| Antibodies and living cells in breast milk help protect your baby against infections. | Infant formula does not contain protective antibodies and living cells. |
| Because breast milk contains antibodies, it is more protective against infections such as gastroenteritis. | Formula may introduce infection through contaminated water or dirty bottles, so ensure that everything is clean. |
| Breast milk contains the fatty acids docosahexanoic acid (DHA) and arachidonic acid (ALA), vital for brain and vision development. | Some formulas do contain these fatty acids. However, they all contain vitamin $B_{12}$, so if you are a vegetarian, your baby is much less likely to develop vitamin $B_{12}$ deficiency, which is found naturally only in foods of animal origin. |
| The iron in breast milk is more easily absorbed than the iron in infant formula. | Formula contains more iron and more vitamin K, which is necessary for blood clotting, than breast milk. |
| A breast-fed baby is unlikely to be overfed because breast milk is supplied on demand. | It is easier to overfeed formula-fed babies because carers may try to get the baby to take more. |
| Your health, your diet, stress levels, any medications, or alcohol intake can affect breast milk. | Quality of infant formula is not affected by your diet or state of health. |
| Breast milk reduces the risk of your child developing asthma, eczema, other allergies, and intolerance to cow's milk later. There is a lower incidence of many other disorders, from ear infections and colitis (inflammation of the colon) to diabetes, immune disorders, sudden infant death syndrome (SIDS), and the cancer lymphoma in breast-fed babies. | Formula has not been shown to reduce the risk of these disorders in babies. |
| Breast milk is always available wherever you are and is at the right temperature. | Formula needs to be prepared, refrigerated for storage, and warmed before giving it to your baby. |
| Breast-feeding does not require time to prepare the milk or special equipment (unless you express milk). | Formula requires equipment and time to prepare. |
| Breast-feeding is usually less expensive than formula. | You have to buy formula. |
| You are the only one who can feed the baby, unless you choose to express milk, in which case your partner or others can also help with feeding. | Others can help with feeding, so you can share feeding with your partner, have more time to yourself, get more sleep, and go back to work without expressing milk. |

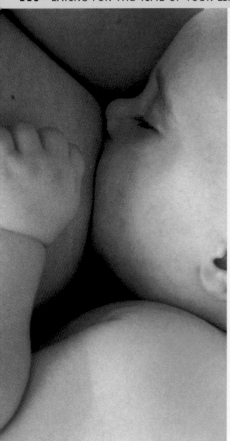

# Benefits of breast milk

## Breast milk is the perfect food for your baby in the first year.

Breast-feeding is recommended as the "gold standard" for feeding babies by all professional groups including the Department of Health and the World Health Organization. This is because of its health advantages for both the baby and mother. Breast milk is considered the ideal source of food to support optimum growth and development in your baby. Complemented by appropriate introduction of solid foods at around six months of age, breast

**Breast-feeding** This provides your baby with the ideal food, which can also protect against infection. In addition, breast-feeding can strengthen the bond between you.

milk is recommended for the entire first year of your baby's life, or longer if desired.

According to the latest Infant Feeding Survey in the UK, 69 per cent of mothers are breast-feeding their babies when they leave hospital after giving birth. This is an increase of three per cent from the previous survey in 1995. Many women stop breast-feeding within the first few weeks or months. The main reasons given for stopping suggest that better breast-feeding support may have made a difference.

### Protection against disease

Breast milk is not only the best source of nutrition for your baby, but it also contains antibodies (disease-fighting proteins) that are transferred from the mother to the baby during the first two weeks of breast-feeding. About

# How do I breast-feed?

When you are breast-feeding, it is important to be comfortable, with your back well supported with cushions. Have a snack and a glass of water by your side because you are likely to be feeding for a while. Over time, you and your baby will become more comfortable as you get to know each other, and both of you can relax and enjoy this bonding experience.

### FEEDING POSITIONS

There is no right or wrong position in which to breast-feed your baby. The cradle position is the most popular, in which you and your baby are "tummy to tummy". You can put a pillow under your baby to raise him or her and to prevent you from leaning forwards. Your baby's body will be in a straight line, with the neck in the proper position to feed. Lying on your side is another common position and can be very

relaxing. Again, you should be "tummy to tummy". The "football-hold" is another position and recommended for mothers of twins who want to feed both babies at the same time. While sitting, place the twins, supported by cushions, on either side of you. Use your arms to support each head, with one arm for each baby.

### LATCHING ON

No matter which position you choose, how your baby's mouth is positioned on to your nipple is very important and will help prevent you from getting sore nipples and improve your success at feeding. It will also ensure that your baby gets plenty of milk and that you produce enough.

To encourage your baby to latch on properly, you will need to touch your nipple to your baby's mouth, tickling the lips at the corners of the mouth. This

action stimulates your baby to open his or her mouth wide. When your baby's mouth is open, bring him or her towards you and on to your breast to begin suckling. The entire areola – the pigmented area surrounding the nipple – should be in your baby's mouth while feeding to ensure that your nipple is in the right position. This is because the action of your baby's lips suckling on the areola stimulates milk production.

### BREAKING THE SUCTION

When your baby has finished feeding, you may need to break the suction by inserting your finger into the corner of your baby's mouth. If your baby pulls away without breaking the suction, it can be painful and cause sore nipples.

Remember, during the first few days breast-feeding may be painful, but as your breasts become accustomed to feeding, it will get easier.

80 per cent of the cells in early breast milk are macrophages (cells that kill viruses and bacteria), and even after these two weeks breast milk remains full of antibodies.

Breast-feeding leads to fewer ear and gastrointestinal infections and respiratory illnesses during the first year of a baby's life, and there is strong evidence that it can help prevent infections such as bacterial meningitis and colitis (inflammation of the colon). Breast milk may also protect your baby against immune system disorders, diabetes, allergies, and sudden infant death syndrome (SIDS).

## Benefits for the mother
Breast-feeding strengthens the bond between mother and baby, helps you to lose the weight gained during pregnancy, and decreases your risk of breast cancer, ovarian cancer, and the bone disease osteoporosis later in life. All in all, breast-feeding is the best possible choice for both you and your baby.

## Breast milk: the perfect food for babies

The human breast produces three types of breast milk: colostrum, transitional milk, and mature milk. Colostrum, which is made during late pregnancy and the first few days of breast-feeding, is high in protein, antibodies, some vitamins and minerals, and hormones. These nutrients encourage the growth of friendly bacteria in the intestine, also known as gut flora (see p.48), and the passage of the baby's first stools.

Transitional milk is produced in the second week; it is higher in fat and the milk sugar lactose and lower in protein and minerals than colostrum. From day 15 onwards, mature milk is produced – this is a blend of fat and sugary (lactose) water and is highly nutritious.

**Mature milk** During each feeding, the composition of mature breast milk changes. Babies get 75 per cent of the milk volume in the first five to ten minutes, but only 50 per cent of the calories. The milk produced after five to ten minutes is richest in fat and is known as the "hind milk". It is therefore essential that your baby is allowed to nurse on each breast until satisfied in order to obtain enough calories for adequate growth.

**Whey and casein** Whey accounts for 60–80 per cent of the total protein in mature breast milk, and it contains the proteins that help babies fight infections. Casein accounts for the remaining 20–40 per cent of mature breast milk's total protein and forms compounds that increase your baby's ability to absorb minerals.

**Lactose** The main carbohydrate found in breast milk is the sugar lactose. Small amounts of other carbohydrates are also present in breast milk, some of which can help fight infection.

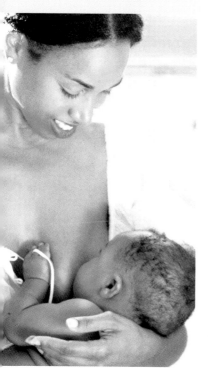

# Feeding on demand

Breast-feeding should occur on demand, whenever your baby is hungry. It may take a few days to get used to your baby's feeding schedule; however, once you have both settled into a pattern, your milk supply will increase and you will be able to satisfy your baby's needs.

### "LET-DOWN" REFLEX
It is best to begin breast-feeding within the first two hours after giving birth. Do not limit the time for each feed in the early stages. You may find it takes two to three minutes of suckling to stimulate the release of oxytocin, a hormone that causes "let-down", a process in which milk begins to empty from the breasts.

**Feeding properly** Babies usually latch on to the breast very naturally. Make sure that you are sitting comfortably before you start, and have a drink and a snack at hand.

### LET YOUR BABY DICTATE
When your baby stops suckling, he or she should be winded and then placed on the other breast for as long as he or she wants. Feeding should be dictated by the baby and not by the clock. If your baby falls asleep during breast-feeding, pause for a short time and resume when he or she is ready again.

### FREQUENT FEEDS
A baby who suckles vigorously usually empties the breast in 10–20 minutes after let-down. It may take up to an hour to empty both breasts. Alternating the breast that your baby starts on each time will help ensure even milk production.

Babies will suckle until satisfied and in the first six weeks should feed eight to 12 times during 24 hours. Frequent feeds reduce the risk of breast engorgement, which can cause you discomfort and increase the risk of breast infection.

# Feeding your baby formula

## Infant formula provides a balanced food source for babies.

Infant formulas for babies have been developed as a substitute for breast milk when a woman is unable to breast-feed because of physical or medical reasons or because she chooses not to.

Infant formulas are made to meet babies' needs and to match the composition of breast milk as closely as possible. They also need to be friendly to your baby's immature intestine. For all these reasons, the composition of infant formulas, including the vitamin and mineral content, is carefully controlled by the Infant and Dietetic Foods Association, which sets strict standards.

Because breast milk contains living cells and other factors that cannot be reproduced artificially, it is impossible to produce a formula equal in all aspects to breast milk. However, formulas do meet the nutritional needs of most babies.

### Types of formulas

Most infant formulas are derived from cow's milk or soya milk. These are known as standard formulas and are generally well tolerated by most babies (below). However, special formulas are available for babies who are not able to digest, absorb, or process standard formulas (below).

### Similar to breast milk

Cow's milk contains most of the nutrients necessary for growth and development, although not in the appropriate proportions that are suitable for human babies. However, cow's milk can be easily modified by formula manufacturers into the right proportions.

Once the milk has been modified, the formula has a similar amount of calories as breast milk and also similar amounts and proportions of proteins, fats, lactose (the sugar that is found naturally in milk), vitamins, and minerals.

Soya milk formulas are modified too. For example, they have certain amino acids (the building blocks of proteins) added to make them more like human milk.

**Bottle-feeding** If you choose to bottle-feed your baby, other members of the family – especially dad – can help with the feeds and increase their bonding with the baby.

# Choosing the right formula

Once you have decided to bottle-feed your baby, you will have to choose a suitable formula. If you are unsure of which type to opt for, your baby's doctor or health visitor will be able to advise you. The most widely used formulas are made from cow's milk, although soya milk formulas are available for babies with milk allergy. Most cow's milk and soya milk formulas are similar and will provide enough calories and nutrients to meet your baby's needs. However, the sources and kinds of nutrients differ between brands.

### STANDARD FORMULAS

Infant milks can be either whey-based or casein-based. In whey-based milks, the cow's milk protein is adjusted so that the casein to whey ratio is similar to that of breast milk. In casein-based milks there is more casein than whey: the ratio remains the same as cow's milk. Whey-based milks are the first choice if a mother does not breast-feed,

whereas the casein-based formulas are generally used if the baby appears not to be fully satisfied on a whey-based infant milk.

### SPECIAL FORMULAS

Your baby will need a special infant formula if he or she is diagnosed with a problem in which certain substances found in breast milk or formula cannot be digested or processed properly. In special formulas, one or more of the basic nutrients – usually the protein and/or carbohydrate – have been modified into an alternative form that your baby can tolerate better.

There are various types of special formulas. Examples include higher-calorie formulas for premature babies; hypoallergenic formulas for babies allergic to cow's milk or soya milk; and predigested formulas for babies who cannot digest proteins, fats, and other substances present in breast milk or standard formula.

## Essential fatty acids and docosahexanoic acid

Essential fatty acids (see p.38) are components of fats that we must get from our diet because our bodies are not capable of making them from other substances in food. They include linoleic acid and are necessary in the body to make cell membranes and many important hormones. They also make other chemical messengers, which "tell" our body how to function properly.

Docosahexanoic acid (DHA) is an important chemical that our body makes from essential fatty acids. It is essential from conception through infancy for the normal growth and development of the brain and vision. DHA is the most abundant fat in breast milk and certain infant formulas now contain this essential fatty acid.

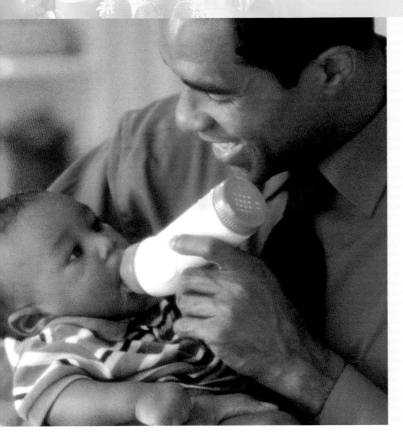

## How much formula?

When preparing formula, always follow the manufacturer's directions carefully. Your baby's daily needs are 500–600ml (18–20floz) until one year – average milk intake is 150ml per kg (5floz per 2.2lb) of body weight. Early on, your baby will only drink 30–60ml (1–2floz) at each feed and will gradually work up to 120–180ml (4–6floz). When starting solid foods, he or she may drink a 180–240ml (6–8floz) bottle after meals and one at bedtime.

Do not enlarge the hole in the teat – this will lead to overfeeding and possibly rapid weight gain, or choking. When your baby refuses the bottle or drops it or stops sucking, he or she has most likely had enough. By recognizing this, you will be less inclined to overfeed. If your baby always seems hungry, discuss it with your health visitor.

# Preparing and storing formula

Make sure you follow safe, strictly hygienic procedure when you are preparing and storing infant formula.

### PREPARING BOTTLES

To reduce the risk of infection and to make sure your baby gets the correct amount of formula, follow these tips:
• Always buy and use formula before its use-by date.
• Use a perfectly clean can opener to open liquid formula. After opening, use the contents straight away.
• Follow the manufacturer's directions precisely. If you do not add enough powder, your baby will not get enough calories. Too little water will cause your baby to get too high a concentration of formula, which may lead to diarrhoea, dehydration, or overfeeding.
• Use fresh boiled and cooled tap water for formula preparation, not water that has been repeatedly boiled. Also do not use artificially softened water, nor water that has been filtered through a jug.

• Wash baby bottles, teats, and any equipment in hot soapy water, then rinse well and sterilize.
• Your baby may like formula warmed to body temperature. You can warm it by standing the bottle in a bowl of warm (not boiling) water.
• Do not use a microwave oven to warm formula. There may be "hot spots" in the formula that burn your baby's mouth.
• Before giving any warmed formula to your baby, make sure you always check the temperature yourself.

### STORING FORMULA

When storing infant formula, you need to be very hygienic to protect your baby from harmful germs.
• Do not use a liquid or prepared formula that has been frozen or stored at temperatures below 0°C (32°F) or heated above 35°C (95°F).
• If preparing formula in advance, store it in the refrigerator, to minimize any bacterial growth.

• Throw away any refrigerated formula that has not been used within 24 hours.
• If you and your baby are going out, put the right amount of powdered formula in a few bottles, then add freshly boiled and cooled water when ready to feed.

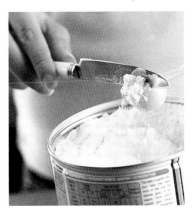

**Preparing infant formula** Always level off the scoop when preparing formula or you will make it too concentrated.

# Introducing first foods

## At about six months your baby is ready to start solid foods.

Recommendations about when to introduce solid foods to your baby's diet have changed considerably over the years. In the past, some doctors advised that children should eat a wide variety of foods as early as the first month of life. Experts now advise delaying the introduction of solid foods until your child is at least four to six months of age. However, breast milk or formula should continue to be the most important source of nutrients throughout the first year of life.

### When to start
The digestive system of a young baby is not developed enough to cope with solid foods until about four to six months of age, and introducing solid foods any earlier can stimulate the development of

**New tastes** At about six months of age, your baby will be ready to be fed with a spoon and you will be able to add cereals, puréed fruits, and vegetables to her diet.

food allergies (*below*). Also, giving solid foods too soon could cause choking (*opposite*). Very young babies have a reflex whereby their tongue naturally pushes the food out of their mouths, but by the age of four to six months they lose this tongue-thrust reflex and so you can begin spoon-feeding. At this age, most babies can sit supported in a chair, and will have developed control and coordination of their head, neck, and mouth muscles. They can eat properly, although they are likely to make a mess, so protect clothes with a bib.

### Spoon-feeding
The introduction of solid foods marks the beginning of a critical period during which a baby learns to eat from a spoon and to accept different tastes and textures. Not coincidentally, a baby's readiness for these experiences generally corresponds to a physical need to supplement the amount of calories and nutrients available from breast milk or formula. However, milk or formula should still continue to be the major source of calories and nutrients during the remainder of the baby's first year. The common belief that solids can "fatten up" the baby or help him or her sleep better is a misconception. Most solid foods have fewer calories than breast milk or formula and should not be the sole nutrient source.

### Gradual introduction
New foods should be introduced gradually – not more often than every three days, or longer if there is a family history of allergies – and no more than one new food at a time. Following these rules will make it easier for you to identify a food that your baby is sensitive to or has an allergic reaction to. The table shown opposite gives general guidelines on when and how to introduce the basic food groups.

## Food allergies

These affect five to eight per cent of children in the UK. Even the tiniest amount of an offending food can be life-threatening. Common foods that cause allergies include cow's milk, gluten (eg wheat and oats), soya, eggs, shellfish, and nuts such as peanuts. If there is a family history of allergies, delay giving gluten until six months, eggs until two years, and shellfish and nuts until three years.

**Recognizing allergy** After giving a new food to your baby, look out for signs of an allergy developing, such

as a skin rash, vomiting, or diarrhoea. If your child's lips and face swell, get an ambulance as this is an emergency. Avoiding the offending food is the only prevention. (*See also pp.252–255.*)

**Check labels** Substances that cause allergies are often hidden in foods – for example, wheat is in processed meats and eggs are in dressings – so check food labels carefully. If you feel your child is falling short on vital nutrients because he or she has to avoid certain foods, consult your doctor or a state-registered dietitian.

# Adding new foods to your baby's diet

During the first four to six months of life, all the food a baby needs is breast milk or formula. After this, you can begin to add solid foods – initially puréed – along with the milk feeds, which should continue until at least 12 months of age. Between seven and 12 months, a baby needs 700–900 calories a day.

No real consensus exists among the experts regarding when and how to introduce solid foods, but you may find the chart below helpful; it shows you when you can add new foods and textures to your baby's diet. It is important not to rush your baby, but to take one step at a time. If he or she

will not eat one particular type of food it could simply be that he or she does not like it – like adults, babies dislike some foods. Pay attention to nutrition labels if you are buying ready-prepared food for your baby: they can be high in salt or sugar. When puréeing vegetables at home, do not add salt.

In terms of drinks, offer him or her occasional drinks of water. Experts feel that there is no specific need for fruit juice in a baby's diet, but if you do decide to give it to your baby, do not give more than 180ml (6floz) of diluted 100 per cent fruit juice per day, and serve it only at mealtimes.

## Foods to avoid

Children under one year are at risk of choking and at higher risk for food allergies. Do not give the following to babies under age one:
- Any milk not designed for human babies, such as cow's, goat's, and soya milk
- Nuts and peanut butter
- Hard sweets and marshmallows
- Whole grapes or cherry tomatoes
- Set and liquid honey
- Ice cream
- Small pieces of raw hard fruits or vegetables
- Popcorn and crisps.

| NEW FOOD | 4–6 MONTHS | 6–9 MONTHS | 9–12 MONTHS |
|---|---|---|---|
| **Milk** | • 4–6 feeds of breast milk/formula per day | • 3–5 feeds of breast milk/formula per day | • 3–4 feeds of breast milk/formula per day |
| **Breads, grains, rice, pasta, and potatoes** | • Rice, barley, or oat iron-fortified cereal mixed thinly with breast milk/formula twice daily<br>• Rusks, toast strips | • Bread and bagels<br>• Small pieces of cooked noodles<br>• Mashed potatoes<br>• Unsweetened, dry cereal<br>• Teething biscuits | • White wheat bread<br>• Rice<br>• Waffles<br>• Pasta and spaghetti<br>• Couscous<br>• Boiled potatoes |
| **Vegetables** | • Puréed, well-cooked dark yellow, orange (but not sweetcorn), or dark green vegetables | • Well-cooked, mashed vegetables such as butternut squash and peas | • Cooked vegetables such as boiled carrots and broccoli<br>• Some raw vegetables, such as tomatoes and peeled cucumber |
| **Fruits** | • Puréed fresh or cooked fruits, unsweetened<br>• Mashed bananas | • Peeled or skinned soft fruit wedges such as bananas, peaches, pears, oranges, and apples | • Any fresh fruit peeled and seeded or canned in juice<br>• Limit juice to 120–180ml (4–6floz) per day |
| **Dairy foods** | • No cow's milk or other dairy foods at this stage | • Cottage cheese<br>• Yogurt<br>• Bite-size strips of cheese | • Slices of cheese, cut up<br>• Cheese on toast, cut into small strips |
| **Protein foods** | • Babies get all the protein they need from breast milk or formula | • Well-cooked and puréed, minced, or finely chopped chicken, fish, and lean meats (without bones, skin, or fat)<br>• Well-cooked and mashed eggs<br>• Well-cooked pulses such as baked beans or chickpeas | • Small tender pieces of chicken, fish, or lean meat<br>• Lean minced beef or minced turkey breast<br>• Chicken nuggets<br>• Ravioli |

# Nutrition for toddlers

In the second year, a child will increase the range of foods he or she eats.

During the second year of life, children show more and more interest in food, and parents may notice that they are more choosy about what they eat. Growth rates slow at this time and toddlers may

**Learning to feed herself** During the second year, toddlers love to sit at the table with the rest of the family and feed themselves. Offer foods that they can pick up easily, and keep a close eye while they are eating.

seem to eat less compared to the first year of life. Those taught to eat wholesome, fresh foods now will be more likely to prefer these foods for life.

### Introducing cow's milk

Children at this age will usually want to eat what the people around them are eating, and will reach out and grab food and drinks. It is therefore the perfect opportunity to set a good example as a role model. At this time, your child will also make the transition from breast milk or infant formula to whole cow's milk and should be drinking out of a cup rather than a bottle. Their expanding palate is ready for new textures, colours,

and flavours, and it is the perfect time to offer a variety of healthy foods, not only for their three meals a day but also for snacks.

### Starting good habits now

Eating habits formed in the first two years of life are thought to persist for years, if not for life, so it is important to establish healthy habits as early as possible.

Children begin expressing personal preferences at an early age. Parents must guide a child's healthy food choices and allow the child to determine what and how much he or she wishes to eat.

At times, it may seem to you that your child is not eating enough food. But forcing children to eat something that they do not want makes them stubborn about their eating habits. By allowing some independence at this age you will be helping to alleviate mealtime problems in the future.

### Serving sizes: 1–2 years

Children aged one to two years need foods from all the food groups, but with fewer and smaller servings than older children. For each food group, the daily number of servings and some examples of an average serving are given below.
- At least 4 servings of starchy carbohydrate foods (at least one serving at each meal): a serving is ¼–½ slice of bread or 2–4 tbsp cooked rice or pasta.
- 2–3 servings of vegetables: a serving is 2 tbsp peas or carrots.
- 2–3 servings of fruits: a serving is ½ apple or a small banana.
- 2 servings of dairy foods or a minimum of 350ml (12floz) milk: a serving is a small pot of yogurt or 40g (1½oz) cheese.
- 2 servings of protein foods: a serving is 30g (1oz) meat, chicken, or fish, or 1 tbsp peanut butter.

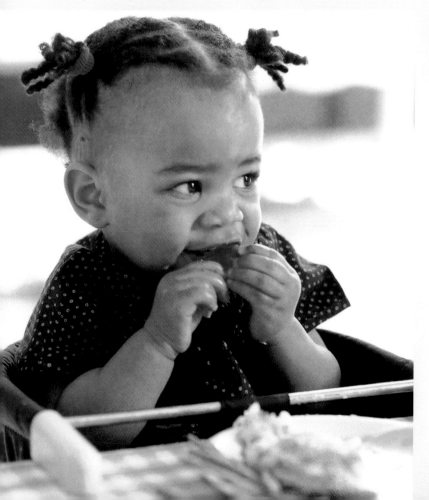

# How much should your child be eating?

It is very important to keep in mind that your child's stomach is much smaller than an adult's and, therefore, he or she does not need as much food as an older sibling does. An example of what a one- to two-year-old child can eat in a day is shown in our sample menu on the right. If your child is particularly energetic, he or she may need another snack after dinner.

Some helpful tips to bear in mind when feeding your young child include:
• Use smaller plates for toddlers and let their appetite regulate how much food they want to eat.

• Do not force, bribe, or nag a child to finish his or her meal or "clean the plate". This negative approach will lead to arguments over food or could result in an overweight child who develops habits that are difficult to break. Your child will let you know when he or she has had enough by clamping his or her lips closed, pushing the plate away, or dropping food on the floor.
• Serve a well-balanced meal that includes foods from all the food groups and offer them in small quantities. There should be no need for second servings. If your child is still hungry and

asks for more, give more vegetables or fresh fruit. He or she may want to eat more at the next meal.
• If your child is cutting back on the amount of milk he or she drinks, offer yogurt or cheese as a snack or dessert.

### SAMPLE MENU: 1–2 YEAR OLD

**Breakfast**
• 30g (1oz) fortified cereal with whole milk and 120ml (4floz) diluted apple juice (half juice, half water)

**Snack**
• 1 small bowl of fruit salad and 120ml (4floz) whole milk

**Lunch**
• 1 small bowl of macaroni cheese with peas, 120ml (4floz) whole milk, and 1 small banana

**Snack**
• 1 digestive biscuit and 120ml (4floz) diluted apple juice

**Tea**
• 50g (2oz) chicken breast with 2–4 tbsp cooked rice and 2 tbsp cooked diced carrots, 2 slices of cucumber, and 120ml (4floz) water

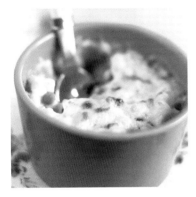

**Macaroni cheese**  This dish is a good source of calcium. You can also add some peas to the cheese sauce to make sure that your child is getting nutrients from vegetables too.

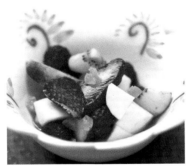

**Fruit salad**  Full of beneficial vitamins, phytochemicals, minerals, and fibre, a small bowl of fresh fruit salad makes an ideal dessert or snack for a young child.

# Introducing new foods

When most of your child's teeth have come through, he or she is ready to chew and try new textures. However, there is still a risk of choking, so you need to avoid certain foods (right).

As you can see from the sample menu above right, children of this age need three meals and at least two snacks a day. You can start to give them family foods, such as baked chicken, but it is very important to cut everything up into tiny pieces so that your child is not at risk of choking.

Since children of this age prefer to grab everything within reach and put it in their mouth all at once, try giving a

few bites at a time so that they learn not to rush when eating. Serve water with meals in order to help your child swallow these new foods.

If your child rejects a new food, remove it without fuss and reintroduce it at a later date. Your child may not be hungry, or may want something else that day. Do not draw attention to the food being new or, even before it is tried, suggest that your child may not like it.

Make the effort to eat with your child often, both at home and in restaurants. This can encourage your child to try new foods. Eating with young friends can also stimulate his or her appetite.

# Preventing choking

The risk of choking is particularly high for young children because they may have problems chewing. It is best to avoid giving young children small pieces of fruit such as whole grapes, raw vegetables, or chunks of cooked meat because they could be a hazard. Instead, cut everything into tiny pieces or short, fine sticks. For very young children, cook food well and then mash or purée it. Wet or juicy foods may slip down a child's throat without being chewed properly, so give these foods one at a time.

# Feeding pre-school children

**Between the ages of two and five, children need plenty of snacks.**

After the rapid growth of early infancy, toddlers' growth rates slow and they tend to eat less, although appetite fluctuations are normal and correspond to growth spurts. Therefore, your child may seem hungry one day and not very interested in food the next.

Learn to recognize when your child is hungry and offer healthy, appetizing meals, a small snack between each meal, and a piece of fresh fruit before bedtime. Keep in mind that giving your child too many drinks between meals will fill up his or her small stomach very quickly, so do not overdo it. This also applies to serving sizes:

children cannot manage adult-sized portions, so offer smaller amounts of food on smaller, child-friendly plates.

## Giving the right food

Because appetites vary from child to child and from day to day, you may worry about your child's eating habits. For example, sometimes he or she may want to eat the same foods over and over again for every meal, and at other times that same food might be rejected outright. Inconsistency when it comes to mealtimes is very common. The way to deal with this is to offer a nutritious selection of foods, to remain patient, and to give your child the freedom to choose what he or she wants to eat – within reason. Over the course of a few weeks, most children's diets will

balance out. If your child is a fussy eater you may need to develop some strategies to help you deal with this (*see p.127*).

## Monitoring your child

By monitoring your child's growth (*see p.112*) and eating habits, and looking for any signs or symptoms of nutritional deficiency, you can assess if he or she is getting the proper amounts of all the essential nutrients. Children who are eating enough will be growing at the appropriate rate. You can keep growth charts (*see pp.111–113*) at home to track your child's height and weight for age.

It is difficult to detect nutrient deficiencies on your own – usually only severe deficiencies can be seen. This is why regular health reviews for your child are vital.

## What can I offer my pre-school child?

Pre-school children need more grain-based foods, vegetables, and protein foods as they get older. Give them semi-skimmed milk and low-fat dairy products instead of whole milk as long as they are not underweight (do not change to skimmed milk until after age five). Children of this age need three meals and at least two snacks during the day plus sometimes a bedtime snack. To prevent a child from eating too much and gaining excess weight, try to serve fresh fruit for snacks. Provide water with at least one meal and one snack rather than fruit juice because juice supplies extra calories and may reduce a child's appetite for the next meal. Pay attention to your child's appetite and use smaller plates with smaller, child-sized portions.

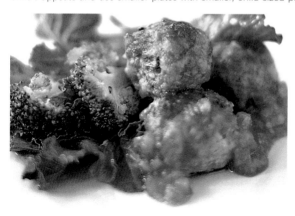

**Tea** Meatballs in a fresh tomato sauce with broccoli is a popular meal for five-year-olds. It is rich in protein, vitamins C and K, iron, and lycopene.

### SAMPLE MENU: 5-YEAR-OLD

**Breakfast**
- 30g (1oz) cereal with semi-skimmed milk and ½ banana

**Snack**
- Apple with a piece of cheese and a glass of water

**Lunch**
- Chicken sandwich, carrots, and 150ml (5floz) low-fat yogurt

**Snack**
- 2 digestive biscuits, a satsuma or kiwi fruit, and 120ml (4floz) semi-skimmed milk

**Dinner**
- 3 meatballs in tomato sauce, 4–8 tbsp noodles, broccoli, and a glass of water

**Snack**
- Cereal with semi-skimmed milk

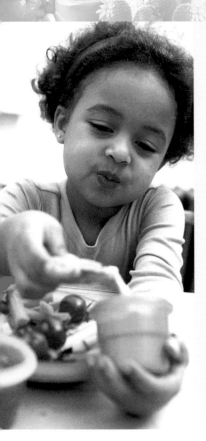

If you are concerned about your child's eating habits, you might want to try recording a "food diary" of everything he or she eats and drinks each day for a week. Record the type of food, its brand, and the amount eaten. Discuss the week's intake with your health visitor.

Computer analysis programmes can be used to show the amount of calories your child is consuming, which of the food groups he or she is getting enough of, and if he or she is at risk of developing any nutritional deficiencies. One of the most common nutrients lacking in a child's diet is iron, especially among fussy eaters, so try to give your child plenty of iron-rich foods, such as meat, dried fruits, poultry, and pulses (*see p.135*).

**Dipping foods** Make mealtimes fun and interesting activities for children. Letting them dip food into tubs is a good way to increase the amount of vegetables they eat.

## Serving sizes: 3–5 years

For three- to five-year-olds, the serving sizes of vegetables and protein foods are about the same as those for one- to two-year-olds, but they will eat more. The number of daily servings and examples of a serving are given below:
- At least 4 servings of starchy carbohydrate foods: a serving is ½–1 slice of wholemeal bread or 4–8 tbsp cooked rice.
- 2–3 servings of vegetables: a serving is 2 tbsp peas or carrots.
- 2–3 servings of fruits: a serving is ½ fruit, such as an apple, pear, or peach, or a small banana.
- 2 servings of dairy foods such as a small pot of yogurt, or at least 350ml (12floz) milk.
- 2 servings of protein foods: a serving is 30–55g (1–2oz) meat, chicken, fish, or tofu, 1 egg, or 1 tbsp peanut butter.

# Making food interesting to eat

An excellent way to get young children to eat nutritious food is to make meals and snacks fun and interesting, and to let children help you prepare them. Try some of the following tips so your child will look forward to mealtimes.
- Cut sandwiches, pizza, and meats into small shapes. By making all the choices nutritious, your child will be eating healthy food no matter which one he or she wants to try.
- Serve sticks of fruit and vegetables, breadsticks, and small biscuits with a tasty dip. Some possibilities for dips include cream cheese or tofu blended with fruit juice or milk, a vegetable or fruit purée, and hummus.
- Involve your child in helping to prepare ingredients – tearing lettuce for a salad, washing vegetables, and sprinkling on grated cheese are all simple tasks for young children.
- Create meals with your child. Mini pizzas are lots of fun for children to assemble, and the bases and toppings

can be very nutritious. Great toppings for mini pizzas include pizza or pesto sauce, grated mozzarella cheese, lots of vegetables (broccoli, tomatoes, asparagus, spinach, and sweetcorn are all delicious), chicken, tuna, or lean minced beef, and canned pineapple chunks (*see p.131*).
- Let your child make his or her own snacks (with a bit of supervision). It's easy to learn how to spread peanut butter or jam on to oatcakes, how to make a banana sandwich, and how to fill celery sticks with cream cheese.
- Offer fruit as a snack. Most children love fruit and, if it is regularly offered, they will ask for it rather than a biscuit or chocolate bar.
- Prepare healthy desserts such as cut-up apples, oranges, and pears, canned fruit in its own juice, and fresh fruit salad. Other healthy ideas include baked custard, rice pudding, bread and butter pudding, fruit sorbet, or angel cake with fresh berries.

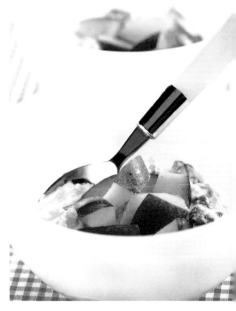

**Fruit and fibre** Adding chopped fresh fruit to a dessert is a good way to get extra nutrients and fibre into your child's diet, especially if he or she is a fussy eater.

# Healthy eating habits

To encourage healthy eating habits in your pre-school child, follow the tips outlined below. Do not worry if you can't do everything at once; just adopting one tip at a time will make a difference to your child's eating habits.

• Serve fruits and vegetables every day, both at mealtimes and also as snacks. Canned fruits in juice, such as peaches, pineapple, or mandarin oranges, are a quick storecupboard standby.

• Provide water or semi-skimmed milk with meals and snacks.

• Don't be afraid to say no to chocolate and other sweets, sugary fizzy drinks, and crisps, especially if your child has already had some of these that day.

• Serve small portions on small plates and in small cups. Giving too much and insisting that your child finishes everything will lead to overeating and will not help your child regulate his or her own eating habits.

• Do not use dessert as a reward. Encouraging children to eat all of their main course to get dessert will make the dessert seem more important than the nutritious part of the meal.

• When your child has finished eating, ask him or her to take the plate to the sink and return to the table to sit with the family. If necessary, use colouring or sticker books to keep the child entertained while the rest of the family finishes their meal. You can also adopt this strategy when you eat out together.

• Keep a stock of healthy snacks to offer when your child is hungry.

• Limit TV and video and computer games to no more than two hours a day. A sedentary lifestyle will lead to weight gain (and overweight children).

• Encourage your child to be active, and exercise regularly as a family.

• Try to gather the family together for meals as often as possible.

## Being a role model

As a parent, you are responsible for setting a good example for your children when it comes to establishing healthy eating habits. From an early age, children usually want to copy what you are doing and will reach out for whatever you are eating or drinking. If you drink a cola with meals and eat in front of the television, your child will be likely to want to do the same thing. However, cola is not appropriate for children – it is high in calories and will reduce room for milk with its much-needed calcium content – and eating in front of the TV does not promote family bonding or socializing. Think about your own food habits and make a conscious effort to eat healthy, well-balanced meals as a family, at the table – without the television on.

# What to give children to drink

The healthiest drinks to give young children are milk and water. Other drinks, such as fizzy colas, juice drinks, and squashes are high in sugar and can cause tooth decay. Although it contains more nutrients, 100 per cent fruit juice is high in natural fruit sugars and calories too. If you do give your child fruit juice, follow these tips:

• Give your child fruit juice only as part of a meal or snack.

• Always dilute fruit juice with water to reduce its high sugar content.

• Limit the amount of fruit juice given to two- to five-year-old children to about 120–180ml (4–6floz) per day.

• Encourage your child to eat fresh fruit in place of fruit juice. This will increase the intake of fibre.

• Do not give your child unpasteurized fruit juices as they may contain bacteria.

**Choose milk** A healthier alternative to sugar-dense juices, milk is rich in calcium, which helps build strong bones.

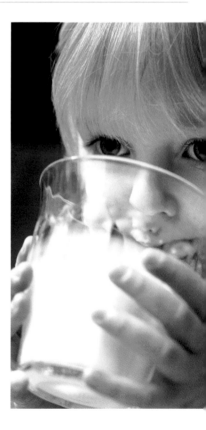

## Keeping teeth healthy

Sugary and starchy foods that stick to teeth feed the bacteria that cause tooth decay. To ensure that your child's teeth develop properly and remain healthy, give a variety of foods to provide all the necessary nutrients for tooth development. Limit the amount of sugary drinks and foods, such as biscuits and sweets, that you provide. Good,

teeth-friendly snacks include cubes of Cheddar cheese, yogurt, fresh fruit, and vegetable sticks with dips. In addition, fluoride (*see p.65*), which is present in many water supplies, helps protect teeth. Once teeth begin to erupt, make sure that your child has regular dental check-ups and brushes his or her teeth in the morning and before going to bed.

# Managing the fussy eater

There are many strategies to help you overcome fussy eating. If you are having problems with your child's eating habits, try following the tips below:

• First of all, be patient. Sit down at the table with your child and have a conversation about his or her day.

• Offer a variety of bite-sized foods in order to allow your child to pick and choose the most appetizing and thus expand his or her diet.

• Present food in small and interesting shapes to make it look more appealing.

• Offer your child foods that pack lots of nutrients in small portions, such as avocados, broccoli, whole grains such as brown rice and porridge, cheese, eggs, fish, red kidney beans, yogurt, pasta, peanut butter, pumpkin, sweet potatoes, and tofu.

• Do not turn each meal into a battle. If your child has developed a "food fad" and insists on eating the same foods every day, keep offering a healthy selection of food at each meal. Your child will eventually tire of eating the same foods. The less pressure you put on your child, the more likely it is that he or she will pass through this stage without problems.

• Do not try to force-feed your child or hover over him or her worrying about what he or she will or will not eat.

• If your child does not like different foods to be touching one another, serve them on separate plates.

• Do not prepare something else for your child if he or she refuses to eat what is on the plate.

• Do not give snack foods if your child refuses to eat his or her meal.

• Do not punish your child for not eating a particular food; it is much better to congratulate him or her for what he or she does eat.

**Finger foods**  Try serving dahl (mashed lentils) or hummus (chickpea purée) in a bowl with cut-up pitta bread or vegetables for dipping.

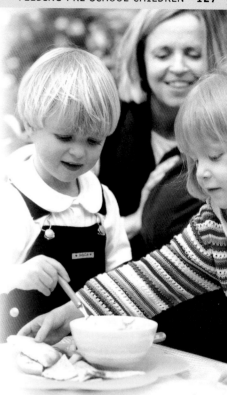

# Case study  Pre-school child who eats only white food

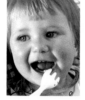

**Name**  Jodie

**Age**  Three years

**Problem**  Jodie will not eat anything green or red and tends to eat the same foods every day for lunch and tea. She mostly eats white foods, such as cheese, yogurt, and pasta.

**Lifestyle**  This toddler's mother is concerned that her child's diet is very limited and she has become a fussy eater. Jodie's mother is also concerned about whether her daughter should take a multivitamin supplement.

Although her appetite varies from day to day, Jodie's evening meal usually consists of chicken nuggets, pasta, and stewed apples with yogurt at least five nights a week. Sometimes she will eat pizza and stewed apples, but she has not been open to trying any other foods that the family is eating, such as chicken, beef, rice, potatoes, or vegetables. She does like some fruits, such as canned mandarin oranges, fresh strawberries, and bananas. In addition, she often takes only a few bites of whatever foods she is offered and announces that she is done. Jodie rarely finishes what is on her plate and frequently returns to the kitchen after an hour or so asking for an ice lolly or other sweets.

**Advice**  It is normal for children at this age to have small appetites, so they may appear to be fussy eaters and may need to eat every few hours. Young children often have "food fads", preferring to eat the same food every day. Then, after a week or so, they move on to other foods or food groups. Jodie's mother should carry on offering the foods Jodie likes, and should avoid forcing her or bribing her with dessert to get her to finish what is on her plate. It is best to let Jodie regulate her own intake. If she usually leaves food, then her mother should serve smaller portions. If Jodie continues to say she is not hungry, her mother should serve only water with meals (and no fruit juice between meals). She can also try to introduce new foods at the beginning of a meal when Jodie is hungry (tell her that her pasta is still cooking). Eventually Jodie will start to eat a more varied diet.

As long as she grows normally and does not lose weight Jodie is eating enough. However, since her diet is so limited and she avoids vegetables, she may benefit from a "complete" vitamin and mineral supplement containing iron, which is suitable for children. Her mother should discuss this with her GP.

# Nutrition for school-age children

## School children need a variety of foods to grow and develop.

Good nutrition is essential for school-age children. They need enough fuel to get them through the day and for their minds to thrive and brains to develop. Start with a healthy breakfast. If they are taking a packed lunch, ensure that it contains a mix of nutritious foods from the five food groups.

### Limiting "junk food"
Foods such as chips, biscuits, and crisps are extremely tempting to children. These are high in sugar,

fat, salt, and calories, but don't offer much in the way of nutrients. Sugary fizzy colas and juice drinks also contain lots of calories.
   Your child's diet can contain some foods that are high in sugar and fat as long as the total diet is well balanced, with foods from all the basic groups eaten in the right proportions.

### Healthy snacking
Snacking is important for children because they usually do not eat enough at mealtime to sustain their blood sugar levels between meals. Snacks prevent children from getting so hungry that they cannot focus on school or other activities

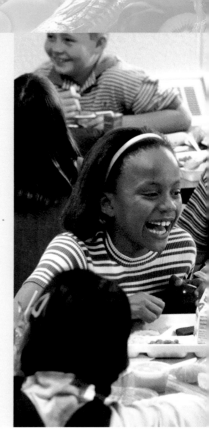

## What to give your school-age child

School-age children need to eat three meals and at least one snack per day. Breakfast is an important meal because it helps minds stay alert until lunchtime. At school, midday meals will include nutritious choices, but children can bypass the healthy option in favour of pizza, sugary drinks, and chips. So you might want to encourage your child to take a packed lunch a few times a week (see p.130). After school, children are hungry, and healthy snacks (opposite), such as fruit, vegetables, yogurt, and cereal with semi-skimmed milk, will keep them going until their tea.

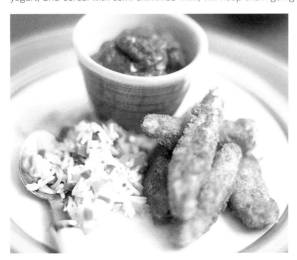

**Chicken dippers**
Full of protein and vitamins, baked egg-and-crumbed chicken strips with a fresh tomato sauce for dipping are fun to eat. Serve them with vegetable rice and a glass of milk.

(see p.130)

---

**SAMPLE MENU: 10-YEAR-OLD**

**Breakfast**
- 3 tbsp low-sugar cereal with semi-skimmed milk and banana, and 150ml (5floz) orange juice

**Snack**
- Wholemeal toast with peanut butter and 4floz (120ml) apple juice

**Lunch**
- Cheese sandwich (2 slices of wholemeal bread and 40g/1½oz cheese), 6 carrot sticks, and 1 medium apple

**Snack**
- 200ml (7floz) fruit smoothie made with yogurt or milk

**Tea**
- 55–85g (2–3oz) baked crumbed chicken breast strips with fresh tomato sauce, 4–8 tbsp cooked rice with vegetables, and 200ml (7floz) skimmed or semi-skimmed milk

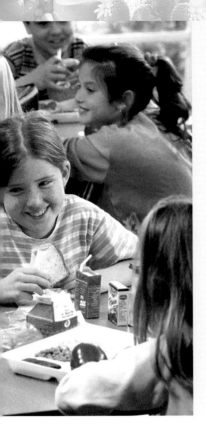

and offers an opportunity, along with meals, for children to get enough calories and nutrients for normal growth and development. Snacks can contribute a significant amount of important nutrients so should be as healthy as possible. If a child does not eat fruits or vegetables at mealtimes, these foods make excellent snacks.

## Empty calories

Most children like to snack on sweets, crisps, biscuits, and other foods low in nutritional value but high in calories. The calories in these snacks are called "empty calories". Such snacks can cause weight gain as your child grows.

**School lunches** The midday meal allows children to have a break, sit down together, and enjoy one another's company while refuelling for the afternoon.

## Serving sizes: 6–12 years

For children aged six to 12 years, the number of daily servings from each food group and examples of a serving are shown below:
- 5–11 servings of starchy carbohydrate foods: a serving is 1 slice of wholemeal bread or 2 heaped tbsp cooked rice.
- 2–3 servings of vegetables: a serving is a medium-sized mixed salad or 3 tbsp cooked vegetables such as carrots or peas.
- 2–3 servings of fruit: a serving is 1 medium apple, 2 small satsumas, or 150ml (5floz) fruit juice.
- 2–3 servings of dairy foods: a serving is 40g (1½oz) cheese or 200ml (7floz) semi-skimmed milk.
- 2–3 servings of protein foods: a serving is 55–85g (2–3oz) cooked lean meat, 2 eggs, or 3 heaped tbsp cooked lentils or other pulses.

# Healthy snacks for children

Children are often hungry, but most especially when they get home from school. If you have healthy snacks ready for them to eat before their tea, and again in the evening, you'll be able to satisfy their snack attacks. Here are some ideas:
- Breakfast cereal
- Rice cakes or pretzels
- Cut-up vegetables, such as carrots, peppers, tomatoes, or cucumbers, with hummus as a dip
- Fresh fruit such as bananas, pears, plums, grapes, oranges, strawberries, peaches, and apples
- Frozen juice cubes or lollies
- Fresh fruit salad
- Fruit smoothie made with yogurt or milk
- Oat cakes with cheese spread
- Low-fat yogurt or fromage frais
- Hard-boiled egg
- Sandwiches, such as tuna, egg and cress, turkey or chicken, cheese and tomato, or peanut butter
- Digestive biscuits
- Home-made trail mix (a mixture of dried fruit such as raisins, cranberries, and apricots, unsalted peanuts, sunflower seeds, and crunchy low-sugar cereal)

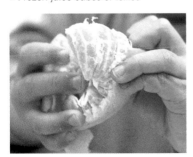

**Appealing fruit** Clementines and satsumas are packed with vitamin C and are a good source of fibre. They are also easy to peel.

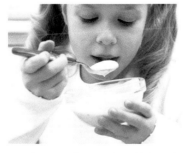

**Superfood** Low-fat yogurt is an ideal snack. It is rich in calcium, protein, and some of the B vitamins, and is easier to digest than milk.

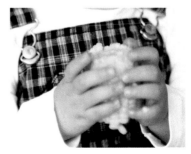

**User friendly** Give your child a section of boiled corn on the cob for a snack. Sweetcorn is a good source of fibre.

# Preventing excess weight in childhood

The number of overweight children in the UK has increased dramatically in the last decade. One of the main reasons for this is that children spend more time watching television and playing video games than they do getting exercise. Children also tend to snack while watching television. It's important for parents to try to limit sedentary activities.

A recent study into the relationship between obesity and television and video game use found that children who were limited to seven hours of television and video games per week had significant decreases in weight and body fat compared to

a control group of children who were allowed to watch TV or play video games as much as they liked. The first group of children also ate fewer meals in front of the television.

To prevent children from becoming overweight, parents should therefore encourage activity – both indoors and out – be it art or crafts projects, creative imaginary play, skipping, throwing a ball, or running in the park. Remember that a large play area and expensive equipment are not essentials for children to be active. For more information on weight management in children, see pages 206–207.

# Lunchbox ideas

When preparing a packed lunch for your child, make sure to include foods from each of the food groups (see p.71) and vary these foods throughout the week. Variety will ensure that you are providing the maximum number of nutrients and will also prevent your child from getting bored with eating the same things.

Prepare foods that are appropriate for your child's age; for example, peeled apple or pear slices are ideal for a young child, while whole fruit is fine for an older child. You could try letting your child make his or her own sandwich, choosing healthy fillings together. If your children buy drinks at school, teach them why it is better to choose semi-skimmed milk or bottled water, both of which are healthier than fizzy colas, sweetened juice drinks, and squashes.

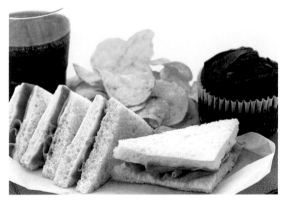

**Unhealthy lunch**
Ham and cheese are high in saturated fat, while white bread is low in fibre. Potato crisps, chocolate chip muffin, and a cola add extra fat, sugar, and calories to this very unhealthy lunch.

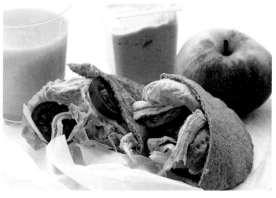

**Healthy lunch**
A wholemeal pitta containing sliced chicken, tomato, and lettuce is a nutritious low-fat lunch. An apple, low-fat yogurt, and orange juice are healthy choices and add vitamins, minerals, and fibre.

## Lunchbox tips

Try some of these suggestions for your child's lunchbox, and make sure you follow the storage tips.

**Packed lunch ideas** Provide a carton of semi-skimmed milk or apple or other 100 per cent fruit juice with each lunch. Also add one or more pieces of fruit, and vary the choices daily.
● Raisin bread or an English muffin spread with reduced-fat cream cheese and topped with low-sugar jam or spread; include a pot of low-fat fruit yogurt.
● Wholemeal pitta pocket filled with tuna, sweetcorn, reduced-fat mayonnaise, and shredded lettuce; include some cherry tomatoes.
● Flour tortilla wrap filled with red kidney beans, grated reduced-fat Cheddar cheese, shredded lettuce, and a mild salsa; include some baby carrots.
● Pasta salad with shredded chicken breast, sweetcorn, diced cucumber, and chopped parsley in a low-fat dressing; include a muesli bar.

**Storage tips** If keeping drinks cool at school is a problem, freeze them at home; by lunchtime they will be thawed.
● Keep cold foods chilled in an insulated lunchbox or pack with a frozen bottle of water.
● Keep hot foods warm in a vacuum flask.

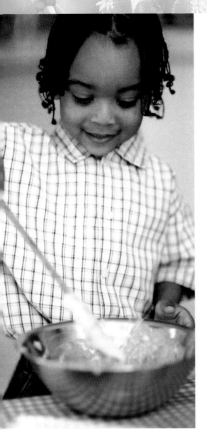

# Cooking with kids

One of the most effective and fun ways to teach children about healthy eating is to involve them in preparing meals for the family. This can begin by planning a menu and going to the supermarket together to shop for ingredients, which will expose children to label reading and the cost of food. Helping you in the kitchen will stimulate their interest in nutritious food and how to cook it.

## SKILLS THAT LAST FOR LIFE

Children develop a sense of pride and ownership as they learn how to cook for the family. Engaging children's interest in preparing healthy meals and snacks will give them skills that will stay with them for life. In addition, cooking can put into practice what they are learning in school, such as reading, science, and mathematics.

**Mixing it up** Teaching children to cook lets them see how ingredients are combined to make healthy dishes. It also gives them an opportunity to practise their maths.

Teach young children about colours, shapes, and sizes, and to recognize the names of fruits and vegetables. Make a guessing game out of mixing a fruit salad and let them help you wash fresh vegetables. As your child grows older, he or she can take over the peeling and cutting up of vegetables and be shown how to prepare other foods.

When you cook together, start with a simple meal such as roast chicken, brown rice or new potatoes, and green beans. Encourage your child to find healthy recipes he or she would like to make. Try to find dishes that combine lots of different colours, such as red (tomatoes), green (peas), orange (carrots), and yellow (sweetcorn).

## SAFE COOKING PRACTICES

Safety is always an issue in the kitchen, but even more so when children are involved. Younger children should never be left unsupervised in case they burn or cut themselves. Older children also need to be monitored as they may be overconfident of their abilities.

# Recipe Children's choice pizza

## INGREDIENTS

**Serves 6**

400g (14oz) can tomatoes

dried oregano

1 pizza base

50g (2oz) sliced ham

½ red pepper

200g (7oz) can artichoke hearts

45g (1½oz) black olives

fresh basil

**1** Drain and chop the tomatoes. Heat a little olive oil in a saucepan, add the tomatoes and a good pinch of oregano, and simmer until the mixture is slightly thickened.

**2** Preheat the oven to 220°C (425°F, gas 7). Brush the pizza base with a little olive oil, then spread the tomato sauce evenly over the surface.

**3** Cut the ham into strips; slice the pepper; quarter the artichoke hearts; and pit the olives. Place these on the pizza base, then drizzle a little olive oil over the top.

**4** Bake the pizza until the crust is just crisp. Garnish with fresh basil leaves and serve.

**Vary the toppings** You can use many other toppings, such as sweetcorn, fresh spinach, broccoli florets, aubergine or courgette slices (lightly fried), pineapple chunks, grated mozzarella cheese, canned tuna, strips of cooked chicken, or anchovy fillets.

### Each serving provides

Calories 215, Total fat 4.0g (Sat. 0.2g, Poly. 0.2g, Mono. 0.6g), Cholesterol 5.0mg, Protein 8.0g, Carbohydrate 40g, Fibre 3.3g, Sodium 465mg. Good source of – Vits: A, C, K; Mins: Ca.

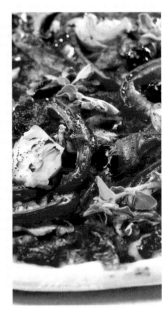

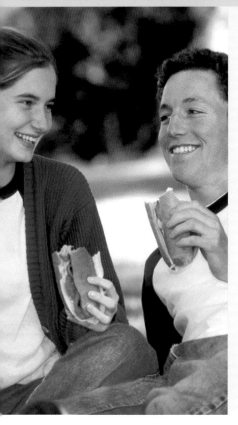

# Dietary needs of adolescents

## Children aged 11–18 years have increased needs for nutrients.

Girls aged 11–14 and boys aged 12–15 undergo major physical and psychological changes (puberty) that affect both their behaviour and what they need to eat. The body changes increase their energy and nutrient needs, which differ in boys and girls, although both sexes require extra calcium and iron at

**Growing up** As they go through major body changes, adolescents often develop ravenous appetites. Make sure they fill up on nutritious foods, rather than empty-calorie snack foods.

this stage. Wanting independence, resisting authority, and developing logical reasoning are characteristics of adolescents that you must keep in mind when you address their nutritional needs and behaviour.

### Becoming adults

Puberty usually starts in girls between 11 and 14 years, earlier than in boys, for whom it most often starts between 12 and 15 years. Girls usually have a rapid period of growth at the onset of puberty, whereas boys grow at their fastest after their sexual development is more advanced.

Growing adolescents have increased energy and nutritional needs to support their rapid

## Encouraging teenagers to eat healthily

Teenagers these days are busier than ever. They often leave the house at 7am and may not return until late afternoon, when they have a quick snack before rushing out to an evening activity or to do their homework. Finding the time to properly nourish an active teenager can be quite a challenge: those involved in sport need more calories and fluids and often complain about being hungry all the time; teenage boys are the biggest consumers of fast food; and more and more teenagers are deciding to become vegetarians or even vegans.

As teenagers will be away from home more and more often when making food choices, it is important to reinforce the healthy eating messages now – this is a "teachable moment" and an opportunity to provide alternatives to less nutritious food, such as the ideas listed on the right. Try to limit the amount of fast food your teenager eats and stock healthy after-school snacks such as fresh fruit, muesli bars, pretzels, and yogurt.

| POOR CHOICE | HEALTHY CHOICE |
| --- | --- |
| Sweetened cereal | Low-sugar cereal or porridge |
| Doughnut | Crumpet with reduced-sugar jam |
| Crisps | Handful of nuts |
| Crumbed chicken nuggets | Chicken fillet |
| Chocolate bar | High-fibre cereal bar |
| Cheeseburger with fries | Veggie burger with salad |
| Ready meal | Low-fat ready meal |
| Milkshake | Yogurt smoothie |
| Ice cream | Frozen yogurt |
| American-style muffin | Wholemeal muffin |
| Chocolate chip cookie | Digestive biscuit |
| Chocolate cake | Malt loaf |
| Tortilla chips and cheese dip | Tortilla chips and salsa |

growth. If your child is physically active, this will further increase his or her energy requirements.

In healthy girls, menstruation usually starts about a year after their growth spurt begins. As they start menstruating, their iron (*see p.66*) and protein needs increase, as do other mineral needs associated with rapid growth (*below*).

As boys enter puberty, their muscle mass increases, and this increases their needs for protein, calories, vitamins, and minerals, with the exception of iron.

## Risk of deficiencies

If your adolescent has a poor diet, he or she may be at an increased risk of several vitamin and mineral deficiencies, most notably calcium and iron. The highest requirements for calcium are during infancy, when the first growth spurt takes place, and during adolescence. The high calcium requirements of adolescents – 1000mg per day for boys and 800mg per day for girls – are needed for bone growth and for depositing calcium within the bones. These bone processes are promoted by hormonal changes that are linked with puberty and its associated growth spurt.

## Preventing overweight

Teenagers have easy access to high-calorie fast foods and may prefer sedentary activities, such as watching television and using the computer. As a result of this they may gain excess weight. If you are overweight, your child is at higher risk of becoming overweight. An overweight teenager may develop high blood pressure and diabetes.

It is therefore critical that you think about your children's future health. Make a commitment for your whole family to eat healthily, to limit the intake of fast food, and to be more physically active.

## Serving sizes: 13–18 years

The nutritional requirements of adolescents are similar to those of adults. For each food group, the daily number of recommended servings and examples of a serving are shown below.

- 5–11 servings of starchy complex carbohydrate foods: a serving is 1 slice of wholemeal bread or 3 tbsp breakfast cereal.
- 2–3 servings of vegetables: a serving is a medium-sized mixed salad or 3 heaped tbsp cooked vegetables such as peas.
- 2–3 servings of fruits: a serving is 1 apple or 2 small satsumas.
- 2–3 servings of dairy foods: a serving is 200ml (7floz) milk or a pot of low-fat yogurt.
- 2–3 servings of protein foods: a serving is 55–85g (2–3oz) cooked lean meat, chicken, or fish, 2 eggs, or 4 tbsp cooked lentils.

# Teens and exercise

Adolescents can improve their overall health by exercising regularly and reducing the amount of television that they watch. Participation in team sports is an excellent way for your teenager to get aerobic exercise and to make new friends. Or it may be that your child would prefer an individual sport.

Invite your teenager to join in any exercise you do as a family, such as going swimming or for a bike ride. You may find, though, that he or she prefers to exercise alone or with friends. At this age many young people prefer to join a gym or sports club independently. If you or another family member are able to make a financial contribution, this would be a great incentive to get fit.

**Be active** Encourage your teenager to take plenty of exercise, either as part of a team, in an individual sport, or with friends at the weekend. Enjoying an active lifestyle now will set a pattern for adulthood.

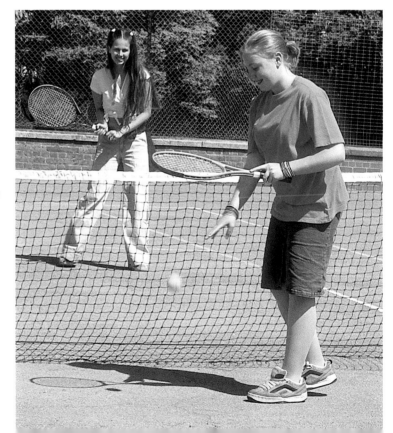

# Calcium needs

Needed for the strength and structure of bones and teeth, calcium is vital in a teenager's diet. Children aged seven to ten years need 550mg of calcium per day. For 11- to 18-year-olds, the daily recommendation goes up to 1000mg for boys and 800mg for girls. However, many teenagers fail to get this amount. This is called the "calcium crisis" as it can lead to osteoporosis (see p.242) in later life.

To make sure your teenager gets enough calcium, encourage him or her to eat or drink plenty of dairy products, which are the most efficient food sources of calcium. Opt for lower fat versions in order to keep down intake of saturated fat. Ideally, teenagers need three to four servings a day of calcium-rich foods. The best sources of calcium are shown in the chart (right). Calcium-fortified orange juice and cereal are good sources too. If a teenager does not get enough calcium, he or she should take a supplement (see p.109).

| CALCIUM-RICH FOOD | SERVING SIZE | CALCIUM |
|---|---|---|
| Tofu | 100g (3½oz) | 510mg |
| Canned salmon (with bones) | 100g (3½oz) | 300mg |
| Milkshake (vanilla) | 300ml (10floz) | 300mg |
| Skimmed milk | 200ml (7floz) | 244mg |
| Low-fat plain yogurt | 150ml (5floz) | 243mg |
| Semi-skimmed milk | 200ml (7floz) | 240mg |
| Buttermilk | 200ml (7floz) | 240mg |
| Whole milk | 200ml (7floz) | 236mg |
| Reduced-fat Cheddar cheese | 28g (1oz) | 235mg |
| Edam cheese | 28g (1oz) | 223mg |
| Low-fat fruit yogurt | 150ml (5floz) | 210mg |
| Cheddar cheese | 28g (1oz) | 207mg |
| Cheese pizza | 100g (3½oz) | 190mg |
| Ice cream | 1 scoop | 60mg |

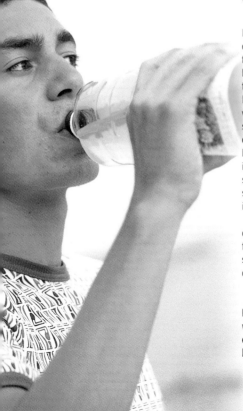

# Why you should limit soft drinks

Ideally, soft drinks should be avoided, or limited to 350ml (12floz) a day for teenagers, as the high sugar levels can lead to excessive calorie consumption, tooth decay, and excess weight gain. Many studies have shown that teenagers who drink a lot of sweetened beverages such as colas, fizzy lemonade, sports drinks, and juice drinks and squashes, have an unnecessarily high calorie intake. This is due to the very high sugar content of these drinks – most soft drinks contain 9 teaspoons of sugar in each 330ml can.

Studies suggest that many teenagers consume twice as much cola and other fizzy drinks as milk – 21 per cent of seven- to ten-year-olds drink an average of ten cans a week. This substitution of soft drinks for milk is one of the factors contributing to the poor intake of calcium among teenagers in the UK.

Drinking healthier beverages, such as skimmed or semi-skimmed milk or water, can help prevent your teenager from becoming overweight. Here are some tips to help you limit the amount of soft drinks your teenager consumes:

● Always keep a range of healthy drinks at home. In this way, even though your teenager might have sweetened drinks when he or she goes out, the intake can be balanced with healthier choices.

● If your teenager doesn't want to drink water when he or she is at a restaurant or party, suggest he or she orders a diet cola. This will address peer pressure to drink fizzy colas but will keep calories and sugar intake under control.

● Try serving your teenager a fruity spritzer – 100 per cent fruit juice mixed with sparkling mineral water. Add a few ice cubes and garnish with a slice of lime or lemon.

**Refreshing water** The ideal thirst quencher, water does not contain any calories. Always encourage your teenager to carry a water bottle in his or her backpack.

# Making sure teenage girls get enough iron

To support their growth, adolescents have increased requirements for energy and nutrients, but most especially iron (*see p.66*). Vigorous exercise, such as running or dancing, further increases these requirements.

Since menstruation begins during adolescence, teenage girls will lose blood and therefore iron on a monthly basis, so have increased iron needs.

## IRON DEFICIENCY
The body needs iron to build red blood cells. When you do not get enough iron from the food in your daily diet, you tire more easily and lack stamina, which can be especially difficult for teenagers involved in sport (*see p.61*).

Many teenage girls skip meals or try unbalanced fad diets in an effort to lose weight, or they may decide to become vegetarian. As a result they may not be getting enough iron for their bodies' needs during these years, which puts them at higher risk for iron-deficiency

anaemia. This condition is common in teenage girls, especially those who have heavy menstrual periods.

Teenage girls between 11 and 18 years of age need 14.8mg of iron each day (teenage boys need 11.3mg of iron per day). To achieve an iron-rich diet, encourage your teenage daughter to eat red meat at least once a week and lots of iron-rich pulses, vegetables, and dried fruits on a regular basis. Starting the day with a breakfast cereal fortified with iron is also a good idea. The recipe (*below*) for an iron-rich bean dish will provide an iron boost.

If your teenage daughter becomes a vegetarian, she can still meet her daily iron requirements, but it will take careful planning and eating a varied diet with foods from the main food groups (*see pp.100–101*). If no one else in the family is a vegetarian, invest in a recipe book to get plenty of new ideas for vegetarian meals. Everyone in the family can enjoy eating vegetarian a few times a week.

## IRON AND VITAMIN C
In order to maximize the amount of iron absorbed from a food, your daughter should also eat foods containing vitamin C (*see p.56*) as part of the meal. These foods aid the absorption of iron.

Citrus fruits or juices, such as orange or grapefruit, tomatoes, and broccoli are all good sources of vitamin C. Non-meat foods that are iron-rich include broccoli, raisins, watermelon, spinach, baked beans, molasses, chickpeas, and pinto beans. Raisins and dried apricots make a convenient iron-rich snack, as well as being good sources of other important nutrients and fibre.

A multivitamin and mineral supplement that contains iron might also be helpful. If you suspect that your daughter is not getting a sufficient amount of iron in her diet (*see p.55*), discuss it with your GP or suggest that your daughter does this. A simple blood test can be done to check for iron-deficiency anaemia, and an iron supplement recommended if needed.

# Recipe Iron-rich bean dish

### INGREDIENTS

1 onion

4 garlic cloves

1 carrot

2 courgettes

2 peppers

2 potatoes

4 ripe tomatoes

400g (14oz) can cannellini beans

2 tbsp chopped fresh basil

### Serves 4

**1** Slice the onion; crush the garlic cloves; and finely chop the carrot and courgettes. Core and seed the peppers and chop them finely.

**2** Heat a little olive oil in a large pan, add the prepared vegetables, and cook over a medium heat until they are soft (about 5 minutes).

**3** Cut the potatoes into 1cm (½in) cubes. Cut the tomatoes into wedges. Add the potatoes and tomatoes to the pan together with 120ml (4floz) water. Cover and simmer for about 30 minutes, stirring occasionally, until all the vegetables are tender.

**4** Drain and rinse the beans. Add to the vegetables in the pan and stir to mix. Cook for a further 5 minutes, until the beans are very hot.

**5** Add the basil and season with black pepper, stirring gently to combine.

**6** Serve hot in warmed bowls, drizzled with a little olive oil and garnished with chopped fresh basil. Serve with crusty whole-grain bread.

### Each serving provides
Calories 260, Total fat 1.1g (Sat. 0.2g, Poly. 0.5g, Mono. 0.1g), Cholesterol 0mg, Protein 13g, Carbohydrate 54g, Fibre 10g, Sodium 37mg. Good source of – Vits: A, Fol, C; Mins: Ca, Fe, K, Mg, P.

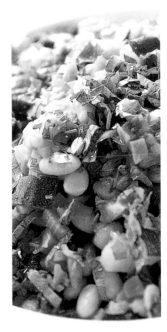

# Nutrition throughout adulthood

## Your food choices throughout adulthood can help ensure good health into old age.

Do you take your good health for granted? If you are like most people 20–50 years old, you have never had to worry about your health. However, you may have noticed that you no longer can eat whatever you want and still stay slim, as you could when you were younger. Maybe you have put on extra weight and have not been able to exercise as much as you used to due to your busy schedule at work or home.

Those of us between the ages of 20 and 50 usually feel that we are healthy. We are too busy to go to the doctor and we really do not think we need to change our diets, or to increase our physical activity.

However, what you eat and how much you exercise can have a significant impact on your current and future health. If you eat lots of fatty and sugary foods and do not move about much, the chances are that you will feel sluggish and not be motivated to exercise. But this stage of life is the most critical time for determining your future health and probably the easiest time for you to adopt healthier dietary habits and a more active lifestyle. And if you smoke, to stop.

By making the effort to eat a well-balanced diet and exercise on a regular basis, you will feel better and have more energy. You will also probably live longer and the years ahead will be healthier.

### Eating for two

Making healthy food choices and gaining enough weight during pregnancy have been shown to improve the health of your baby. In this chapter we discuss which nutritional needs are increased during pregnancy (see pp.138–141) and while you are breast-feeding (see pp.142–143), as well as how to meet those needs with food and vitamin and mineral supplements. Since breast-feeding is the best for your baby, we describe the benefits for you and explain how to breast-feed with success.

### Nutrition for athletes

The nutritional needs of athletes vary depending on the amount and type of physical activity they are involved in. We describe the specific requirements for both

## Do men have specific dietary needs?

Due to a larger muscle mass, men have a higher metabolic rate than women. This means they need more calories and also more of certain vitamins and minerals, specifically those involved in releasing energy from food.

Men's larger bodies contain more water, bone, muscle, organ tissue, and fat than women's, and their increased muscle mass requires more protein for its maintenance. Therefore, men tend to eat more food than women.

Each day, men burn up about 600 calories more than non-pregnant women do. Men's needs for carbohydrate are the same as women's and they need the same amount of fibre – 18g. There is no recommended amount of dietary fat, but men require 60 per cent more essential fatty acids than women (see p.38). While men's daily recommended intake of protein is the same as that for women, at 0.75g per 1kg (2¼lb) of body mass, men's intake needs to be 10g per day higher on average due to their greater muscle mass. Dietary and health recommendations for men include:
- Eat lots of fruits and vegetables. Rich in nutrients, the health benefits of these foods cannot be overstated.
- Avoid saturated fats. Keep intake of red meat to a minimum. Use low- or reduced-fat dairy products. Limit ice cream and fatty foods such as chips.
- Drink alcohol in moderation – up to three to four units per day (two to three units for women).
- Manage stress. Stress is unavoidable and not necessarily bad for you – it is how you react to stress that determines its effects on your health. Techniques such as yoga or meditation can help.
- Do not smoke cigarettes and cigars, and try to avoid passive smoking.
- Maintain a healthy weight. Excess weight, especially round the abdomen, is a risk for heart disease and diabetes.
- Make exercise a priority. Get plenty of physical activity to stay healthy.
- Have regular medical check-ups.

## Nutrients for men

The nutrients below are thought to have an impact on fertility, prostate health, and the prevention of cancer and cardiovascular disease.

**Lycopenes** These nutrients occur in tomatoes, watermelon, and pink grapefruit. They may lower the risk of prostate and lung cancers.

**Vitamins $B_6$, $B_{12}$, and folate** These B vitamins lower blood levels of homocysteine, thus lowering the risk of cardiovascular disease.

**Selenium and vitamins C and E** These antioxidants are necessary for normal fertility in men, and adequate intake or supplements may help to improve fertility.

**Zinc and folate** A combination of zinc and folate supplements may improve fertility in men.

endurance and non-endurance athletes, focusing on supplements and sports drinks, and provide suggestions for meals and snacks for active people (*see pp.146–149*).

## Menopause and older adults

The population of older adults is rapidly expanding worldwide. In the second half of this chapter we address the nutritional needs for optimum health of men and women as they age – through the menopause, over the age of 50, and after 70 years (*see pp.154–155*). Lifestyle changes, such as taking part in regular physical activity, can ease the effects of ageing and help your sense of well-being as you advance into the senior years.

**Healthy choices** Try to make healthy eating a priority, even when you are dining out. Order two starters or a starter and salad. Or share a starter or main course.

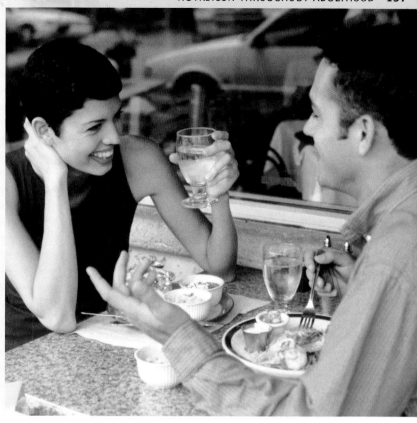

# When do women's dietary needs change?

Because women are generally smaller than men and have less muscle mass they require fewer calories. However, women will need more calories during pregnancy (when eating for two), and if a woman decides to breast-feed she will need extra calories and nutrients to produce enough breast milk. Athletic women also need more calories than those with sedentary lifestyles.

### IRON FOR BLOOD LOSS

Throughout the reproductive years women need more iron in their diet to replace the iron in the blood lost as a result of menstruation. Otherwise they could be at risk of iron-deficiency anaemia (*see p.55*). So it is important to eat plenty of iron-rich foods (*right*).

### FOLATE FOR PREGNANCY

During pregnancy, women need extra calories and nutrients and more of most of the vitamins and minerals (*see pp.50–67*). The B vitamin folate is very

important: an increased intake of folate before conception and in early pregnancy prevents neural tube defects such as spina bifida in babies (*see p.139*). For this reason women who are thinking of having a baby, and women who are pregnant, should take a supplement.

New mothers need extra calories and nutrients (*see pp.142–143*). A woman's body needs to recover after delivery. Increased amounts of iron and various vitamins and other minerals are vital for returning to normal health.

## Which foods are good for women?

Folate, calcium, and iron are key nutrients for women. Try to eat foods rich in these nutrients.

**Folate** Good sources of folate include green vegetables, such as cabbage and spinach, and pulses such as chickpeas and kidney beans.

### CALCIUM FOR BONE HEALTH

Breast-feeding is recommended as the best way to feed a baby for the first six months of life. Breast-feeding mothers need a balanced, nutritious diet, not just for themselves but to produce the nutrient-rich milk for their baby. Since calcium is lost from the bones to make breast milk, mothers will need extra calcium. By restoring the lost calcium, they will protect themselves from the degenerative bone disease osteoporosis (*see p.242*) in later years.

**Calcium** This mineral is naturally abundant in dairy products, canned fish eaten with bones, and spinach.

**Iron** Foods that are naturally rich in iron include red meat and offal; spinach; dried fruits; and pulses such as soya beans and kidney beans.

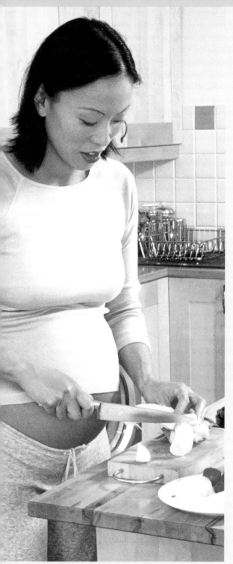

**Increased needs** During pregnancy you need more calories than usual – for yourself and for your growing baby. Make sure you choose nutrient-rich foods to get your extra calories.

## Jargon buster

**Neural tube defects** Abnormalities in a foetus's brain and spinal cord and their protective coverings. Neural tube defects can be mild (meningoceles – opening of the spinal cord that can be surgically repaired) or severe (anencephaly – lack of brain). The best known neural tube defect is spina bifida.

# Eating for two

## When pregnant, you need to eat for yourself and your baby.

Good nutrition is vital for both normal pregnancies and those considered high risk, such as in a woman who is carrying twins or has gestational diabetes.

Pregnant women require more calories and nutrients than other women to provide for their growing baby (*opposite*). To achieve this, a pregnant woman should consume an extra 200 calories per day during the second and third trimesters of her pregnancy. This is about a ten per cent increase in calorie intake. Healthy pregnant women need few or no additional calories during the first trimester.

Increased demands put pregnant women and their unborn babies at risk of nutritional deficiencies if these demands are not met by the diet (*opposite*) or by ante-natal supplements (*see p.140*).

### Key nutrients

Taking a supplement of folic acid (commonly known as folate) one to three months before conception and for the first three months of pregnancy will reduce the risks of neural tube defects by 20 per cent. Folate also works with vitamin $B_{12}$ to form healthy red blood cells. Other key nutrients needed during pregnancy are iron, which is used to make red blood cells for both the growing baby and mother, whose blood volume increases by 50 per cent during pregnancy, and calcium for the baby's skeleton.

### Health problems

Changes in your body during pregnancy may result in temporary health problems. These include gestational diabetes, constipation, heartburn and indigestion, and nausea and vomiting. In gestational diabetes, body cells have difficulty absorbing glucose from the blood during pregnancy due to resistance to the hormone insulin (*see p.141*).

The intestinal muscles are more relaxed during pregnancy. This can cause constipation because of the slower movement of food through the body and the increased amount of water absorbed from the food by the intestine.

Heartburn and indigestion occur when the stomach contents flow up into the oesophagus, causing discomfort in the chest. During pregnancy, it is usually due to the shift of organs in the abdomen to accommodate the growing baby.

Nausea and vomiting (morning sickness) are due to increased levels of the pregnancy hormone human chorionic gonadotropin, levels of which peak at about 12 weeks into a pregnancy. Tips to manage these disorders through dietary means are discussed on page 141.

### Weight gain

If you do not gain enough weight during pregnancy, you could put your baby at risk of being born prematurely or underweight. On the other hand, excessive weight gain can increase the risk of your having problems such as back ache and varicose veins, as well as complications such as pre-eclampsia, and it will make it more difficult for you to lose the weight once the baby is born.

• If your weight is in the normal or healthy range before you become pregnant, you should ideally gain about 11–16kg (24–35lb) during your pregnancy.

• If you are underweight at the start of pregnancy, you'll gain a little more – 12.5–18kg (28–40lb).

• If you are overweight at the start of pregnancy, your ideal weight gain is 7–11.5kg (15–25lb).

# Increased needs during pregnancy

Eating for two does not mean eating twice as much. During pregnancy the expectant mother's metabolic rate is reduced and the body becomes more energy efficient, which explains why the calorie requirements of pregnant women do not increase dramatically. The need for several vitamins and minerals is increased slightly.

Pregnant woman must get enough fats. Two fatty acids – docosahexanoic acid and arachidonic acid – are vital for the development of the baby's brain and vision. The best source of these fatty acids is oil-rich fish. Increasing water and fibre will help prevent problems like constipation.

Extra needs for nutrients can be met through the diet (*below*) or by taking ante-natal supplements (*see p.140*). The table (*right*) shows the recommended daily intakes of key nutrients for pregnant and non-pregnant women aged 19–45.

| NUTRIENT | NON-PREGNANT | PREGNANT |
|---|---|---|
| Protein | 45g | 51g |
| Vitamin A | 600mcg | 700mcg |
| Vitamin $B_1$ | 0.8mg | 0.9mg |
| Vitamin $B_2$ | 1.1mg | 1.4mg |
| Niacin | 13mg | 13mg |
| Vitamin $B_6$ | 1.2mg | 1.2mg |
| Vitamin $B_{12}$ | 1.5mcg | 1.5mcg |
| Folate | 200mcg | 300mcg |
| Vitamin C | 40mg | 50mg |
| Calcium | 700mg | 700mg |
| Iron | 14.8mg | 14.8mg |
| Magnesium | 270mg | 270mg |
| Selenium | 60mcg | 60mcg |
| Zinc | 7.0mg | 7.0mg |

# Foods to eat during pregnancy

The best foods to eat during pregnancy are those that supply essential vitamins, minerals, lean protein, and energy.

**Protein** Every day eat two to three servings of protein-rich foods such as lean red meat, poultry breast, fish (cooked only), eggs, and pulses.

**Calcium** Adequate calcium intake during pregnancy is very important to prevent osteoporosis later in life. Eat or drink at least three servings of calcium-rich foods every day.

**Folate** Increased folate is required in early pregnancy to prevent neural tube defects (*see p.56*). Folate is found in fresh green vegetables, pulses, liver, oranges, and poultry. So make time for breakfast; add beans and lentils to your diet; and eat at least five servings of fruits and vegetables each day.

**Small meals** You may find it easier to eat small carbohydrate-rich meals, such as pasta with vegetables, to maintain energy levels.

**Iron** Necessary for the production of red blood cells in both you and your unborn baby. Iron-rich foods include red meat, pulses, raisins, spinach, black-eyed beans, dried fruits, and green vegetables. Vitamin C helps your body absorb iron from plant sources.

**Fibre** Increased intake of high-fibre foods, such as vegetables and whole grains, is recommended for the prevention of constipation.

**Fluids** Drink at least 2 litres (3½ pints) of water each day to provide fluids for blood production and to aid digestion.

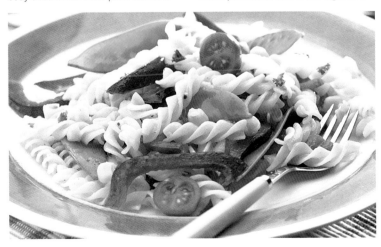

# Foods to avoid during pregnancy

The chances of your unborn child becoming infected during pregnancy are small, but you should be aware of potentially risky foods to avoid.

**Listeriosis** The bacterium *Listeria monocytogenes*, which causes listeriosis, can cross the placenta and may be fatal for the baby. To prevent infection, avoid eating unpasteurized dairy products, especially soft mould-ripened cheeses such as camembert and blue-veined cheeses.

**Liver** Because of high levels of vitamin A, liver and liver products such as pâté should be avoided.

**Toxoplasmosis** This protozoal infection, which can be harmful to an unborn baby, is caused by *Toxoplasma gondii*. Cysts (dormant stages) of *T. gondii* are excreted in the stools of infected cats and can be passed to humans by handling cats or cat litter, by fruit or vegetables contaminated with cysts, or by eating the meat of animals that feed on food contaminated with cysts. Minimize the risk of infection during pregnancy by avoiding cats, by washing fruits and vegetables before eating, by avoiding any undercooked meat, and by wearing gloves when gardening.

**Salmonella** This common type of food poisoning, due to *Salmonella* bacteria, does not usually harm the baby, but if severe in a pregnant woman it can lead to miscarriage or pre-term labour. You should avoid raw and undercooked eggs and undercooked poultry.

**Other infections** You should avoid raw seafood, such as sushi and oysters, during pregnancy as they carry a risk of hepatitis and intestinal parasites.

**Heavy-metal poisoning** Remove heavy metals from vegetables by washing them thoroughly with water or by removing their skin. Because they contain high levels of mercury, avoid eating shark, swordfish, and marlin. The mercury levels in tuna are lower, so the advice is to limit the amount of tuna you eat to no more than two steaks a week.

## Alcohol and caffeine

It is best to moderate your alcohol and caffeine consumption during pregnancy. Excessive alcohol can lead to your baby being born with foetal alcohol syndrome and learning difficulties. A high intake of caffeine may increase the risk of miscarriage in early pregnancy.

The effects of alcohol are most severe in the first two months of pregnancy, when your baby's organs are developing. Just one episode of binge drinking at this stage of pregnancy is now thought to be as harmful to your baby as excessive drinking throughout pregnancy.

Pregnant women should reduce their intake of caffeine from all sources – coffee, tea, cocoa, and cola drinks – to 300mg per day (*see p.97*). More than this amount may interfere with your baby's growth and development and increase the risk of low birth weight.

# Do you need ante-natal supplements?

Many doctors prescribe an ante-natal multivitamin and mineral supplement because many pregnant women do not eat enough to meet their increased nutritional needs, especially with regard to the B vitamin folate.

## NEED FOR CALCIUM

Even though your calcium needs do not increase with pregnancy, your baby needs calcium as early as four to six weeks after conception, when teeth and bones begin to form. By 25 weeks, your baby's needs are even higher due to significant bone growth at this time. During pregnancy, your body adapts to absorb more calcium from food, but it is still important to eat plenty of calcium-rich foods. If you do not include dairy products in your diet you may need to take a calcium supplement. As the amount of calcium you absorb depends on your levels of vitamin D, you should try to spend at least 10 minutes a day in the sun when you are pregnant.

## NEED FOR IRON

Iron is necessary for the production of red blood cells in both the mother and her growing baby. A mother's blood volume increases by up to 50 per cent during pregnancy, requiring an extra 500mg of iron. The foetus requires an additional 300mg of iron, accumulating most of its iron stores during the third trimester. The body absorbs iron more efficiently from foods when you are pregnant, so if you have good stores of iron at the beginning of pregnancy it should not be necessary to increase your iron intake. If you had low iron stores at the outset, due to heavy blood loss from menstrual periods or a low dietary intake, an iron supplement may be needed to prevent anaemia. Vitamin C helps the body absorb iron.

## Special need for folate

Supplementation with the B vitamin folate decreases the risk of neural tube defects in your baby (*see p.139*). Therefore, women who are planning a pregnancy should take a folate supplement. In fact, since about half of all pregnancies are unplanned, all young women could benefit from taking a multivitamin with folate. From the time of conception and for the first three months of pregnancy women are now advised to take a daily supplement of 400mcg folate. Thereafter the recommended intake of folate throughout pregnancy is 300mcg per day (it is 200mcg for non-pregnant women).

Women who have already had a pregnancy affected by a neural tube defect are advised to take a higher dose folate supplement, which their doctor will prescribe.

# Minor ailments during pregnancy

Common ailments during pregnancy include nausea and vomiting (also known as morning sickness), which are most common in the first three months of pregnancy; heartburn and indigestion; and constipation. The suggestions below may help ease these symptoms. Tips for dealing with constipation, such as drinking plenty of water and eating lots of fibre, can be found on page 229.

## MORNING SICKNESS

If you are experiencing morning sickness, try some of the following suggestions to ease your discomfort:
• Eat some dry crackers or toast first thing in the morning.
• Avoid strong food odours by eating food cold or at room temperature and using good ventilation while cooking.
• Avoid fragrances that might trigger nausea, such as perfume, household cleaners, and air fresheners.
• Drink a cup of ginger tea. Make it yourself by steeping one teaspoon of ground or grated ginger in boiling water in a teapot for a few minutes. Strain and add honey or brown sugar to taste.

## HEARTBURN AND INDIGESTION

Try some of the following tips if you are suffering from heartburn and indigestion during pregnancy:
• Eat small, low-fat meals and snacks, such as fruits, pretzels, crackers, and low-fat yogurt, slowly and frequently.
• Drink fluids between meals.
• Avoid foods that may irritate the stomach, such as caffeine, spearmint, peppermint, citrus fruits, spicy foods, high-fat foods, and tomato products.
• Take a walk after meals.
• Avoid eating or drinking for one to two hours before lying down.

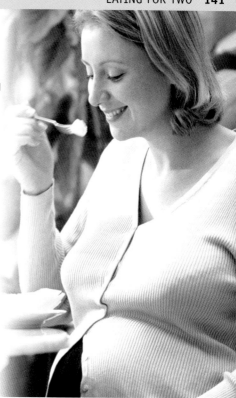

**Relieving heartburn** Slowly eating a bland snack such as a watery melon or low-fat yogurt can help ease heartburn. Yogurt is also a good source of calcium.

# Dealing with gestational diabetes

In gestational diabetes, the levels of blood sugar glucose are raised during pregnancy. The disorder occurs in about four per cent of all pregnancies. It is usually diagnosed during the second or third trimester of pregnancy when the body may become resistant to the hormone insulin, which is what enables body cells to take up glucose from the blood. The resistance occurs because hormones produced by the placenta have an anti-insulin effect. Symptoms can include excessive thirst, passing large amounts of urine, and fatigue, but often there are no symptoms.

In about 90 per cent of cases, blood glucose levels return to normal after delivery, but these women remain at increased risk of developing diabetes in later life (see pp.246–247).

## NUTRITION GOALS

The aims of treating gestational diabetes through nutrition are to provide enough calories for the appropriate weight gain in pregnancy, to achieve and maintain normal levels of glucose in the blood, and to avoid the production of chemicals known as ketones.

## KETONES

Because in diabetes the body cannot use glucose efficiently as a source of energy, it derives energy by breaking down fats instead. This produces waste products called ketones. The build-up of ketones (ketosis) in the body causes symptoms such as nausea, abdominal pain, and fruity-smelling breath.

If you are diagnosed with gestational diabetes, you will be asked by your doctor to monitor your blood glucose levels via a finger stick test and to test your urine or blood for ketones. Most women who have gestational diabetes will be referred to a state-registered dietitian for nutritional counselling and for the design of a meal plan that will be adjusted through pregnancy based on levels of glucose in the blood.

## MEAL PLANNING

Generally, 40–45 per cent of calories in the diet should come from carbohydrates, eaten throughout the day. An evening snack is recommended to prevent ketosis overnight. Carbohydrate is not as well tolerated at breakfast as at other meals, possibly due to the levels of certain hormones, so an initial meal plan may limit carbohydrate in the morning.

## INSULIN INJECTIONS

If your blood sugar levels are persistently high, you will most likely have to have insulin injections. This is the best thing for your baby, and with the help of your ante-natal care provider, you can have a healthy pregnancy. The main goal of this therapy is to prevent complications associated with gestational diabetes developing in both the mother and baby. If your blood sugar levels are not treated, your baby might gain too much weight and then might need to be delivered by caesarean section.

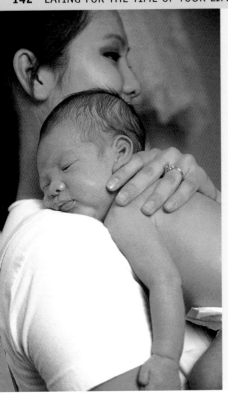

# Nutritional needs of new mothers

## After giving birth, women still need extra calories and nutrients.

Most women want to know how to lose the weight they gained during pregnancy as soon as possible. For some, it disappears in weeks, for others years. Without eating well-balanced meals and exercising, you may find it difficult to lose weight.

**Mother and child** After giving birth, a woman must consume more calories and nutrients, not only for her body to recover but also to produce milk if she decides to breast-feed.

### Calories for breast-feeding
Taking drastic measures to slim down after the birth of your baby will not help you to keep up your strength, nor will it give you the important nutrients you need for healing. And if you plan to breast-feed, your body will require more calories than you needed when you were pregnant. If you decide not to breast-feed your baby, your nutritional needs will return to normal after a few weeks.

### Don't skip meals
Because this is a stressful period – having a newborn and not getting enough sleep – it is important to

## Requirements for breast-feeding

Mothers who are breast-feeding should be encouraged to obtain their nutrients from a well-balanced, varied diet and to drink about 2 litres (3½ pints) of fluid per day to maintain their milk production. As with pregnant women, breast-feeding women have an increased requirement for calories and essentially all nutrients, especially protein, vitamins A and C, and calcium.

**Calcium** Mothers who are producing milk should make sure that they get 1250mg of calcium each day. About two to eight per cent of total body calcium is used for production of breast milk. Mothers usually replace this calcium after a pregnancy; however, women who have several children or short intervals between their pregnancies may not be getting enough calcium to replace the loss, putting them at risk of developing the bone disorder osteoporosis later in life (see p.242).

**Vitamin and mineral supplements**
Requirements for almost all nutrients are increased during lactation. For example, an extra 350mcg vitamin A

is needed every day, as well as an extra 30mg of vitamin C, an extra 2mg of niacin, an extra 60mcg of folate, and an extra 50mg of magnesium; an extra 6mg of zinc is needed for the first four months and thereafter an extra 2.5mg. Ante-natal vitamin supplements (see p.140) are often prescribed to breast-feeding women in order to ensure they have an adequate intake of the required vitamins and minerals.

**Foods to avoid** Substances from some foods that a mother eats while breast-feeding may pass into her milk and affect the baby in adverse ways. In many cases, this will first be noted by the mother whose baby seems to be suffering from colic or having abdominal bloating and wind. Other symptoms may include diarrhoea, vomiting, bronchitis, wheezing, runny nose, and skin rashes.

Foods eaten by the mother that may cause these symptoms in breast-fed babies include cow's milk and other dairy products, eggs, wheat products, citrus fruits, caffeine, chocolate, garlic, cabbage, and cucumber.

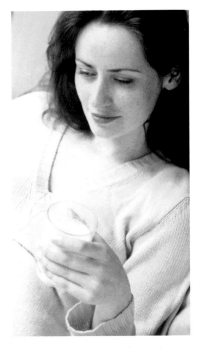

**Calcium-rich diet** A new mother needs to ensure she gets plenty of calcium, especially if she is breast-feeding, to keep her bones strong. Milk is an excellent source.

keep your immune system strong. To do this, it is essential for you to eat three meals every day. Try to avoid skipping meals, no matter how busy you may be (or in an effort to lose weight). Even a high-fibre muesli bar and a piece of fruit for breakfast, eaten on the run, is better than nothing. You are the most important person in your baby's life. It's vital for you to take care of yourself so you will be able to take care of your child.

A good strategy to adopt is to plan ahead. For example, if you are packing a bag to go out with your baby, put in some nutritious snacks for yourself, such as fresh fruit and rice cakes with peanut butter, and drinks such as water or 100 per cent fruit juice. Also, plan healthy meals that can be prepared quickly so you are able to eat on a regular schedule.

## Weight loss after pregnancy

You should not go on a slimming diet immediately after pregnancy, particularly if you are breast-feeding. Weight loss after giving birth should be gradual. This is particularly true for breast-feeding women, who burn more calories than other women in order to support the production of breast milk.

A woman should not expect to return to her pre-pregnancy weight immediately after giving birth. On average, a new mother will lose 6.8kg (15lb) within the first week after her baby is born.

Many mothers are concerned about their weight gain during pregnancy and worry that they may not return to their original weight. This concern is real as some women retain 2.3–4.5kg (5–10lb) for each of

their pregnancies. Breast-feeding women who eat nutritionally well-balanced diets will typically lose 450–900g (1–2lb) per month during the first four to six months of breast-feeding. This weight loss is more rapid than for mothers who bottle-feed their babies from the start.

A weight loss of more than 700g (1½lb) per week can decrease the production of breast milk and put both the mother and baby at risk nutritionally. However, there are some mothers who maintain or gain weight during breast-feeding but lose the additional weight after they have weaned their infants.

The best way to return to your pre-pregnancy weight is to exercise every day, such as walking with your baby in a sling or pushchair.

## Case study  New mother losing too much weight

**Name** Suzie

**Age** 26

**Problem** Suzie is very busy with her young baby and finds it hard to sit down for a meal. Yesterday Suzie ate cornflakes with semi-skimmed milk for breakfast, half of a cheese and pickle sandwich and orange juice for lunch, and some chicken breast with a baked potato and diet cola for her dinner. She likes ice cream at night if she has time between feeds.

Suzie says she is now hungrier than she was during her pregnancy, but cannot find time to eat. She knows she is not drinking enough as her mouth is dry. She is afraid that she is not producing enough milk because her baby always appears hungry and is not as chubby as her friend's bottle-fed baby. Her mother told her not to eat vegetables and

chocolate because they would upset the baby and produce wind.

**Lifestyle** Suzie had a healthy 3.7kg (8lb 2oz) baby boy, now six weeks old and weighing 5kg (11lb). This was her first pregnancy. She has lost 9kg (20lb) since giving birth and currently weighs 63.5kg (140lb). She is 1.7m (5ft 6in) tall and weighed 59kg (130lb) before she was pregnant.

**Advice** Suzie is not getting enough calories to maintain her weight and produce enough breast milk for her baby. Her requirements when she is breast-feeding are increased by about 550 calories per day. She specifically needs more protein, vitamins A, $B_{12}$, and folate, calcium, and zinc.

To increase her intake of calories, Suzie should follow the recommended servings from the main food groups (*see pp.70–72*) and eat a number of servings towards the higher end of the range given for each food group.

Since she lacks the time to prepare and eat balanced meals, she should buy healthy ready meals that can be cooked quickly in the microwave. Suzie can also increase her intake of whole grains by eating microwaved instant porridge with semi-skimmed milk and a sliced banana or berries for her breakfast. She can add some carrot sticks and a glass of milk to her sandwich at lunch, and include a piece of wholemeal bread and fresh fruit salad with her dinner. These are healthy additions that are quick and easy to prepare.

Semi-skimmed milk or low-fat yogurt and iron-rich dried fruit can be added as snacks. She should also take a multivitamin. To increase her fluid intake, she should drink more of the nutritious fluids (up to 3 litres/5¼ pints every day), such as milk, 100 per cent fruit juices, and water with meals and snacks. To make this easy, Suzie should keep a large bottle of still water and a glass to hand at all times.

# During and after the menopause

## Lifestyle changes can ease the symptoms of the menopause.

The menopause is a natural part of ageing that occurs when a woman's ovaries dramatically reduce their output of sex hormones, especially oestrogen. The change often occurs over a few years, usually between the ages of 45 and 60, but it can happen at an earlier age in some women. As hormone levels drop, a woman's menstrual periods end.

### What are the symptoms?
Menopausal symptoms vary greatly. Some women experience significant discomfort, while others have no symptoms. Typical symptoms are hot flushes (sudden intense waves of heat and sweating), depression, anxiety, and mood swings. There may also be urinary and vaginal problems, such as atrophy (where the vaginal tissue becomes thinner, drier, and more delicate), irregular or heavy periods until menstruation finally stops, infections, urinary incontinence, and inflammation of the vagina. Many women also notice changes to the condition of their skin and hair.

### Making lifestyle changes
To prevent the consequences of low oestrogen levels and ease the transition during the menopause, there are lifestyle changes you can

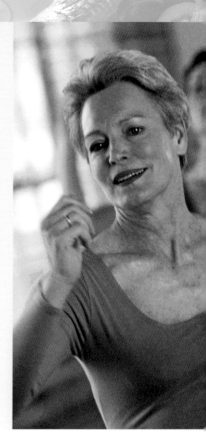

## Foods that reduce symptoms

Studies show that certain dietary changes during the menopause may help ease symptoms. Generally, eating a healthy, balanced diet that includes moderate amounts of fat and plenty of fruits and vegetables and whole grains will make you feel better. More specifically, soya is known to contain chemicals that can ease symptoms. Calcium is also vital, not so much to reduce symptoms, but to keep bones strong and prevent or delay the onset of osteoporosis.

**Soya products**  Foods that naturally contain soya include soya milk, soya beans, tofu, edamame, soya nuts, and tempeh. These foods are good sources of protein and phytochemicals called isoflavones. Interest has centred on two specific isoflavones – genistein and daidzen, which are similar in structure to the sex hormone oestrogen. They mimic the activities of oestrogen in the body and may help reduce menopausal symptoms that occur due to reduced levels of oestrogen, such as urinary and vaginal problems and menstrual irregularities. In addition, isoflavones have anti-cancer properties.

**Calcium-rich foods**  The decline in oestrogen levels during the menopause increases the rate of mineral loss from bone and as a result post-menopausal women are more vulnerable to the bone disorder osteoporosis. This makes it even more important to ensure that your calcium intake is adequate. The recommended daily amount (RDA) for calcium for women aged over 50 is the same as that for women 19–50 years – 700mg. Good sources of calcium are dairy foods, dark green leafy vegetables, and canned fish such as salmon that are eaten along with their bones.

### Herbal supplements

Various herbal supplements, such as black cohosh, may help reduce the symptoms of the menopause.

**Black cohosh**  This woodland plant has large leaves and a thick knotted root system. It has been used for more than 100 years to help reduce the symptoms of the menopause. Scientific studies have shown that this herbal supplement can reduce hot flushes, vaginal dryness, and depression. However, do not use black cohosh for more than six months or if you are taking hormone replacement therapy (HRT) or any medications for high blood pressure.

**Other herbal remedies**  Dong quai, evening primrose oil, and wild yam can also be used to ease the symptoms of the menopause, but, as yet, there is not sufficient evidence to support their effectiveness.

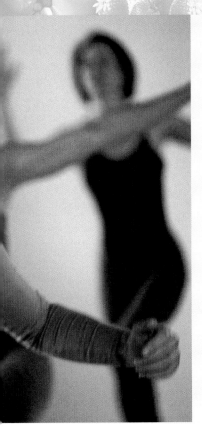

make. These include eating plenty of the nutrient-rich foods that may help reduce symptoms and prevent post-menopausal problems, such as the bone disease osteoporosis (*see p.242*). Evidence has shown that soya products and herbal supplements, as well as certain nutrients can also help (*below*).

### Physical activity

Exercise can reduce menopausal symptoms. For the greatest effect on the health of your heart and lungs, try to do at least 30 minutes of moderate aerobic exercise, such as walking, cycling, or swimming, each day. Weight-bearing exercise, such as playing tennis, walking, and lifting weights can help delay

**Keeping bones strong** Together with a healthy diet rich in calcium, weight-bearing exercises, such as dancing and jogging, keep bones strong and help prevent bone loss.

or prevent bone loss. Regular exercise will also help prevent overweight – studies have shown that women who have successfully lost weight, and kept it off, are more likely to participate in some type of physical activity every day.

### After the menopause

Reduced levels of the hormone oestrogen puts post-menopausal women at risk of osteoporosis. This disease may develop because oestrogen helps maintain normal bone density.

Before the menopause, women are at lower risk of cardiovascular disease (*see pp.214–221*) compared to men because oestrogen helps lower "bad" LDL-cholesterol levels in the blood and raise "good" HDL cholesterol. However, as oestrogen declines with the menopause, a woman's risk of cardiovascular disease increases and becomes the same as that of a man.

# Nutrients that help ease menopausal complaints

To ensure that you get plenty of the nutrients that can help ease troubling menopausal complaints (*below*), eat a varied diet and try these tips. For breakfast, add ground linseeds to your whole-grain cereal. For lunch, try eggs, canned fish, or a vegetable source of protein – such as soya beans or a mixture of other pulses with grains like wholemeal bread or brown rice – plus a big mixed salad. For dinner, have lean meat, poultry, or fish with a dark green leafy vegetable such as spinach, kale, or spring greens. For snacks, enjoy fruit and nuts – be sure to eat a minimum of two pieces of fruit each day and a handful of almonds at least every other day. In addition, drink two glasses of skimmed or semi-skimmed milk every day.

| COMPLAINT | NUTRIENT | TOP SOURCES |
|---|---|---|
| **Depression, mood swings** | • Omega-3 fatty acids<br>• Folate<br>• Vitamin D | • Linseeds, oily fish<br>• Whole grains, green leafy vegetables, orange juice<br>• Oily fish, enriched dairy products |
| **Breast soreness and lumps** | • Vitamin E | • Almonds, avocado, vegetable oil, linseeds |
| **Heavy menstrual bleeding** | • Iron | • Red meat, pulses, spinach, raisins, bran cereal |
| **Hot flushes** | • Calcium<br><br>• Exercise | • Low-fat dairy products, green leafy vegetables, canned oily fish eaten with bones (salmon, sardines)<br>• 20 minutes per day, such as dancing, swimming, or walking |
| **Osteoporosis** | • Vitamin D<br>• Calcium | • Oily fish, enriched dairy products<br>• Low-fat dairy products, green leafy vegetables, canned oily fish eaten with bones (salmon, sardines) |

# The extra needs of athletes

## When exercising, we need extra calories and nutrients.

Proper nutrition is not only essential for the growth, maintenance, and repair of your body's tissues, but it also provides fuel for exercise. The fuel that your body uses is known as ATP (*below*).

### Adjusting your diet

If you are an athlete, the best diet you can have is similar to the best diet for a non-athlete: obtaining enough calories while limiting how much saturated fat you eat.

### Jargon buster

**ATP** This chemical, which is short for adenosine triphosphate, is a product of the breakdown of carbohydrates, proteins, and fat in the body. Whenever your body needs energy for chemical reactions and processes, it uses ATP.

To achieve an athlete's diet, you do not need to change the food you eat; you need to adjust the amount of food and fluids, the number of meals, and timing of meals (before, during, and after competition).

### The need for extra calories

Calorie needs vary widely among athletes as body size, age, gender, and environment all influence the number of calories burned during exercise. The intensity, duration, and mode of exercise, your level of conditioning, and how efficiently you move also influence how many calories you burn up.

The basic energy requirement per day for a sedentary or overweight person is 20 calories per 1kg (2¼lb) of body weight. Moderately active people need 25–35 calories per 1kg (2¼lb) of body weight, with women at the lower end and men at the higher end of the scale. Very active people require more: male athletes need 37–51 calories and female athletes 41–58 calories per 1kg (2¼lb) of body weight per day.

### The fuel of choice

Carbohydrate is the fuel of choice for exercise. Compared to fat, it is more easily converted into ATP, providing energy for all working muscles and the rest of the body. At rest, when plenty of oxygen is available, the body burns mostly fat. When you begin to exercise, less oxygen becomes available, and carbohydrates become a more important energy source, especially for short, intense exercise.

Protein is stored in the body as muscle, and fat is stored as body fat. Carbohydrates are only stored in tiny amounts in the body – in the liver and muscles as a molecule called glycogen – so it is important to eat carbohydrates before you exercise. If you exercise for a long time or at a moderate pace, you exhaust glycogen stores, and the body breaks down fat for energy.

**Burning up fuel** Carbohydrates provide the fuel needed for the energy muscles expend during intense exercise such as sprinting.

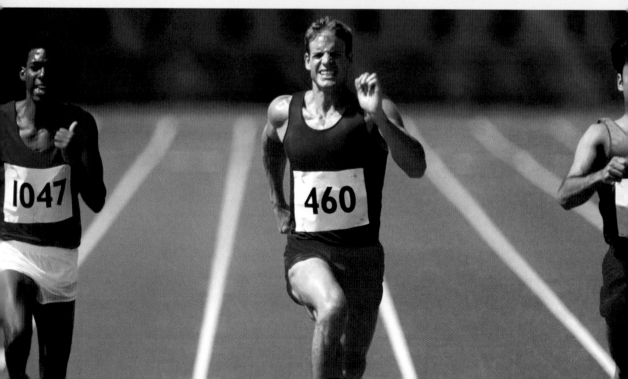

# Very active people need more protein

The protein needs of athletes depend on the type of exercise (resistance or endurance) and its intensity and duration. During rest, protein can supply as much as five per cent of the energy the body burns up. During aerobic exercise, such as jogging, protein may then account for as much as 15 per cent of the energy used. Hardly any protein is used during resistance, or strength, training.

When exercise is extremely intense or if there is no fat or carbohydrate available for the body to use as fuel, muscle will then be broken down.

People who play a sport that requires muscle building, such as wrestling and rugby, need more protein in their diet than sedentary people. If you start a programme of resistance training, the current recommendations are that you increase protein intake during the initial weeks of your training programme.

- Moderately active men and women need 0.35g of protein per 450g (1lb) of body weight per day.
- Men who do endurance sports, such as long-distance cycling and marathons, need to increase their protein intake to 0.65g per 450g (1lb) per day.
- Men who do resistance training, such as weightlifting, need 0.7g of protein per 450g (1lb) per day.
- Women athletes, participating in either endurance or resistance exercise, need 0.5g of protein per 450g (1lb) of body weight per day.

## Healthy protein sources

The best food sources of protein should also be low in fat. About 225–300g (8–10oz) per day of the following should meet the protein needs of most athletes:
- Low-fat dairy products
- Lean beef
- Poultry
- Eggs
- Fish
- Shellfish
- Tofu
- Kidney beans
- Lentils
- Nuts
- Sesame seeds
- Soya beans

# Making sure you get plenty of fluids

Water accounts for 80 per cent of our bodies. During exercise, our muscles generate internal heat. In order to prevent the body temperature from rising too high, we sweat – water and salts are excreted through pores in the skin to cool the body.

**Dehydration**  If excess sweating occurs during exercise without replacing the fluid you have lost, you can become dehydrated. Symptoms of dehydration include general discomfort, headache, exhaustion, and apathy.

**Keeping hydrated**  Because a loss of three per cent of body weight as water can decrease athletic performance, it is vital to drink enough before, during, and after an event, especially with the meal eaten prior to exercise.

- The day before a competition try to drink at least 225ml (8floz) of fluid at each meal and at least 1 litre (2 pints) of fluid between meals.
- Avoid drinking large amounts of tea, coffee, and alcohol because they have a diuretic effect – that is they increase the amount of urine produced by the body.
- During exercise, have a drink at regular intervals – about 225ml (8floz) every 30 minutes. Fluid intake following physical activity can also be critical in helping athletes recover quickly between bouts of training and competition.
- Take carbohydrate drinks before a competition, then isotonic drinks for carbohydrates during exercise, and hypotonic drinks to avoid dehydration.

**Don't drink too much water**  It is very important to follow the recommendations above because drinking too much water can cause problems. If you drink more than 3.5 litres (6 pints) while sweating profusely, you are at risk of low blood sodium levels (hyponatremia). This is a risk for athletes who participate in endurance events, such as triathlons or marathons. Symptoms include headache, nausea, fatigue, drowsiness, muscle weakness, muscle twitching or cramping, confusion, seizure, and possibly coma.

## Sports drinks

There are three basic types of sports drinks, each for a different need:

**Carbohydrate drinks**  Rich in carbohydrate, these sports drinks should be taken before an event in order to replenish glycogen reserves in the muscles and liver.

**Isotonic drinks**  Designed to be taken while exercising, isotonic drinks quickly deliver glucose to the muscles for extra energy.

**Hypotonic drinks**  These drinks contain little carbohydrate. They replenish water and salts lost from the body and prevent dehydration.

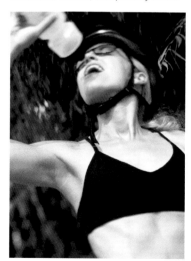

**Preventing dehydration**  Make sure you drink plenty of fluids during prolonged exercise to prevent dehydration, especially if you are outdoors in hot weather.

**Strength training** During intense short-burst exercise, such as weightlifting, muscles burn up glucose anaerobically (without oxygen).

# Needs of non-endurance athletes

For non-endurance athletes, such as footballers, tennis and rugby players, and weightlifters, the bulk of their calorie intake (55–60 per cent) should come from carbohydrates – mainly starches and a small proportion from sugars. No more than 30 per cent of their calories should come from fat and the remainder (10–15 per cent) from protein. As with any diet, it should be well-balanced and provide all the necessary nutrients.

## GLUCOSE AND GLYCOGEN

When starches or sugars are eaten, the body changes them to glucose, which is the only form of carbohydrate used directly by muscles for energy. Glucose is also stored in the liver and muscles as glycogen. During exercise, glycogen is broken down to provide energy. There is usually enough glycogen in the muscles for 90–120 minutes of exercise. Most exercise and sport do not use up your glycogen stores so eating carbohydrates during the activity is not necessary.

Here are a few tips for non-endurance athletes about what to eat and drink before, during, and after exercise:
**Before** Have some high-carbohydrate foods like a banana, bagel, or fruit juice. These foods are broken down quickly and provide glucose. Researchers have found that eating something between one and four hours before exercise keeps glucose available for working muscles. It is also critical to drink plenty of water beforehand to keep muscles hydrated.
**During** Perspiration and exertion deplete the body of the fluids necessary for optimum performance and lead to dehydration. Drink plenty of water – at least 120ml (4floz) every 20 minutes of exercise. Replace carbohydrates with a sports drink (see p.147) if the exercise lasts over 90 minutes.
**After** If the exercise was strenuous and lasted a long time, glycogen stores may need refuelling. Foods and drinks high in carbohydrates right after exercise will replenish glycogen stores.

# Do performance enhancers work?

Any substance that can improve the performance of a sport is known as an ergogenic aid. These aids include sports drinks (see p.147), caffeine, and creatine (right).
**Caffeine** Found naturally in tea, coffee, and chocolate, this stimulant is often added to soft drinks as a performance enhancer. Caffeine is a controlled, or restricted, drug during competition. It should be avoided before competition and training due to its diuretic (urine-producing) effect, as this can contribute to the risk of dehydration.
**Supplements** To prevent fatigue, some athletes use alkaline salts such as sodium bicarbonate to neutralize the build-up of lactic acid. This acid is a waste product of anaerobic respiration, in which the muscles burn glucose without using oxygen. Many athletes use creatine to enhance muscle activity and increase muscle mass (right).

Professional athletes need to be very careful when taking any supplement or

ergogenic aid, unless it is approved by a sports governing body. In some cases, supplements that are not banned or restricted may be chemically converted in the body into ones that are.
**Vitamins and minerals** Most athletes have lower blood levels of vitamins than non-athletes, regardless of whether they are taking any supplements. However, while it is true that physical activity may increase the need for some vitamins and minerals, the athlete's increased needs generally can be met with a well-balanced and varied diet. Studies have shown that vitamin supplements do not improve athletic performance. However, there may be situations where vitamin intake should be increased, such as restriction of food to maintain weight, by altering the diet or supplements.

Some female athletes may develop an iron deficiency and so should eat iron-rich foods, such as red meat, pulses, and spinach, or take a supplement to prevent anaemia (see p.271).

# Creatine supplements

Studies have shown that creatine – an amino acid present in some proteins – may be beneficial for athletes who participate in sports that involve short bursts of intense exercise, such as weightlifting and sprinting.

Creatine works by providing quick energy for the initial phase of muscle contraction. It can also increase muscle mass and strength, necessary for these kinds of sports. It works by pulling water into muscle cells from the surrounding fluid, resulting in a larger muscle and, eventually, a stronger muscle.

Creatine occurs naturally in the body – it is manufactured by the liver – but it can also be obtained in the diet from fish and red meat. It is marketed as a supplement in the form of creatine phosphate, which is more bioavailable, or easier for the body to use.

# Needs of endurance athletes

Carbohydrates are the most important nutrient for endurance sports, such as marathons and long-distance cycling, swimming, or cross-country skiing.

## CARBOHYDRATE LOADING

Before an event, some athletes practise "carbohydrate loading", an approach that maximizes stores of muscle glycogen, which is the first fuel to be used during intense exercise. To achieve this, you limit your intake of carbohydrates for a few weeks before eating a lot of them in the days before the event. The initial reduction in carbohydrates makes the body extremely sensitive to them when they enter the body, allowing glycogen stores to be replenished. See below for a healthy carbohydrate-rich meal to eat the day before an event.

## DAY OF THE EVENT

It is best to eat a light breakfast, such as cereal or toast and fruit juice. After breakfast, drink water in small amounts at regular intervals to ensure you start the race fully hydrated. Since the body's carbohydrate stores become depleted during the exertion of an endurance event, replace them whenever possible. Sports drinks (see p.147) help maintain diminishing stores of energy, water, and nutrients, especially salts lost in sweat, throughout the event. Up to 4–5 litres (7–9 pints) of sweat may be lost when running a marathon. After the event, the body's water and energy levels need to be restored as soon as possible.

## WHAT TO AVOID

Endurance athletes should avoid coffee, tea, and alcohol because they might lead to dehydration. Some athletes, however, do take caffeine just prior to a race to enhance performance.

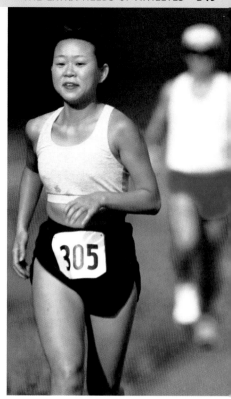

**Running a marathon** Always begin an endurance event fully hydrated and with replenished glycogen stores.

# Recipe  Carbohydrate meal for endurance athlete

### INGREDIENTS

**1 large onion**

**4 garlic cloves**

**2 tbsp olive oil**

**1 aubergine**

**1 tbsp reduced-salt soy sauce**

**400g (14oz) can tomatoes**

**225g (8oz) plum tomatoes**

**fresh thyme**

**400g (14oz) fusilli pasta**

**Serves 6**

1 Finely chop the onion and crush the garlic cloves. Heat a little olive oil in a frying pan, add the onion and garlic, and fry until the onion is softened.

2 Cut the aubergine into 1cm (½in) cubes. Add to the pan and cook until tender. If the mixture becomes too dry, add a little water.

3 Add the soy sauce to the vegetable mixture, stir gently to mix, and cook for a further 1–2 minutes.

4 Add the canned tomatoes to the pan with their juice. Stir, then cover the pan and cook for about 20 minutes.

5 Skin, seed, and finely chop the plum tomatoes. Add to the frying pan together with a little chopped thyme. Simmer for a further 2 minutes.

6 Cook the pasta in a large pan of fast-boiling water, until just firm to the bite. Drain.

7 Season the sauce with freshly ground black pepper before spooning over the pasta. If you like, garnish with chopped fresh flat-leaf parsley.

**Each serving provides:**
Calories 294, Total fat 5.2g (Sat. 0.8g, Poly. 1.0g, Mono. 2.8g), Cholesterol 0mg, Protein 9.0g, Carbohydrate 56g, Fibre 4.0g, Sodium 117mg. Good source of – Vits: A, Fol, C; Mins: Ca, K, Mg, P.

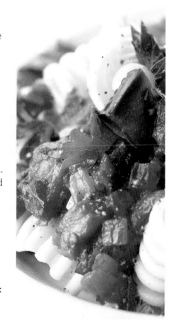

# The middle to later years of life

## Good food choices and exercise between 50 and 70 years can help you defy ageing.

As people age, they tend to eat less, and therefore take in fewer calories and smaller amounts of important nutrients. In addition, it becomes more difficult for the body to digest and absorb certain vital nutrients. For example, in older people the amounts of calcium, vitamin $B_{12}$, and folate in the diet often fall well below the recommended daily intakes.

For good health over 50, it is important to make sure that you eat nutrient-dense foods and that you remain physically active.

### Changing calorie needs

Your body changes as you get older and these changes affect your nutritional needs. There is a reduction in muscle, an increase in body fat, and your total body water decreases by up to 20 per cent. You need fewer calories than you did when you were younger since your basal metabolic rate (BMR; see p.26) decreases as muscle mass declines with age.

The good news is that moderate exercise helps preserve muscle mass and can thereby slow the rate at which this process occurs.

**Gentle exercise** Walking is an excellent excercise, so playing golf is an ideal activity that helps improve stamina, flexibility, and muscle and bone strength.

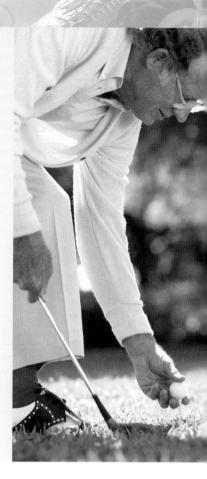

# Do you need to take supplements?

If you are over the age of 50, the key nutrients you should get enough of are vitamins $B_6$, $B_{12}$, folate, and D, and the mineral calcium. It is better to try to meet your daily needs through a healthy well-balanced diet, but these nutrients are so important that you might need to take a supplement.

See your doctor for advice before you start to take a supplement because high doses of certain vitamins and minerals can be harmful, and taking a high dose of one vitamin or mineral can interfere with the absorption of others. For most older adults, a multivitamin and mineral supplement will be sufficient.

**Vitamin $B_6$** Older people who suffer from depression or women taking hormone replacement therapy have lower blood levels of vitamin $B_6$. Post-menopausal women with osteoporosis (see p.241) have also been shown to have low levels of this vitamin.

**Vitamin $B_{12}$** Most people who eat animal products get sufficient vitamin $B_{12}$ from their diet, but about 10–15 per cent of those who are over the age of 60 have lost the ability to absorb this vitamin properly. This is due to a reduction in the secretion of acid and pepsin (which break down proteins in food) in the stomach. Many experts recommend that people over age 50 meet most of their dietary requirement for vitamin $B_{12}$ with synthetic vitamin $B_{12}$ because this is easier for the body to absorb and is used in fortified foods or supplements.

**Folate** Older adults who are prescribed a folate supplement must also take a vitamin $B_{12}$ supplement, because too much folate may mask a vitamin $B_{12}$ deficiency. This can result in anaemia and damage to the nervous system.

**Vitamin D** This vitamin aids calcium absorption and helps maintain healthy bones, both very important for older adults, but it may be difficult for them to get enough. For adults under the age of 65 there is no recommended daily amount (RDA). For adults over 65 years the RDA is 10mcg per day. Those who have limited exposure to sunlight and who eat or drink very few dairy products would benefit from taking a vitamin D supplement (see p.269), as they are at risk of the bone diseases osteomalacia (see p.241) or osteoporosis.

**Calcium** Osteoporosis is a major health risk for both older women and men. The daily recommended amount of calcium is 700mg for men and women. This amount of calcium should help retain the mineral in the bones, keeping them strong and making them less susceptible to fracture. If you have difficulty getting enough calcium through your diet, see your GP or a state-registered dietitian about taking a supplement (see p.267).

Regular exercise has other benefits too – it keeps your bones strong, enhances mobility and flexibility, and increases your sense of well-being (*see p.153*).

## The digestive system

Digestion and absorption of food appear to be well preserved as people age. However, some of the digestive processes are affected. Saliva production decreases, which may affect how food is broken down in the stomach to prepare for digestion and absorption in the intestine. The stomach reduces its secretion of acid and pepsin, which may lead to decreased absorption of vitamins $B_{12}$, folate, and D and the mineral calcium. The smooth muscles in the intestine become less efficient, resulting in slower movement of food through the intestine and often constipation.

As you age, there is also a decline in the skin's production of vitamin D, which is necessary for the body to use calcium, making it more difficult for the body to meet its calcium needs. Calcium is especially important for women during and after the menopause (*see p.144–145*). For all of these reasons, older adults should eat nutrient-dense foods and may also need to take supplements.

## Health problems

Chronic disorders, such as arthritis, diabetes, cardiovascular disease, and osteoporosis, are more likely to develop after the age of 50. The risk of other serious disorders such as cancer, heart attack, and stroke is also increased. You can reduce the risk or minimize the effects of many disorders by avoiding or eating certain foods (*see Food as Medicine, pp.210–271*).

In addition, if you have been prescribed any medications, they may affect your appetite or even prevent, or in some cases enhance, absorption of certain nutrients, vitamins, or minerals from the stomach or intestine (*see p.153*).

## Drinking alcohol

Recent studies have suggested that moderate drinking (up to three to four units a day for men and up to two to three units daily for women) may have health benefits for older adults. These include improving mood, mixing socially, maintaining mental faculties, enhancing bone-mineral density, and improving cardiovascular health. For people with little interest in food, a small sherry before meals can stimulate appetite. However, many older people drink more than this, often due to depression or loneliness.

Too much alcohol can drain the body of water-soluble vitamins and decrease the absorption of other vitamins and minerals. It can also displace more nutritious foods. If you do consume alcohol, stay within the guidelines, remembering that home-poured measures are often larger than those on which the guidelines are based.

# Easing constipation with diet

A slower intestine is one of the most common changes experienced by older people. The smooth muscles of the gut contract more slowly and thus food moves more slowly through the intestine. This can lead to constipation – difficult and infrequent passage of small, hard stools. It can usually be corrected by increasing fibre and fluid intake. High-fibre foods include whole grains, pulses, fruits, and vegetables. A bowl of porridge or whole-grain cereal each day is often enough to achieve bowel regularity.

Try to achieve a routine in which you go to the toilet at the same time each day. If you ignore the urge to go, stools remain in the gut longer, becoming dry and hard, and you will strain more when you do go.

### DRINK PLENTY OF WATER

Try to drink at least six to eight glasses of water daily, even if you are not thirsty. As you age, your thirst response may decrease, so you may not always recognize when you need fluids. Keep a bottle of water and a glass handy to remind you to drink regularly through the day and ensure that you get enough fluids, which will help stools stay soft, bulky, and easy to eliminate.

### TRY TAKING A NATURAL LAXATIVE

If water and fibre are not sufficient, try taking a gentle laxative. Laxatives cause the stools to retain water as they pass through the intestine, so they remain soft and bulky.

Drink several glasses of water with the laxative, and choose a sugar-free variety if you are diabetic. It's best to avoid mineral oil laxatives as they can interfere with the absorption of the fat-soluble vitamins. Persistent use of stimulant laxatives should be avoided because your colon will eventually be unable to function without them.

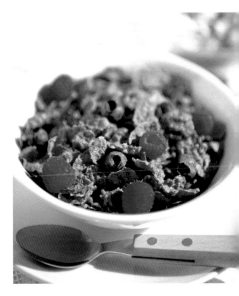

**Fibre can prevent constipation** Enjoying a bowl of whole-grain cereal topped with fruit for breakfast each day will boost your fibre intake and help prevent constipation.

# Which foods can fight ageing?

Certain foods are rich in antioxidants. These are substances that neutralize free radicals – chemicals that damage cells in the body and thus aggravate ageing and disease.

The main antioxidants are vitamin A (*see p.52*), vitamin C (*see p.56*), vitamin E (*see p.58*), beta-carotene (a precursor of vitamin A), and the minerals selenium (*see p.67*) and zinc (*see p.67*). Some phytochemicals, such as lycopene (*see p.59*), are also antioxidants. You can try the following tips to get the maximum benefit from antioxidants:

- Make sure you eat plenty of fresh fruits and vegetables.
- Since vitamin E is one of nature's best antioxidants, do not eliminate olive and rapeseed oils from your diet.
- Try to reduce the amount of work antioxidants have to do by preventing the build-up of free radicals. Do not smoke, spend too long in the sun, or let yourself get too stressed, and keep away from polluted areas.

## ANTIOXIDANT-RICH MEALS

Ideas for modifying a snack or a meal to pack a powerful antioxidant-rich punch include the following:

- Cubes of orange-fleshed melon
- Strawberry smoothie (*see p.81*)
- Mashed avocado on a toasted bagel
- Grilled salmon on a bed of salad leaves, red peppers, tomatoes, and mango, sprinkled with ground linseeds
- A mixture of broccoli, peas, and cauliflower, served hot or cold
- A handful of baby carrots or almonds
- Spinach sautéed in olive oil with garlic, then sprinkled with lemon juice and Parmesan cheese
- A mixed salad with tomatoes, celery, sweetcorn, and broccoli added
- A jacket-baked sweet potato topped with low-fat yogurt
- Flaked almonds sprinkled over green beans or peas
- Sliced oranges for dessert
- Fresh berries on your cereal
- Bread sticks with tomato salsa.

## Age spots

When free radicals – damaging chemicals in the body (*see p.58*) – build up they can produce a substance known as lipofucsin. This substance is deposited in the skin, most commonly on the face and back of the hands, in the form of brown spots or patches. These areas are commonly known as "age spots" or "liver spots". The number of age spots that you have is thought to indicate the total amount of damage that your body has suffered from free radicals.

Eating foods that are rich in antioxidants (*left*), especially those that are good sources of vitamins A, C, and E and selenium, can prevent the formation of liver spots by breaking down the lipofuscin before it is deposited. In addition, using creams that contain vitamin C may eventually make age spots disappear from the skin.

# Recipe Antioxidant-rich fish with salsa

| INGREDIENTS |
| --- |
| 2 lemons |
| 4 cod steaks |
| 1 yellow or red pepper |
| 1 stick celery |
| 4 plum tomatoes |
| 1 onion |
| 2 chillies |
| fresh flat-leaf parsley |
| 1 garlic clove |

**Serves 4**

1 Grate the zest of one lemon into a shallow dish; add the juice of both of the lemons and ground black pepper to taste.

2 Add the cod steaks to the lemon juice. Leave to marinate in the fridge for 30 minutes, turning once.

3 Core and seed the pepper. Chop it finely, together with the celery, tomatoes, onion, chillies, and some parsley. Crush the garlic and add to the other ingredients, mixing together to make a salsa.

4 Preheat oven to 220°C (425°F, gas 7). Lightly brush a baking dish with olive oil and arrange the fish steaks in it. Cover each steak with a few spoonfuls of the salsa mixture. Pour the marinade juice over the salsa and add a little more olive oil.

5 Bake the cod steaks for about 20 minutes or until they are cooked through.

6 Garnish with more chopped flat-leaf parsley. Serve with a green salad or green beans, broccoli, or spinach for an antioxidant-rich meal.

**Each serving provides:**
Calories 159, Total fat 1.5g
(Sat. 0.3g, Poly. 0.8g, Mono. 0.3g),
Cholesterol 64mg, Protein 29g,
Carbohydrate 7.5g, Fibre 2.0g, Sodium
69mg. Good source of – Vits: A, Fol,
C, K, Mins: Ca, Mg, P.

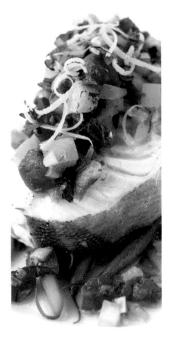

# The importance of keeping fit

Regular exercise significantly slows the effects of ageing. Not only does physical activity give you more energy and make you feel relaxed, but it also enables you to meet new people, boosts your self-esteem, and maintains a feeling of independence. It also reduces the risk of many age-related disorders, including diabetes, cardiovascular diseases such as stroke and heart attack, and the bone disease osteoporosis.

Exercise for people over 50 should aim to maintain strength, bone density, balance, flexibility, mobility, and general well-being. You can increase your bone strength and density by weight-bearing exercises, such as tennis, jogging, or brisk walking. In addition, you should increase your calcium and vitamin D intake and expose your skin to sunlight, which allows the body to make vitamin D, to maximize bone strength.

You can increase your flexibility and mobility in the following ways:
- Be active and do plenty of walking.
- Practise yoga or simple stretches.
- Try body-weight exercises, such as squats, leg lifts, and arm raises.
- Do exercises that increase muscular strength, such as weight-training.
- Take up activities that are good for the heart and lungs, such as swimming or gardening. Remember to begin any new exercise gently to avoid injury.

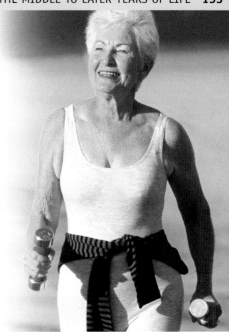

**Out and about** Exercising outdoors – in a park or on the beach – is beneficial for your health and well-being. Exposure to the sun also allows your body to make vitamin D.

# Do your medications affect your diet?

Many people over the age of 50 have long-term, or chronic, disorders, such as high blood pressure and arthritis, and need to take daily medications to control their symptoms. These medications may interact with the foods that you eat. Some medications can block the absorption or processing of a nutrient in the body, while others enhance it. Conversely, some nutrients block or improve the effects of a medication. Taking medications may affect your appetite, and there is also greater risk for missing out on a key nutrient due to an interaction. If you take any medication, your GP or chemist should be able to tell you which foods or nutrients may cause interactions. The most common interactions are listed below.

| DRUG GROUP | REACTS WITH | EFFECT | WHAT YOU CAN DO |
|---|---|---|---|
| **Analgesic drugs** | • Alcohol | • Increases risk for liver damage | • Avoid alcohol |
| **Antibiotic drugs** | • Calcium and biotin<br>• Vitamin K | • Reduces absorption of drug<br>• Drug interferes with manufacture of vitamin K in the intestine | • Take drug on an empty stomach<br>• Take a multivitamin supplement |
| **Anti-coagulant drugs** | • Foods rich in vitamin K<br>• Vitamin E supplements | • Decreases drug effectiveness<br>• Increases drug effectiveness | • Limit foods high in vitamin K<br>• Avoid vitamin E supplements |
| **Anti-hypertensive and diuretic drugs** | • Potassium and magnesium | • Some of these drugs increase potassium and magnesium losses | • Eat plenty of potassium- and magnesium-rich foods |
| **Anti-inflammatory drugs** | • Alcohol | • Can aggravate bleeding from the stomach | • Avoid alcohol |
| **Cholesterol-lowering drugs** | • Any food | • Enhances drug absorption | • Take with food |
| **Steroid drugs** | • Sugar<br>• Sodium (Salt) | • Drug elevates blood-sugar levels<br>• May cause fluid retention | • Reduce sweets and colas<br>• Limit sodium (salt) intake |

# Feeling good into old age

## It is essential to eat healthily as you advance in age.

People aged 70 years and over are the rapidly expanding sector of the British population. In general, their nutritional needs are the same as those of adults aged 50–70 (see pp.150–154), but deficiencies are more common, especially in frail or house-bound older adults who rely on others for their basic needs. In addition, older people often have small appetites, which is why it is important that they try to eat nutrient-dense foods.

### Changes in senses

The taste buds deteriorate with age. To compensate, many older people prefer very sweet or salty foods. Adding sugar contributes empty calories (those with no nutritional value) to the diet, and adding salt to food can worsen high blood pressure. The senses of smell and sight may also deteriorate, resulting in a preference for strong-smelling foods or a loss of interest in food.

### Health problems

Most older people have at least one long-term disorder, such as cardiovascular disease, arthritis, or diabetes. In addition, some are affected by dementia, which is a reduction in mental capacity due to a disorder that affects the brain. These and other disorders affect what you eat, and they may require dietary restrictions such as a low-fat or low-salt diet. The chapter Food as Medicine provides more information about which foods to eat if you are ill (see pp.210–271).

Physical disabilities can affect nutritional health. For example, being unable to walk to the kitchen or go food shopping without help can result in poor eating habits. Emotional changes resulting from depression, grief, and loneliness can lead to loss of appetite.

### Difficulty chewing

Dental problems are common in older people. Loose, decaying, or missing teeth, dentures that do not fit properly, and gum disease make it difficult to chew food and increase the risk of poor nutrition. Regular dental check-ups are vital to help detect these problems before they become a nuisance.

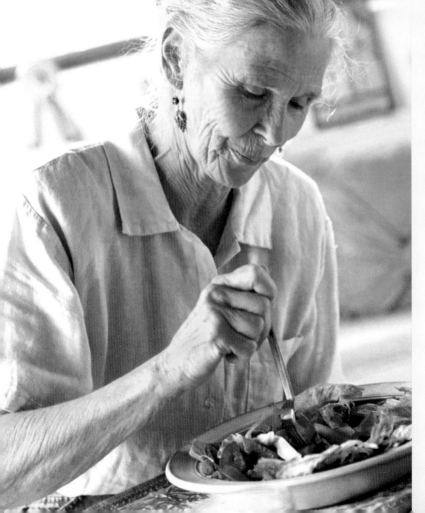

**Continuing healthy eating** As you age, it becomes more difficult to digest and absorb certain nutrients. Therefore, it is vital to have a varied diet of easy-to-digest, nutrient-dense foods such as the salad shown here.

## Staying active

It is important to keep as active as possible later in life as this will benefit your health and well-being. Gentle activities such as walking, swimming, and neck and shoulder exercises are excellent. Even a short walk round the garden, or moving around in the house during the day is beneficial. If you cannot walk easily or have difficulty moving about, think about installing or using mobility aids in your home, such as a walker.

# Flavourful meals and snacks

Scientists refer to those 85 years and over as the "old-old", and for this fast-increasing group weight maintenance is the biggest issue, with the focus on maintaining muscle mass and preventing weight loss. Therefore, making sure that you have access to meals and snacks that taste good and are easy to chew and swallow will help you feel good on a daily basis.

These meals should also be packed with nutrients and calories, such as the soup, scrambled eggs, and fruit with yogurt that are shown below. Frozen ready meals are a good choice too, because they can be quickly microwaved and require very little washing up – a key factor for older people who may also have difficulty preparing and cooking food.

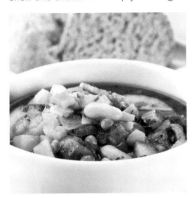

**Spicy bean soup** Home-made or from a can, hearty soups like this are an excellent source of protein, vitamins, minerals, and fibre.

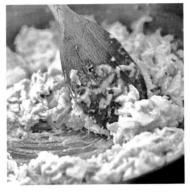

**Scrambled eggs** A quick and nutritious snack, well-cooked eggs can be livened up by adding chopped herbs and grated cheese.

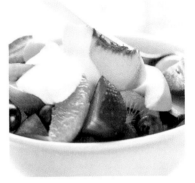

**Fruit and yogurt** Add low-fat yogurt – a great source of calcium – to mixed fresh fruits for a fibre- and calcium-rich dessert.

# Case study House-bound senior with a hip fracture

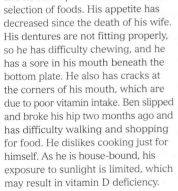

**Name** Ben

**Age** 85 years

**Problem** Ben's diet is low in calories and he eats a poor selection of foods. His appetite has decreased since the death of his wife. His dentures are not fitting properly, so he has difficulty chewing, and he has a sore in his mouth beneath the bottom plate. He also has cracks at the corners of his mouth, which are due to poor vitamin intake. Ben slipped and broke his hip two months ago and has difficulty walking and shopping for food. He dislikes cooking just for himself. As he is house-bound, his exposure to sunlight is limited, which may result in vitamin D deficiency.

**Lifestyle** Ben lives alone. His wife died three months ago. He does not drink or smoke. He rarely sees his children, who live some distance away. Yesterday for his breakfast, Ben had a couple of biscuits, a slice of white toast with jam, and a cup of coffee. For lunch, he had a bowl of chicken and rice soup with a few cream crackers and two biscuits. For dinner, he had a jam sandwich on white bread with a few more biscuits. He does not usually snack between meals. Ben takes an iron supplement that was prescribed for anaemia. He has constipation but uses laxatives.

**Advice** Ben's family should be made aware of his current problems so that they can visit him and arrange for his health and diet to be monitored more closely. Ben will need physiotherapy to improve his mobility.

With regard to nutrition, Ben's diet needs to be higher in calories as well as protein, fibre, vitamins, and calcium. In addition, he should continue taking his iron supplements.

For breakfast, Ben could have instant porridge with milk and orange juice, to give him calories, vitamin C, folate, and calcium. For his lunch, he could have a hot meal delivered from a social services agency. Alternatively, he could try prepared foods, such as a tuna sandwich. Adding a simple dessert such as canned rice pudding or custard to his dinner will give him more calories, as would fruit (fresh or canned in its own juice). He could also try high-calorie, high-protein drinks in order to increase his intake of calories and protein, as well as vitamins and minerals.

Ben should make arrangements to have his dentures adjusted. His GP can prescribe a multivitamin and mineral supplement for him. In addition, the local authority can help him get in touch with community resources that benefit elderly people who have trouble with food shopping, such as a Meals on Wheels service.

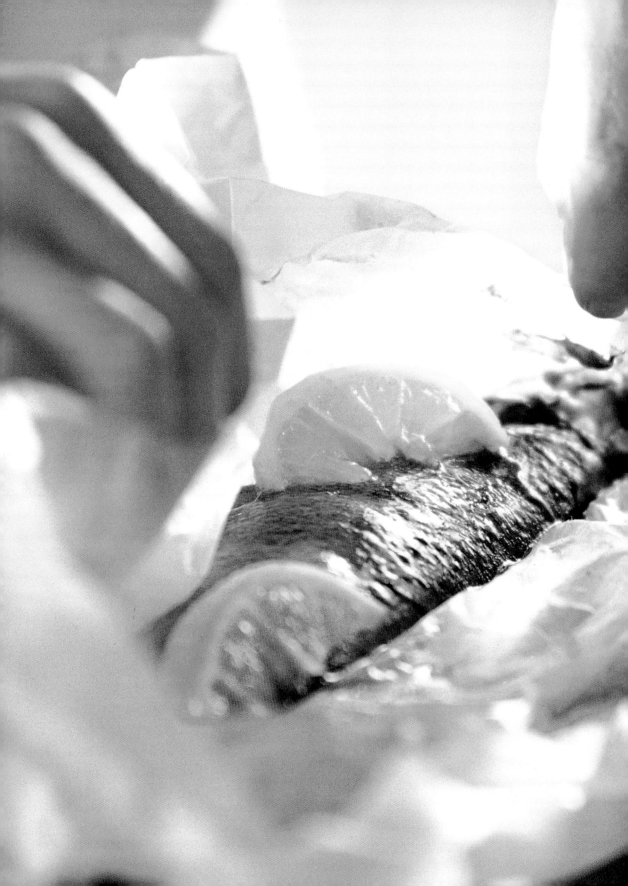

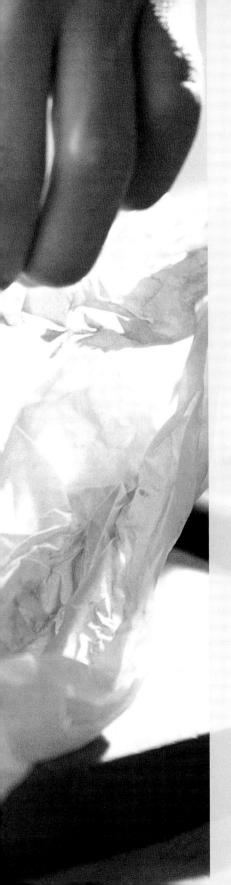

# The truth about weight control

Not only does controlling your weight make you feel and look better, but there is also abundant evidence to show that keeping your weight within healthy limits decreases your risk of developing a variety of serious medical conditions, including high blood cholesterol, high blood pressure, other cardiovascular diseases, diabetes, and cancer.

# Why weight control is important

**Weight control means maintaining a healthy weight that is just right for your body.**

If advertising for weight-loss diets and equipment is to be believed, weight control is primarily about improving your appearance. While it is true that keeping your weight in check can make you look better, it is even more important for your health and life expectancy. Being overweight increases your risk of developing a number of serious medical conditions (*right*).

**Build activity into daily life** Regular exercise is one of the keys to weight control for adults and children alike. Walking is a great activity for the family to enjoy together.

In 2002 the Health Survey for England found that between 1993 and 2002 the proportion of men who were overweight or obese rose from 62 to 70 per cent; in the same period the proportion of overweight or obese women rose from 56 to 63 per cent. These kinds of statistics highlight the importance of weight control.

## Changing your "set point"

To maintain a healthy weight for your height and frame, you need to adopt a strategy that will work for you in the long term. Many slimming diets promise quick results, and while these may help you "kick start" weight loss, they are not suitable for long-term weight control. The reason for this is what scientists identify as "set point" – the level at which your body defends its current weight.

If you consume extra calories (for a short period), your body will use these by generating more heat. If, on the other hand, you use more calories than you consume, your body will become more efficient at turning those calories into energy, to prevent short-term weight loss. This means that if you are trying to lose or gain weight, you have to make a serious commitment over a long period of time in order to retrain your body and readjust your set point.

## Weight control for life

But where you do you start? In this chapter, we will guide you through the maze of diet plans, pointing out their strengths and weaknesses, and help you develop your own long-term weight-control strategy through good nutritional choices and regular exercise.

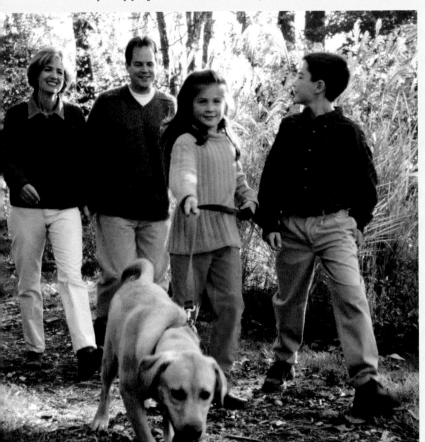

## Health risks of obesity

The more overweight you are, the higher your risk of disease and premature death.

- Carrying too much weight places greater strain on your heart and other organs as well as on weight-bearing joints, and puts you at greater risk of developing a range of serious medical conditions, including cardiovascular disease such as high blood pressure, respiratory disease, osteoarthritis, gall stones, and certain cancers.
- Being obese increases your risk of complications during surgical procedures as well as creating extra difficulties for the surgeon performing the operation.
- Since being overweight makes it more difficult to engage in regular exercise, a downward spiral into increased health risk and lack of fitness is likely to ensue. A weight loss of just ten per cent can reduce the risk and improve your health.

# The benefits of controlling weight

Keeping your weight in check is critically important for your health. The more overweight you are, the higher your risk of developing various medical conditions (*opposite below*) and the more probable that your excess weight will shorten your life. Conversely, if you are overweight, losing weight will greatly benefit your health and well-being.

• Research shows that losing just ten per cent of excess body weight lowers blood pressure, thereby reducing the risk of cardiovascular disease such as stroke (*see pp.214–215*).

• Losing weight lowers blood cholesterol and triglyceride levels, both of which are associated with increased risk of cardiovascular disease (*see pp.214–215*).

• Overweight people are twice as likely to develop type 2 diabetes as those who maintain a healthy weight. Losing weight reduces blood glucose levels and decreases the risk of developing diabetes (*see pp.246–247*).

• Losing weight will not only reduce your risk of developing osteoarthritis (*see p.245*), but will also reduce the stress on weight-bearing joints, such as the hips, knees, and lower spine, that are already affected by osteoarthritis.

• If you are considering surgery to replace arthritic hip or knee joints, you will almost certainly be advised to lose weight before the operation and to control your weight afterwards to optimize the chances of a successful outcome.

• Obesity and being overweight are major risk factors for certain cancers. These include cancer of the uterus, cervix, ovary, breast, gall bladder, and colon in women, and cancer of the colon, rectum, and prostate in men. Losing weight will produce a corresponding reduction in those risks (*see pp.258–259*).

• Sleep apnoea is a serious condition that is closely associated with being overweight. A weight loss will usually improve this condition (*see p.225*).

• In addition, controlling your weight leads to enhanced self-esteem and a sense of well-being, as well as improving your appearance.

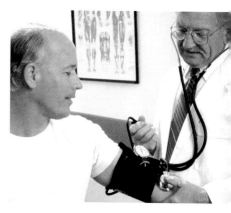

**Weight and blood pressure** If you are overweight, even a small reduction in weight will lower your blood pressure, which in turn reduces your risk of cardiovascular disease.

---

# Questionnaire Are you controlling your weight?

Circle the letters that accompany your answers to these simple questions, then check your score.

**1 Do you usually finish what is on your plate?**
a  No, I usually don't try to finish.
b  Yes, and then I am done.
c  Yes, and then I have seconds.

**2 Do you always have three courses when eating in a restaurant?**
a  Rarely.
b  Sometimes, but not often.
c  Always.

**3 Do you exercise at least three times a week?**
a  Yes, and sometimes more.
b  No, but I lead an active lifestyle.
c  No, I rarely exercise.

**4 Do you eat fruits and vegetables every day?**
a  Yes, about five servings a day.

b  Yes, a few servings a day.
c  No, only a few times a week.

**5 Do you eat low-fat dairy products?**
a  Yes, I always choose low-fat dairy.
b  Yes, a few servings a day.
c  No, or only a few times a week.

**6 Do you try to eat low-fat meals and snacks?**
a  Yes, I always choose low-fat foods.
b  Yes, but I frequently cheat.
c  No, I choose high-fat foods.

**7 How much TV do you watch?**
a  I usually watch less than one hour a day.
b  I watch two to three hours a day.
c  I watch over four hours a day.

**8 Do you limit your intake of sweets and desserts?**
a  Yes, I choose fruit instead.
b  Yes, but I occasionally indulge.
c  No, I eat sweets almost every day.

**9 Do you have water instead of sweetened drinks?**
a  Yes, I drink water or diet cola.
b  Yes, but I also have sweetened drinks and fruit juices.
c  No, I prefer cola and juice drinks.

**Score a** 1 **b** 2 **c** 3

**9–13 points** You are doing well and making a lot of effort to control your weight. Keep up the good work!

**14–20 points** Good job: you are really trying and your efforts will pay off over time. Look at the areas where you scored high and think about making some extra effort.

**21–27 points** Your score indicates that you are making choices that may lead to weight gain. These are just a few of the many small changes that you can make that will help you control your weight. Start slowly.

# Tips for successful weight control

Maintaining a healthy weight is all about balancing your total food intake, and the energy (calories) this provides, with the energy you expend in the course of your daily life. It's a simple equation – but not so simple to follow. We develop habitual ways of behaving in all areas of life, including what and how we eat and how active or sedentary our lives are. These habits build up over many years, so it is no easy matter to change them. But if you find it difficult to control your weight, then you must make a serious commitment to change these habits. Here are some tips to help you.

### EAT ONLY WHAT YOU NEED
The key to controlling your weight is to balance the calories you consume with the number you expend in the course of your daily activities (*see p.34*). Many people eat much more than they need and the excess calories are stored as fat. The more active you are, the more you can eat – and still maintain a healthy weight. You will benefit from both the physical activity and the weight control.

### FILL UP ON FRUIT AND VEG
Since there is a limit to the number of calories you can consume in a day if you want to maintain or lose weight, it is best to concentrate on those foods that supply your body with essential vitamins and minerals, such as fruits and vegetables, rather than on so-called "empty calorie" or junk foods (*see p.99*). Simply eating two servings of vegetables with a meal will help to fill you up and so reduce your desire to snack on less valuable foods. Similarly, eating an apple an hour before a meal will help you eat less at mealtime.

### CUT OUT FATTY FOODS
Fat has more than twice the number of calories by weight as carbohydrate or protein. Therefore, if you want to cut down on calories and still eat enough to feel satisfied, you should eat fewer fatty foods. Even the healthy oils contain 99 calories per tablespoon. So aim to limit the amount of fried food you eat and replace full-fat dairy products with low- or reduced-fat varieties.

### REDUCE CALORIE-DENSE SNACKS
Many people eat sensibly and healthily at mealtimes, but then consume high-calorie snacks in between. If you are hungry and want a snack, make it a healthy choice, such as raw vegetables or fruits. If you snack out of boredom, try to identify the situations that trigger this impulse and devise alternative strategies for dealing with the impulse – for example, go for a walk or ring a friend for a chat.

**Eating healthily**
The sensible approach to controlling weight is to eat vegetables, fruits, and low-fat proteins. This woman may think her salad is healthy, but salami is high in saturated fat. She would also be better off eating wholemeal bread.

## Exercise and weight control

Regular exercise is vital for long-term weight control. People who have some physical activity at least three times a week are more likely to lose weight and keep it off than those who do not exercise at all. Strength training, such as lifting weights, is also helpful, since this type of activity increases muscle mass, which helps the body to burn more calories, even at rest.

To make exercise work, select an activity that you enjoy, start slowly, and stick with it. The great thing about exercise is that it makes you feel good, so it is self-reinforcing.

Exercise also combats one of the complaints that people most commonly consult their doctor about – fatigue. Once you start to exercise, you will find you sleep better, your aches and pains will lessen, your outlook on life will improve, and fatigue will vanish.

Any food that has sugar first in the list of ingredients on the nutrition label (*see p.277*) is likely to be high in calories, and may contain very little of nutritional value. Despite the notion that some people have a "sweet tooth", anyone can get used to less sugar in food. If you find this difficult, try to retrain your palate by gradually eating fewer sweets and sugary desserts.

### BEAT THE FATIGUE TRAP
Feeling tired can lead people to eat foods that give a quick burst of energy, such as chocolate. A well-balanced diet and a multivitamin supplement will help you maintain energy levels through the day.

### JOIN A SUPPORT GROUP
Weight-loss groups offer sensible dietary advice, regular weigh-ins, and group support, which can really help with long-term motivation when you are trying to lose or control weight. Choose a group that offers free weigh-ins once you have reached your target weight and, ideally, an exercise session.

# Avoiding weight gain as you age

Getting older is often accompanied by steady weight gain because your body starts to digest food more slowly. For each decade between the ages of 20 and 60, scientists estimate that we gain 4.5kg (10lb) in weight. It used to be believed that this kind of weight gain was normal, but we now know that it is unhealthy and brings an increased risk of developing a variety of serious medical conditions, such as diabetes and stroke.

The main reasons for weight gain in middle age are a decrease in physical activity and eating too much. In order to maintain a healthy weight you need to recognize that your energy needs may be considerably less now than they were when you were younger, and that you must tailor your nutritional intake to your current requirements.

## KEEP MOVING

Whatever your level of fitness, you should try to incorporate as much exercise into your life as possible. It may be that you

have an illness, injury, or condition such as osteoarthritis (*see pp.240–241*) that makes it more difficult to continue with the level of activity or type of exercise that you enjoyed in the past. If necessary, consult your doctor for help finding an exercise programme that suits your age and ability, and takes into account any medical condition from which you suffer.

It is never too late to start something new, and the benefits of embarking on a fitness programme, such as improved flexibility and energy levels, and loss of excess weight, will quickly become apparent. Joining a group programme can make exercise more enjoyable and help keep you motivated.

## MODIFY YOUR DIET

Maintaining a healthy, balanced diet is important throughout life, but as energy requirements decrease with ageing, it is even more important that you choose wisely, cutting down on sugary and fatty foods, and opting instead for a diet of

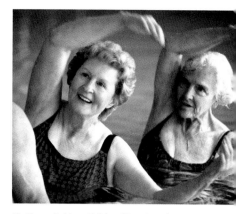

**Finding suitable activities**  Water-based exercises are particularly beneficial for older people, allowing a good workout without putting undue strain on weight-bearing joints.

nutrient-dense fruits and vegetables, whole grains, and low-fat sources of protein and calcium. If you are trying to lose weight, make sure that you do not miss out on important nutrients. Taking a multivitamin supplement is advised.

# Case study  Older adult eating the same yet gaining weight

**Name**  Marilyn

**Age**  65 years

**Problem**  For most of her life, Marilyn has been able to control her weight, but recently it has become difficult. She has suffered from back pain for several years and has tried numerous treatments. Most recently Marilyn underwent surgery and her pain has lessened. However, she has not been as active and has gained 4.5kg (10lb) since last year. She finds this weight gain depressing. In addition, she has borderline high blood pressure, which did not need medication, but now her blood pressure is rising.

**Lifestyle**  Marilyn has always led an active life. She raised three children and now spends time with her six

grandchildren. She is 1.57m (5ft 2in) tall and weighed 50kg (110lb) for most of her life. Now she weighs 54.4kg (120lb) and complains that all her clothes are too tight. She eats small portions and snacks on fresh fruit or sometimes yogurt. She drinks cola or iced tea with meals, always has dessert with dinner, and has a small snack before going to bed. She does not drink alcohol. She and her husband frequently eat out and have begun to travel quite a bit.

**Advice**  Gaining weight as you get older is a very common problem. Marilyn cannot eat as many calories as she did when she was younger because she is not as active. Because of her surgery, her activity is limited and this is the most likely explanation for her weight gain. In addition, she has also been eating out more, and this often means larger portions.

There are a number of measures that Marilyn can take. The most important for her overall health as well as for the strength of her back – and to prevent her feeling depressed about her weight gain – would be for her to begin a daily exercise programme such as walking or swimming. This will also help maintain her overall muscle mass, which declines as we age. Since Marilyn already eats small portions, the most significant change in her diet would be to switch to fresh fruit for dessert at dinner, and to substitute water or diet cola for regular cola and sweetened iced tea. She should avoid using salt when cooking and eating out because of her raised blood pressure.

Marilyn does not get sufficient calcium, so she should either drink more milk or eat more low-fat yogurt. If she cannot do this, then she may need to take a calcium supplement.

# Looking at diet plans

There is a proliferation of weight-loss diets, not all of which are good for you.

Many of us have attempted to lose weight at one time or another, and the natural tendency is to look for a fast and easy way to shed that extra weight. As a result, weight loss is now a multi-billion-pound industry, encompassing everything from diet books and slimming clubs to weight-loss programmes selling specially formulated foods and medications.

## Think long-term
Weight loss is difficult and there are no miracle solutions. To lose weight and keep it off takes time

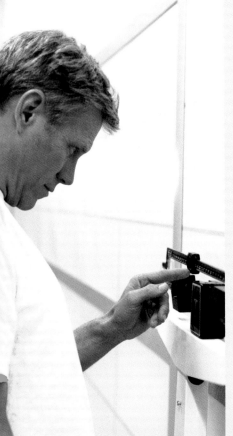

**Monitoring your weight** When you are trying to slim, weighing yourself is one way of monitoring your progress – but do it just once a week, always at the same time of day.

and commitment. Many popular programmes appear to fulfil their promises in the short term by restricting certain food groups. However, these sorts of plans rarely teach you how to establish and maintain healthy eating habits in the long term and, once you have returned to your old eating habits, your lost weight quickly returns.

## Changing your behaviour
Regardless of which type of weight-loss diet you choose to follow, there are guidelines that can help you succeed in changing your eating habits.
• Try to avoid exposing yourself to situations where uncontrolled eating is likely to occur.
• Alter unhealthy eating habits, such as skipping meals or filling up on snacks.
• Change behaviour chains: for example, if you like to eat ice cream late at night, don't buy it – or go to bed earlier.
• Monitor yourself: it has been proved that keeping a food diary helps change eating behaviour.
• Think about how you will address problems and difficult situations before they arise.
• Change the way you think about your weight and your efforts to change it.
• Provide yourself with non-food rewards for accomplishing your weight-loss goals.

## Seeking medical advice
Before beginning any slimming diet, especially very low calorie or quick weight-loss plans, it is a good idea to talk to your GP. This is especially important if you are on any medication as the dose may have to be adjusted. Your

doctor will help you monitor your progress and also determine how much and what type of exercise is appropriate for you. Your GP may also advise you to take vitamin and mineral supplements while you are on the diet.

In general, women who are pregnant or breast-feeding or anyone under the age of 18 should not go on a weight-loss diet. If you are in one of these categories and are concerned about your weight, seek advice from your GP first.

## The diet directory
On the following pages, you will find information on the most popular slimming diets currently available, and guidance about what to expect if you choose a particular plan, including a sample day's menu from each one. We also look at the potential health benefits or hazards of each diet.

There are many types of diets. Some limit certain macronutrients, such as fat or carbohydrates; others limit types of food, such as starchy carbohydrates. Some promote specific foods, such as grapefruit or cabbage soup, while others attempt to regulate your intake according to a strict formula, such as 40 per cent carbohydrate, 30 per cent protein, 30 per cent fat.

Other diet programmes are based on theories that our bodies do not tolerate certain foods and that these have to be eliminated entirely. Most diets are aimed at helping you to lose weight, but others promise a disease-free life to those who follow the plan. When evaluating each of these diets, consider what it promises.

We firmly believe that there is no single best way for everyone to lose weight: most weight-loss diets work for some people; none works for everyone. However, with a little trial and error, everyone should be able to find a weight-loss diet that is effective for them.

| DIET TYPE | UNDERLYING THEORY | DIET PLAN |
|---|---|---|
| **Low-fat** | Weight loss occurs on these very low-fat, high-fibre, mainly vegetarian diets because much less of such foods is required in order to feel satisfied. | • Ornish Diet (see p.164)<br>• Pritikin Diet (see p.164)<br>• Rosemary Conley's Low-fat Diet (see p.165)<br>• Low-fat Living (see p.166)<br>• fatmanslim (see p.167) |
| **Carbohydrate-controlled** | Based on a strict ratio of carbohydrate, protein, and fat, these diets aim to maintain stable blood sugar levels, which helps the body break down fat, work within its "peak performance zone", and maximize weight loss. | • Atkins Diet (see p.167)<br>• Carbohydrate-Addict's Diet (see p.169)<br>• Protein Power Lifeplan (see p.169)<br>• Sugar Busters (see p.170)<br>• Zone Diet (see p.171)<br>• Life Without Bread (see p.172)<br>• Scarsdale Diet (see p.172)<br>• Food Doctor Diet (see p.173)<br>• South Beach Diet (see p.174) |
| **Controlling portion sizes** | Based on the principle that eating large portions is a major factor in becoming overweight, these diet plans promote weight loss by controlling portion sizes. | • Picture Perfect Weight Loss (see p.175)<br>• Volumetrics Weight-control (see p.176)<br>• 90/10 Weight-loss Plan (see p.177)<br>• Change One Eating Plan (see p.177) |
| **Glycaemic index** | These diets are based on the theory that insulin levels and weight can be controlled by eating low-glycaemic-index foods. | • Glucose Revolution (see p.178)<br>• Montignac Method (see p.179)<br>• GI Point Diet (see p.180) |
| **Food-combining** | Based on the belief that different food types are digested in different ways and should not be eaten together; weight loss results from correct combining of food types. | • Hay Diet (see p.180)<br>• Somersizing (see p.181)<br>• New Beverly Hills Diet (see p.182)<br>• Fit for Life (see p.183) |
| **Metabolic typing** | Different blood types affect digestive processes; weight loss occurs when only correct foods for blood type are consumed. | • Eat Right 4 Your Type (see p.184)<br>• Body Code (see p.184)<br>• Metabolic Typing (see p.185) |
| **Quick weight loss** | Based on severe calorie restriction, these plans produce specific weight loss over a very short time period. | • Cabbage Soup Diet (see p.186)<br>• 5-Day Miracle Diet (see p.187)<br>• Grapefruit Diet (see p.188)<br>• Rotation Diet (see p.188)<br>• 14-day Beauty Boot Camp (see p.189) |
| **Low-calorie, liquid meal replacement** | Weight loss based on very low-calorie meal replacements supplying 100 per cent of recommended daily vitamins and minerals. | • Cambridge Diet (see p.189)<br>• Herbalife (see p.190)<br>• SlimFast (see p.190) |
| **Detox** | Programmes aimed at eliminating toxins from the body, since a healthy liver burns fat more efficiently and therefore aids weight loss. | • Fat-Flush Plan (see p.191)<br>• Juice Fasts (see p.192)<br>• Living Beauty Detox (see p.192)<br>• Detox Diet (see p.193) |
| **Weight-loss centres** | Weight-loss programmes supported by regular weigh-ins, advice, and group support; these work on the basis that slimmers find it easier to maintain a diet plan in which they are accountable to others. | • Weight Watchers (see p.194)<br>• National Slimming Centres (see p.195)<br>• Slimming World (see p.196)<br>• LA Weight Loss (see p.196)<br>• Nutrisystem (see p.197) |

# Diet directory

There is a huge variety of diet plans and weight-loss programmes – some sensible, some bizarre, and a few that are potentially dangerous. The most widely used are reviewed here.

## Ornish Diet

*Low-fat*

* ⊗ **Are special products required?**
* ✅ **Is eating out possible?**
* ⊗ **Is the plan family-friendly?**
* ✅ **Do you have to buy a book?**
* ⊗ **Is the diet easy to maintain?**

Dr Dean Ornish is a cardiologist who has demonstrated that the build-up of fatty plaques in the arteries, which causes heart attacks (*see p.215*), is preventable and reversible by following his programme. In addition to the diet, the plan covers regular exercise, anger management, meditation and relaxation exercises, and stopping smoking.

### HOW IT CLAIMS TO WORK
This diet works on the principle that by virtually eliminating fat from your diet, you get fewer calories without eating less. It is a plant-based diet that excludes all cooking oils and animal products, except skimmed milk and low-fat yogurt. It also excludes plant foods that are high in fat, such as nuts and seeds, avocados, and olives. Less than ten per cent of calories from fat is allowed, which amounts to only about 15–25g (½–1oz) of fat per day. The diet is high in fibre and allows moderate use of salt, sugar, and alcohol.

Although this diet does not restrict total calories consumed, when you eat less fat you tend to eat fewer calories. The diet allows you to eat plenty of food and to eat frequently.

### THE REGIMEN
Three meals and one or two snacks per day are allowed, of mostly fat-free foods such as pulses, fruits, grains, and vegetables. These foods can be eaten at any time of day, in fairly unrestricted quantities. Fat-free products and egg whites are allowed in moderation, as are certain commercially available low-fat products such as yogurt. The diet also advocates snacking throughout the day to maintain energy levels rather than eating three large meals at long intervals, and lists ideas for healthy snacks. It recommends eating high-fibre fruits, vegetables, grains, and pulses, which help lower levels of cholesterol (*see p.40*) and the hormone insulin and contribute to weight loss.

### ORNISH DIET

**Breakfast**
* Glass of orange juice
* Bowl of cereal with fresh berries and low-fat plain yogurt

**Lunch**
* Cubes of firm tofu with cooked broccoli florets, potatoes, and chickpeas
* Garlic bread
* Green salad
* Apple

**Dinner**
* Bruschetta with sun-dried tomatoes and capers
* Pasta shapes tossed with red peppers, greens such as spinach, cannellini beans, a little chopped garlic, and grated lemon zest
* Grilled asparagus dressed with lemon and caper vinaigrette, and freshly ground black pepper
* Green salad
* Peaches poached in red wine

**Snacks**
* 1–2 snacks of fresh fruit or raw vegetables

### IS IT HEALTHY?
Research shows that the low-fat, low-cholesterol Ornish Diet can reverse cardiovascular disease (*see pp.214–221*) by lowering blood cholesterol levels and reducing blood pressure (*see p.215*). However, some critics argue that the diet is too low in fat and does not provide sufficient amounts of essential fatty acids (*see p.40*). The diet excludes fish and oil, despite evidence that fish, fish oil, and olive oil provide a protective effect against cardiovascular disease.

Dr Ornish's patients were treated in a spa-like environment where all of the meals were prepared by chefs. For people trying to follow the diet at home, the plan may be difficult to maintain.

## Pritikin Diet

*Low-fat*

* ⊗ **Are special products required?**
* ✅ **Is eating out possible?**
* ✅ **Is the plan family-friendly?**
* ✅ **Do you have to buy a book?**
* ⊗ **Is the diet easy to maintain?**

This low-fat plan was developed in the 1970s by Nathan Pritikin as a means of treating cardiovascular disease. The work is continued today by his son Robert.

### HOW IT CLAIMS TO WORK
This is a low-fat, primarily vegetarian diet based on whole grains, fruits, and vegetables. The author argues that you can eat a much greater volume of low-fat foods and feel satisfied, without taking in too many calories. This diet requires no calorie counting or portion control. Foods are ranked according to their caloric density, and slimmers are encouraged to create a healthy balance of low- and medium-ranked foods. The diet encourages the consumption of healthy fats that are high in omega-3 fatty acids (*see p.40*).

### THE REGIMEN
Processed foods, eggs, and most types of fat are eliminated in favour of whole grains, fruits, and vegetables, and low-fat carbohydrates such as brown rice and wholemeal pasta. The diet is

## PRITIKIN DIET

### Breakfast
- Bowl of cinnamon-flavoured porridge cooked with skimmed milk, topped with sliced banana and blueberries

### Lunch
- Grilled chicken breast with steamed corn-on-the-cob
- Green salad with a fat-free dressing

### Dinner
- Fat-free vegetarian chilli with steamed brown rice
- Tomato and cucumber salad with a balsamic vinegar dressing
- Fresh pineapple slices or pineapple canned in juice

### Snacks
- Baked tortilla chips with a tomato salsa

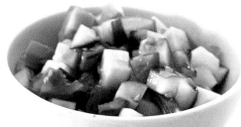

**Pritikin Diet** This spicy and satisfying dish of mixed beans and vegetables, served with brown rice and accompanied by a tomato and cucumber salad, is a typical low-fat, high-fibre, and high-carbohydrate meal from the Pritikin Diet.

therefore high in fibre, low in cholesterol, and low in saturated and total fat. The programme is based on three meals a day with snacks between meals. Less than ten per cent of total daily calories is allowed to come from fat. About 75 per cent of calories should come from carbohydrates and about 15 per cent of calories from protein.

### IS IT HEALTHY?
Although very low-fat diets are often unsatisfying, leading some slimmers to overeat or give up, the health benefits of eating less fat and more fruits, vegetables, and whole grains are well documented – especially their role in the prevention of many long-term diseases. No food groups are entirely eliminated in the Pritikin Diet, and the sample menus provide a large variety of nutritional choices. The revised Pritikin Diet encourages the limited use of fats that are high in omega-3 fatty acids. Overall, we feel that the Pritikin Diet is safe and effective.

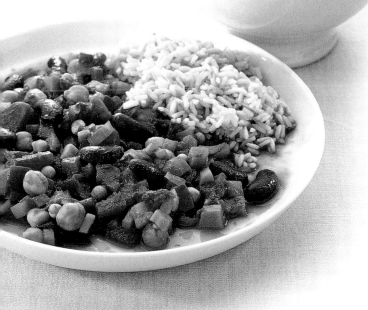

# Rosemary Conley's Low-fat Diet

*Low-fat*

- ✖ Are special products required?
- ✔ Is eating out possible?
- ✔ Is the plan family-friendly?
- ✖ Do you have to buy a book?
- ✔ Is the diet easy to maintain?

The author promotes this diet through various books as well as an online internet site (slimwithrosemary.com) and a bimonthly magazine. There are also Rosemary Conley Diet and Fitness classes that are run under franchise (currently over 180 franchisees run 2000 classes each week throughout the UK). In addition, the author has produced several exercise videos.

## HOW IT CLAIMS TO WORK
The diet works on the principle that because fat contains twice as many calories as protein or carbohydrates, restricting fat will lead to a reduction in the total number of calories consumed. Regular exercise is a very important part of the plan. Exercise helps to burn calories but it also has the advantage of helping to increase lean body mass and increase the metabolic rate. The combination of reduced energy intake and increased energy expenditure helps produce a slow but steady weight loss.

The author advises that most of the food eaten should contain no more than five per cent fat (or 5g fat per 100g/3½oz of food). Notable exceptions are oily fish, which is recommended once a week, and the "150 calorie treat". The regimen recommends eating breakfast, lunch, and dinner with a dessert each day, as well as drinking 300ml (½ pint) of semi-skimmed milk.

## THE REGIMEN
While reducing fat intake, the diet allows unlimited quantities of vegetables – including potatoes – and specified portions of meat and dairy foods in three meals a day. Snacks can be included if the meal quantities are redistributed to accommodate them.

## ROSEMARY CONLEY

**Breakfast**
- Bowl of high-fibre cereal with skimmed milk

**Lunch**
- Grilled chicken breast and mixed salad with a little fat-free dressing
- Wholemeal roll
- Low-fat yogurt

**Dinner**
- Grilled monkfish with lemon and dressing
- Boiled new potatoes
- Steamed French beans
- Fresh fruit salad

**Snacks**
- Banana or other fruit
- Low-fat yogurt

You do not need to count calories and can eat unlimited quantities of some foods to keep hunger at bay. Calorie-counted balanced meal ideas, along with recipes, are provided. Within the personal calorie allowance, a 150-calorie "treat" can also be eaten daily (or saved up for a special occasion each week). The diet provides good advice on subjects such as choosing a balanced diet, eating at least five portions of fruit and vegetables each day, low-fat shopping and cooking, fitting in with family meals, eating out, developing will power, and coping with lapses. Once slimmers reach their target weight, they are advised on how to maintain their weight loss. Regular exercise is advised as part of the plan. For people who don't have the time or don't feel comfortable attending a class, advice is given for exercising at home.

### IS IT HEALTHY?
Weight loss can be impressive with this diet. However, slimmers are encouraged to focus on inches lost from areas such as hips and thighs too. Although the diet is low in fat, an exception is made for healthy sources of fat, such as oil-rich fish. On the whole the regimen is a healthy one and people should lose

weight if they follow it. The fact that it is low in fat can help reduce the risk for health problems such as heart disease and cancer. The emphasis on exercise is good. But being so low in fat the diet may become monotonous after a while.

# Low-fat Living

*Low-fat*

- ⊗ **Are special products required?**
- ⊘ **Is eating out possible?**
- ⊘ **Is the plan family-friendly?**
- ⊘ **Do you have to buy a book?**
- ⊗ **Is the diet easy to maintain?**

This programme is based on four small, low-fat meals and three low-fat, high-fibre snacks per day. The plan also advocates daily exercise.

### HOW IT CLAIMS TO WORK
According to Dr Robert Cooper, the author of this programme, you start to burn fat the moment you get up in the morning. He recommends five minutes of easy physical activity every morning, followed by a low-fat breakfast rich in protein and carbohydrates. Dr Cooper claims that eating low-fat, high-fibre snacks between meals increases your energy and metabolism, and reduces the urge to overeat, especially at night. The book categorizes low-fat, high-fibre snacks, exercise, and drinking water as fat-burners, whereas high-fat, low-fibre meals or snacks and skipping meals are regarded as fat-makers.

Each meal provides fewer than 500 calories, with a maximum of 20–25 per cent of those calories from fat. Snacks should be lower in calories than meals. All recommended meals need to be prepared according to recipes found in the book. Artificially sweetened foods and drinks are not permitted, since they may stimulate an appetite for fats in some people and there is no evidence that they contribute to weight loss.

### THE REGIMEN
The regimen consists of four meals and three snacks daily, which should be eaten at specific times. You should eat breakfast at 7am, snack one at 10am,

lunch at midday, snack two at 3.15pm, pre-dinner appetizer at 5.30pm, dinner at 6–7pm, and snack three at 8.45pm.

Examples of foods on the Low-fat Living programme include: wholemeal breads and crackers, pastas, fat-free dairy products, tomatoes, including pasta sauce, canned foods packed in water, eggs (yolks and whites), fresh vegetables, herbs, spices and dry seasonings, and sweeteners such as brown sugar, honey, maple syrup, molasses, and sugar.

Because this is a low-fat programme, no fatty foods or all-fat dressings are permitted. Fat-free processed products should be consumed sparingly since they may trigger an unusually high insulin response if they are eaten in large quantities. In addition to the type of foods permitted on this diet, the timing of meals and snacks is important. Also low-intensity exercise, especially aerobics, is strongly recommended during the programme.

### IS IT HEALTHY?
Overall, this diet is very healthy since it is low in fat and high in fibre, and can help reduce your blood pressure and cholesterol levels, thus reducing your risk of diabetes (*see p.246–249*) and

## LOW-FAT LIVING

**Breakfast (7am)**
- Boiled egg with toasted wholemeal bread
- Glass of skimmed milk

**Lunch (12pm)**
- Bowl of gazpacho
- Low-fat whole-grain crackers, plain or flavoured with chilli and cheese

**Dinner (5.30–7pm)**
- Green salad with a creamy garlic dressing
- Grilled chicken breast fillet with linguine or other pasta (served without sauce)

**Snacks (10am, 3.15pm, 8.45pm)**
- 3 low-fat, high-fibre snacks such as whole-grain crispbread

cardiovascular disease (*see p.214–221*). You are likely to have more energy and feel good when you follow this diet, since it offers plenty of food and high-fibre snacks, and encourages daily physical activity. Since the diet is very low in fat, however, it may be difficult to follow, especially if you often eat out. Recipes for the suggested meals and snacks are helpful, but might require considerable preparation. You should be careful to stick to the portion sizes.

# fatmanslim

*Low-fat*

⊗ **Are special products required?**
⊘ **Is eating out possible?**
⊘ **Is the plan family-friendly?**
⊗ **Do you have to buy a book?**
⊘ **Is the diet easy to maintain?**

This 12-week programme, presented on an interactive website (fatmanslim.com) based in the UK, has been popular with men since it was launched in 2002. It is founded on the principle that men who want to lose weight also want to remain in control, and make their changes in private and on their own time rather than attending group classes or seeing a nutritionist.

## HOW IT CLAIMS TO WORK
Dr Ian W Campbell, the author, wanted to reach those men whom he knew needed help to lose weight but who were likely to be reluctant to attend his medical clinics or a weight-loss group. The fat that accumulates around a man's waist is, medically speaking, the most dangerous, so the plan focuses on reducing girth size – calling itself a "waist-loss programme". The principle of the plan is long-term lifestyle change.

## THE REGIMEN
An assessment of motivation and long-held habits is followed by a balanced, nutritious diet that encourages eating plenty of fruits and vegetables and reducing fat intake. Absolutely nothing is forbidden, because Dr Campbell recognizes this as a quick way to lose a slimmer's new-found commitment. Daily

## FATMANSLIM

### Breakfast
• Glass of fresh fruit juice
• Low-sugar cereal with banana

### Lunch
• Whole-grain sandwich with low-fat meat or cheese and salad
• Apple

### Dinner
• Grilled chicken breast with rice
• Green salad with fat-free dressing
• Low-fat yogurt or fruit

### Snacks
• If you're hungry, eat fresh fruit ideally
• Low-fat low-sugar snack bar

exercise, which is a major element of the programme, is introduced gradually over the 12 weeks. All forms of physical activity are encouraged, and practical tips on how to increase exercise at a safe rate are given.

Written by men, for men, fatmanslim is direct and practical – and humorous. The medical benefits of modest but sustained weight – and waist – loss are explained, and new techniques are explored to enable a man to find the drive and determination for life-long changes. The programme incorporates medical, psychological, social, and practical information to help.

The website allows for direct access to Dr Campbell's advice, and provides an interactive forum for members to discuss issues and gain support from other men on the programme. The weight-loss principles are traditional, and suitable for the whole family, but the style of delivery makes it ideal for men who want to lose weight at their own pace, and keep it off long-term.

## IS IT HEALTHY?
The benefits of eating a diet that is rich in fruits and vegetables, while low in fats and sugars, are well proved. The diet is balanced and nutritionally sound and will most likely promote weight loss. The added benefits of incorporating

extra physical activity into the daily routine include a reduction in the risk of heart disease, high blood pressure, and diabetes, as well as an increase in self-esteem and energy level, and an overall feeling of well-being.

# Atkins Diet

*Carbohydrate-controlled*

⊗ **Are special products required?**
⊘ **Is eating out possible?**
⊗ **Is the plan family-friendly?**
⊘ **Do you have to buy a book?**
⊗ **Is the diet easy to maintain?**

By severely limiting carbohydrate intake, the Atkins Diet produces ketosis, a state in which the body uses up its stored carbohydrate and begins to burn fats for energy (*see p.168*).

## HOW IT CLAIMS TO WORK
Dr Atkins believed that weight gain is the result of fat synthesis from excess ketones (*see p.168*). He claimed that fat loss occurs when the body changes from using carbohydrates for fuel to using fats. This change requires a period on a low-carbohydrate diet.

The Atkins Diet is organized into different stages. The first stage limits carbohydrates such as bread and pasta, fruits, and some vegetables and includes high-fat food to encourage your body to become ketotic and start using ketones for energy. Some carbohydrates can be reintroduced later, in the maintenance stages of the diet.

## THE REGIMEN
The Atkins programme begins with a 14-day induction phase to place your body into ketosis. During this period, your daily diet consists of 100g protein, which is the equivalent of eating about 400g (14oz) of meat, 75g fat, and less than 20g carbohydrates, totalling 1500–3500 calories per day.

The induction phase is followed by an on-going weight-loss phase, during which you continue to limit your intakes of carbohydrates to less than 30g per day – the amount of carbohydrate in two slices of bread or 225ml (8floz) cola.

## ATKINS DIET: INDUCTION PHASE

**Breakfast**
- Omelette with ham, cheese, bacon, and mushrooms

**Lunch**
- Chef's salad of ham, chicken, cheese, and eggs, with a creamy Italian dressing

**Dinner**
- Grilled salmon
- Steamed kale tossed with finely chopped garlic, lemon juice, and sesame seeds

**Snacks**
- Berries with cream
- Cheese sticks

The programme is then modified to pre-maintenance and maintenance phases, when your carbohydrate intake can be increased up to 120g (4oz) or eight servings per day. (For comparison, note that a typical "balanced" diet would include more than 300g/10oz or 16 servings of carbohydrate per day.)

### IS IT HEALTHY?

Reducing your calorie intake by cutting carbohydrates is a good slimming principle, but not when taken to this extreme. You will lose weight, but the long-term health effects are not known.

Some 3.6–4.5kg (8–10lb) of weight loss during the first week or so on a low-carbohydrate diet such as this is due to water loss associated with using up stored glycogen. However, while such an immediate result provides a psychological boost to a slimmer, once you start eating carbohydrates again this weight will return.

Another criticism of the diet is that glycogen stores are needed for exercise, and exercise is a key to long-term weight maintenance. For example, scientific studies of athletes show that dietary carbohydrate is essential for optimum athletic performance.

Dr Atkins claimed that you can eat as much as you want on his diet; however, like any other diet, this works only to the extent that your calorie intake is less than your calorie expenditure. Ketosis does tend to reduce appetite but, more importantly, eliminating an entire food group is a significant dietary change that may be enough to help you begin to lose weight. For example, many combination foods are eliminated including pizza (because of the crust), hamburgers (because of the bun), and all sandwiches (because of the bread). These foods can be high in fat, and can come in large portion sizes. Many convenience and snack foods such as biscuits, crisps, and pasta are excluded, and instead structured meals and low-fat snacks are eaten, resulting in a lower total calorie intake than usual.

## Jargon buster

**Ketones** These chemicals, also referred to as ketone bodies, are produced by your body when it does not get enough calories from carbohydrates and burns fats for energy instead.

**Ketosis** This is a state in which the body has used up its store of carbohydrates and is producing ketones from the breakdown of fat.

**Ketogenic diet** A diet that causes your body to produce ketones. This involves limiting your intake of carbohydrates. Examples include the Aktins Diet and Scarsdale Diet.

Some people find the metabolic changes that result from this diet uncomfortable. Carbohydrate cravings, for example, may or may not disappear with time. Some people develop blood pressure problems, which can lead to dizziness on rising from a seated position, and some complain of bad breath. The lack of fibre in the Atkins Diet may lead to constipation and an increase in the risk of certain illnesses, such as colon cancer, while the restricted intake of dairy products, fruits, and vegetables may lead to deficiencies in calcium, the B vitamins, vitamin C, and certain important minerals including iron.

In order to counteract these potential deficiencies, Dr Atkins recommended the consumption of specific supplements available from his website. His claims that significant calories will be lost through excreting ketones in urine have been disproved. However, when ketones are excreted, they remove water and the minerals sodium and potassium from the body, which means that people on this programme must drink plenty of water, diet cola, tea, or coffee (but not fruit juices) to avoid dehydration.

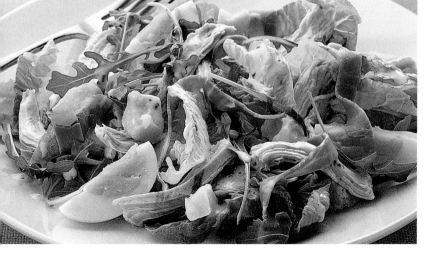

**Atkins Diet** High in protein and saturated fat from ham, chicken, cheese, and eggs, but low in carbohydrate and fibre, this salad is typical of meals from the induction phase of this weight-loss programme.

# Carbohydrate-Addict's Diet

*Carbohydrate-controlled*

⊗ **Are special products required?**
⊘ **Is eating out possible?**
⊘ **Is the plan family-friendly?**
⊘ **Do you have to buy a book?**
⊗ **Is the diet easy to maintain?**

This diet is based on the theory that many people have an exaggerated insulin response to carbohydrates, which creates an addiction to them.

## HOW IT CLAIMS TO WORK

This diet is a modification of the low-carbohydrate programmes such as the Atkins Diet (*see p.167*). Its authors claim that as many as 75 per cent of us are carbohydrate-sensitive. This creates an exaggerated insulin response to carbohydrate intake, leading to hunger and cravings after their consumption. Instead of limiting carbohydrates completely to create ketosis – as in the Atkins Diet – this plan recommends limiting carbohydrate consumption to one hour each day, in order to balance insulin responses. The programme recommends that two out of three meals each day be carbohydrate-free. These are called "complementary" meals. Unlike the other restricted carbohydrate diets, which can lead to carbohydrate craving, this diet allows one "reward" meal each day, during which any foods can be eaten, including carbohydrates, as long as they are part of a balanced meal and are consumed within a one-hour period.

## THE REGIMEN

The diet is somewhat complicated because it is divided into an entry plan and four different diets. Everyone on the diet uses the entry plan and then, once it is completed, you determine whether you will follow plan "A", "B", "C", or "D", according to how much weight you have lost and whether or not you wish to lose more. This is not as difficult as it sounds, since the different regimens are very similar. For example, plan "B"

is the same as plan "A", except that you do not eat the snack.

There are also five guidelines for following the regimen:
● Eat two complementary meals daily.
● Eat one reward meal daily.
● Complete your reward meal within one hour.
● Consume any alcoholic beverages with your reward meal.
● Drink plenty of water, vegetable or fruit juices, or coffee during the day.

## IS IT HEALTHY?

Many of us would probably lose weight if the only time we drank alcohol was with our evening meal and we cut out snacking between meals. If you are the type of person who feels tired an hour after having a piece of cake, or if you get hungry soon after having a carbohydrate-based meal, then this diet will teach you a lot about managing your appetite and avoiding cravings.

On the down side, it is difficult to confine all your carbohydrates to one hour-long period each day and it is not obvious that this provides any benefit over avoiding simple sugars altogether. The authors ran a weight-loss clinic for

### CARBOHYDRATE ADDICT'S DIET

**Breakfast**
● Omelette with steamed spinach and soured cream

**Lunch**
● Big bowl of green beans cooked with olive oil, spring onions, fresh basil, cloves, and chili powder, and topped with soured cream

**Dinner (reward meal)**
● Chicken cooked with 1 tbsp olive oil, lemon juice, garlic, rosemary, salt, and pepper
● Broccoli florets
● Steamed rice
● Cucumber salad dressed with salt, white wine vinegar, soured cream, sesame oil, spring onions, and ginger

**Snacks**
● Only on some plans

years and presumably had good results with their regimen, but there is no data on its long-term health effects or its effectiveness in maintaining lost weight.

The plan is promoted as a lifelong solution to yo-yo dieting; however, there is no evidence as yet that being allowed to eat whatever you like for one hour each day will enable you to maintain the diet and lose weight.

# Protein Power Lifeplan

*Carbohydrate-controlled*

⊗ **Are special products required?**
⊘ **Is eating out possible?**
⊗ **Is the plan family-friendly?**
⊘ **Do you have to buy a book?**
⊗ **Is the diet easy to maintain?**

This high-protein, low-carbohydrate diet claims to help you lose weight, lower cholesterol and blood pressure levels, feel fitter, and restore your health – all in just a few weeks.

## HOW IT CLAIMS TO WORK

The authors believe that eating more protein than is normally recommended will help balance the body's hormonal response to other foods. The plan is more detailed than the Atkins Diet and somewhat more difficult to follow, since protein requirements must be calculated and daily protein intake divided among your meals and snacks. There are no food groups to avoid, so you have to make more decisions.

## THE REGIMEN

Carbohydrates are restricted to between 30–55g per day, which is slightly more than allowed during the middle phases of the Atkins Diet (*see p.167*). This is low enough to induce ketosis. However, this plan does not allow an unlimited intake of fat, and the authors do advise slimmers to seek their doctor's advice before they begin the programme. The plan focuses on a high protein intake, including eggs, cottage cheese, tofu, lean meat, poultry, pork, and seafood. It recommends three meals a day with

## PROTEIN POWER LIFEPLAN

### Breakfast
● Boiled egg with a slice of buttered toast
● Fresh strawberries or raspberries

### Lunch
● Steamed pumpkin
● Fresh spinach salad with vinaigrette or blue cheese dressing
● Fresh blueberries
● Low-fat cottage cheese

### Dinner
● Steamed prawns
● Steamed broccoli and sautéed red or yellow peppers with a low-fat vinaigrette
● Mixed fruit salad

### Snacks
● Sliced raw vegetables, including peppers, carrots, and tomatoes

regular snacks in order to avoid hunger. Carbohydrates are permitted at every meal. In addition to recommending lots of exercise, the plan also suggests taking vitamin and mineral supplements.

### IS IT HEALTHY?
While this diet plan does a better job of explaining the low-carbohydrate approach than the Atkins Diet, it creates the same potential problem of calcium excretion

## Jargon buster

**Aerobic exercise** Any repetitive exercise, such as jogging, in which the body uses oxygen to burn fat. To be effective, it needs to be sustained for at least 15 minutes while you maintain 65–85 per cent of your maximum heart rate.

**Anaerobic exercise** Any vigorous, short-burst exercise that causes your muscles to work without oxygen. Glycogen is burnt for energy. This type of excercise can cause fatigue, but if you exercise regularly your anaerobic fitness will improve.

due to excessive intake of protein. It also requires more work by the liver and the kidneys, which is not advisable for those with liver or kidney problems (see pp.236–239).

The authors of this plan claim that the body has no need for carbohydrate, but if that were true then muscle would store only fat and not glycogen. Glycogen is required for the generation of energy in muscles. If there is no carbohydrate in the diet, the authors claim energy will come from protein.

As yet, no studies have been carried out on the long-term effects of this diet, which may be high in saturated fat and low in many vitamins and in calcium. Recent research has demonstrated that people are more likely to lose weight when their intake of protein is higher than normal, but there is no reason to eliminate carbohydrates in order to do this. While it is true that insulin promotes fat storage, insulin production can be limited by eating complex carbohydrates (see p.46–47) and by eating balanced meals and snacks.

## Sugar Busters

*Carbohydrate-controlled*

✖ **Are special products required?**
✔ **Is eating out possible?**
✖ **Is the plan family-friendly?**
✔ **Do you have to buy a book?**
✖ **Is the diet easy to maintain?**

The authors of this plan believe that we eat too much sugar and refined carbohydrates and that this has contributed to the current increased prevalence of obesity and diabetes.

### HOW IT CLAIMS TO WORK
The authors of this diet recommend that by balancing the proportion of carbohydrate to protein that you eat, you will lose weight because this will increase glucagon production. Glucagon is a hormone that stimulates the release of glucose into the bloodstream.

They suggest that to achieve this, 45 per cent of calories should come from high-fibre carbohydrate sources, 30–35 per cent of calories from fat, and

20–25 per cent from protein. This is based on the idea that eating foods high in sugar causes an overproduction of insulin and also a suppression of glucagon, thus promoting fat storage in the body and inhibiting weight loss.

In addition, the authors emphasize that exercise is important because it lowers insulin levels and increases insulin sensitivity.

### THE REGIMEN
The authors recommend eating more unrefined foods, high-fibre vegetables, stone-ground whole grains, lean meats, fruits, and, if you choose, alcohol in moderation. Excluded vegetables (those containing less than 2.5g of fibre) include beetroot and carrots. The diet plan also recommends eliminating refined sugar, such as is found in cakes, biscuits, sweets, and fizzy drinks, as well as high-glycaemic-index foods (see p.47) such as white flour, pasta, and potatoes.

You are allowed three meals a day, made up of moderate-sized portions, and the authors suggest that you limit the volume of fluids that you drink with each meal. However, they recommend that you drink at least six to eight glasses of water a day, in addition to coffee, tea, and diet cola. You are allowed to snack on all types of fruits.

## SUGAR BUSTERS

### Breakfast
● Glass of orange juice
● Bowl of porridge made with skimmed milk

### Lunch
● Turkey sandwich on whole-grain or wholemeal bread with mustard, lettuce, and tomato

### Dinner
● Grilled or baked pork fillet
● Brown rice cooked with sliced onions in fat-free, unsalted chicken or vegetable stock
● Steamed green beans

### Snacks
● Apple or other fruit
● Small handful of nuts

## IS IT HEALTHY?

While this theory has some scientific rationale, there is no evidence that the proportion of carbohydrate to protein to fat does what the authors claim. However, the focus on high-fibre carbohydrates is healthy, and there are significant potential benefits from reducing our intake of simple carbohydrates such as sugar. While there is no direct evidence that diabetes results from sugar intake, diabetes risk is related to obesity. In turn, obesity is related to calorie intake – and excess calories are often consumed in the form of simple carbohydrates such as soft drinks, juices, sweets, cakes, biscuits, and other snacks. All of us can benefit from reducing the amount of sweet foods we eat, and a period of time following this diet might change a few of your dietary habits.

Some of the ideas presented in this plan – such as that digestive juices are diluted by drinking fluids with your meals – have no scientific evidence to support them. Also, there is certainly no health risk from reducing your intake of simple carbohydrates, but most of us are not likely to give up our sweetened drinks and desserts completely.

More seriously, the plan's emphasis on monitoring precise proportions of carbohydrate, fat, and protein is the kind of inappropriate focus that can result in the development of eating disorders.

# Zone Diet

*Carbohydrate-controlled*

⊗ **Are special products required?**
⊘ **Is eating out possible?**
⊘ **Is the plan family-friendly?**
⊘ **Do you have to buy a book?**
⊗ **Is the diet easy to maintain?**

The aim of this carbohydrate-controlled diet is to make the body work within its peak performance zone for maximum energy, "fat-burning", and weight loss.

## HOW IT CLAIMS TO WORK

According to the Zone Diet plan, what is important is not what you eat, but the balance between what you eat and the hormonal response it creates. In particular, the author looks at food's impact on the body's ability to influence eiconsanoids – chemical messengers derived from dietary fats that control various metabolic processes.

The author states that people can be divided into those who produce enough insulin and those who produce too much of the hormone. He prescribes a very simple test to find out which group you fall into: have pasta for lunch at noon and see how you feel at 3pm. If you can barely keep your eyes open and you are feeling hungry, you are among the 75 per cent of people who have a genetic predisposition to over-produce insulin. The diet plan is designed to limit this and any subsequent overeating.

## THE REGIMEN

Meal plans are tailored to gender, activity level, and current percentage of body fat, but all are based on 40 per cent of calories from carbohydrate, 30 per cent from protein, and 30 per cent from fat. All meals and snacks follow this ratio. The typical British diet generally gets as much as 50–60 per cent of its energy from carbohydrates and about 35–40 per cent from fat. The author believes that a high intake of dietary carbohydrate leads to hyperinsulinism and obesity, while a high intake of dietary protein leads to high glucagon and ketosis.

The diet calls for the consumption of a specific number of small portions of carbohydrate, fat, and protein at regular intervals throughout the day (roughly four and a half hours apart). For most people this means eating three meals a day, and two substantial snacks. The snacks should follow the same ratio of carbohydrate to protein to fat (40:30:30) as your main meals.

The plan suggests that you divide your plate into three equal sections. On one third put low-fat protein, no bigger and no thicker than the palm of your hand. The remaining two thirds of the plate should be filled to overflowing with fruits and vegetables.

## IS IT HEALTHY?

There is no scientific evidence that this plan, which is based on a combination of combating insulin resistance and altering eiconsonoid levels, will produce

---

### ZONE DIET

**Breakfast**
● Flour tortilla wrap filled with grated reduced-fat Cheddar or other cheese, grilled and chopped lean bacon or lean cooked ham, and chopped spring onions, green pepper, and tomato, served with reduced-fat guacamole
● Grapes

**Lunch**
● Open face sandwich of whole-grain or wholemeal bread topped with sliced reduced-fat cheese and grilled lean bacon, with lettuce and sliced tomato
● Low-fat plain yogurt with chopped peaches

**Dinner**
● Pork medallion and sliced apple sautéed in white wine with Dijon mustard and chopped fresh rosemary
● Steamed broccoli
● Large green salad with an olive oil and vinegar dressing

**Snacks**
● Small cooked chicken breast, slice of melon, and a few nuts
● Low-fat cheese and a small orange

---

the health effects claimed. It is more likely that your response to dietary carbohydrates is influenced by your usual diet and activity levels than by some genetic predisposition. While it is true that refined foods or those with a high glycaemic index (*see p.47*) may overstimulate insulin secretion, this can be avoided by consuming low-glycaemic-index carbohydrates.

This is a complicated regimen that few can follow accurately. The diet may be high in saturated fat, depending on the types of proteins selected. There are also potential problems linked to high protein intake, such as bone loss.

The author sells specific "zone" food products such as snack bars that claim to slow ageing. However, there is no evidence to support such claims.

# Life Without Bread

*Carbohydrate-controlled*

⊗ **Are special products required?**
⊘ **Is eating out possible?**
⊘ **Is the plan family-friendly?**
⊘ **Do you have to buy a book?**
⊗ **Is the diet easy to maintain?**

This diet is based on the clinical experience of Dr Lutz, an Austrian physician who claims to have helped thousands of patients to lose weight and achieve health by following low-carbohydrate diets.

## HOW IT CLAIMS TO WORK

Life Without Bread is based on eating a low-carbohydrate, high-fat, high-protein diet. The authors claim that this was what humans ate during evolution, and it is what we are suited to. Today's typical high-carbohydrate, low-fat diet, they claim, is alien to our species.

The authors also describe the benefits of low-carbohydrate diets in relation to disorders such as cardiovascular disease, diabetes, gastrointestinal disorders,

### LIFE WITHOUT BREAD

**Breakfast**
• Scrambled eggs with wholemeal bread (no spread)
• Glass of orange juice

**Lunch**
• Grilled chicken breast with boiled fresh or frozen peas
• Large green salad with olive oil and vinegar dressing

**Dinner**
• Grilled tuna steak
• Steamed green beans and steamed brown rice

**Snacks**
• Plain whole-milk yogurt
• Nuts
• Piece of cheese
• Apple

obesity, and cancer. In the section on cardiovascular disease, they claim that saturated fats and cholesterol from animal foods do not contribute to cardiovascular disease, and argue that current nutritional advice on this topic is flawed.

## THE REGIMEN

This diet restricts carbohydrates, of which no more than 72g (or six bread units, each containing 12g carbohydrate) per day should be consumed – hence the name of the diet. Examples of what one bread unit consists of include:
• ½ cup dry pasta
• 1 slice of bread
• Half grapefruit
• 225ml (8floz) milk or yogurt
• 225ml (8floz) beer.
Foods restricted in the diet include most that contain carbohydrates (breads, pastries, cereals and grains, pasta, potatoes) as well as sweet fruits, dried fruits, and sweetened foods of any kind (yogurt, drinks, desserts, sweets).

You can eat all the protein foods, cheese, non-starchy vegetables, and healthy fats you want from a variety of plant and animal sources, along with moderate amounts of nuts, yogurt, and whole milk. Protein foods (meat, poultry, and fish) can be fried, baked, roasted, grilled, or steamed.

The diet does not provide any specific menu plans, but it does explain how to work the low-carbohydrate eating plan into meals and snacks. A table listing grams of carbohydrate for a variety of items allows the reader to plan full menus containing a wide variety of foods.

## IS IT HEALTHY?

The Life Without Bread programme is a moderately low-carbohydrate, rather than an extremely low-carbohydrate, diet. By limiting carbohydrates to less than 72g per day, you can follow this programme without severe restrictions on healthy foods such as fruits and dairy products, both of which are permitted in limited amounts.

Although this book is entitled *Life Without Bread*, meal planning is based on "bread units", each of which contain 12g of carbohydrate. So this diet is not really about eliminating carbohydrates or bread, but limiting intake and finding

alternatives to form the basis of your meals. The diet promotes a healthy weight loss because you are reducing calories but still consuming a variety of carbohydrates.

Compared to some other plans, the book is complicated and technical, which may be difficult for the average reader to follow every day.

The authors of Life Without Bread claim that low-carbohydrate diets can help or cure diabetes, gastrointestinal disorders, cardiovascular disease, and even cancer. They do not accept that saturated fat contributes to increasing blood cholesterol or LDL levels (*see p.38–40*). On the contrary, they urge the consumption of foods high in saturated fat, such as cheese, cream cheese, soured cream, and whole milk. As there is a huge amount of evidence that limiting saturated fat is important for the prevention of these chronic diseases, this is a major flaw in the diet.

# Scarsdale Diet

*Carbohydrate-controlled*

⊗ **Are special products required?**
⊘ **Is eating out possible?**
⊗ **Is the plan family-friendly?**
⊘ **Do you have to buy a book?**
⊗ **Is the diet easy to maintain?**

In common with other high-protein, low-carbohydrate diets, this plan claims to produce weight loss by forcing the body into ketosis (*see p.168*).

## HOW IT CLAIMS TO WORK

This very high-protein, low-carbohydrate, short-term, calorie-restricted diet claims to alter your metabolism and produce a 450g (1lb) a day weight loss, with up to 9kg (20lb) or more in two weeks.

Because the Scarsdale Diet is very low in fat and carbohydrates, it is claimed that the body will be forced into ketosis and begin to burn stores of fat rather than carbohydrates for energy. The metabolism of fat produces ketone bodies, and the greater the amount of ketone bodies produced by the body, the more body fat is broken down, and the more weight is lost.

## THE REGIMEN

The Scarsdale Diet allows 1000 calories or fewer per day, and averages 43 per cent protein, 22.5 per cent fat, and 34.5 per cent carbohydrates. The calories are distributed among three meals, spaced throughout the day. The only between-meal snacks permitted are carrots and celery. Oil, mayonnaise, and other salad dressings are not permitted; salads are dressed only with vinegar and lemon juice. Vegetables are eaten without butter or oil; lemon juice or vinegar can be used instead. Skin is removed from chicken and turkey before eating and all meats must be lean. Alcoholic beverages are not allowed, but you are encouraged to drink plenty of water. Decaffeinated coffee, tea, diet cola, and soda water are permitted when on the diet.

Because the diet is so low in calories, it is limited to 14 days at a time. It may last five, nine, or 14 days, depending on how much weight you want to lose. After two weeks, you have to switch to the "Keep Trim Program", which offers an expanded list of foods and drinks. It includes one alcoholic drink daily, all lean meats including chicken and turkey, fish, eggs, cheeses, soups, vegetables, fruits, nuts, bread, condiments, and herbs, seasoning, and spices. Bread is

### SCARSDALE DIET

**Breakfast**
● Grapefruit half
● Slice of toasted bread (no spread)

**Lunch**
● Assortment of lean cooked meats (eg sliced chicken, turkey, tongue, and beef)
● Sliced raw, grilled, or stewed tomatoes

**Dinner**
● Fish or shellfish salad
● Slice of toasted bread (no spread)
● Grapefruit half

**Snacks**
● Carrots or celery

still limited to two slices per day. Sugar, pasta, potatoes, sweets and desserts, cream, whole milk, dairy products made with whole milk, and fatty meats are not permitted.

### IS IT HEALTHY?

An older version of the Atkins Diet (*see p.167*), this diet is dangerously low in carbohydrates and is lacking in many key vitamins and minerals found in

**Scarsdale Diet** This platter of lean meat and tomatoes is typical of the high-protein meals allowed during the initial phase of the diet.

carbohydrates and dairy products. If followed, it will promote weight loss, but it is a very difficult diet to maintain, as it is highly restrictive and has very limited snacks. If you follow this diet, you are likely to be hungry between meals and need to eat a more substantial snack to satisfy your cravings. In addition, because of the Scarsdale Diet's high-protein content, it is not appropriate for people with kidney disease and may pose serious health risks if followed for more than the recommended 14 days.

# Food Doctor Diet

*Carbohydrate-controlled*

⊗ **Are special products required?**
⊘ **Is eating out possible?**
⊘ **Is the plan family-friendly?**
⊘ **Do you have to buy a book?**
⊘ **Is the diet easy to maintain?**

The Food Doctor Diet is written by Ian Marber, a graduate of the Institute for Optimum Nutrition. Marber is head of the Food Doctor clinic in London, where he advises clients on a wide range of nutrition problems. This simple and straightforward programme promises to help you achieve a healthy digestive system, good health, and lifelong weight control, without your feeling hungry or having to count calories.

## HOW IT CLAIMS TO WORK

This plan focuses on achieving good health, especially for your digestive system. The author suggests that a healthy digestive system will enhance the absorption of nutrients, and reduce cravings for sugary and processed foods and for sweet, fizzy drinks. In the book he educates readers about the normal physiology of digestion, absorption, and intestinal bacteria.

The programme recommends including lean proteins, complex or starchy carbohydrates that are broken down slowly, monounsaturated fats, and a variety of healthy foods in the daily diet. Regular exercise is also recommended, and the author states that the plan is safe, sustainable, and simple to follow.

## THE REGIMEN

The Food Doctor Diet places a great deal of emphasis on intestinal health. The author believes that a diet high in saturated fats, processed foods, and /or sugar can lead to the growth of yeasts and unfriendly bacteria in the gut, which can cause bloating, food cravings, and problems such as thrush. The Food Doctor plan focuses on lean proteins, essential fats, fibre, and carbohydrates that are absorbed slowly.

The book begins with an initial seven-day plan designed to improve digestion and reduce fermentation in the gut. The plan is based around small meals and regular snacks. Fruit is forbidden in the first week because it contains fructose, which the author believes encourages the growth of unfriendly bacteria. Meat is also forbidden in this initial stage as are tea, coffee, and alcohol. This initial phase is followed by ten principles on how to achieve a long-term healthy eating programme, which the author refers to as a "Plan for Life".

The plan places a lot of emphasis on selecting carbohydrates that have a low glycaemic index (see p.47) and then

### THE FOOD DOCTOR DIET

**Breakfast**
- Glass of hot water with lemon juice
- 2 eggs, poached or scrambled
- Slice of rye bread, lightly toasted

**Lunch**
- Bowl of home-made soup
- Grilled turkey breast
- Brown rice
- Salad that contains 5 different vegetables and salad leaves

**Dinner**
- Stir-fried mixed vegetables such as carrots, courgettes, asparagus, and baby corn, with strips of skinless chicken breast or prawns
- Glass of mineral water

**Snacks**
- Oatcakes with sliced turkey or guacamole
- Apple or pear with 5 Brazil nuts

combining them with lean protein foods and fibrous vegetables to slow absorption of their sugars into the bloodstream. The author suggests that the ideal ratio of nutrients for lunch will come from a meal in which 40 per cent of the food on the plate is lean protein, such as a grilled skinless chicken breast, 20 per cent is complex carbohydrate, such as brown rice, and the remaining 40 per cent is vegetables. If you eat late in the evening the author recommends that you aim for a meal in which 50 per cent of the food on the plate is lean protein, such as grilled fish, and the remainder is filled with vegetables.

Numerous recipes are included to help you succeed during the initial phase, including broth-based vegetable soups, which are an integral part of the menus. A food diary is also supplied to enable you to track what you eat and drink as well as how you feel during the first three days of the initial week. A shopping list for the seven-day menu plan is also provided.

The Plan For Life section of the book supplies useful information about food shopping and healthy ways to cook. In addition, the author sets out specific principles, such as the importance of eating protein with carbohydrates and drinking adequate fluids. The book also includes ideas for meal planning and a lot of healthy recipes that appear quite tasty and easy to prepare.

### IS IT HEALTHY?

The principles of the Food Doctor Diet are sound. In both the initial seven-day menu plan and the Plan for Life, portion sizes are small and many will be hungry trying to follow the programme, but almost everyone should lose weight. While we are not convinced of the validity of the healthy digestive system concept, the diet recommended is healthy and the "principles" proposed will help many to achieve their dietary goals. Many interesting recipes are included, which adds to the value of this book. We do not agree that many patients' weight problems are related to intestinal inflammation, but this book may be especially helpful for patients with digestive problems such as gluten enteropathy (coeliac disease).

# South Beach Diet

*Carbohydrate-controlled*

- ⊗ Are special products required?
- ⊘ Is eating out possible?
- ⊘ Is the plan family-friendly?
- ⊘ Do you have to buy a book?
- ⊘ Is the diet easy to maintain?

This programme is another modification of the low-carbohydrate diets and was developed by a prominent Miami cardiologist as a means of improving the health of his patients.

## HOW IT CLAIMS TO WORK

The author of this diet believes that other low-carbohydrate diets, such as Atkins (see p.167), neglect the healthy aspects of carbohydrates by limiting intake of this food group. He also claims that other low-carbohydrate diets encourage the intake of saturated fats and proteins, which can lead to high triglycerides and cholesterol (see pp.39–41). This diet, in contrast, limits "bad" carbohydrates, such as white bread and other refined wheat products, potatoes, and white rice, while maintaining the consumption of "good" carbohydrates such as brown rice and wholemeal pasta.

For the first phase of the diet, which lasts for two weeks, carbohydrates are completely eliminated, including fruits and alcohol. The author claims that this alters the way the body processes carbohydrates and reverses or prevents insulin resistance, the precursor to diabetes (see pp.246–251).

On completion of the first phase, carbohydrates are gradually reintroduced, along with fruit and wine. The staple of this diet becomes lean meats, vegetables, low-fat dairy products, and eggs. The diet is claimed to be easy to maintain since it allows slimmers to eat until their hunger is satiated. It also encourages both midday snacking and an evening dessert in addition to a filling breakfast.

The theory of the South Beach Diet is that the structured meals and snacks prescribed in the book will maintain satiety and prevent you from snacking on bad carbohydrates, such as crisps, cakes, and biscuits.

## SOUTH BEACH DIET: PHASE I

### Breakfast
- Glass of vegetable juice
- Western egg white omelette, made with liquid egg substitute mixed with chopped red pepper, chopped green pepper, chopped spring onion, and grated reduced-fat cheese

### Lunch
- Chef's salad of mixed greens topped with cooked ham and turkey, low-fat cottage cheese, and 2 tbsp balsamic vinaigrette
- Sugar-free fruit jelly

### Dinner
- Grilled salmon with steamed asparagus and mashed potatoes
- Green salad with olive oil and vinegar dressing
- Virtually-fat-free fromage frais flavoured with a few drops of vanilla extract and sweetened with a sugar substitute

### Snacks
- Reduced-fat mozzarella cheese
- Celery stick with reduced-fat cream cheese

## THE REGIMEN

The diet is divided into three phases. In each one you can eat three meals and a mid-morning and afternoon snack. The lists of permitted foods change in each phase. Phase I, which lasts for two weeks, excludes all carbohydrates, including fruits, sweets, and alcohol.

In Phase II, the diet becomes more liberal, with the reintroduction of fruits and one forbidden food. For example, if you love chocolate you can add chocolate to your second two weeks of the diet. Phase III of the diet serves as a maintenance phase, when more portions of forbidden foods are added – in moderation.

Most of the weight loss occurs during the first two phases of this programme, and the author claims that the diet is very flexible. If you go on holiday and gain weight, for example, you would simply revert to the initial phase for

another two weeks when you return home. Recipes are provided for each phase of the diet, including several from restaurants in the Miami area.

## IS IT HEALTHY?

Certain aspects of this diet are extremely logical and probably helpful for people trying to lose weight. For example, eating until you are full will help you maintain the diet for the necessary period of time. The diet is also positively healthy, because it encourages the abundant consumption of vegetables and, unlike the Atkins Diet (see p.167), does not allow unlimited intake of fats and proteins. Slimmers are encouraged to use monounsaturated oils, such as olive oil, when cooking and to stick to moderate portions of lean meats such as fish and poultry. This advice should help dieters improve their cholesterol and lipid profiles as well as lose weight.

However, it is difficult to completely give up carbohydrates, even for two weeks, and those who are not used to following recipes and preparing foods every day may find it difficult to follow this diet. The absence of fruit in the first phase is also questionable.

The book is practical – it dedicates a chapter to eating out and makes many suggestions for foods that could be ordered at a restaurant. The book describes the glycaemic index – how the carbohydrates affect blood glucose levels (see p.47). For example, a baked potato is different to mashed or boiled potato, since the body will process the former much more quickly. The author suggests that if you must eat a baked potato, top it with some grated cheese: this will make it healthier by slowing the body's absorption of carbohydrate.

This diet claims to be scientifically proved, but no real data is presented, apart from the results witnessed by the author. The idea that snacking will be prevented simply by maintaining satiety is also unproved. Finally, although the author addresses the use of medication in weight control, he neglects to cover the benefits of exercise, implying that the South Beach Diet itself is enough to maintain health. This is a serious omission, since exercise is an essential component of weight control.

# Picture Perfect Weight Loss

*Controlling portion sizes*

- ⊗ **Are special products required?**
- ⊘ **Is eating out possible?**
- ⊘ **Is the plan family-friendly?**
- ⊘ **Do you have to buy a book?**
- ⊗ **Is the diet easy to maintain?**

This plan, which was devised by Dr Shapiro, gets its name from the pictorial comparisons of foods that it employs to show the calculated calorie content of different food choices.

## HOW IT CLAIMS TO WORK

Drawing on his years in clinical practice counselling those who wish to lose weight and keep it off, Dr Shapiro has developed a programme that he calls "Food Awareness Training", to teach his clients how to make mindful choices about food. His principle is that people must change their relationship with food and learn to select low-calorie foods that can be eaten in filling, satisfying portions, rather than high-calorie alternatives that result in weight gain.

Successful weight loss following this plan comes from applying Dr Shapiro's principles to adhere to a reduced-calorie diet and also by increasing your levels of physical activity.

## THE REGIMEN

Dr Shapiro has developed a flexible, non-restrictive programme in which no food is taboo, and no prescription is offered for when to eat or for "correct" portions. When beginning this diet, you are asked to keep a food diary faithfully for at least a week, detailing when and what foods you ate along with the degree of hunger and the situation in which eating occurred. Keeping the diary serves as an awareness tool to increase forethought and responsibility for food choices and to highlight pitfalls in your eating habits. Once conscious of your current eating habits, you will make healthier choices and modify your eating behaviour. To assist you in making better choices, Dr Shapiro provides pictures that graphically demonstrate the number of calories in various portions of foods. Dr Shapiro also includes a list of foods that you should stock to eat at any time, a supermarket shopping guide, an exercise guide, and a selection of menus from restaurants, with options highlighted.

## IS IT HEALTHY?

The strength of Dr Shapiro's plan is its emphasis on a healthy, reduced-calorie diet and regular exercise. He offers good advice on how to rethink your relationship with food, and diets in particular. The food diary is an important tool for success, especially if you have someone you can share it with in order to establish support and accountability.

If you use it correctly, this programme will accomplish reduction of calories without feelings of deprivation. Calorie counting is not necessary, but some people may find it difficult to visualize the calorie and portion comparisons. In this respect, the lone slimmer may have a more difficult time than those people who can visit Dr Shapiro's clinic on a weekly basis in order to meet with his nutritional counsellors and dietitians.

### PICTURE PERFECT WEIGHT LOSS

**Breakfast**
- Small bowl of chopped banana and melon
- Smoked salmon
- Pumpernickel bread

**Lunch**
- Tossed salad with prawns and a light dressing
- Sourdough bread

**Dinner**
- Bowl of Manhattan clam chowder
- Pasta primavera
- Mixed berries with raspberry sorbet

**Snacks**
- Low-fat yogurt
- Piece of fruit
- Rice cakes
- Handful of almonds

# Volumetrics Weight-control

*Controlling portion sizes*

- ⊗ **Are special products required?**
- ⊘ **Is eating out possible?**
- ⊘ **Is the plan family-friendly?**
- ⊘ **Do you have to buy a book?**
- ⊘ **Is the diet easy to maintain?**

The concept of satiety, or feeling of fullness after a meal, forms the basis of this weight-loss and maintenance programme. The authors believe that the fuller you feel at the end of a meal, the less you are likely to eat between meals or at the next meal.

## HOW IT CLAIMS TO WORK

The aim of this programme is to create satiety by choosing low-calorie foods in quantities that make you feel full, rather than eating the same volume of high-calorie foods. Successful weight loss on the plan occurs by reducing calorie intake through food choices that satisfy your appetite and meet the American daily nutritional requirements, as well as by increasing the amount of exercise you do. The authors claim that you can expect to lose 450–900g (1–2lb) per week. Subsequent weight maintenance is achieved by making the same food choices, but balancing consumption of calories with calorie expenditure.

## THE REGIMEN

During the weight-loss phase, which should not exceed six months at a time, the authors suggest reducing calorie intake by 500–1000 calories per day. Three meals each day plus snacks are recommended, and the proportions should follow those of the United States Department of Agriculture's Food Guide Pyramid. This suggests that 20–30 per cent of total calories should come from fat; 55 per cent from carbohydrates, in the form of whole grains, vegetables, and fruits (aiming for 20–30g of fibre daily); and 15 per cent of total calories from proteins, including lean meats, low-fat fish, and poultry without the skin. Moderate amounts of sugar and

### VOLUMETRICS WEIGHT-CONTROL

**Breakfast**
- Citrus fruit salad
- English muffin with low-calorie spread and low-sugar jam or fruit concentrate
- Glass of semi-skimmed milk

**Lunch**
- Mexican mixed bean and cheese wrap with baked tortilla chips and tomato salsa
- Peaches

**Dinner**
- Steak and vegetable kebabs with asparagus
- Cos salad with a low-calorie dressing
- Cubes of watermelon with a scoop of fat-free frozen yogurt or sorbet

**Snacks**
- Handful of mini pretzels

alcohol are allowed in this diet, as are tea and coffee. Water (2.2 litres/72floz per day for women and 2.9 litres/96floz a day for men) may come from food or drinks. No foods are eliminated from Volumetric Weight-control, but those that are high in calories are limited.

## IS IT HEALTHY?

The Volumetrics Weight-control plan is based on sound, sensible principles for weight loss and maintenance and is backed by short-term studies that confirm its potential for success. Long-term studies are underway. The book provides a clear explanation of the diet's underlying principles as well as comprehensive guides for choosing low-calorie, low-energy-dense foods. Sample menu plans and recipes are also included.

Followed correctly, weight loss is safely accomplished by making wise food choices, reducing calories while still meeting nutritional needs, and increasing physical activity. Because no food is eliminated, the feeling of deprivation is avoided, which makes this programme sustainable.

This is a safe and effective weight-control programme for everyone from the moderately overweight to the obese. If you follow it, try to keep your calorie intake to at least 1000 calories per day and eat a wide variety of foods.

# 90/10 Weight-loss Plan

*Controlling portion sizes*

* Are special products required?
* Is eating out possible?
* Is the plan family-friendly?
* Do you have to buy a book?
* Is the diet easy to maintain?

This is a low-calorie plan, high in fibre, phytochemicals, and antioxidants and low in saturated fat. The title refers to the concept of eating healthily 90 per cent of the time, while for the other ten per cent you can enjoy "fun foods".

## HOW IT CLAIMS TO WORK
On this 14-day plan, which may be repeated until you achieve your goal weight, you lose weight by limiting your calorie intake to between 1200 and 1600 calories daily, depending on your current weight and activity level. Ninety per cent of each day's calories should come from the menus provided, and the remaining ten per cent from a list of "fun foods". The programme relies on portion control, and by allowing the foods we often crave, encourages you to eat those foods in moderate amounts. Physical activity is emphasized as an important component in losing weight and in keeping it off.

The author, Joy Bauer, claims that you may lose up to 4.5kg (10lb) in the first two weeks but admits that much of that is usually water loss; in subsequent weeks, 250–900g (½–2lb) is average. The author discourages quicker weight loss as being unsafe and running the risk of losing lean muscle mass.

## THE REGIMEN
In the 90/10 Weight-loss Plan, you follow a daily menu, which includes breakfast, lunch, dinner, and snacks.

Each day, you choose one item from the list of fun foods or snacks. This may be eaten at any time during the day. Calorie counting is not necessary if you follow the menus, but the calorie range for each meal is given in case you are not able to follow the menus provided. The plan offers menus for 14 days, and additional main course alternatives are suggested to lend diversity to the plan. Multivitamin and calcium supplements are recommended, and the programme encourages you to drink plenty of water, coffee, tea, and soda water.

Before you begin the diet, the author suggests taking a "before" photograph, writing down your clothing size and body measurements, and, if possible, having your body fat measured. She then recommends repeating this two weeks later, so that you can track your progress in other ways besides weight.

## IS IT HEALTHY?
The 90/10 Weight-loss Plan is based on the interesting concept of eating healthily for 90 per cent of the time, then being allowed to "cheat" for the remainder. The menus are designed to be low in saturated fat and high in fibre, phytochemicals, and antioxidants.

Even if you substitute some of the other dinner plans provided, this diet may become monotonous, since you are asked to repeat the menu repertoire every two weeks for as long as it takes to achieve your target weight loss. The

### 90/10 WEIGHT-LOSS PLAN

**Breakfast**
* Whole-grain waffle with fresh berries

**Lunch**
* Cottage cheese with a fresh fruit salad

**Dinner**
* Spinach lasagne
* Green salad with olive oil and vinegar dressing

**Snacks**
* Muesli bar or cereal bar
* Crisps (fun food)

1200-calories-per-day diet included in the book is very restrictive; few will be able to follow it successfully for extended periods of time. The book includes tips for subsequent weight maintenance, but it could be more instructive in teaching you how to determine sensible portion sizes and how to make healthy meal choices, especially when you are eating out.

# Change One Eating Plan

*Controlling portion sizes*

* Are special products required?
* Is eating out possible?
* Is the plan family-friendly?
* Do you have to buy a book?
* Is the diet easy to maintain?

Based on the idea that it takes time to adjust to new habits, this 12-week plan advises making just one change to your eating habits each week. Online support and information are available.

## HOW IT CLAIMS TO WORK
The plan starts by overhauling your breakfast routine and then, over the first month, works through lunch, snacks, and dinner. Each chapter provides a guide to staying within 1300 calories a day (or up to 1600 calories a day for the active or significantly overweight) by focusing on portion control. Change One is based on the principle it is not what you eat, but how much you eat that is at the root of weight problems. The menus provide reduced calories without compromising nutritional value or fibre intake. Since exercise is included as part of the programme, you can expect to lose weight in safe amounts (450g to 1.35kg/1–3lb per week) and maintain weight loss. A limited trial showed that volunteers who followed the programme over the 12-week period lost an average of 7.7kg (17lb).

## THE REGIMEN
In the first week of the diet, the focus is on breakfast. Lower-calorie, nutritionally balanced meals begin the day, but you

## CHANGE ONE EATING PLAN

### Breakfast
• Plain yogurt layered with crunchy cereal, fruit, and coconut

### Lunch
• Chef's salad with cooked turkey breast, ham, grated cheese, and a low-fat dressing
• Whole-grain roll
• Cubes of orange-fleshed melon such as cantaloupe

### Dinner
• Grilled halibut steak with grilled onions and spring onions, ziti or other small pasta shapes, and steamed courgettes
• Blueberry mousse

### Snacks
• Baked tortilla chips with salsa

are encouraged to eat as you usually would for the rest of the day. In the following three weeks, changes are gradually made to lunch, snacks, and dinner, until you have totally overhauled your daily eating habits.

In the last eight weeks, you focus on how to make good choices when eating out and at weekends and holidays, how to stock a healthy kitchen, and how to incorporate other good habits, such as regular exercise, to help you keep on track towards your goal. All foods are allowed in appropriate amounts, and moderate amounts of good fats are also included in the plan.

Change One offers meal suggestions and recipes. It also covers potential pitfalls, and slimmers are encouraged to keep a food diary. Each chapter has a guide suggesting optimum strategies for speeding up weight loss.

### IS IT HEALTHY?
The Change One Eating Plan offers a sensible, sound regimen that will lead safely to weight loss and weight control without compromising good nutrition. The recipes, meal plans, and shopping guides provide helpful tools and structure throughout the 12-week plan. The online support and additional information may

also prove valuable, since those who have the backing of a support group tend to be more successful in their weight-loss efforts than those people who try to go it alone.

# Glucose Revolution

*Glycaemic index*

- ⊗ **Are special products required?**
- ⊘ **Is eating out possible?**
- ⊘ **Is the plan family-friendly?**
- ⊘ **Do you have to buy a book?**
- ⊘ **Is the diet easy to maintain?**

Based on the glycaemic index (GI; *see p.47*), diets such as this were developed originally to help people with diabetes, but the emphasis on unrefined grains and other useful carbohydrates, low-fat foods, and plentiful fresh fruit and vegetables will aid healthy weight loss for a wide range of people.

### HOW IT CLAIMS TO WORK
The Glucose Revolution is based on extensive research of the glycaemic index, which is a numerical way of describing how the carbohydrate in individual foods immediately affects blood-sugar levels. High-GI foods

increase blood-sugar levels, causing a rapid rise and subsequent fall in blood sugar, stimulating a counter-regulator response and possibly an increased appetite. This diet claims to ensure that you eat enough and eat the right kind of carbohydrates. It is directed at helping people with diabetes and those with excess fat in the abdominal area.

### THE REGIMEN
The diet is based on a selection of low-GI foods. These have the advantage for weight loss of containing more fibre, so they fill you up and satisfy your hunger. In addition, such foods tend to be less processed and contain less sugar than high-GI foods. Suggestions include eating five servings of vegetables and pulses every day, two servings of fruits, and four servings of bread and cereals; eating regularly; and decreasing your intake of total fat and saturated fat.

### IS IT HEALTHY?
The concept of a glycaemic index has been controversial for a number of years because of variations in the technology used to measure the speed of the

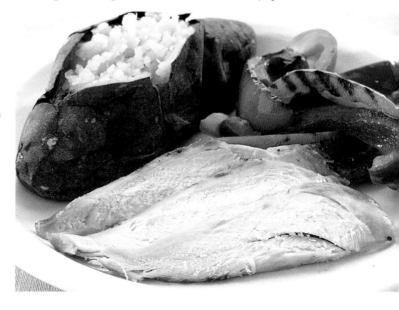

**Glucose Revolution** Roast chicken breast, baked sweet potato, and grilled peppers provide a typical low-fat, low-GI, high-fibre meal on this programme.

glucose response. However, with more modern methods and standardization of measurements, GI is one way to evaluate how carbohydrates can affect blood-sugar levels, either when eaten alone or with meals. This concept is particularly important for people with diabetes and abdominal obesity, since the insulin resistance that accompanies these conditions makes it difficult for their bodies to metabolize large amounts of carbohydrates. The glycaemic index has also been distorted to form the basis of other well-known diets, and this has created some misunderstanding of the concept. This book recommends a more balanced long-term approach that can be successfully maintained.

The plan advocates eating plenty of fibre-rich vegetables and pulses every day. Maximizing fresh fruits, whole-grain breads, and cereals that have a low-GI value, and minimizing saturated fat intake, this programme will promote a sensible, well-balanced, healthy weight loss. The Glucose Revolution diet may be especially helpful for people with type 2 diabetes (see pp.246–251).

Specific advice on quantities, for both small and average eaters, is supplied in the book's weight-loss section.

## GLUCOSE REVOLUTION

### Breakfast
● Bran cereal with skimmed or semi-skimmed milk
● Whole-grain bread with low-sugar jam

### Lunch
● Chicken, turkey, or ham sandwich on whole-grain or wholemeal bread
● Green salad

### Dinner
● Roast chicken with baked sweet potato and grilled green and red pepper strips
● Low-fat ice cream with sliced fresh pears or canned pears in fruit juice

### Snacks
● Fresh fruit

# Montignac Method

*Glycaemic index*

⊗ **Are special products required?**
✔ **Is eating out possible?**
✔ **Is the plan family-friendly?**
✔ **Do you have to buy a book?**
✔ **Is the diet easy to maintain?**

Developed by Michel Montignac, this diet plan combines a reduction in high glycaemic-index (GI) foods (see p.47) with recommendations for specific combinations of foods.

## HOW IT CLAIMS TO WORK
The diet is based on reducing high-GI foods and increasing low-fat, high-fibre, low-GI foods, along with some specific food combinations. The diet does not require calorie-counting and you can eat as much as you wish, as long as it is the right kind of food.

Foods are categorized in the diet as carbohydrates (good and bad), lipids (meat, dairy, and oils), carbohydrate-lipids (nuts, avocados, and offal), and fibre (vegetables and whole grains). Combinations of carbohydrates and lipids in the same meal are not allowed.

## THE REGIMEN
The diet is divided into two phases:
● Phase I of the diet consists of three meals per day, following the food-combining principles (fruits – which are classified as good carbohydrates – must be eaten alone, not with or close to any other meal).
● Phase II allows you to gradually reintroduce some "bad" carbohydrates. You can begin to drink some wine and eat a little unsweetened dark chocolate.

You should minimize drinking with a meal, but can drink plenty of water at other times. Aim to avoid coffee and tea altogether.

## IS IT HEALTHY?
Weight loss on this diet is promoted by the reduced calorie intake that occurs when you give up foods such as chips and pastries. The fact that you can eat

## MONTIGNAC METHOD

### Early morning
● Grapes

### Breakfast
● Porridge (instant or regular) with skimmed milk

### Lunch
● Roast chicken with whole-grain (brown) rice, tomatoes, and courgettes
● Fat-free cheese
● Apple purée

### Dinner
● Chicory salad with sliced hard-boiled eggs, sliced tomatoes, grated hard cheese, and a sugar-free dressing

### Snacks
● Not allowed in Phase 1. Dark chocolate in Phase 2.

some chocolate and drink a little wine in Phase 2 may explain the popularity of the diet. However, the author is not a health-care professional and makes claims that are unscientific and even wrong. For example, he claims that North Americans have reduced their caloric intake by 30 per cent in the last hundred years while becoming more obese. In fact, over the past 20 years, Americans have increased their caloric intake by about 200 calories per day.

Montignac fails to consider levels of physical activity, which are also markedly lower now than a century ago, but it is our sedentary lifestyle, combined with increased calorie intake, that is leading to the increase in excess weight in both adults and children.

Montignac also believes that bad carbohydrates – those with a high GI – interfere with the absorption of fats when they are consumed together, resulting in fats being stored. But if absorption is blocked, then fats cannot be stored. The best way to prevent fats from being stored is to avoid eating them in the first place. If you follow this diet, make sure you also take a vitamin and mineral supplement every day.

# GI Point Diet

*Glycaemic index*

⊗ **Are special products required?**
⊘ **Is eating out possible?**
⊘ **Is the plan family-friendly?**
⊘ **Do you have to buy a book?**
⊘ **Is the diet easy to maintain?**

The plan is written by State-Registered Dietician Azmina Govindji and life coach and NLP trainer Nina Puddefoot. It is based on the glycaemic index (GI) (*see p.47*), but also guides people towards a diet that is low in fat and contains plenty of fruit and vegetables.

## HOW IT CLAIMS TO WORK

The authors allocate a certain number of points (GiP's) to each of hundreds of different foods. The number of points given is determined by the GI as well as the calorie content of the food in question. For example, low-fat protein foods and most fruits have a low GiP. The GiPs are given in tables in the book. The authors claim the diet works because it keeps you feeling full while you lose weight. This will certain help make it easier for people to stick with the plan. But the fact that this diet also encourages you to make low-fat choices and controls portion sizes will contribute to weight loss by restricting the total number of calories consumed.

## THE REGIMEN

In the introductory two weeks, which is called the "start-it" phase, men are allowed 22 GiPs (GI Points) and women 17 GiPs each day. This is a "kick start" for the diet when you are likely to lose weight reasonably quickly. Following this is the "lose-it" phase, when men are allowed 25 GiPs each day and women 20 GiPs. Although this means eating more than during the "start-it" phase, the authors claim there will be a steady and sensible weight loss of 450–900g (1–2lb) per week.

During each of the first two phases both men and women also have a daily allowance of 200ml (⅓ pint) of semi-skimmed milk, and diet soft drinks, and sugar-free flavoured water and squash are unlimited. In addition, women are allowed up to seven units of alcohol per week and men up to ten units. There is no restriction on the amount of vegetables that can be eaten. Once slimmers have achieved their goal weight they are encouraged to follow the third phase – the "keep-it" phase – which is designed to help maintain the weight loss achieved.

The guidelines for the diet are to eat three meals and three snacks each day, comprising a variety of foods from all the different food groups. There are recipes and menu plans in the book, as well as advice for eating out. The plan also encourages people to take exercise every day – at least two ten-minute bursts of reasonably intense physical activity – and suggests some tips to get you started.

## IS IT HEALTHY?

The GI Point Diet falls in line with current guidelines on healthy eating, and it includes advice on behavioural modification techniques along with motivational tips, to enable people to make permanent changes to their eating habits. There is some evidence that choosing a diet based on low-GI carbohydrate foods and whole-grain cereals can help protect against health problems such as heart disease and diabetes. The diet may be difficult to follow as slimmers must carry around the food lists and count points all day (or know in advance what they are going to eat). Also, during the start-up phase hunger is likely to be a problem.

---

**GI POINT DIET**

**Breakfast**
● Tomato juice cocktail
● A bowl of bran flakes with semi-skimmed milk

**Lunch**
● Bowl or mug of cream of tomato soup
● Greek salad (feta cheese, olives, tomatoes, cucumber, and onion) with oil-free dressing
● Sugar-free jelly and strawberries

**Dinner**
● Stir-fried ginger chicken and vegetables (green and red peppers, courgettes, broccoli florets, and mushrooms)
● Basmati rice
● Grapes

**Snacks**
● Fresh or dried fruit, biscuits

---

# Hay Diet

*Food combining*

⊗ **Are special products required?**
⊘ **Is eating out possible?**
⊘ **Is the plan family-friendly?**
⊘ **Do you have to buy a book?**
⊗ **Is the diet easy to maintain?**

The Hay Diet was introduced in the 1930s by Dr William Hay, who believed that eliminating refined foods from the diet and avoiding eating protein and starch at the same meal allows the body to heal itself. Loss of excess weight is an additional benefit.

## HOW IT CLAIMS TO WORK

This diet is based on the belief that weight gain stems from a metabolic imbalance resulting from poor digestion. According to this theory – which was based on experiments conducted in the 1920s, using techniques that are now outdated – the imbalance occurs because we eat a mixed diet, and the enzymes required for the digestion of carbohydrate and protein operate optimally in different chemical environments. Eating foods in the wrong combinations, therefore, causes the body to be in an acidic rather than an alkaline state. Dr Hay states that protein and starch foods need different conditions in the digestive tract for digestion and should never be combined at the same meal, with four hours between each meal. In the diet, food is classified according to its chemical requirements for efficient digestion:
● Fruits and vegetables are alkali-forming foods and are good for us.
● Most protein foods (meats, fish, eggs, poultry, and cheese) are acid-forming foods and should be limited.

## HAY DIET

**Breakfast**
- Plain yogurt with sliced apple and flaked almonds

**Lunch**
- Toasted banana sandwich
- Mixture of grapes, hazelnuts, and raisins
- Fresh pear

**Dinner**
- Grilled cod with carrots, peas, and cauliflower
- Fruit salad of pineapple and fresh orange

**Snacks**
- Fresh fruit
- Chopped vegetables

- Starchy foods are also considered to be acid-forming and, as with protein foods, should be limited.

### THE REGIMEN
This diet prescribes completely natural whole foods, with at least 50 per cent from fresh fruit, vegetables, and salad. No processed foods, such as white flour and sugar, are permitted. The "food combining" element of the diet means that concentrated proteins, such as meat and cheese, should be eaten at separate meals from carbohydrates.

The rules for a healthy diet include eliminating processed and refined foods, eating only whole grains, minimizing milk intake, and avoiding combinations that clash. Neutral foods, which include vegetables, nuts, seeds, and oils, form the foundation of the diet. These can be eaten with either proteins or starches.

### IS IT HEALTHY?
While there is no scientific basis for the claim that an acidic condition counteracts the body's healthy alkaline state, this diet promotes weight loss by decreasing your intake of calories. Eating more fruits and vegetables, whole grains rather than refined and processed foods, and limiting protein intake is a healthy idea.

# Somersizing

*Food combining*

- ⊗ **Are special products required?**
- ⊘ **Is eating out possible?**
- ⊘ **Is the plan family-friendly?**
- ⊘ **Do you have to buy a book?**
- ⊗ **Is the diet easy to maintain?**

Suzanne Somers, the author of this diet plan, incorporates ways to splurge and enjoy foods into her own version of a food-combining programme.

### HOW IT CLAIMS TO WORK
Somersizing claims to reprogram your metabolism to burn fat by providing a constant source of energy, with frequent small meals and plenty of fresh fruit and vegetables throughout the day. No portion monitoring or calorie counting is required, but you do need to think about which types of food to eat at any one time. The plan advocates eating proteins and fats with vegetables and no other carbohydrates, and eating carbohydrates with vegetables and no fat. It also eliminates sugar, white flour, alcohol, and caffeine and suggests that fruit should be eaten on its own or on an empty stomach.

### SOMERSIZING

**Breakfast**
- Whole-grain toast with fat-free cottage cheese

**Lunch**
- Grilled fish with lemon-butter sauce and mange-tout tossed in butter
- Green salad with a sugar-free dressing

**Dinner**
- Beef pot roast with onions, sliced fresh tomatoes, and steamed asparagus
- Green salad with vinaigrette dressing

**Snacks**
- Peaches

### THE REGIMEN
Somersizing prohibits all alcoholic and caffeine-containing drinks (decaffeinated coffee is allowed). So-called "funky" foods, such as sugar, honey, beetroot, carrots, white flour, pasta, white rice, sweetcorn, bananas, potatoes, sweet potatoes, and pumpkin are discouraged. Nuts, olives, avocado, liver, coconuts, milk (other than skimmed), tofu, and soya milk are also restricted because they are "combination foods" that contain both carbohydrates and proteins, which the diet claims should not be eaten together.

The main points of the Somersizing diet to remember are:
- Fruits should be eaten alone or on an empty stomach.
- Carbohydrates should be eaten only with other carbohydrate-rich foods.
- Proteins and fats can be eaten together.

### IS IT HEALTHY?
By following the rules of this diet, you are likely to be successful in losing weight because you are cutting out food groups and reducing your daily calorie intake. With exercise, this combination does promote weight loss.

Reducing some processed foods that are low in fibre and high in sugar, and eating plenty of fresh vegetables is a healthful approach, but restricting foods that contain both carbohydrate and protein (such as avocados) makes no sense, since that is the way they are available in nature. We also know that nuts, olives, and avocados are excellent sources of monounsaturated fats, which are helpful in preventing cardiovascular disease (*see pp.214–221*).

However, it does not make any sense to suggest that fat and protein can be eaten together while carbohydrates and protein cannot. The author claims that when carbohydrates and protein are eaten together, their enzymes cancel each other out, halting the digestive process and causing weight gain. The fact is that most foods naturally contain all of the three macronutrients (proteins, fats, and carbohydrates) in various combinations, so there is no reason to believe that they cannot be digested together in the body successfully.

# New Beverly Hills Diet

*Food combining*

⊗ Are special products required?
✔ Is eating out possible?
⊗ Is the plan family-friendly?
✔ Do you have to buy a book?
⊗ Is the diet easy to maintain?

According to the author of this diet, which claims to be a 35-day lifestyle eating plan rather than a diet, the key to losing weight and feeling healthy is to improve digestion by combining fats, proteins, and carbohydrates correctly.

## HOW IT CLAIMS TO WORK

The author, Judy Mazel, believes that when carbohydrates are eaten with proteins, they become trapped and are not digested properly. She goes on to claim that when carbohydrates are not digested, they are stored as fat. The premise is that proteins are the most difficult foods to digest, carbohydrates are easier, and fruits are the easiest. Fats do not interfere with the digestion of either protein or carbohydrates, but must not be eaten with fruit. Since fruits are digested very quickly, they have to be eaten alone, or they will become trapped in your stomach by other foods. Ideally, proteins should be eaten with other proteins, carbohydrates with carbohydrates, and fruit eaten alone.

## THE REGIMEN

Unlike the first edition of the book, this New Beverly Hills Diet includes foods from all food groups, including animal protein, for the first ten days. The plan recommends beginning each day with fruit: you may eat as much fruit as you want, but should avoid mixing fruits. After eating proteins or carbohydrates, you should not eat fruit.

If you eat a carbohydrate food (such as starches, vegetables, salads, cereals, or grains) after eating fruits, you may eat carbohydrates without restriction until you eat a protein.

Once you eat protein (such as meat, fish, milk, yogurt, cheese, nuts, seeds, or ice cream), then 80 per cent of what you eat for the rest of the day should be protein only.

If you want to eat what the author calls your "open meal" (in which you combine carbohydrates and proteins, such as a hamburger and chips), you have to eat only carbohydrates for lunch and snacks that day.

Fats (such as butter, mayonnaise, oil, soured cream, and double cream) can be combined with carbohydrates or proteins. Diet colas and artificial sweeteners are not permitted in the diet. Most alcoholic drinks are considered carbohydrates and should be consumed only with other carbohydrates. However, wine is considered a fruit and must be combined only with other fruits.

The plan also includes antidotes and precedotes to offset the negative side effects of eating foods that are difficult to digest. Antidotes are foods eaten for breakfast the day after you eat food that is difficult to digest. Precedotes are foods eaten for breakfast the day you know you are going to eat a difficult-to-digest food. For example, before you eat fatty, creamy, or cheesy foods, you have to eat plenty of pineapple or strawberries as a precedote. Alternatively, you can eat one of these fruits as an antidote for breakfast the day after you have consumed a difficult-to-digest food.

Supplements are not essential for the diet, but nutritional yeast flakes mixed with water can be taken in order to supply B vitamins, sesame seeds as a calcium source, and blue-green algae as a source of natural nutrients. Also, a supplement of 1000mg of vitamin C with bioflavonoids is recommended.

## NEW BEVERLY HILLS DIET

**Breakfast**
● Dried apricots

**Lunch**
● Spinach salad with leeks, mushrooms, and Mazel dressing (rice vinegar, sesame oil, cloves, garlic, ginger, and pepper)

**Dinner**
● Pasta with marinara sauce and broccoli

**Snacks**
● All carbohydrates, protein, or fruit, depending on the day

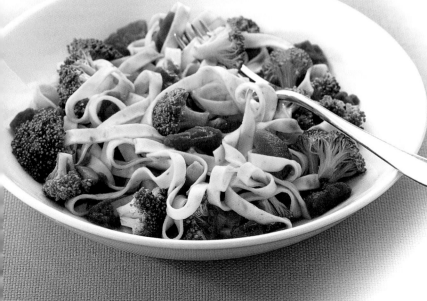

**New Beverly Hills Diet** Pasta tossed with a fresh vegetable-based sauce is a typical "carbohydrate meal" you can look forward to in this food-combining programme.

## IS IT HEALTHY?

This diet is based on the concept of food combining – a theory that has no scientific evidence to support it. The idea that carbohydrate is stored as fat because it is improperly digested makes no sense from a medical perspective.

There is no scientific evidence that food composition affects the way in which enzymes digest food. In any case, most foods found in nature contain some proteins, fats, and carbohydrates, making it very unlikely that our bodies are not adapted to dealing with combinations of nutrients. It is true that the absorption of carbohydrates will be delayed if they are combined with other foods, but no matter what we eat with carbohydrates, they will always be absorbed. If you select high fibre, complex carbohydrate sources, such as wholemeal bread, they will take longer to be absorbed by the body than simple carbohydrates such as sweets or fizzy drinks.

You may lose weight with the New Beverly Hills Diet due to a significant reduction in the calories you consume, but trying to remember which foods to eat when, and in what combination, can be confusing, time-consuming, and often very frustrating, especially when you are eating out or preparing meals for a family.

The New Beverly Hills Diet is an improvement on the old version, but in our opinion it is still nutritionally unbalanced and restrictive.

# Fit For Life

*Food combining*

⊗ **Are special products required?**
⊘ **Is eating out possible?**
⊘ **Is the plan family-friendly?**
⊘ **Do you have to buy a book?**
⊗ **Is the diet easy to maintain?**

Fit For Life is another diet claiming that combining food in certain ways improves digestive processes and thereby leads to successful weight loss.

## HOW IT CLAIMS TO WORK

This is essentially a no-processed-food regimen. The diet is high in fruits and vegetables and limited in dairy products and meats. It also recommends that foods be eaten in specific combinations at certain times of the day. The goal is rapid weight loss based on when and how you eat. It draws on various theories, including natural body cycles, water content of food, food combining, "proper" fruit eating, and detoxification.

The theory behind this food-combining diet is that the body is not designed to digest more than one "concentrated" food in the stomach at the same time. (Any food that is not a vegetable or a fruit is considered concentrated.) The authors cite research carried out in the 1940s suggesting that carbohydrate and protein cannot be digested when consumed together. In addition, they suggest that eating two concentrated foods together will cause the food to rot because it cannot be digested properly.

The idea behind high-water-content foods such as fruit is to maintain and replenish the body's water content to prevent waste accumulation.

The book also espouses "natural hygiene" – a theory that the body is constantly seeking to clear itself of waste, and that helping this process along will improve health.

According to the authors, the body operates in cycles:

### FIT FOR LIFE

**Breakfast**
● Fruit salad of banana, grapefruit, and apple

**Lunch**
● Vegetable salad of chopped lettuce, tomatoes, cucumber, olives, Brussels sprouts, and sunflower or sesame seeds
● Whole-grain bread

**Dinner**
● Bowl of creamy cauliflower soup
● Roast chicken breast with steamed green beans
● Green salad
● Glass of vegetable juice

**Snacks**
● Handful of almonds

● Noon to 8pm is for appropriation (eating and digestion).
● 8pm to 4am is for assimilation (absorption and use).
● 4am to noon is for elimination (of body waste and food debris).

## THE REGIMEN

This diet advises that in the mornings you eat only fruits; for lunch you eat raw vegetables with some whole-grain bread or vegetable soup; and for dinner you have salad with grain and meat. The authors are against cooking where possible, as they claim it removes water from food and destroys its natural enzymes. If your diet does not include enough high-water-content foods, they recommend drinking distilled water, since the minerals in natural water are presumed to bind with cholesterol and form plaques. Eating fruit is highly recommended, but it should be eaten separately and never immediately following any other foods.

## IS IT HEALTHY?

By restricting certain foods at each meal, you will take in fewer calories overall and you will lose weight. The scientific basis for food combining is unfounded, and there is no reason for most people to avoid combining foods. However, if you often have difficulty digesting certain foods, or experience abdominal discomfort after eating, it may be worth following this regimen for a few weeks to see if you feel better.

Most foods promoted on this diet are healthy, but the rules do not promote flexible, long-term habits that are easy to maintain. The concept of daily cycles is based on normal hormonal changes in the body, but there is no scientific evidence to support the claim that these fluctuations influence nutritional requirements and how and when you should eat specific types of food.

In addition, the authors argue that calories are the enemy only if they are consumed in foods that are highly processed or ill-combined, rather than encouraging sensible portion control. Overall, this diet has serious flaws and if followed for more than several weeks could lead to deficiencies of vitamin D, calcium, and iron.

# Eat Right 4 Your Type

*Metabolic typing*

- ✖ Are special products required?
- ✔ Is eating out possible?
- ✖ Is the plan family-friendly?
- ✔ Do you have to buy a book?
- ✖ Is the diet easy to maintain?

This diet is based on the idea that your blood type reflects your anthropological background and that this influences your body's reaction to food.

## HOW IT CLAIMS TO WORK
The author of this diet plan claims that people's metabolic profiles differ and that these can be matched to specific dietary constituents. In order to avoid the complexity that renders some metabolic-profiling systems useless, this plan categorizes all people by their blood type. The author proposes that your anthropological background – whether your ancestors were hunters, cultivators, enigmas, or nomads – is reflected in your blood type; that the antibodies on the outside of blood cells vary with blood type; and that these react in varying ways to food antigens, causing intolerance and illness. If you eat the right foods for your type you will lose weight and have more energy.

### EAT RIGHT 4 YOUR TYPE: TYPE O

**Breakfast**
- Cinnamon and raisin toast with cream cheese

**Lunch**
- Grilled chicken with green salad and a low-fat dressing

**Dinner**
- Grilled lamb chops with asparagus, green beans, and carrots

**Snacks**
- Slices of tofu or tofu-based low-fat dessert

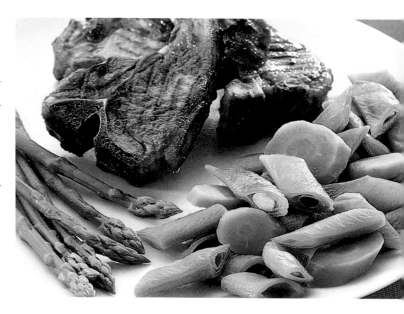

**Eat Right 4 Your Type** Lamb with vegetables is a high-protein meal recommended by this programme for people with blood group O.

## THE REGIMEN
Lists of permitted and non-permitted foods are available for each blood group. The recommended diets range in calorie value from about 1500 to 1800 a day.
- Persons with Type O blood are believed to be the oldest in evolutionary terms and are therefore more adapted to a red-meat-based, low-carbohydrate diet, with few grains and no wheat.
- Type As are younger evolutionarily, as humans moved from being hunter-gatherers to a more agrarian lifestyle. This group tolerates vegetables better and are advised to follow a vegetarian, high-carbohydrate, low-fat diet.
- Type Bs emerged when the races were merging from Africa, Europe, Asia, and America. According to this plan, Type Bs tolerate a more balanced diet that includes a variety of vegetables, fruits, dairy products, grains, and meats.
- Type ABs represent the newest group from interbreeding. They have fewer restrictions and tolerate more foods.

## IS IT HEALTHY?
The idea of basing your dietary needs on your blood type has no scientific foundation. Neither has the premise

that your risk of certain diseases is based on your blood type. If it were, people's blood types would be tested as routine when they are admitted to hospital or for surgery visits.

A serious drawback of the diet plan for Type A and O blood types is that dairy products are limited and, consequently, the diets are low in calcium.

# Body Code

*Metabolic typing*

- ✖ Are special products required?
- ✔ Is eating out possible?
- ✔ Is the plan family-friendly?
- ✔ Do you have to buy a book?
- ✖ Is the diet easy to maintain?

This plan is based on the theory that humans can be classified into different genetic types, with different dietary requirements. For every type, however, the focus is on a nutritious diet and regular exercise.

## HOW IT CLAIMS TO WORK
According to the authors, not every diet, lifestyle, or exercise plan is suitable for all people. They classify the human body into two basic genetic types – strong and sleek. Strong types are generally more solid and muscular than

sleek types and require a low-protein, plant-based diet as well as plenty of physical activity. Sleek types, on the other hand, are generally leaner and more delicate than strong types. They need less physical activity and more protein in their diets.

Each of these two body types is subdivided into two further categories. Strong body types may be "warriors" or "nurturers", while sleek types may be "communicators" or "visionaries".

According to the authors of this plan, the four body types are influenced by a specific gland that governs food intake and energy balance. Your diet and exercise plan depend on what body type you are:
• Warrior-type people are healthiest on a plant-based diet that includes whole grains, fruits, and vegetables.
• Nurturers need to eat plenty of soya and linseeds, and minimize their intake of meat and fish.
• Communicators need a diet high in leafy vegetables, monounsaturated fats, and lean protein, including all white meats, fat-free dairy products, eggs, some nuts, and soya protein.
• Visionaries need an Asian-style diet that includes lots of cooked vegetables, whole grains, and protein, especially those derived from soya.

## THE REGIMEN

The Body Code embraces a holistic philosophy, founded on a balance of body and spirit. Unlocking the "Body Code" enables people to define their types, which are characterized by prototypical physical features and personal attributes:
• Warriors need a diet based on plant foods. This is because animal foods over-stimulate their dominant adrenal glands, leaving them out of balance. Their everyday diet should include plenty of vegetables, fruits, roots, and grains to stimulate the non-dominant glands and to create energy balance. Higher-calorie plant foods, such as nuts and seeds, should be restricted if weight loss is desired. Warriors should avoid consuming saturated and hydrogenated fats including red meats in favour of white meats, alcohol, salts, and refined grains and flour, and include herbs,

---

### BODY CODE: WARRIOR TYPE

**Breakfast**
• Whole-grain cereal, cherry sauce, and skimmed milk

**Lunch**
• DeLayne's tomatoes and rice (recipe in book)

**Dinner**
• Chicken Parmesan with wholemeal pasta tossed in a red sauce
• Green salad

**Snacks**
• Fat-free yogurt
• Vegetable crudités
• Unlimited fruits, vegetables, whole grains, white and pink fish, white poultry, egg whites and substitutes, fat-free dairy, ginger tea, linseeds, and alfalfa

---

teas, and condiments that will help control their appetite and balance the biochemical reactions in the body.
• Nurturers are curvy and pear-shaped; charismatic, compassionate, and selfless. They need a diet based on plants and high-water-content foods. Their everyday diet should include plenty of plant foods, especially fruits and vegetables. Since the nurturer's appetite is stronger in the evening, they should eat a substantial meal at this time of day.
• Communicators are lanky, long-limbed, lively, creative, and unpredictable. They need a diet based on monounsaturated fats, vegetables, protein, and small amounts of carbohydrate. They can eat as much protein as they like, including red meat, as long as they are careful to limit saturated fat.
• Visionaries are thin and youthful, calm, intellectual, and reserved. Their basic diet is based on proteins, whole grains, and cooked vegetables. The best foods for the visionaries' diet are soya proteins and vegetables.

## IS IT HEALTHY?

The positive aspects of the Body Code diet are that it teaches a way of life, rather than a quick fix. The programme

---

states that weight loss and health maintenance require a nutritious diet complemented by regular exercise, which we support. They also stress that healthy eating requires a commitment and perseverance for success and that physical and emotional fitness need to be part of your lifestyle.

However, there is little evidence to support the idea of a dominant gland leading to physiological imbalance as a principle factor in weight management. There are many glands at work in the body and, in good health, these glands work in synchrony and harmony. In a few cases, glandular disease is a relevant consideration, but it is not a basic tenet of weight management, and it is not appropriate for most people. Omitting or favouring entire food groups can lead to deficiency in essential vitamins and minerals, including iron.

# Metabolic Typing

*Metabolic typing*

⊗ **Are special products required?**
✓ **Is eating out possible?**
⊗ **Is the plan family-friendly?**
✓ **Do you have to buy a book?**
⊗ **Is the diet easy to maintain?**

This diet is based on the belief that people vary in their nutritional needs according to their body types, which reflect their unique ancestral histories.

## HOW IT CLAIMS TO WORK

The Metabolic Typing diet proposes that our unique body types derive from variations in our ancestors' diets, which were determined by diverse geographic and environmental circumstances. It is suggested, for example, that people with tropical ancestral origins have different nutritional needs from those originating from temperate zones.

The authors of Metabolic Typing assert that universal diets are ineffective for the varied physiologies and nutritional needs of different populations. Instead, they identify individual biochemical profiles and nutritional needs in order to produce customized diets designed to promote vigour and well-being in the individual.

## METABOLIC TYPING: PROTEIN TYPE

### Breakfast
• Scrambled eggs with a bacon rasher and potatoes sautéed in butter

### Lunch
• Chicken thigh or leg with sliced carrots, cauliflower florets, and olive spread

### Dinner
• Grilled steak with peas and sweetcorn
• Avocado dressed with olive oil and vinegar

### Snacks
• Full-fat plain yogurt sprinkled with sunflower seeds and cashew nuts

## THE REGIMEN

The first step in this programme is to establish your type by completing a 65-point questionnaire that evaluates physical appearance, anatomical and structural characteristics, psychological characteristics, behavioural habits, and food preferences and reactions. Specific combinations of carbohydrate, fat, and protein for optimum nutrition are then recommended, according to your classification as a "Protein Type", "Carbohydrate Type", or "Mixed Type".
• Protein Types are advised to include meat, seafood, and dairy at every meal. Offal (such as beef or chicken livers), sardines, anchovies, caviar, and whole-fat dairy foods are particularly recommended. Sprouted-grain breads are the only breads allowed; unripe apples and pears are acceptable but in moderation. All nuts and oils are allowed, but alcohol, caffeine, and fruit juices should be avoided by people who are Protein Types.
• Carbohydrate Types are advised to base their meals on high-starch vegetables, such as potatoes and sweet potatoes, as well as on whole grains. Nuts and oils should be eaten sparingly and only light meats and fish, such as chicken breast and white fish, should be included. Dairy products must be fat-free or low-fat and all pulses should be avoided. Alcohol and caffeine are restricted.
• Mixed Types must include ample foods from both the Protein- and Carbohydrate-Types regimens.

## IS IT HEALTHY?

Few people can claim to have a single ancestral lineage. Most of us are a mix of races, ethnicities, and genes, and this complicates any historical correlations between geography and optimum nutrition. However, it is important to remember that the foods our ancestors ate were natural, and natural foods contain all three macronutrients in variable proportions. Fats, proteins, and carbohydrates are essential for life, and we are all equipped with the genetic tools to digest and benefit from these macronutrients. On the positive side, this diet may encourage you to eat more natural, unprocessed foods.

In addition, human nutrition must adapt to and accommodate changes in our lifestyle due to new developments in technology, wider availability of foods from around the world, prosperity, illness, and level of physical activity. These factors affect our nutritional status and demand a diet designed to suit individual needs.

**Cabbage Soup Diet** Unlimited quantities of home-made vegetable soup form the basis of this short-term, quick-weight-loss programme.

# Cabbage Soup Diet

*Quick weight loss*

⊗ **Are special products required?**
⊗ **Is eating out possible?**
⊗ **Is the plan family-friendly?**
⊘ **Do you have to buy a book?**
⊗ **Is the diet easy to maintain?**

This extremely low-calorie diet should be followed for only seven days at a time. It is not nutritionally sound nor is it a safe way to lose weight.

## HOW IT CLAIMS TO WORK

The authors of the diet claim that you can lose 4.5–6.8kg (10–15lb) by eating as much cabbage soup as you want to for seven days. The cabbage soup includes a variety of low-calorie vegetables with canned tomatoes, flavoured onion soup mix, and stock or vegetable juice.

## THE REGIMEN

In addition to eating unlimited amounts of home-made cabbage soup, this plan allows combinations of foods each day, such as fruit and milk one day, vegetables and milk the next day, and beef on the following day. No bread, alcohol, or fizzy drinks are allowed.

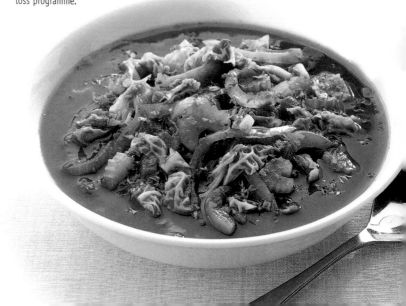

## CABBAGE SOUP DIET

### Unlimited cabbage soup plus:

**Day 1**
● Any fruit except bananas

**Day 2**
● Unlimited vegetables
● Baked potato with butter

**Day 3**
● Any fruit except bananas
● Unlimited vegetables

**Day 4**
● Up to 8 bananas, plus unlimited skimmed milk

**Day 5**
● Large quantity of beef with canned tomatoes
● 6–8 glasses of water

**Day 6**
● Unlimited beef and vegetables

**Day 7**
● Brown rice
● Unsweetened fruit juices

### Snacks
● Cabbage soup

**Recipe: Cabbage Soup**  This recipe makes about six servings of soup. You can eat as much of the soup as you like throughout the day.
● 6 large onions, chopped
● 2 green peppers, seeded and chopped
● 2 cans (400g/14oz each) tomatoes
● 1 bunch celery, chopped
● ½ cabbage, chopped
● 1 packet dry onion soup mix
● 1–2 stock cubes (optional)
● 3 litres (5¼ pints) vegetable juice with 1 litre (1¾ pints) of water, or just use 3 litres (5¼ pints) of water.

Soften the onions and peppers, then add the other vegetables. Add the soup mix, stock cubes, and liquid. Bring to the boil, then simmer for up to 2 hours. Season to taste with salt and freshly ground black pepper and your choice of chopped parsley or curry powder.

### IS IT HEALTHY?
The diet offers quick weight loss, most of which is water weight. It is neither nutritionally balanced nor a safe method for achieving long-term weight reduction and is likely to promote cravings as soon as you come off the diet. If you do decide to try it, be sure to eat sensible, well-balanced meals once you have completed the seven days.

# 5-Day Miracle Diet

*Quick weight loss*

⊗ **Are special products required?**
✓ **Is eating out possible?**
✓ **Is the plan family-friendly?**
✓ **Do you have to buy a book?**
✓ **Is the diet easy to maintain?**

This programme aims to control the food cravings that often cause people to abandon their attempts to lose weight by maintaining stable blood-sugar levels throughout the day.

### HOW IT CLAIMS TO WORK
The author claims that a drop in blood-sugar levels results in uncontrollable cravings, often for foods such as sweets and alcohol. After you eat, insulin levels rise to reduce blood-sugar levels, and this leads to a drop in blood sugar, which prompts the urge to eat more. This diet recommends eating at specific, regular times during the day, and advocates consuming certain types of foods in specific combinations.

### THE REGIMEN
According to this programme, breakfast should be eaten within 30 minutes of waking up, a snack within two hours of breakfast, lunch by 1pm, followed by an afternoon snack three hours later, and dinner several hours after having the snack.

In addition to specifying the times of the meals, specific types of foods to be eaten at each meal are listed.
● Breakfast: protein and bread.
● Lunch: protein and fresh vegetables with optional fruit.
● Dinner: a variety of vegetables, protein, and bread.

Men can eat three starchy foods per day, while women can eat these foods only on alternate days.

Recommended snacks include fresh fruits and vegetables. Plenty of water is advised and coffee is allowed. Pasta is limited to twice a week and consumed only at dinner, but you are allowed to eat one or two foods a week that you "absolutely adore".

### IS IT HEALTHY?
This is a sensible diet that does not advocate any bizarre eating habits. It is essentially a calorie-controlled plan that will help you lose weight by reducing portion sizes and limiting your intake of carbohydrates. Starches are permitted only twice a day, mostly at breakfast and at lunch or dinner, but not both. If your eating habits are very different from this, such that you skip meals and eat a lot of sweets, you may feel better and be able to regulate your blood-sugar levels by eating at specific times each day. However, there are no miracles when it comes to dieting and losing weight, and you will certainly need to follow this plan for longer than five days in order to see long-term results.

### 5-DAY MIRACLE DIET

**Breakfast (½ hour after waking)**
● Egg
● Slice of toast with spread

**Lunch (by 1pm)**
● Tuna with spinach and tomato salad with a balsamic vinegar dressing
● Orange

**Dinner**
● Grilled chicken with steamed spinach
● Salad of chopped tomatoes, chopped red or green pepper, chopped lettuce, and a balsamic vinegar dressing
● Slice of bread

**Snacks (2 hours after breakfast; 3 hours after lunch)**
● Nectarine, grapefruit, carrots, or raw cauliflower

# Grapefruit Diet

*Quick weight loss*

⊗ **Are special products required?**
⊘ **Is eating out possible?**
⊗ **Is the plan family-friendly?**
⊘ **Do you have to buy a book?**
⊗ **Is the diet easy to maintain?**

This diet is based on the idea that eating grapefruit with every meal helps you to lose weight by burning fat.

## HOW IT CLAIMS TO WORK
The theory behind the diet is that grapefruit contains enzymes that make the body burn fat for energy. Calories are limited to fewer than 800 per day, which promotes quick weight loss – primarily due to loss of body water.

## THE REGIMEN
The Grapefruit Diet advocates eating half a grapefruit before every meal and before any caffeinated drinks. The diet restricts dairy products, other fruits, and most vegetables. You can drink black tea or coffee with meals.

## IS IT HEALTHY?
There is no evidence to support the idea that eating grapefruit helps burn fat. Any weight loss that occurs is due to the extremely low calorie intake. If

---

### GRAPEFRUIT DIET

**Breakfast**
• ½ grapefruit

**Lunch**
• ½ grapefruit
• Egg and mixed salad with tomatoes and carrots
• Slice of wholemeal toast

**Dinner**
• ½ grapefruit
• Eggs, lettuce, chopped tomatoes, and dressing
• Black tea or coffee

**Snacks**
• Not allowed with this diet plan

---

you like grapefruit, you may be able to stay on this diet for about a week, but with fewer than 800 calories daily, any weight loss that occurs will be mostly due to loss of water weight.

This diet is not nutritionally balanced. It is low in fibre, essential vitamins, and minerals such as iron and calcium. Because the calorie intake is so low, causing you to be in a ketotic state (*see p.168*), you are likely to lack energy, and any attempt to exercise may make you dizzy or light-headed.

# Rotation Diet

*Quick weight loss*

⊗ **Are special products required?**
⊘ **Is eating out possible?**
⊗ **Is the plan family-friendly?**
⊘ **Do you have to buy a book?**
⊗ **Is the diet easy to maintain?**

This diet is designed to reduce overall calorie intake without causing the body to go into "starvation mode", which leads to additional weight gain when normal eating is resumed.

## HOW IT CLAIMS TO WORK
This plan recommends a rotation of diets of varying calorie levels that will create a calorie deficit great enough to produce significant weight loss, without causing the body to lower its metabolic rate as it does in fasting. The author recommends two cycles of rotation diet, each followed by no dietary restriction for one to four weeks. The author's rationale is that low-calorie diets cause a reduction in the body's metabolic rate, which sets the slimmer up for rebound weight gain when he or she stops slimming and reverts to a normal calorie intake.

The author describes the "starvation response", which is the body's response to caloric restriction. To preserve essential functions, the body lowers its metabolic rate – the rate at which calories are burned at rest (*see p.34*).

## THE REGIMEN
The diet advocates different calorie levels for men and women, and recommends an extremely low-calorie regimen for

---

### ROTATION DIET: 1,200 CALORIES

**Breakfast**
• ½ grapefruit
• Slice wholemeal bread with slice of cheese
• Non-calorie drink

**Lunch**
• Salmon with unlimited "free" vegetables
• Wholemeal crackers
• Non-calorie drink

**Dinner**
• Baked chicken with cauliflower and beetroot
• Apple
• Non-calorie drink

**Snacks**
• Any from the list of "safe" fruits, such as apples, oranges, and berries

---

three days, followed by a more modest calorie restriction for four days, and then a week of mild calorie restriction.
• Women are allowed:
600 calories per day for 3 days
900 calories per day for 4 days
1200 calories per day for 7 days.
• Men are allowed:
1200 calories per day for 3 days
1500 calories per day for 4 days
1800 calories per day for 7 days.

This level of caloric restriction is likely to cause more hunger than most of us are willing to tolerate. To compensate, the diet recommends filling up on "free vegetables", such as asparagus, celery, chicory, Chinese leaves, endive, lettuce, cucumber, radishes, courgettes, spinach, and watercress.

The diet recommends "safe" fruits for snacking on when you are hungry; these include apples, berries, grapefruit, melon, oranges, peaches, and pineapple. It also recommends standard serving sizes, based on the American Food Guide Pyramid, and there is no specific restriction on caffeine and alcohol.

## IS IT HEALTHY?
This extremely low-calorie programme should be attempted only under medical supervision. The claim that

it prevents rebound weight gain is not proved. Because the diet produces a deficit of 7200 calories in the first week and then 6300 calories in the second week, it is designed for men or women to lose 2.7–3.2kg (6–7lb) in two weeks. However, what the diet actually claims to produce is weight losses of 6.4kg (14lb) in three weeks, which does not seem possible. The diet will result in significant weight loss if it is followed, but will also result in severe hunger and dehydration, which is likely to cause people to stop following the programme.

The rotational aspect of this diet seems like a gimmick, but people who are able to tolerate this level of caloric restriction will lose a significant amount of weight in a short period. However, whether or not they maintain the weight loss in the long-term is more likely to be due to what they eat after reverting to normal eating than to the diet they followed while losing the weight.

A psychologist and obesity expert has devised this plan, and its strength lies not in the actual diet recommended but in the many suggestions given for behavioural management in relation to eating and appetite. This section of the book is the most helpful.

# 14-day Beauty Boot Camp

*Quick weight loss*

⊗ **Are special products required?**
⊘ **Is eating out possible?**
⊘ **Is the plan family-friendly?**
⊘ **Do you have to buy a book?**
⊘ **Is the diet easy to maintain?**

Developed by a former model, this is an intensive 14-day programme that aims to provide a total body makeover in just two weeks. As well as weight loss, the programme focuses on self-esteem, hair, and wardrobe.

## HOW IT CLAIMS TO WORK
This diet is low in sugar and high in protein, complex carbohydrates, fibre, and vegetables. Drinking water is an important element in the programme.

According to the author, water helps convert food to energy and drinking plenty of cold water can burn up to 250 extra calories each day as well as giving a feeling of fullness.

## THE REGIMEN
In addition to eating three times a day, plus a snack, which will provide about 1000–1200 calories, you are advised to drink eight to ten glasses of iced water daily, flavoured with lemon or lime juice. Drinking three cups of green tea daily is also recommended for its antioxidant effect (*see p.20*) and some coffee is allowed. You should not eat dinner after 8pm or in the three hours before going to bed, to prevent overeating and to help you feel more alert in the morning. Eating high-fibre foods is also recommended to satisfy hunger and suppress appetite.

## IS IT HEALTHY?
Of all the quick weight-loss diets, this offers the most healthful suggestions. Eating high-fibre foods and plenty of

### 14-DAY BEAUTY BOOT CAMP

**Breakfast**
- Bowl of bran flakes topped with blueberries
- Glass of skimmed milk or soya milk

**Lunch**
- Pitta pizza: pitta pocket filled with grated mozzarella cheese and chopped tomato flavoured with oregano, garlic powder, Italian seasoning, and black pepper
- Mixed salad of leafy greens, carrots, tomatoes, and celery, with a fat-free dressing or balsamic vinaigrette

**Dinner**
- Grilled chicken or fish with cooked vegetables drizzled with lemon juice
- Small baked potato topped with plain yogurt

**Snacks**
- Apple
- Reduced-fat peanut butter

vegetables, including semi-skimmed and skimmed milk and soya milk, and drinking eight to ten glasses of water every day will all definitely help you feel good and probably look better.

This diet allows only 1000–1200 calories per day. Since this is likely to be less than your usual intake, the diet will promote weight loss, assuming you follow the plan and limit portion sizes. Drinking lots of water and eating plenty of high-fibre foods may help curb your hunger, although it is unlikely that water actually burns calories.

You should keep in mind that any weight loss you experience during the first two weeks of any diet is usually water weight, so you would need to continue to follow this programme for more than two weeks to see any more permanent changes in your weight.

You should also take a multivitamin and mineral supplement, as well as calcium, while following this diet.

# Cambridge Diet

*Low-calorie, liquid meal replacement*

⊘ **Are special products required?**
⊗ **Is eating out possible?**
⊗ **Is the plan family-friendly?**
⊗ **Do you have to buy a book?**
⊗ **Is the diet easy to maintain?**

This weight-loss programme is based on eating only specially manufactured, low-calorie foods that are designed to be nutritionally complete.

## HOW IT CLAIMS TO WORK
The Cambridge Diet is a very low-calorie plan – intake is only about 400 calories a day. The diet involves drinking shakes instead of eating meals for at least the first two weeks. This "sole source" period is marked by rapid weight loss because of the ketosis that results from the low-carbohydrate content of the shakes and severely restricted calories (*see p.168*).

## THE REGIMEN
For the first two weeks, you are allowed to drink three or four shakes every day (they are available in eight flavours). You

## CAMBRIDGE DIET: SOLE SOURCE

**Breakfast**
- High-protein shake

**Lunch**
- High-protein shake

**Dinner**
- High-protein shake

**Snacks**
- Not allowed

are also encouraged to drink 2 litres (3½ pints) of calorie-free fluids daily. After the initial two weeks, you can introduce the specially formulated bars and soup.

The diet recommends remaining on the 400-calorie regimen for a maximum of eight weeks. After achieving your target weight, you follow a maintenance plan, which can include varying calorie levels (from 800–1500 calories daily) and incorporates regular foods.

### IS IT HEALTHY?

Very low-calorie diets with liquid meal replacements are effective for weight loss because of the dramatic reduction in calories, but these diets are particularly ineffective in promoting long-term weight maintenance. In fact, once they return to eating regular food, most people regain all the weight they have lost – and in many cases more.

Very low-calorie diets have been shown to create mineral imbalances that can result in sudden death. They should therefore be undertaken only under the supervision of a medical professional. Currently, the products associated with this diet are available via independent counsellors who will provide screening, monitoring, and advice. However, it is unlikely that the counsellors are medically qualified as most health professionals do not advocate such diets for weight loss.

If you decide that you want to try to follow this programme, make sure that you discuss it first with your GP. It may be better to drink shakes for two meals a day and to eat a well-balanced third meal plus some healthy snacks to help decrease hunger cravings.

# Herbalife

*Low calorie, liquid meal replacement*

- ✓ **Are special products required?**
- ✓ **Is eating out possible?**
- ✗ **Is the plan family-friendly?**
- ✗ **Do you have to buy a book?**
- ✗ **Is the diet easy to maintain?**

This is another weight-loss programme based on replacing meals with specially manufactured, low-calorie replacements and supplements, including shakes, soups, and bars.

### HOW IT CLAIMS TO WORK

The Herbalife diet promotes weight loss by limiting your intake of calories to about 1000 calories per day, with meal replacement drinks and bars. The authors of this programme claim to have helped many people lose significant amounts of weight.

### THE REGIMEN

Herbalife sells products designed for people following their "Green" and "Gold" weight-loss plans. Both plans require replacements of two meals a day with liquid supplements, soups, or bars. Both also prescribe specific vitamin, mineral, herbal, and fibre supplements. The Gold plan offers a

## HERBALIFE (GOLD PLAN)

**Breakfast**
- Herbalife protein bar
- Piece of fruit

**Lunch**
- Herbalife shake
- Large green salad

**Dinner**
- Herbalife shake
- Large green salad
- Steamed vegetables

**Snacks**
- Herbalife soup mix
- Herbalife roasted soya nuts
- Piece of fruit

high-protein, low-carbohydrate shake for people who are carbohydrate-sensitive. In addition to the shakes and soups, slimmers are encouraged to eat steamed vegetables and/or green salad at mealtimes, and to snack on fruit once or twice a day.

### IS IT HEALTHY?

This programme is an expensive way to lose weight, and it does not teach you how to eat sensibly in the long-term. You are required to buy not only drinks or shakes, but also bars, soups, and an array of vitamins, minerals, and fibre supplements.

# SlimFast

*Low-calorie, liquid meal replacement*

- ✓ **Are special products required?**
- ✓ **Is eating out possible?**
- ✗ **Is the plan family-friendly?**
- ✗ **Do you have to buy a book?**
- ✗ **Is the diet easy to maintain?**

This plan is based on reducing total calorie intake by replacing two meals and snacks each day with specially manufactured, low-calorie products including SlimFast shakes in various flavours, soups, and bars.

### HOW IT CLAIMS TO WORK

The diet is based on a daily intake of 1200–1500 calories, which should promote weight loss in most people. The plan comprises two meal replacements with one sensible meal each day and emphasizes portion control when planning your main meal as well as following standard nutritional guidelines. SlimFast also advocates 30–60 minutes of exercise per day. The associated website gives information on lifestyle changes, exercise plans, healthy meal and snack ideas, and achieving long-term weight maintenance.

### THE REGIMEN

The SlimFast plan does not advocate using their products as the sole source of nutrition, but instead

## SLIMFAST

### Breakfast
- SlimFast shake or bar
- Glass of orange juice

### Lunch
- SlimFast shake or bar
- Piece of fresh fruit

### Dinner
- Lean meat (grilled or baked) with a medium baked potato, steamed vegetables, and a salad
- Piece of fresh fruit

### Snacks
- Air-popped popcorn
- Piece of fresh fruit
- Fresh vegetables
- SlimFast bar

recommends eating at least 1200 calories per day, since fewer calories than this may cause unhealthy, rapid weight loss. They recommend losing no more than 900g (2lb) per week after the first week. The diet plan suggests limiting alcohol consumption and how often you eat out, as well as controlling portion sizes.

### IS IT HEALTHY?
This plan will promote weight loss, and it may be helpful for people who eat on the run and need quick meals but want to avoid fast-food restaurants. The soups and shakes are quick and easy to prepare. However, drinking the shakes and eating bars every day will become monotonous after a while, making the diet difficult to maintain.

Essentially, the SlimFast diet promotes weight loss by cutting down on calories. The key to long-term success with this diet is the sensible evening meal, which limits portion sizes and does teach you how to eat healthily, at least at dinner. SlimFast has data showing successful weight loss and effective management from people who have followed this diet for a number of years.

# Fat-Flush Plan

*Detox*

- ✅ **Are special products required?**
- ✖ **Is eating out possible?**
- ✖ **Is the plan family-friendly?**
- ✅ **Do you have to buy a book?**
- ✖ **Is the diet easy to maintain?**

This is a detox diet aimed at cleansing your liver of toxicity, which contributes to weight gain and other conditions, including cellulitis, high blood pressure, and mood swings.

## HOW IT CLAIMS TO WORK
Claiming to melt fat from the hips, waist, and thighs in just two weeks, this diet's underlying theory is that "hidden weight gain" is caused by five factors:
- Liver toxicity
- Waterlogged tissues
- Fear of eating fat
- Excess insulin
- Stress fat.

The author claims that liver toxicity (caused by caffeine, sugar, trans fatty acids, medications, certain herbs, and lack of dietary fibre) is responsible for weight gain, cellulitis, bloating, elevated blood pressure and blood cholesterol levels, mood swings, and skin rashes.

The author also claims that fear of eating fat results from consuming the wrong types of fat (saturated), while excess insulin results from excessive intake of refined carbohydrates.

The book also states that some medical researchers have suggested high levels of cortisol (a hormone that is produced in stressful situations) in the blood is linked to abdominal obesity, which they refer to as stress fat.

## THE REGIMEN
The plan recommends special fat-flush supplements and a drink claimed to cleanse the system, enable natural weight loss, and help melt away accumulated fat. The drink is made from unsweetened cranberry juice with purified water and psyllium or ground linseeds, hot water, and lemon juice. You have the drink when you rise, mid-afternoon, and 20 minutes before lunch and dinner.

Other foods are included for claimed detox properties, such as red meat for l-carnitine; eggs for taurine, cysteine, and methionine; and cruciferous vegetables, garlic, onions, and some specific herbs (dandelion root, milk thistle, turmeric, and Oregon grape root).

Flour, sugar, margarine, shortening (and all products containing these), artificial sweeteners, and caffeinated drinks are not allowed.

The diet is divided into three phases:
- Phase 1 – during which the liver detoxification is primary and about 1200 calories a day are consumed – is the weight-loss phase.
- Phase 2 – during which 1200–1500 calories are allowed – is a transition to a more long-term diet.
- Phase 3 – when 1500 calories are allowed – is a long-term lifestyle diet.

## IS IT HEALTHY?
If you decide to go on the Fat-Flush Plan because you are looking to "flush" or "melt" fat from your body, you are likely to be disappointed. Aerobic exercise, such as running, cycling, swimming, and aerobic dancing, is the only proven way to burn body fat.

## FAT-FLUSH PLAN

### Breakfast
- Scrambled eggs with spinach, green peppers, spring onions, and parsley

### Lunch
- Grilled salmon with lemon juice and steamed asparagus
- Salad of mixed green leaves, broccoli florets, and sliced or diced cucumber dressed with linseed oil

### Dinner
- Grilled pork chop seasoned with a pinch of mustard powder, with steamed kale
- Baked pattypan squash dressed with linseed oil

### Snacks
- ½ large grapefruit
- Apple

The concept of liver toxicity is often used by alternative practitioners to explain a variety of common problems, but there is little evidence to support the idea that the liver is responsible for "hidden weight gain". The regimen proposed to improve liver toxicity is an extreme diet and may be beneficial to only a very small number of people, although the drink may provide some vitamins and minerals.

Eliminating dairy, wheat, sugar, and yeast-containing foods may be helpful for people who are affected by food sensitivities or food allergies, but how this relates to weight loss is questionable. It is difficult to eliminate these foods entirely from your diet, so if this is necessary because of allergies you may lose weight simply because you have cut your calorie intake.

The most beneficial advice that this diet offers is to increase water and add linseed oil because of its high content of omega-3 fatty acids.

# Juice Fasts

*Detox*

- ⊗ **Are special products required?**
- ⊗ **Is eating out possible?**
- ⊗ **Is the plan family-friendly?**
- ⊘ **Do you have to buy a book?**
- ⊗ **Is the diet easy to maintain?**

This diet claims that fruit- and vegetable-juice fasts cleanse the body of harmful toxins. Juice Fasts recommends freshly squeezed juice from organic produce rather than pasteurized varieties, which should be avoided.

## HOW IT CLAIMS TO WORK

This plan claims to offer a safe and easy way to detoxify the body and lose weight. It claims that fruit and vegetable juices are concentrated nutritional elixirs easily assimilated and that the nutrients present in juices bind with harmful toxins and carry them out of your body.

## THE REGIMEN

You are allowed to drink as much fruit and vegetable juice as you like, made from a range of produce, at any time of day. The recommended amounts vary from 240–500ml (8–16floz), but not more than 600ml (1 pint) in one serving.

Fruits such as apples, pears, grapes, and watermelon contain high amounts of water and this, it is claimed, will flush your digestive tract and kidneys and purify your bloodstream.

Advocates of juice fasting also claim that fruits have a purging effect on the liver and gall bladder. Pineapple, for example, contains the enzyme bromelian, which encourages the secretion of hydrochloric acid from the body and helps digest protein. Many other claims are made for the detoxifying effect of fruit and vegetable juices. For example, grapes and apples are potent cleansing agents; watermelon juice is a diuretic (increases urine production); prune and apricot juice are natural laxatives that help promote bowel movement; and cabbage juice is soothing for intestinal wind and ulcers.

Some fruits, such as papaya, coconut, banana, strawberry, peach, cantaloupe, honeydew, plum, and avocado, do not release water when they are blended so they are better eaten whole. Dried fruits can be added to improve the nutritional content of juice.

Vegetable and fruit juices can be combined. For example, carrot can be combined with apple, alfalfa, ginger, watermelon, and lemon zest.

You can also prepare green juices, which are claimed to heal, stabilize, and calm the body and give energy by relaxing and centring. Examples of green juice combinations include celery and spinach; celery, spinach,

---

### JUICE FASTS

**Ingredients for one day's juice:**
- 120ml (4floz) grape juice
- ½ cup beetroot (about 70g/2½oz)
- 2 bunches carrots
- 1 red pepper
- 4–5 sticks celery
- Handful of spinach
- 1 garlic clove
- ⅕ habanero chilli

**Snacks**
- Fruit or vegetable juice

---

and tomato; cabbage, celery, and tomato; and celery, spinach, cabbage, dill, tomato, lemon, garlic, ginger, cayenne, and tamari. Only one green juice should be consumed per day.

## IS IT HEALTHY?

Fasting has been recorded throughout history as part of many different religious practices. However, fasting to detoxify your body or to get you started on a quick weight-loss programme has become popular only in recent years. Juice fasting should not be continued for more than three days because you will not take in adequate protein and may become light-headed and dizzy as a result of the low calorie level and inadequate sodium intake. Because of the high carbohydrate content, juice fasting is not an appropriate diet for people with diabetes.

A number of weight-loss programmes advocate a juice fast combined with high-protein foods to help achieve immediate weight loss. However, such diets should not be followed by people with high blood pressure, diabetes, cardiovascular disease, kidney stones, gout, or high uric-acid levels in the blood because of the high protein and carbohydrate intake.

# Living Beauty Detox

*Detox*

- ⊘ **Are special products required?**
- ⊗ **Is eating out possible?**
- ⊗ **Is the plan family-friendly?**
- ⊘ **Do you have to buy a book?**
- ⊗ **Is the diet easy to maintain?**

This detox plan, aimed specifically at women, proposes internal cleansing as a means of achieving exterior beauty. It claims that the body's appearance is a reflection of inner well-being.

## HOW IT CLAIMS TO WORK

According to Living Beauty Detox, a woman's physiology fluctuates daily, weekly, monthly, and annually, and the programme provides seasonal guides

## LIVING BEAUTY DETOX: TYPE I

### On rising
- Living Beauty Elixir
- 2 high-fibre supplements
- 2 glasses of water

### Before breakfast
- Large cup of dandelion root tea

### Breakfast
- ½ grapefruit
- Boiled eggs
- Steamed kale and red peppers seasoned with chopped fresh thyme

### Lunch
- Grilled spring lamb burger
- Watercress and beansprout salad with a dressing of linseed oil, fresh lemon juice, and chopped fresh chives

### Mid-afternoon
- 2 glasses of water

### 4 pm
- Strawberries

### Dinner
- Poached salmon with steamed Brussels sprouts
- Tomato salad with parsley and spring onions with a dressing of linseed oil, fresh lime juice, and chopped fresh mint

### Mid-evening
- Living Beauty Elixir
- 2 high-fibre supplements
- 2 glasses of water

### Snacks
- As specified

for hormonal, nutritional, emotional, and spiritual balance throughout her life. Seven elements are proposed as the foundation of the programme:
- a cleansed, detoxed system to maintain liver function
- purified water to dilute toxins and flush the body
- powerful proteins to maintain healthy skin, hair, and nails
- beautifying oils, such as omega-3 in order to stabilize blood sugar and suppress appetite
- energizing, immune-boosting organic fruits and vegetables to limit bloating
- revitalizing vitamins, minerals, and protective antioxidants
- balanced hormones.

Living Beauty Detox makes the claim that by including the seven elements in their diets and eliminating sugar, caffeine, alcohol, refined white flour products, and manufactured and/or hydrogenated oils (see p.38), women will rejuvenate their inner wellness and reveal their outer beauty.

### THE REGIMEN

Lasting from three days to two weeks, this diet of balanced fruits, vegetables, and lean protein with supplements of vitamins, minerals, antioxidants, herbs, and spices is complemented by a specially made elixir that is designed to cleanse the body of harmful pollutants. You are encouraged to drink plenty of water and dandelion tea.

Each season, women should analyze their appearance to identify their type and discover sources of underlying internal imbalance. The appropriate detox diet should be maintained during each season of the year.
- Type 1 manifests symptoms of toxin-overload in the spring.
- Type 2 will be susceptible in the summer months.
- Type 3 is vulnerable in autumn.
- Type 4 exhibits imbalance in the winter months.

### IS IT HEALTHY?

This plan is time-intensive and it may be costly to follow. In addition it is low in carbohydrates, which makes it quite difficult to maintain.

The human body is designed to maintain a balance between internal and external environments. The skin, lungs, and immune system provide an external barrier, while the liver, kidneys, and gastrointestinal tract cleanse the body of metabolic wastes or toxins. A diet that is rich in fruits, vegetables, whole grains, lean protein foods, and low-fat dairy products, complemented by regular exercise, should be adequate to maintain normal, healthy physiological function. If your body's innate detox systems are compromised by illness or disease, an extreme or alternative dietary regimen may do more harm than good by placing your organ systems under further stress. In such circumstances, you should consult your GP or a state-registered dietitian, who will formulate an appropriate diet for your needs.

# Detox Diet

*Detox*

- ✖ **Are special products required?**
- ✔ **Is eating out possible?**
- ✖ **Is the plan family-friendly?**
- ✔ **Do you have to buy a book?**
- ✖ **Is the diet easy to maintain?**

According to Dr Elson M. Haas, the author of this plan, detoxification is the missing link in the North American diet and she recommends this diet as a way of losing weight and improving health.

### HOW IT CLAIMS TO WORK

This detoxification plan claims to renew health and increase energy and vitality, as well as promote weight loss. Dr Haas is a practicing physician of integrated medicine and the founder and medical director of the Preventive Medical Center in California. She believes that health problems often arise from nutritional deficiencies, or from congestion resulting either from a reduced ability to eliminate toxins from the body or from the over-consumption of substances such as caffeine, alcohol, nicotine, refined sugar, and food chemicals.

Dr Haas claims that people who are deficient in a variety of nutrients may experience problems such as fatigue, coldness, hair loss, or dry skin. Such people need to be nourished with wholesome foods and to follow a detox diet to aid healing.

Congestive problems include acute and chronic diseases that result from clogging of tissues and tubes and the suffocating of cells and vital energy. Colds and flu, cancer, cardiovascular diseases, arthritis, and allergies are all examples of congestive disorders.

Dr Haas claims that such problems may be prevented or treated, at least in part, and often dramatically improved by cleansing and detoxification.

Dietary changes, including more fruits, vegetables, and water, fewer animal fats and proteins, and the elimination of damaging substances from the body, mark the beginning of a rejuvenation process for the human body.

## THE REGIMEN
The plan includes three meals a day, with drinks including vegetable water and water with lemon juice in place of snacks. Special guidelines include:
• Chewing your food thoroughly and taking time when you are eating
• Relaxing a few minutes before and after a meal
• Eating in a comfortable sitting position
• Consuming plenty of steamed fresh vegetables and some fresh greens
• Drinking only herbal teas after dinner.

Dr Haas recommends following this diet for five to seven days and explains

### DETOX DIET

**Breakfast**
• Piece of fresh fruit

**15–30 minutes later**
• Bowl of cooked whole grain sweetened with freshly squeezed fruit juice

**11am**
• 1–2 glasses of vegetable water with a little sea salt

**Lunch**
• Steamed mixed vegetables, including carrots, green beans, and broccoli

**3pm**
• 1–2 glasses of vegetable water with a little sea salt

**Dinner**
• Steamed mixed asparagus, courgettes, and onions

**Snacks**
• Not allowed

that although you may feel a little weak or have a few symptoms for the first couple of days, this stage will pass. Symptoms may include irritability, fatigue, flu-like feelings, headaches, and mild sinus congestion. Clarity and feeling good should appear by the third or fourth day, if not before.

If you start to feel weak or hungry while you are following this diet, assess your intake and elimination of fluids. If necessary, you can eat a small portion of protein food (85–115g/3–4oz) in the mid-afternoon. This could be fish, free-range organic chicken, chickpeas, lentils, mung beans, or black beans.

## IS IT HEALTHY?
The claim that medical problems may be prevented or improved by cleansing and detoxification is not based on any sound scientific evidence. The Detox Diet is very low in calories, protein, fat, and carbohydrates. It is therefore rather difficult to maintain and may promote nutrient deficiencies if followed for more than a few days. It is true that making the suggested dietary changes – such as eating more fresh vegetables and fruits, drinking more water, limiting animal fats and animal-based protein sources, and eliminating caffeine, alcohol, nicotine, and refined sugars – will help you feel better and lose weight, but it is questionable whether following the Detox Diet menu several times a year is necessary for optimum health.

# Weight Watchers

*Weight-loss centres*

⊗ **Are special products required?**
⊘ **Is eating out possible?**
⊘ **Is the plan family-friendly?**
⊘ **Do you have to buy a book?**
⊘ **Is the diet easy to maintain?**

This popular and comprehensive weight management programme is based on a points system for choosing food that promotes healthy weight loss and long-term weight maintenance. In addition, Weight Watchers provides group support and professional counselling, and it encourage regular physical activity.

### WEIGHT WATCHERS

**Breakfast**
• Small glass of fruit juice
• Sugar-free cereal with skimmed milk from daily allowance and a chopped banana

**Lunch**
• Medium-sized baked jacket potato
• Low-fat coleslaw
• Spoonful of grated Cheddar cheese
• Green salad with an oil- and fat-free dressing
• Apple

**Dinner**
• Grilled or baked chicken breast with couscous and steamed broccoli florets
• Peaches canned in juice with a scoop of low-fat ice cream
• Small glass of wine

**Snacks**
• 300ml (½ pint) skimmed milk (daily allowance)
• Pot of low-fat plain yogurt
• Small handful of pistachio nuts

## HOW IT CLAIMS TO WORK
Weight Watchers' aim is to teach people how to modify their lifestyles, with the help of trained counsellors and group support. A "Winning Points Plan" assigns every food a number of points based on its fat, fibre, and calorie content. There are no forbidden foods, which allows for flexibility and encourages healthy menu selections. This plan facilitates immediate weight loss and enables life-long maintenance of a healthy diet. Weight Watchers At Home and Weight Watchers Online are available for those who are unable or choose not to take part in the weekly group sessions.

## THE REGIMEN
There is no weighing or measuring of foods on this programme. Instead, each weight-watcher is assigned a daily point quota, to which every food and drink that is consumed contributes. To help the slimmer, Weight Watchers has also

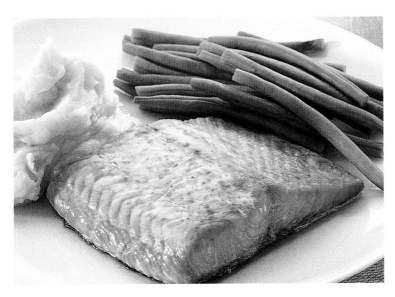

**Weight Watchers** Eating well-balanced, nutritious meals, such as grilled salmon with mashed potato and green beans, is encouraged by this points-based diet programme.

developed special products, ranging from soups and yogurts to ready meals, but they are not an essential part of the diet. Individual quotas are based on BMI (*see pp.26–27*) and the amount of weight to be lost. Slimmers may satisfy their daily point quotas by consuming any combination of foods and drinks, but high-calorie foods have higher point values, while healthful foods have lower values. For example:

- 1 chicken breast = 2.5 points
- 1 crispy spring roll = 5 points
- 1 medium apple = 0.5 points
- 175ml (6floz) wine = 2 points.

The plan encourages drinking plenty of water, and allows tea and coffee (with skimmed milk) and low-calorie drinks.

Encouragement to exercise regularly, routine weight plotting, and counsellor support are all offered by this plan, which teaches life-long habits for healthy eating and exercise.

### IS IT HEALTHY?

Weight Watchers allows people to be flexible in their choices of food while it teaches healthy habits for weight loss and long-term weight maintenance. The programme offers professional advice

on the behavioural aspects of weight control and encourages personal accountability for the lifestyle choices that you make. The regimen thus promotes permanent changes in behaviour, which contribute to its resounding success. The menus and recipes incorporate foods from all food groups in balanced proportions, and the meals are easy to prepare, which promotes long-term maintenance of the goal body weight.

Weight Watchers is ideal for people who wish to lose weight steadily and derive benefit from long-term lifestyle reforms. The group sessions are helpful for support and offer an opportunity to meet new people. This programme is sensible and highly recommended.

# National Slimming Centres

*Weight-loss centres*

- ⊗ **Are special products required?**
- ⊘ **Is eating out possible?**
- ⊘ **Is the plan family-friendly?**
- ⊗ **Do you have to buy a book?**
- ⊘ **Is the diet easy to maintain?**

This programme, which promotes weight loss and long-term management in the context of a healthy lifestyle, is

supported in the United Kingdom by a widespread network of centres with counsellors and doctors.

### HOW IT CLAIMS TO WORK

The plan is based on lowering daily calorie intake and encourages regular exercise to help achieve weight loss. It endorses adopting modified eating habits for long-term weight and health maintenance, and promotes a reduced fat and low sugar intake along with the avoidance of alcohol. Lessons in food preparation and checking food labels make the adoption of healthy nutritional habits easier, leading to permanent, health-promoting lifestyle changes and maintenance of a healthy weight.

### THE REGIMEN

Anyone who contacts a centre is offered a free consultation with a counsellor or doctor in order to determine whether the plan is the best choice for that individual. If you choose to participate in the plan, a low-calorie diet with reduced fat and sugar is formulated. Suggestions include using low-fat spread (rather than butter or margarine), choosing lean meats and low-fat dairy products, and using fewer processed foods and condiments. Slimmers consume three meals a day, each of which contains equal shares of lean

### NATIONAL SLIMMING CENTRES

**Breakfast**
- Scrambled egg
- Toast with low-fat spread
- Glass of grapefruit juice

**Light meal**
- Sliced ham with lettuce
- Whole-grain bread
- Low-calorie yogurt
- Piece of fruit

**Main meal**
- Spaghetti with bolognese sauce
- Large green salad with oil and vinegar dressing

**Snacks**
- Dried apricots

proteins (meat, fish, chicken, and eggs), starchy carbohydrates (bread, potatoes, rice, and pasta), and fruits and vegetables. Slimmers can drink tea, coffee, and low-calorie drinks.

National Slimming Centres offer vitamin supplements and supervised swimming and cycling classes to provide a comprehensive healthy living plan. Adherence to diet and exercise plans is facilitated by complimentary diet sheets, diaries, and guides.

## IS IT HEALTHY?

This programme emphasizes changes in behaviour as the cornerstone of long-term success. Lifestyle modifications in diet and exercise are the most reliable means of achieving immediate weight loss and long-term weight management. National Slimming Centres endorse this philosophy and offer excellent options for people committed to changing habits and embracing healthy living.

# Slimming World

*Weight-loss centres*

⊗ **Are special products required?**
⊘ **Is eating out possible?**
⊘ **Is the plan family-friendly?**
⊗ **Do you have to buy a book?**
⊘ **Is the diet easy to maintain?**

Slimming World was founded in 1969 by Margaret Miles-Bramwell, who remains the driving force behind the company to this day. Currently there are over 5500 Slimming World groups held on a weekly basis throughout the UK. Groups are run by consultants, all of whom are former members of Slimming World who have successfully lost weight and undergone training at the Slimming World head office. There is a one-off membership fee and then a small fee to pay for each class.

## HOW IT CLAIMS TO WORK

The programme is based on a principle called "Food Optimising", which is designed to guide members towards making food choices that are beneficial for weight loss and good health. Foods are divided into three groups: free

foods, healthy extras, and "syns". Free foods are those that can be eaten in unlimited quantities. The healthy extras group includes calcium- and fibre-rich foods. These are "portion controlled" – members are given a daily allowance from this group to ensure that their overall diet is well balanced. Syns are foods such as chocolate, crisps, and alcohol. Members are allowed to eat a certain number of syns every day, depending on their present weight and activity levels, and weight-loss goals.

## THE REGIMEN

Within the Food Optimising programme, members can select either the "green choice" or the "original choice". On the green choice plan, the free foods are fruits, vegetables, certain low-fat dairy products – such as low-fat yogurt and cottage cheese – and carbohydrates

---

### SLIMMING WORLD

**Breakfast**
• Half a small melon such as cantaloupe or Ogen
• Fresh strawberries and raspberries
• Slices of wholemeal bread toasted and topped with lots of baked beans
• A poached egg

**Lunch**
• A large jacket baked potato filled with canned tuna in brine mixed with sweetcorn and reduced-calorie mayonnaise
• Large mixed salad
• Fresh pineapple and mango with very-low-fat plain yogurt

**Dinner**
• Fusilli pasta with a chunky sauce made with tomatoes, aubergines, courgettes, peppers, celery, garlic, herbs, and spices

**Snacks**
• Fresh fruit
• Crackers with cheese triangles
• Fun-size chocolate bar
• 2 measures of any spirit, served with diet mixer if wished

---

such as pasta, rice, and potatoes. On the original choice plan, the free foods are fruits, vegetables, low-fat dairy products, meat, poultry, and fish, and carbohydrates are allocated to the healthy extras group.

Members can choose to follow just the green plan or they can alternate between the green plan and the original plan. The Food Optimising programme automatically limits calorie intake by guiding slimmers towards selecting those foods that will make them feel full and satiated.

## IS IT HEALTHY?

Slimming World offers a flexible and easy-to-follow weight-loss programme. It enables its members to make healthy choices that will help them to manage their weight without having to follow a restrictive diet. It doesn't involve any calorie counting or weighing of food. Because the foods that are designated free foods can be eaten in unlimited quantities, slimmers should never need to feel hungry.

In addition to dietary management, the programme includes advice about behavioural modification and increasing activity levels. Members attending the classes have the added benefit of group support and motivation.

# LA Weight Loss

*Weight-loss centres*

⊘ **Are special products required?**
⊘ **Is eating out possible?**
⊗ **Is the plan family-friendly?**
⊗ **Do you have to buy a book?**
⊗ **Is the diet easy to maintain?**

This is essentially a calorie-restricted weight-loss and maintenance plan, tailored to individual activity levels, and offering personal counselling during the weight-loss phase. It is not currently available in the UK.

## HOW IT CLAIMS TO WORK

The programme, which is individualized according to weight, weight-loss goals, level of exercise, lifestyle, and medical issues, promises that you can eat the

## LA WEIGHT LOSS: RED PLAN

### Breakfast
- Egg white substitutes
- Low-calorie bread
- Small orange

### Lunch
- Grilled chicken breast with lettuce, celery, and tomato salad dressed with oil
- Rice cake

### Dinner
- Grilled halibut with steamed broccoli florets, cucumber slices, and steamed whole-grain (brown) rice

### Snacks
- LA Lite bar
- LA Lite shake made with skimmed milk
- Small apple

foods you like and still lose weight. An extensive medical history questionnaire is completed at the outset, which offers a three-step guide to weight management. This programme consists of weight loss (without loss of lifestyle), weight stabilization, and weight maintenance. Specially formulated bars, shakes, and supplements are available to facilitate the programme's sequential process.

### THE REGIMEN
The programme begins with a three-day high-protein food plan, followed by a calorie-restricted diet aimed at a weight loss of 700–900g (1½–2lb) per week. All the foods allowed are available in supermarkets so it is quite easy for you to prepare your own meals. In addition, the programme offers ideas for when you are eating out.

Depending on your level of physical activity, you will be prescribed one of three levels of calories; the red, gold, and yellow plans. LA Weight Loss does not advocate exercise, but it does suggest that vitamin and mineral supplements are mandatory for weight loss and long-term maintenance. The plan also offers counselling throughout the weight-loss phase of the programme.

### IS IT HEALTHY?
LA Weight Loss provides a reduced-calorie meal plan to help control weight. This plan consists of high-protein, low-carbohydrate foods along with food supplements. Personalized counselling is available several times each week, but most counsellors have no medical or nutritional training and are really just selling supplements, bars, and shakes.

This programme is a good option for individuals who may be sensitive to a high-carbohydrate, low-fat diet, but its maintenance requires continued supplementation with expensive products and nutrient bars. Weekly weigh-ins are helpful for accountability during all phases of the programme.

# Nutrisystem

*Weight-loss centres*

- ✔ **Are special products required?**
- ✖ **Is eating out possible?**
- ✖ **Is the plan family-friendly?**
- ✖ **Do you have to buy a book?**
- ✖ **Is the diet easy to maintain?**

This weight-loss plan provides nutritionally balanced, portion-controlled, prepacked meals for slimmers. In addition, the plan offers both online and telephone counselling as and when required.

### HOW IT CLAIMS TO WORK
The plan revolves around ready-prepared meals that are in line with traditional guidelines for balanced nutrition, being made up of 60 per cent carbohydrate and 20 per cent each fat and protein, in addition to controlling portion sizes. This leads to weight loss as calories are controlled. Currently an online weight-management programme, Nutrisystem offers slimmers telephone, email, and chat-room consultations with agents or diet counsellors. At present it is not available in the UK.

### THE REGIMEN
Ready-made Nutrisystem meals offer choices for three meals a day, including breakfast, lunch, and dinner. The plan also suggests snacks. This eliminates personal choice in menu planning and standardizes the quantity of food consumed, which reduces deviation from a balanced diet and limits the daily calorie intake. Exercise is strongly encouraged, and regular contact with personal counsellors is recommended for successful and steady weight loss. Both online and telephone support are available as required.

### IS IT HEALTHY?
This plan encourages the purchase of most meals online, which may not be possible or appropriate for everybody. Prepackaged meals may contain high amounts of additives, such as sodium, that are restricted for some individuals. The reliance on prepackaged foods makes this a high-cost programme, which is not conducive to long-term slimming. Nor does it teach people how to eat a healthy diet and control portion sizes for themselves.

The long-term effectiveness of the system may also be compromised by the elimination of individual choice in food planning during the weight-loss period. This may cause difficulties for slimmers in developing and maintaining balanced diets once they start preparing their meals themselves.

## NUTRISYSTEM

### Breakfast
- Nutrisystem blueberry muffin with banana
- Glass of skimmed milk

### Lunch
- Nutrisystem Chicken Cacciatore and salad with fat-free dressing
- Grapes

### Dinner
- Nutrisystem Fettuccine Alfredo and salad with fat-free dressing
- Steamed broccoli with a little margarine
- Nutrisystem Chocolate Decadence
- Glass of skimmed milk

### Snacks
- Fat-free yogurt
- Apple

# Extra help with weight loss

## Some people may need extra help to regain control of their weight.

Research shows that weight-loss plans that include behaviour-change counselling are the most effective at helping people lose weight. The success of these is probably due to the accountability involved – you know you are going to be weighed at each visit and you will most likely be keeping a food diary, recording everything you have consumed.

### Weight-loss centres
Group programmes, such as Weight Watchers, and individual counselling centres, such as the National Slimming Centres, can provide you with the opportunity for support and monitoring (*see pp.194–197*). The best programme for you depends on when you would like to attend sessions and your level of comfort at sharing your experiences with a group. For example, if you like meeting people and do not mind talking about your progress and pitfalls, a group plan is a good choice.

The important considerations for sticking to a programme include convenience of location; finding a counsellor who will listen and get to know you, rather than just try to sell you products; and ensuring the programme includes a maintenance plan for at least one year after you have achieved your goal weight. Remember, with any weight-loss centre, even if you

do not lose weight every week, at least you are focusing on healthy eating and feeling better.

### Seeing a dietitian
If you want to have professional help and advice with weight loss, seeing a state-registered dietitian (SRD) is a good option, especially if you have a medical condition such as diabetes or cardiovascular disease. Ask your GP to refer you to an SRD. He or she will be able to help you plan a diet suited to your individual needs.

Two other ways you could seek help with weight loss include medically supervised residential programmes and weight-loss camps for children (*opposite*). Both of these options are expensive, but they can be effective in helping people lose weight.

### Is there a fat gene?
We have all heard that obesity runs in families: children with two obese parents are almost twice as likely to become obese as children with one obese parent.

The genetics of obesity, however, are very complex. What your genes determine is your metabolism – the rate at which your body burns calories. We all know someone who can eat whatever they want and never gain weight, while for others just looking at sweets seems to add weight. Only some of this difference is determined by genes.

Despite recent news heralding the discovery of the "fat gene", genetics accounts for no more than one third of variations in body weight. Since there has been no change in the human gene pool over the past decade, the dramatic increase in the prevalence of obesity in North America – and now in the United Kingdom – is more likely to be a reflection of environmental rather than genetic influences.

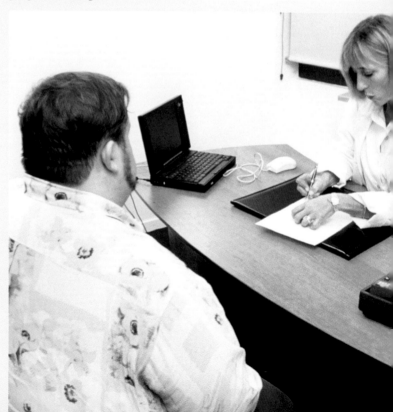

**Seeking medical advice** When excess weight or obesity is seriously undermining health, a dietitian can help formulate the most appropriate therapeutic approach.

# Where can I go for help?

If you know that your weight has become out of control, but you cannot find the motivation and commitment to change your eating and activity patterns in the long-term way that is essential for real weight control, you may look for outside sources of help. For those who can afford it, a personal trainer will create a tailor-made exercise programme and coach you as you achieve your goals.

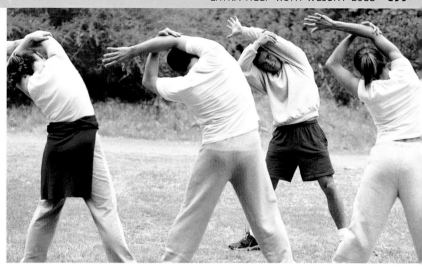

## MEDICALLY SUPERVISED CENTRES

Staying at a health farm or spa for a week to a month may be helpful if you have severe health problems and need to get motivated. What and how much you eat is strictly controlled and your time is taken up with a wide variety of activities, including exercise, relaxation therapy, and beauty treatments. You will lose weight and your health will improve, but unless you continue the regime once you are back home, it is likely to rebound quickly. Serious weight loss requires long-term commitment to a change of lifestyle, involving eating healthily and exercising regularly.

## CHILDREN'S WEIGHT-LOSS CAMPS

Eating healthy food for six to eight weeks, having limited access to junk food, and being physically active all day has been shown to produce 0.9–1.8kg (2–4lb) weight losses per week for children who

**Intensive programme** A stay in a health farm or spa may help get you started on a weight-loss programme, but the lessons learned must be continued in normal life.

attend weight-loss camps. Parents must also show commitment to their children's eating and lifestyle habits in order for them to carry forward into normal life the lessons they learned at the camp.

# Surgical and pharmacological treatment of obesity

When conventional diet and exercise approaches have failed, medication and – in particularly severe cases – surgery may be considered for treating obesity. These are undertaken under the strict supervision of doctors.

**Surgical treatment** To qualify for a surgical option to treat obesity, you must have a BMI of more than 35 (*see pp.26–27*), a history of failed weight loss, and no history of substance abuse or psychiatric disorders.

The most common surgical method for treating obesity in the UK is called laparascopic banding. This procedure limits and controls intake of food, and typically results in a weight loss of between 25 and 50 per cent of body weight, which is generally well maintained. Patients must be able to follow a strict post-surgical diet that includes eating very small amounts of food, mostly protein, for the first six weeks, and taking vitamins and minerals daily.

Side effects include malabsorption of nutrients, undernutrition, and dumping syndrome – a condition in which food passes too rapidly from the stomach to the intestine, causing sweating, fainting, and palpitations.

**Prescription medication** The two medications that are approved for use in the UK and available on prescription are sibutramine and orlistat. Sibutramine is a serotonin and norepinephrine/noradrenaline reuptake inhibitor (SNRI) that works by decreasing food intake. It should not be taken by people who are also taking selective serotonin reuptake inhibitors (SSRI), such as Prozac. Nor should it be taken by those with a history of cardiovascular disease or those taking monoamine oxidase inhibitors (MAOI).

Orlistat blocks the breakdown of triglycerides in the stomach and in the intestine. This results in about 30 per cent of ingested fat remaining unabsorbed, to be excreted in the stool. People taking orlistat have to follow a low-fat diet to minimize side effects. The drug is not suitable for pregnant or breast-feeding women, nor for those who have problems absorbing nutrients or with liver problems such as cholestasis.

**Over-the-counter products** Many weight-loss products are available over the counter, but their safety and effectiveness have not been confirmed by clinical trials.

**Planning ahead** If you are trying to lose weight, make a list of your goals before you start. In addition, keep a food diary to help you identify your habits.

# Your personal diet plan

## Set realistic goals that you can achieve and maintain over time.

Many people lose weight by going on a very low-calorie diet for a short period; but once they start eating normally, the weight piles back on. This is because they have not changed their eating habits or tastes, their activity level, or reset their "set point" (see p.204).

### Setting realistic goals

When you decide it's time to make a change (see pp.30–31) and start a new diet or exercise programme, try to set realistic targets. The key to losing weight and then keeping it off is to set goals that you can achieve and maintain. Once you have achieved these goals – one step at a time – and they have become established, you can raise your sights higher. When you are trying to slim, one per cent of your body weight per week is a safe, steady amount to lose. If you lose more weight than this, you may be losing muscle or fluid and so may become weak or dehydrated.

### Focus on how you feel

If you are eating less and exercising more, and yet not losing weight, do not give up. There are numerous benefits to eating healthily and being more active. You will have more energy, feel better, and have lower levels of cholesterol in your blood. In addition, you will also have a reduced risk of diabetes, cardiovascular disease, and cancer.

# Keys to safe weight reduction

The secret of lifetime weight control is to eat sensibly and maintain an active lifestyle. Here are some tips to help you.

**Lead an active lifestyle** Aim to be more active in your daily life. Participate in exercises that you enjoy, and aim for variety so you do not get bored.

**Follow a balanced diet** Do not skip meals: eat three balanced meals a day, including foods from each food group (see pp.72–73). Many diets advocate eliminating one or two food groups, but they do not teach you how to control your eating habits in the long term.

**Eat a healthy breakfast** Have a low-fat, high-fibre breakfast, such as whole-grain cereal with skimmed or semi-skimmed milk and orange juice. Studies show that people who skip breakfast are more likely to eat fatty foods all day long.

**Cut back on calories** High-protein, high-fat, and high-carbohydrate diets work only because they force people to eat fewer calories. If you want to lose weight you have to eat fewer total calories than you do normally.

**Eat healthy fats** Most of us eat too much saturated fat. Instead of fatty cuts of meat and meat products, high fat dairy products, and cakes and biscuits, choose poultry (particularly breast), fish, shellfish, pulses, eggs, low- or reduced-fat cheeses, and tofu, all of which are excellent sources of protein, nutrients, and healthy fats.

**Eat smaller portions** Learn to eat until you are satisfied, and then stop. Don't have seconds.

**Snack only when you are hungry** If you are hungry between meals, eating a small snack will keep you from making poor food choices at your next meal. Choose healthy snacks like fruits or nuts.

**Drink plenty of water** Sometimes thirst is misinterpreted as hunger, so you may end up eating when all you really need is a drink. Drinking a large glass of water half an hour before eating will help you eat smaller meals.

**Compensate for overindulgence** If you eat too much one day, make a conscious effort to eat less for the next few days and try to increase your activity level.

**Stop late-night snacking** This bad habit can add hundreds of extra calories at a time when you are least likely to burn them off.

• Do the washing up right after dinner and avoid going back in the kitchen.

• If you find yourself drawn to the kitchen during TV adverts, look at a book or magazine instead.

• Exercise often reduces your hunger and will help you sleep better; take a short walk after dinner, ride an exercise cycle, or walk on a treadmill.

• If you are so hungry that you cannot sleep, eat a piece of fruit, then a glass of skimmed or semi-skimmed milk.

# Everyday changes for weight loss

To lose weight, you have to consume fewer calories and exercise more, but it is important that you still obtain the nutrients you need. This means thinking very carefully about what you eat, filling up on nutritious but low-calorie foods, and avoiding high-calorie low-nutrient foods such as sweets, crisps, biscuits, and sugary drinks.

Here are some guidelines to help you achieve a balanced diet that will allow you to lose weight while maintaining your health. Every day you need:

**Two to three servings of vegetables**
Vegetables are filling, low in calories, and a valuable source of phytochemicals, which have many health benefits (*see pp.76–77*). Eat vegetables raw or cook using healthy methods such as steaming or microwaving, and skip added fat such as butter, margarine, or cheese. Alternatively, you can stir-fry or sauté, using a small amount of olive or rapeseed oil or a vegetable spray.

**Two to three servings of fruits** Fruits make great between-meal snacks when you are hungry, and are ideal as desserts

(*see pp.78–79*). If you like fruit juice, be sure to choose 100 per cent juice and limit it to 120ml (4floz) servings diluted with water.

**At least five servings of breads and cereals** Select whole-grain varieties, which have more fibre and fill you up more than refined grains (*see pp.74–75*). Include grains at breakfast, lunch, and dinner and mix with pulses or vegetables for protein-rich meals.

**Two to three servings of dairy foods**
High calcium intake has been shown to aid weight loss and prevent weight gain (*see p.63*), but choose low- or reduced-fat dairy products. If you have trouble tolerating milk, look for products with lactase enzyme added (*see p.232*).

**Two to three servings of protein foods**
There is no need to eat meat every day. Fish and shellfish, eggs, dairy products, soya products, pulses, and nuts are all good sources of protein too and most of them are low in unhealthy saturated fat. To help you lose weight, choose poultry breast without skin, fish, and lean cuts of meat (*see pp.86–91*).

## Tips for eating out

There is no reason to avoid eating out if you are trying to lose weight, but you will need to think carefully about what you order, and about how to avoid consuming more calories in the course of one meal than you really need.

● Have a small snack before setting out for the restaurant so you will not feel hungry when you arrive. You will then be less likely to want bread or a starter.

● Listen to your stomach and stop eating when you are full. Ask the waiter to remove your plate once you have finished.

● Order wine by the glass instead of the bottle and learn to make one glass last for the entire meal. If you are thirsty, drink water.

● Ask the waiter not to bring you any bread, or to remove it if it is already on the table. Most people do not eat bread with their meal at home, so there is no need to do so when eating out.

# Lunch makeover

Going out for lunch often means a visit to a café for a sandwich where there is a mouth-watering array of meats and other fillings to choose from. However, many of these fillings are very high in saturated fat and calories, and need to be limited if you are trying to lose weight.

It is still possible to enjoy the café experience by making some judicious changes in what you normally order.

● Choose a whole-grain or wholemeal bread or roll for your sandwich, rather than white or brown. In this way, you are adding essential fibre and other nutrients to your lunch.

● Opt for lean meats such as turkey or chicken breast or seafood such as prawns rather than sausages or salami, which are high in saturated fat.

● Add healthy fillings such as lettuce, avocado, and tomato slices rather than high-fat cheese, and mustard instead of mayonnaise or sweet pickle.

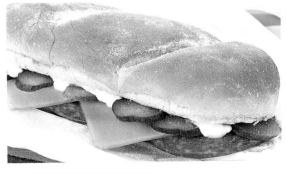

**High-fat option**
This white bread roll filled with salami, processed cheese, gherkins, and mayonnaise has over 800 calories with over 50g of fat, 30g of which is saturated.

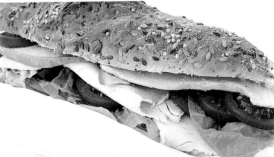

**Healthier choice**
With 500 calories, this rustic whole-grain roll with turkey breast, avocado, lettuce, and tomato has 30g of fat, of which just 7.0g is saturated.

# Regular exercise and weight loss

## Exercise is a vital component of any weight-loss plan.

A recent survey revealed that only 36 per cent of men and 26 per cent of women in the UK meet the current Department of Health recommendation for a minimum of 30 minutes moderate physical activity at least five days a week. Such inactivity carries with it a list of life-threatening ramifications; it is also a major factor in the current levels of overweight and obesity.

If you are trying to lose weight, increasing your level of physical activity is as important as how much you eat. Physical activity refers to all the bodily movements that result in energy expenditure and includes routine activities such as gardening and walking as well as structured exercise and sport.

### Begin gradually

If you have been sedentary for a while, it is advisable to start by gradually increasing the amount of activity in your daily life. For example, walking round your

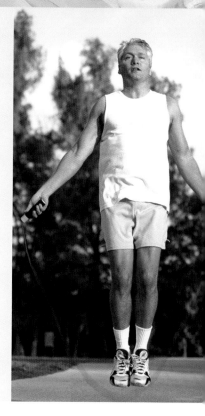

**Aerobic exercise** Skipping is a great workout for the cardiovascular system as well as helping to burn calories. It is even more enjoyable and beneficial if done outdoors.

## How to get started

Once you have been cleared by your GP to begin your exercise programme (*opposite above*) and have planned a balanced routine that includes a mixture of aerobic exercise, strength training, and stretching, there are a few points to bear in mind to help you get the most out of your new routine.

### SET REALISTIC TARGETS

Remember to start any new exercise programme slowly and to increase your efforts gradually. The same holds true when using new exercise equipment. If you start a programme that pushes you too hard, you increase risk of injury and will be less likely to persevere.

Set short- and long-term goals that are based on your current activity level. If you have not exercised for some time, aim to introduce a little exercise two or three times a week, such as a walk or swim during your lunch break. You can then gradually increase the intensity, duration, or frequency of your exercise sessions as you become more active.

### PLAN YOUR PROGRAMME

Select an activity you enjoy, get started slowly, and stick with it. The great thing about exercise is that it makes you feel good, so once it becomes a habit you will not want to miss the opportunity to do it. Aim for a variety of exercises so you stay motivated.

Choose exercises that will work all your major muscle groups, burn calories, and improve your flexibility. Swimming, cycling, running, and other aerobic exercises will raise your heart rate, improve your cardiovascular fitness, and burn calories.

When you lose weight, the body tends to lose fat and muscle, so it is important for you to preserve muscle mass as you burn calories. Strength training with free weights or resistance machines will help increase your muscle mass and raise your metabolic rate. It also will improve the appearance of your body by toning the underlying muscles.

You should always allow at least five minutes before and after each exercise session for stretches. This activity will help prevent injury and complete your balanced work-out.

### DON'T EXPECT INSTANT CHANGE

Do not give up exercising before the benefits start to kick in. People tend to lose motivation at about the two-month mark: they think they should see an improvement in the way they look and feel and, when they do not, they give up, thinking all that sweat and hard work did not make a difference.

In reality, most people will not see a significant improvement until they have been exercising regularly for at least three months. So do not give up. Be patient and keep going; it is worth the wait and the effort.

And remember, as you build muscle and lose fat, your weight may not change initially but you will know that you are shaping up when your clothes start to fit better. You will also be feeling better after about three months, even if the bathroom scales do not change.

neighbourhood or in a local park is a great way to work your body and enjoy the outdoors at the same time. When you do start on an exercise regimen, do so slowly and increase your effort gradually. If you push yourself too hard you risk injury and are more likely to give up. While exercise should be challenging, it is more important that you design for yourself an enjoyable programme that you will continue and develop.

## Exercises for weight loss

There are many forms of exercise, but if you are trying to lose weight the perfect regime includes both anaerobic and aerobic exercise. Anaerobic exercise refers to those activities that use resistance, such as lifting weights. This type of exercise strengthens, tones, and conditions your muscles, and it improves your endurance. It also increases your lean muscle mass and, as a result of this, raises your metabolic rate, which affects the rate at which your body uses up calories. Because your body tends to lose fat and muscle when you lose weight, it is very important to include anaerobic exercise in your exercise programme.

Aerobic exercise, such as dancing and swimming, raises your heart rate and burns calories, especially from fat. Therefore it should form an important component of your weight-loss programme.

## Maintaining flexibility

While stretching exercises do not directly affect weight, they are an important part of physical fitness. Be sure to include five to ten minutes of warm-up and cool-down before and after exercising. This will help you avoid injury and improve flexibility.

## Seeking medical advice

If you have any medical problems, are overweight, are over the age of 50, or have not done any exercise for some time, it is important for your GP to give you a physical examination before you start an exercise programme.

Your doctor may recommend a stress test to check the blood flow to your heart. During this test, you ride a stationary bike or walk on a treadmill, gradually increasing the effort, while your heart rhythm and blood pressure are monitored. This test is a good indication of any potential problem in the blood supply to your heart, such as a blockage in the arteries. If your stress test is abnormal, you will be advised not to exercise until further tests are performed, in order to avoid any risk of heart attack.

# Tips on incorporating activity into your daily routine

In addition to starting on an exercise programme at a gym or health club, it is important to start incorporating more physical activity into your daily routine. As with all behavioural changes, the aim is to make changes gradually (*see pp.30–31*). Choose just one new activity that you think you can succeed in building into your regular schedule. Only when that has been established should you try to include another one.

• Schedule a 30-minute walk at the same time each day. It may help if you can arrange to walk with a friend or a family member, or make a special time to take the dog for a walk.
• Take the stairs instead of the lift at work or when shopping.
• Walk whenever you can instead of driving, including when going to work.
• Get off the bus at the stop before your office and walk the rest of the way.
• Park in the space farthest away from the shops so you have to walk there.

• Do more housework yourself, such as cleaning the house, washing the car, raking leaves, or gardening.
• Invest in some exercise equipment to use at home, such as a stationary bicycle.
• Make time to exercise and schedule it as you would an appointment; many people find that exercising in the morning before the day gets too busy helps them accomplish this goal.
• Buy a fitness video or DVD and get the whole family to join in the routine as a change from watching TV or playing computer games.
• Accustom children to the idea of walking to school or to the bus stop; use the time to talk about what you see and where you are going.

**Start them young**  Get children used to walking places. You can make it fun by playing games such as "I Spy" or "Hop, Skip, and Jump" as you go along.

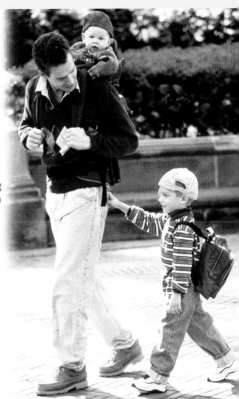

# Calories expended in different activities

There are tremendous benefits, both mental and physical, to getting even a small amount of physical activity each day. All activity is good for you (and will burn calories), but it is worth noting that you do not have to be an athlete to be active. Regular activities such as mowing the grass and playing football with the children all count towards keeping fit.

The amount of calories expended during exercise varies according to your gender and weight. Because of their greater muscle mass, men burn more calories than women while doing the same activity; and the heavier you are, the more calories you will burn. Conversely, when you lose weight your calorie requirements decrease, even if you continue with the same level of physical activity.

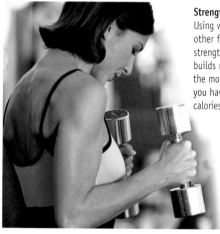

**Strength training** Using weights and other forms of strength training builds muscles; and the more muscle you have, the more calories you burn.

| ACTIVITY 30 MINUTES | CALORIES MAN (80kg/175lb) | CALORIES WOMAN (60kg/135lb) |
|---|---|---|
| Badminton | 180 | 135 |
| Basketball | 280 | 225 |
| Cycling | 334 | 258 |
| Dancing | 188 | 145 |
| Football | 292 | 225 |
| Gardening | 209 | 161 |
| Golf | 180 | 135 |
| Hiking | 251 | 193 |
| Horseriding | 167 | 129 |
| Housework | 188 | 145 |
| Jogging | 292 | 225 |
| Mowing grass | 251 | 193 |
| Playing with kids | 167 | 129 |
| Skating | 292 | 225 |
| Skipping | 400 | 300 |
| Step aerobics | 180 | 140 |
| Stretching/yoga | 167 | 129 |
| Swimming | 334 | 258 |
| Tennis | 292 | 225 |
| Walking | 167 | 129 |
| Weight training | 162 | 127 |

# How to increase metabolic rate

Metabolic rate is the rate at which your body uses energy to keep it functioning, and it varies among people.
• The more you weigh, the higher your metabolic rate will be.
• Metabolic rate increases during rapid growth periods, such as adolescence.
• People with a high proportion of body muscle to fat have a higher metabolic rate than those with a lower proportion of muscle to fat.

### FALSE CLAIMS

Many diets claim to increase metabolic rate through special fat-burning foods and exercises. In fact, your metabolic rate falls if you start losing weight.

### INCREASING EXERCISE

Exercise is the only effective way to increase your metabolic rate. Not only do we use up energy (calories) during exercise, but the increased metabolic rate that occurs while we exercise will continue for several hours afterwards. The amount of increase in the metabolic rate varies from person to person, but even a modest increase should help to counteract the body's natural tendency to decrease metabolic rate.

It is not known why exercise has this effect, but some researchers believe that exercise preserves more of our lean body tissue as fat tissue is lost during weight loss.

# What is "set point"?

Short-term diets are doomed to fail. You may lose some weight but when you return to your usual diet your weight will return to its usual level. This is due to what scientists call "set point" – the level at which the body defends its current weight. If you burn more calories than you eat, your body will become more efficient at converting those calories into energy, so that you will not lose weight. If you are trying to slim, you have to make a serious commitment over a long period in order to retrain your body and readjust your set point.

# Benefits of different types of exercises

Whereas physical activity refers to all the body movements that result in energy expenditure, exercise refers to planned and structured repetitive movements designed specifically to improve fitness and health. These include activities you can do at home, in the gym, or outdoors. Whether you do exercise indoors or out, however, it is also categorized according to whether it is aerobic or anaerobic.

## AEROBIC EXERCISE

This is defined as any activity that uses large muscle groups, can be maintained continuously, and is rhythmic in nature. It is a type of exercise that overloads the heart and lungs and causes them to work harder than when at rest. Examples of aerobic exercise include running, swimming, dancing, skipping rope, and cycling. This type of exercise has many health benefits, which include:
• Improved cardiovascular function
• Lowered blood pressure

• Increased HDL and decreased LDL
• Reduced body fat and improved weight control
• Improved glucose tolerance and reduced insulin resistance.

## ANAEROBIC EXERCISE

In contrast to aerobic exercise, anaerobic exercise involves short bursts of exertion followed by periods of rest, as a result of which you develop muscle strength. Although anaerobic exercise does not burn fat, it contributes to weight loss since bigger muscles burn more calories. Examples of anaerobic exercise include press-ups, stomach crunches, curl-ups, and lifting weights.

## FOLLOW A TAILORED PROGRAMME

Before starting on an exercise regime, it is essential to discuss your aims with a professional who will assess your level of fitness and plan an appropriate programme. As you progress, this should be reviewed and adjusted as necessary.

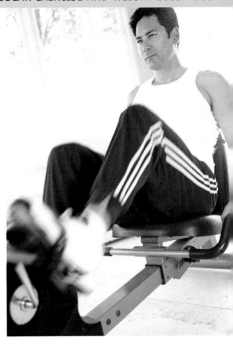

**Indoor rowing**  An ideal aerobic exercise, rowing strengthens the muscles of both the upper and lower body, as well as improving your cardiovascular function.

# Case study  Overweight middle-aged man needing exercise

**Name**  Danny

**Age**  45 years

**Problem**  Danny is 23kg (50lb) overweight and his GP has recently told him that he needs to exercise in order to improve his overall health. He has a family history of cardiovascular disease and diabetes – his mother is obese and has type 2 diabetes and his father has cardiovascular disease.

**Lifestyle**  Danny is a regional manager for a pharmaceutical company, and he travels a lot. He says he does not have time to exercise and believes that he is active enough with his job. Danny is 1.8m (5ft 8in) tall and weighs 104kg (230lb). His weight has been steadily increasing by about 2.3kg (5lb) each year since he was at college. Because

Danny is on the road, driving to visit his sales representatives, he spends most of his day sitting. At night he spends time with his children, then returns to his computer in order to check emails and his schedule for the next day. Danny does not own any exercise equipment and he does not belong to a gym.

**Advice**  In order for Danny to begin a regular exercise regime, he needs to understand the benefits and decide that he is going to make the effort to change his behaviour. But first, his doctor should give him a check-up, to clear him for exercise. The next step is for Danny to figure out when, where, and how he could be more physically active. For example, since he is travelling and staying in hotels at least once a week, he could bring his exercise clothes and shoes, and schedule time to work out while he is

away from home. If joining a gym near his house is feasible, an effective method to get more active would be to go at least once a week to start with, before or after work. When he is at the gym, he could walk on the treadmill for about 20–30 minutes and lift weights for about 10–15 minutes. This will help him feel better and give him more energy as well.

If Danny does not think that he has time to go to the gym, before or after work or at lunchtime, it might be better for him to buy a treadmill or exercise cycle to use at home. He could then exercise at his convenience, either before or after work, and also at the weekends.

As both Danny's parents are ill, he should be motivated to listen to his doctor's advice or Danny too is likely to develop health problems. This is an opportune time for him to begin an exercise programme.

# Children and weight management

## Overweight in children and adolescents is becoming a serious problem in the UK.

According to official figures, since the 1980s the number of children and teenagers who are overweight has increased dramatically: today, one in three children is overweight, while almost nine per cent of six-year-olds and 17 per cent of 15-year-olds are obese.

These increases are thought to be due to a variety of cultural factors, including easier access to high-calorie foods, decreased opportunities for exercise, and increased interest in sedentary activities, such as watching TV or sitting in front of a computer. Overweight children are likely to remain overweight as adults and are at risk of the same health problems as adults.

### What causes obesity?

Studies suggest that genetics plays a major role in the incidence of obesity. According to current estimates, a child with two obese parents has an 80 per cent chance of becoming obese, while a child with just one obese parent has a 40 per cent risk.

Children who lead an inactive life – especially those who watch more than two hours of TV each day – are at risk of obesity. The large amount of food advertising aimed at children during television programmes may be one factor, along with the increase in fast food and soft drink consumption.

### Is my child overweight?

In order to check whether your child's weight is within healthy limits, plot his or her BMI score (*see p.113*). A score in the 85–95th percentile indicates that your child is overweight; a score above the 95th percentile indicates that

### Health risks of obesity

Numerous tracking studies have demonstrated that an obese child runs an increased risk of becoming an obese adult. Obese children may be even more obese as adults than they would have been if they had first become overweight in adulthood. Thus, preventing or treating childhood obesity should significantly decrease the likelihood of adult obesity and its associated medical problems.

Overweight and obese children and adolescents are at risk from the same health problems as adults who are overweight (*see p.158*). These problems include diabetes, high blood pressure, high blood cholesterol levels, sleep apnoea, asthma, gall bladder disease, bone and joint disorders, and liver problems (*see pp.214–251*).

he or she is obese. Your child's progress should be tracked over time because it is normal for overweight pre-pubertal children to be taller than their counterparts of average weight. Overweight children enter puberty and have their growth spurt earlier.

Weight management rather than dieting is usually the way forward, and there are a number of changes that can be made to cut down on calories and to increase physical activity. However, the greatest influence on a child's habits is his or her parents, so the best thing you can do is lead by example.

### Underweight children

Adolescents in particular are also susceptible to eating disorders. These may develop into serious medical problems that require professional help (*opposite*).

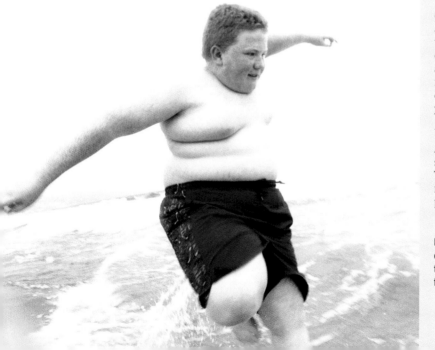

**Enjoying physical activity** If your child is overweight, help him find physical activities that he enjoys. It will help him if the whole family can join in and participate with him.

# Focus on eating healthy and being active

The best way you can help your child maintain a healthy weight is to make healthy eating and exercise a normal part of your daily lives.

• Focus on healthy eating, not slimming. Provide interesting, varied food that all the family will enjoy and be sure to serve fruits and vegetables every day.

• Provide an environment that includes only healthy food choices. Cut down or stop buying unhealthy food, such as crisps and fizzy drinks. It is unfair to expect your child not to eat a food that you or other family members are eating.

• Make eating a sociable and enjoyable occasion; try to eat together, without the television on in the background.

• Drink water or skimmed milk with meals and snacks, rather than cola.

• Serve smaller portions using small plates and glasses, and provide more vegetables or a fruit dessert for people to fill up on if they are still hungry.

• Don't force your children to clean their plates: let them be guided by their appetite and stop eating when they are fully satisfied.

• Limit fast food to less than once a week, and choose carefully. Children who eat a lot of fast food will be eating too much saturated fat, and they may be missing out on important nutrients such as fibre, vitamins, and minerals, especially calcium.

• If your child suffers from allergies or food intolerances, you should consider working with a state-registered dietitian for ideas and nutritional advice.

• Encourage your children to find physical activities that they enjoy and take an interest in their progress.

• Look for activities that you can do together as a family.

• Try to build exercise and physical activity into your daily routine.

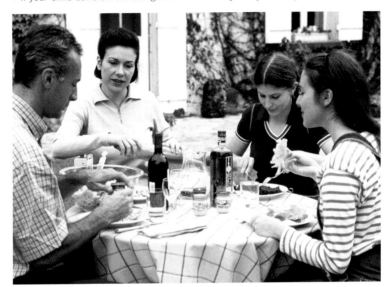

**Eating together** To encourage healthy eating habits in children, eat together as a family. Offer nutritious food and treat mealtimes as a chance to enjoy one another's company.

# Warning signs of eating disorders

Eating disorders most commonly affect adolescents and young women, and occur across all the social groups. Figures suggest that about 20 per cent of teenagers engage in abnormal eating behaviour, while about three per cent have a diagnosed disorder.

Those with anorexia nervosa typically have an altered perception of their own body image (*right*) that leads to severe restriction of calories and a resulting loss of weight. Parents should look out for changes in eating behaviours, such as skipping meals and exercising for at least three hours every day. Because anorexia nervosa often leads to the cessation of menstrual periods, it is important for parents to be aware of changes in their daughter's cycle.

Another type of eating disorder, bulimia nervosa, is characterized by episodes of binge eating followed by purging (*right*). Those affected tend not to lose weight so the problem may be less obvious. Look for damage to the enamel of your daughter's teeth. She may complain of heartburn from vomiting and spend a lot of time in the bathroom after meals.

## WHERE TO GET HELP

Eating disorders are considered to be psychiatric conditions. Treatment for such disorders is complex and requires a team approach combining medical management, psychological intervention, and nutritional counselling. It is crucial to get a diagnosis first from a doctor who is familiar with eating disorders.

## Jargon buster

**Anorexia nervosa** This condition, which occurs mainly, though not exclusively, in adolescent girls, involves an intense fear of gaining weight or becoming fat, a disturbed perception of body weight or shape, and doing intensive exercise. The condition leads to changes in hormone levels that affect growth and menstruation.

**Bulimia** Like anorexia sufferers in terms of concern with weight and body shape, people with bulimia alternate periods of binge eating with strategies to avoid weight gain, such as forcing themselves to vomit and using laxatives.

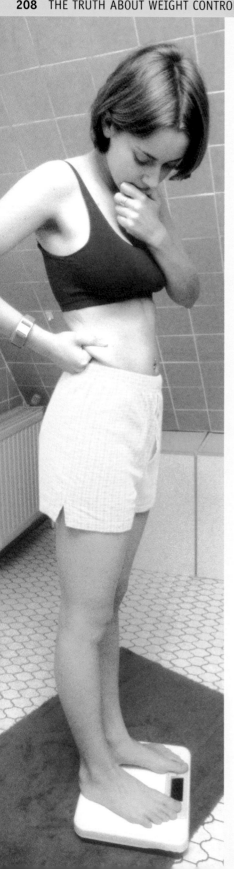

**Weight check** Being underweight, especially resulting from an unplanned weight loss, may be a cause for concern. Weigh yourself and then see your GP if necessary.

# When you need to gain weight

Being underweight has as many health implications as being overweight or obese.

Obesity may be getting all the headlines, but there are also many people who exhibit varying degrees of underweight. For example, adults and teenagers with a BMI below 18.5 (*see pp.26–27 and p.113*) are considered underweight, as are children with a BMI for their age below the 5th percentile (*see p.113*).

As with overweight and obesity, being underweight has many health consequences, including impaired wound healing, higher incidences of infection, and possibly pressure sores. If you lose too much weight, you may develop heart problems since heart function declines with severe malnutrition.

## Causes of underweight

Unplanned weight loss is often a problem in older people; it is also frequently a sign of serious illness. Some of the most common causes of weight loss include:
• Cancers of the colon, lung, and pancreas, and leukemia.
• Gastrointestinal disorders such as peptic ulcer, inflammatory bowel disease, chronic pancreatitis, and coeliac disease.
• Endocrine diseases, such as diabetes and thyroid conditions.
• Infections, such as tuberculosis, fungal disease, parasites, and HIV.
• Psychiatric conditions such as depression, schizophrenia, and Alzheimer's disease often cause weight loss because of poor appetite or forgetting to eat.
• Some medications because they cause loss of appetite, nausea, and diarrhoea (*see p.153*).

## Treating underweight

The aim of nutritional therapy is to increase energy intake and to provide essential vitamins and minerals, without increasing the overall volume of food eaten.

## Nutritional reasons for failure to thrive in infants

Children whose weight or rate of weight gain is significantly below that of other children of similar age and gender are considered to be failing to thrive. Medical problems could be the cause and you should talk to your GP or health visitor; however, 80 per cent of cases are the result of diet. If not caught early, failure to thrive may lead to loss of muscle mass, impaired respiratory and heart function, and a weakened immune system. If caught early, delayed growth can be resolved with diet. The main reasons are:

• Being fed over-diluted or incorrectly prepared formula
• Being given skimmed or semi-skimmed milk instead of full-fat milk between 12 and 24 months of age
• Inappropriate feeding practice for children, such as the consumption of 350ml (12floz) or more fruit juice every day
• Being fed foods low in nutrients and high in calories instead of age-appropriate nutrient-dense foods between 12 and 24 months of age
• Being fed puréed or liquid food at a stage when ready to eat solid food.

# How to gain weight

The first step in treating people who are underweight is to identify and address the underlying specific causes of unplanned weight loss. This may involve taking nutritional supplements or medication or undergoing psychosocial therapy.

## DEALING WITH WEIGHT LOSS
Weight gain can be much harder to achieve than weight loss, particularly if your appetite is poor or you are feeling nauseous. The target is to increase energy intake and to provide essential vitamins and minerals, without increasing the overall volume of food consumed. Eating frequent, smaller, high-calorie nutritious meals and snacks throughout the day allows a greater intake and should prevent further weight loss and promote weight gain if needed.

Nutritional therapy, including dietary education and/or the use of liquid supplements supervised by a dietitian, is usually beneficial. The severity of weight loss should be determined by a nutritional evaluation, which includes laboratory tests combined with a dietary history and evaluation of a person's psychosocial situation.

The goal of nutrient intake in people with low body weight and pronounced weight loss is 30–35cal per 1kg (2¼lb) of body weight per day. At least 20 per cent of the calories consumed should come from protein. Malnourished older people and those with mild to moderate illness need to consume 40cal per 1kg (2¼lb) of body weight per day in order to treat underweight.

## HELP WITH WEIGHT GAIN
Here are some tips on dietary changes that may help you gain weight:
● Serve butter or margarine with vegetables and use oil-based dressings.
● Add cheese to egg dishes such as omelettes and scrambled eggs.
● Add cream, evaporated milk, or whole milk to soups, sauces, and desserts.
● Add fish or minced meat, chicken, or turkey to tomato-based pasta sauces.
● Use butter, full-fat margarine, or mayonnaise in sandwiches.
● Choose full-fat dairy products rather than low-fat or fat-free varieties.
● Eat at least three times a day, and use a clock to remind you when to eat.
● Snack between meals on slices of cheese, peanut butter sandwiches, avocado or cream cheese dips, whole milk puddings, and yogurts.
● Drink whole milk or juices with meals.
● Don't drink too much before eating since this can reduce your appetite.

## Liquid supplements
Nutritional supplement drinks can be beneficial for people who are trying to gain weight. They are available with different calorie and protein quantities to suit different needs and may be bought without a prescription in chemists and supermarkets, although your doctor can also prescribe them.

Liquid supplements usually provide 100 per cent of the recommended daily amount of vitamins and minerals. The drinks are available in a variety of flavours, such as vanilla and chocolate. You can also get savoury flavours. To enhance their taste, supplements with sweet flavours are usually best served chilled.

Liquid supplements should be used only as part of a balanced diet – they are not intended to provide all your nutritional needs. Most types contain little or no fibre, so they will not improve bowel function or prevent constipation. In addition, they do not contain the phytochemicals that occur in fruits and vegetables, which can help in reducing the risk of cancer and cardiovascular disease.

# Tips to boost your appetite

Loss of appetite is a common problem following illness or while taking certain medications or undergoing various therapies. However, these are also the times when your body has most need of good nutrition, to help you regain your strength and boost your immune system. Here are some suggestions for ways to boost your appetite and help you look forward to mealtimes.
● Choose different foods each week at the supermarket to add interest and variety to your diet.
● Arrange to go out for lunch or dinner once a week and try new dishes.
● Get together to eat with your family and friends.
● Even if you do not feel very hungry, try to eat something at every mealtime.
● In the summertime, eat outside in the garden, have a picnic, or eat by an open window.
● Make your food look appetizing with different colours and textures on the plate, attractively presented.
● Take time to arrange the table with your best cutlery, dishes, and place mats. Add flowers too.
● Take a short walk in the fresh air before sitting down to a meal.

**Regaining your appetite** Eating with friends and family may help you regain your appetite after a debilitating illness. Sharing a meal remains a pleasant social experience.

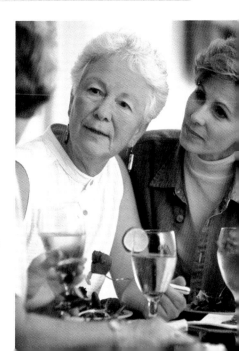

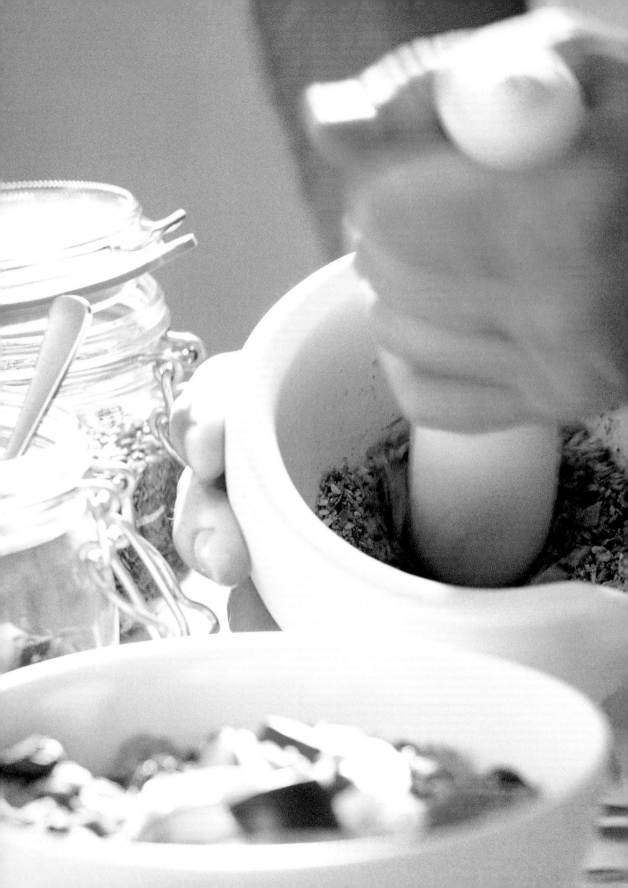

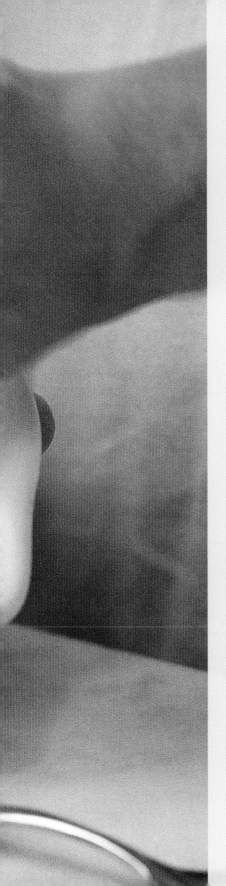

# Food as medicine

There is no doubt that healthy eating can make you feel better, improve your quality of life, and even help you to live longer. This chapter looks at the key role that food can play in the prevention and treatment of a variety of diseases and medical conditions.

# Improving health through diet

**The foods you eat are critical in determining both your current and future health.**

This chapter presents an overview for anyone who is interested in preventing health problems. But more important, it is a starting point for improving health if you already have one of the disorders discussed in this chapter.

### Protection against disease

Each week, more proof emerges showing that a healthy diet and regular exercise help ward off cardiovascular disease, diabetes, cancer, and osteoporosis. Those who eat healthily throughout their lives are more likely to remain disease-free than those who follow the typical North European diet, which is high in artery-clogging fat and low in nutrients.

Healthy eating can help treat health-related problems. For example, the risk of death from cardiovascular disease is starting to fall in the UK, thanks to medical advances. However, people are still eating more fat than they should and exercising less, which is resulting in a rise in rates of obesity. As we gain weight the risk of cardiovascular disease rises. We need to increase our exercise levels and control our fat intake to continue to reduce this risk.

### Maintain a healthy weight

Research shows that if you are overweight and lose weight, your life expectancy increases. It also shows that by improving your diet and exercise habits to lose weight, your health will also improve.

Regular exercise, combined with a well-balanced, nutritious diet, is the key to managing many of the diseases discussed in this chapter.

### Ageing and diet

As we age, our bodies and our dietary needs change. Ongoing research looking at the impact of calorie restriction on health and longevity indicates that adults can improve their health by eating less. If you are overweight, the reasons for losing weight are clear. But even if you are a "healthy" weight, it may be possible to live longer and live better by eating less. This does not mean starvation, it means making smart choices and eating foods that give maximum nutritional benefit for the calories.

### Talk to your doctor

Your doctor is your best source of reliable health advice. The information given here should not be used to prescribe or provide treatment for yourself. Instead, this chapter should be a starting point to help you determine the most important dietary changes you can make to improve your health. Seeing a state-registered dietitian can also help you make the dietary and lifestyle changes your doctor recommends to you.

**Healthy choices** At any stage of life, a nutritious, balanced diet can help prevent and, in many cases, treat existing disorders.

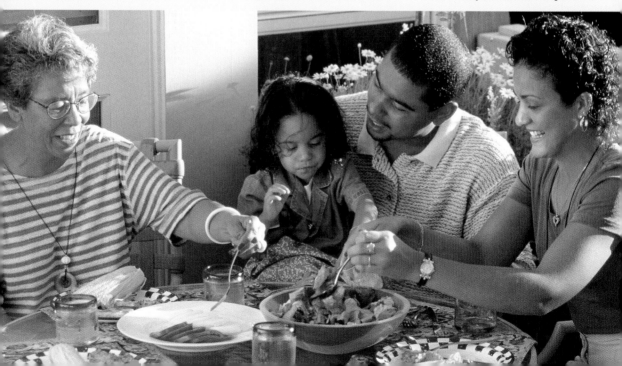

# The top 15 super foods

These foods are highly valued for the health-giving, disease-preventing properties of the nutrients they supply.

**Blueberries** These contain valuable amounts of fibre, vitamin C, and B vitamins. They also contain flavonoids that improve the circulation and aid the body's defenses against infection.

**Broccoli** This is a star ingredient, rich in vitamins and minerals, particularly vitamin C and beta-carotene, as well as folate, all of which can protect against cardiovascular disease and cancer.

**Linseeds** Rich in omega-3 fatty acids, which is beneficial in treating high blood cholesterol and high blood pressure.

**Low-fat yogurt** Rich in calcium, which is vital for bone health, and protein.

**Nuts** Packed with selenium and vitamin E, nuts can help lower cholesterol levels. Recommended as part of the DASH diet to reduce high blood pressure (*see p.220*).

**Oil-rich fish** Tuna, salmon, mackerel, and trout are all oily fish that are rich in omega-3 fatty acids, which may help control cholesterol levels.

**Olive oil** An excellent source of healthy monounsaturated fat, which is good for maintaining levels of "good" cholesterol in the body (*see p.40*).

**Oranges** This fruit is one of the best-known sources of vitamin C, which may help prevent free-radical damage to the cells and tissues.

**Peppers** Peppers are a great source of beta-carotene and vitamin C, both of which are antioxidants that can help ward off cancer.

**Pulses** A significant source of soluble fibre, which can help lower cholesterol levels if eaten regularly. Pulses are also high in iron, folate, and potassium.

**Porridge oats** Oats are a great source of soluble fibre and can help lower blood cholesterol levels. They are also a useful source of magnesium and zinc.

**Quinoa** Originating in South America, this "super" grain is part of the traditional Andean diet. It is gluten-free, and high in fibre and protein.

**Red grapes** These contain antioxidants that can protect against cancer.

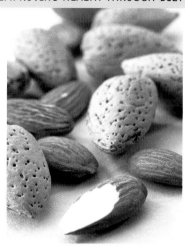

**Almonds** Considered by many to be the most nutritionally balanced nut, almonds are a good source of protein, vitamin E, and selenium.

**Spinach** This folate-rich vegetable is also rich in lutein and vitamin E and has antioxidant properties.

**Tomatoes** Rich in the antioxidant lycopene, tomatoes can help in the fight against cancer. Absorption of lycopene is improved by cooking tomatoes in oil.

# Healthy habits to adopt now

Eating a varied diet, based on a wide range of nutritious ingredients, can help control your weight, reduce cholesterol levels, treat infections, and ensure that you get an adequate intake of vital vitamins and minerals.

**What you eat and drink** Planning your meals is one of the best ways of ensuring that you eat a healthy, well-balanced diet:
• Aim to eat at least five servings of fruits and vegetables every day.
• Cut back on the amount of fat you eat, especially your intake of saturated fat; use monounsaturated or polyunsaturated fats instead.
• Base meals and snacks around whole grains, including wholemeal bread, brown rice, and wholemeal pasta – these are low in fat and high in fibre, which will fill you up.

• Choose foods that are a rich source of soluble fibre, such as oats, lentils, peas, sweetcorn, and pulses.
• Eat fish regularly – aim for at least two servings a week; one of these should be an oil-rich fish (*above*).
• When buying meat, choose lean cuts of meat and poultry.
• Drink or eat at least two servings of low-fat dairy foods a day, such as skimmed milk and low-fat yogurt.
• Reduce your sodium intake and use fresh herbs or ground spices instead to add flavour to your food.
• Drink six to eight glasses of water every day. Carry a bottle with you.

**How you eat** Thinking carefully about your eating habits and behaviours will help you pinpoint areas where changes could be beneficial to your present and future health:

• Instead of eating on the run, sit down and eat your meal at the table; eating with your family at mealtimes will enhance your enjoyment of food and prevent digestive problems.
• Get into the habit of eating smaller portions and stop eating when you are full – you don't have to finish everything (nor do your children).
• Snack on healthy foods, such as fruit or a handful of nuts or seeds; eat less junk food and sweets, which provide only "empty" calories with no useful nutrients.
• Eat less fast food (no more than once or twice a week), and when you do have it, modify your choices to include healthier options.
• If you love cakes or other sweet treats and find it difficult to eliminate these from your diet, look for low-fat versions and buy small portions.

# Cardiovascular disease

## The heart and blood vessels can be affected by several disorders.

Cardiovascular disease, which affects the heart and blood vessels, describes any of several disorders, including high levels of cholesterol in the blood (hyperlipidaemia), high blood pressure (hypertension), heart attack, and stroke.

### What can go wrong

In cardiovascular disease, there is a disruption of the heart's pumping action or the flow of blood through the blood vessels. Arteries can be damaged by high blood pressure and be narrowed by fatty deposits, especially cholesterol, restricting blood flow. A heart attack occurs if the coronary arteries, which supply the heart muscle with blood, become narrowed (coronary artery disease) and blocked. If the flow of blood in the brain is disrupted, it will cause a stroke.

### Common disorders

Two very common cardiovascular disorders that can lead to other more serious problems are high blood pressure and high blood cholesterol. If you are at risk of developing or already suffer from persistent high blood pressure – greater than 140mmHg (systolic) over 90mmHg (diastolic) – then you are putting strain on your heart and arteries.

Elevated levels of total cholesterol (greater than 5.0mmol per litre), LDL cholesterol, or triglycerides in the bloodstream (see p.23) is known as hyperlipidaemia. This can lead to a build-up of plaque (deposits of lipids) in the arteries, increasing the risk of inadequate blood supply to parts of the body.

### Major cause of death

Cardiovascular disease is one of the major causes of premature death in the UK, despite advances in medical treatment over the last 20 years, more screening, and

## The circulatory system

This includes the heart and blood vessels: arteries, shown in red, carry oxygenated blood; veins, shown in blue, carry de-oxygenated blood.

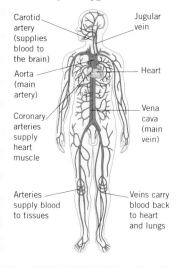

Carotid artery (supplies blood to the brain)

Jugular vein

Aorta (main artery)

Heart

Coronary arteries supply heart muscle

Vena cava (main vein)

Arteries supply blood to tissues

Veins carry blood back to heart and lungs

improvements in diet, all of which have helped reduce the number of deaths. You can significantly reduce your risk of cardiovascular disease by making lifestyle changes such as losing weight if you are overweight, exercising more, and quitting smoking.

# Who is most at risk for cardiovascular disease?

Most at risk of cardiovascular disease (and diabetes) is anyone diagnosed with metabolic syndrome, which is a precursor of cardiovascular disease.

### METABOLIC SYNDROME

It has been estimated that up to 20 per cent of people in the UK suffer from metabolic syndrome (syndrome X). It may be diagnosed if you have at least three of the following five factors:
• Elevated fasting blood sugar levels of 6.7mmol per litre, or diabetes
• Blood pressure above 130/85mmHg, indicating pre-hypertension
• Triglyceride levels in the blood greater than or equal to 2.0mmol per litre

• Low HDL blood levels, defined as less than 1.0mmol per litre for men and 1.4mmol per litre for women
• A waist circumference greater than 102cm (40in) for men and 88cm (35in) for women.

### CORONARY ARTERY DISEASE

This form of cardiovascular disease can result from metabolic syndrome or any of the following nine factors. If you are at risk, changing your diet and lifestyle can help (opposite).
• Elevated LDL blood levels (greater than 3.0mmol per litre)
• Elevated homocysteine or C-reactive protein levels

• High blood pressure, defined as greater than 140/90mmHg, or taking antihypertensive medication
• Low HDL cholesterol (If HDL levels are greater than 1.0mmol per litre for men and 1.4mmol per litre for women, this counts as a "negative" risk factor – its presence removes one risk factor from the total count.)
• A family history of early cardiovascular disease (a heart attack before age 55 for men and 65 for women)
• Age (men older than 45 years; women older than 55 years)
• Diabetes
• Cigarette smoking
• Obesity: BMI over 30 (see pp.26–27).

# What is cardiovascular disease?

Cardiovascular disease covers a range of disorders in which strain is put on your arteries, other blood vessels, or the heart, leading to narrowed or blocked arteries and preventing the heart from pumping blood efficiently.

Lifestyle and diet have a large part to play both in the prevention and treatment of cardiovascular disease. Changing the way you eat, from cutting out saturated fat and increasing omega-3 fatty acids and monounsaturated fats to eating more fruits and vegetables, can make a big difference to your health and well-being. The table below defines each cardiovascular disorder and outlines the main dietary and lifestyle changes you can make to treat the condition.

In addition to the advice given below, it is very important to give up smoking if you are a smoker; avoid exposure to cigarette smoke; limit your intake of alcohol (or avoid it completely if your triglyceride levels are high); lose weight if you are overweight; and increase your level of physical activity.

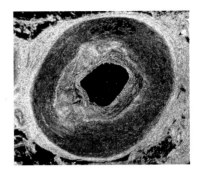

**Atherosclerosis** This cross-section of an artery shows its thickened walls, caused by a diet high in saturated fats.

| DISORDER | WHAT IS IT? | HOW YOU CAN HELP |
|---|---|---|
| Hyperlipidaemia | A combination of high levels of cholesterol, LDL, and/or triglycerides in the blood (*see p.23*), which can lead to narrowing of the blood vessels and clogged arteries. If untreated, you could develop angina and eventually suffer a heart attack. | • Reduce dietary saturated fat, trans fats, and cholesterol<br>• Increase monounsaturated fats and omega-3 fatty acids<br>• Avoid alcohol if triglycerides are high |
| High blood pressure (hypertension) | Persistent blood pressure above 140mmHg (systolic) and 90mmHg (diastolic), which may increase the risk of most other cardiovascular diseases. | • Reduce sodium and alcohol intake<br>• Increase dietary intake of fruits, vegetables, and low-fat dairy products |
| Coronary artery disease | This occurs when the arteries surrounding the heart become clogged and narrowed by plaque (deposits of lipids such as cholesterol). This build-up is known as atherosclerosis, and can restrict blood flow to the heart, potentially causing angina or a heart attack. | • If you have hyperlipidaemia, see above<br>• Eat whole grains for magnesium and fruits and vegetables for potassium<br>• Get regular exercise; limit alcohol<br>• Take one low-dose aspirin daily |
| Angina | Chest pain that occurs when the heart muscle does not receive enough oxygenated blood due to the narrowing of the coronary arteries. It is triggered by exercise or stress. | • Consult your doctor before starting an exercise regime if you are over 50<br>• Reduce stress and saturated fat |
| Heart attack | A heart attack (myocardial infarction or MI) occurs when one or more of the coronary arteries become blocked by a combination of plaque (deposits of lipids such as cholesterol) and/or a blood clot (coronary thrombosis). | • Eat a low-fat diet and reduce dietary saturated fat, trans fats, and cholesterol<br>• Increase monounsaturated fats and omega-3 fatty acids |
| Stroke | A stroke can be caused by a blood clot blocking a blood vessel in the brain; by a blood vessel breaking (interrupting the flow of blood to an area of the brain and destroying brain cells); or by bleeding into the brain from a broken blood vessel. Stroke can lead to a loss of abilities, such as speech, movement, and memory. | • If you have hyperlipidaemia, see the above entry for advice<br>• If you have high blood pressure, see the above entry for advice<br>• Anticoagulation medication may be prescribed for high-risk patients |
| Heart failure | Heart failure occurs when there is a reduced efficiency of the heart, which is defined as the amount of blood pumped by the heart in one minute. The disorder is characterized by the pooling of fluid in the extremities, especially in the legs and ankles, sodium retention, organ failure, and undernourishment caused by loss of appetite. | • Reduce your sodium intake<br>• Increase protein-rich foods if you are underweight<br>• Avoid stress<br>• A medically supervised exercise programme can be beneficial |

# Cardiovascular disease and nutrition

**There is a strong link between diet, exercise, and the development of cardiovascular disease.**

Nutrition plays an essential role in the treatment of cardiovascular disease, especially in high blood pressure and coronary artery disease, which are very common problems in the UK.

## Cholesterol levels

Because an excessive amount of cholesterol in the blood is a major risk factor for other cardiovascular diseases – causing narrowing of the arteries – your first priority is to lower cholesterol levels.

You should reduce your intake of saturated fats and increase your intake of polyunsaturated and monounsaturated fats, which can actually help lower your blood cholesterol levels (*see pp.40–41*). A diet high in monounsaturated fats lowers LDL-cholesterol and triglyceride levels in the blood without lowering beneficial HDL-cholesterol levels. See the table opposite for more information.

## High blood pressure

Another major contributor to other types of cardiovascular diseases is high blood pressure (*see pp.214–215*). As the pressure exerted on blood vessels increases, they narrow, making it more difficult for the blood to get through, thereby increasing the strain on the cardiovascular system.

Diet and exercise are critical in the effective treatment of high blood pressure; in some cases, changing your diet and increasing your activity level can eliminate the need for medication or reduce the dosage required.

## Changing your diet

There is a clear link between the consumption of saturated fats, which will raise LDL levels in the blood, and cardiovascular disease.

## Does my food contain cholesterol?

Dietary cholesterol is present only in foods of animal origin, such as meat, poultry, fish and shellfish, eggs, and whole milk and other dairy products. Cholesterol is not found in foods of plant origin, which include vegetables, fruits, grains, pulses, nuts, and seeds.

The highest amounts of dietary cholesterol come from egg yolks, caviar, and liver and other offal. For example, the yolk of one medium-sized egg contains about 200mg of cholesterol. In the US, the National Cholesterol Education Program recommends limiting your dietary intake of cholesterol to 200mg per day for a heart-healthy diet.

The British Heart Foundation recommends limiting dietary saturated fat intake to less than ten per cent of total calories.

You should also reduce sodium in your diet, particularly if you have high blood pressure or suffer from heart failure, and increase your intake of potassium- and calcium-rich foods (*see p.220*).

## Changing your lifestyle

Lifestyle changes, such as giving up smoking, losing weight, and increasing your exercise level, will help ease the burden on your cardiovascular system and reduce the effects of high blood pressure and high cholesterol. If you have angina, however, check with your doctor before embarking on an exercise programme.

If you suffer from heart failure, make sure you eat enough to achieve and maintain optimum weight, limit sodium intake, and maintain a tolerable activity level.

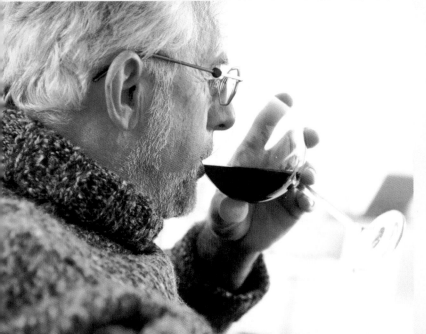

**Red wine can be beneficial** Red wine has been shown to increase HDL, or "good", cholesterol levels, but drink in moderation.

# Reducing total cholesterol, LDL, and triglyceride levels

The first step in treating cardiovascular disease is to lower LDL-cholesterol and triglyceride levels in the blood. LDL cholesterol is usually the primary target and lowering its levels in your blood entails making changes to what you eat, specifically by reducing the amount of saturated fat in your diet. Other lifestyle behaviours, such as weight loss, taking regular exercise, and stopping smoking can also significantly reduce your risk of cardiovascular disease. In addition to lowering LDL and triglyceride levels through nutrition, raising beneficial HDL levels through diet can also reduce the risk.

| GOAL | HOW TO ACHIEVE GOAL | NUTRITIONAL AND LIFESTYLE ADVICE |
|---|---|---|
| **Decrease LDL-cholesterol levels** | • Decrease intake of saturated fat<br>• Use mono- and polyunsaturated fats<br>• Limit dietary cholesterol<br>• Increase soluble fibre<br>• Limit intake of trans fatty acids | • Chose lean meats and low- or reduced-fat dairy foods<br>• Use only rapeseed or olive oil for cooking and baking<br>• Limit egg yolks, butterfat, and fatty meats<br>• Add oats, pulses, and apples to your diet<br>• Use soft, trans-fat-free margarine; limit pastries and other items made with partially hydrogenated oils |
| **Decrease triglyceride levels** | • Use mono- and polyunsaturated fats<br>• Include omega-3 fatty acids<br>• Avoid high-carbohydrate diets<br>• Eliminate alcohol<br>• Lose weight if overweight | • Use only rapeseed or olive oil in cooking and baking<br>• Eat more cold-water fish, linseeds, and linseed oil<br>• Cut down on high-carbohydrate foods<br>• Reduce alcohol intake as much as possible<br>• Exercise, limit saturated fat, and reduce portion sizes |
| **Raise HDL-cholesterol levels** | • Use mono- and polyunsaturated fats<br>• Limit intake of trans fatty acids<br>• Lose weight if overweight | • Use only rapeseed or olive oil in cooking and baking<br>• Use soft, trans-fat-free margarine; limit pastries and other items made with partially hydrogenated oil<br>• Cut out saturated fat, reduce portion sizes, and exercise to help weight loss |

# Case study  Busy accountant with metabolic syndrome

**Name**  Harry

**Age**  52 years

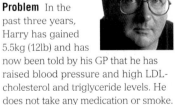

**Problem**  In the past three years, Harry has gained 5.5kg (12lb) and has now been told by his GP that he has raised blood pressure and high LDL-cholesterol and triglyceride levels. He does not take any medication or smoke. He drinks three large cups of coffee each morning and a litre (2 pints) of beer each evening.

**Lifestyle**  Harry is an accountant and has a high level of stress at work and at home. Work commitments mean he often orders a pizza for lunch and eats at his desk. After work and his commute home, Harry is too tired to exercise. He often eats a steak for supper and snacks on ice cream and crisps at night. He rarely eats fruit.

**Advice**  Harry has metabolic syndrome (see p.214), which places him at risk for cardiovascular disease. He needs to lose weight and take some exercise. Based on blood tests (see p.23), his goal is to lower total cholesterol, LDL cholesterol, and triglycerides, and to raise his level of HDL cholesterol. He can achieve this by following the Therapeutic Lifestyle Change Diet (see p.218) and reducing his total intake of calories.

Harry's diet is high in saturated fat and cholesterol. He should substitute monounsaturated fat and omega-3 fatty acids for saturated fat (see p.39), cut back on his portion sizes, and increase his activity level. Eating more fruits and vegetables, whole grains, pulses, low- or reduced-fat dairy products, fish, chicken breast without skin, and lean meats will help. If he likes eggs, he can include two in his diet each week.

For breakfast, Harry could have porridge with skimmed milk and an orange. For lunch, he could order a salmon or turkey salad sandwich or have two slices of vegetable pizza. For dinner, he could have fish and chicken more often and limit red meat to less than once a week.

Harry could increase his daily intake of soluble fibre from oats, oat bran, pulses, and fruits. Cholesterol-lowering margarines could replace other spreads to further lower his LDL-cholesterol levels. He may also benefit from reducing his intake of salt (see p.221).

# Therapeutic lifestyle changes (TLC) diet

If you have cardiovascular disease you need to think carefully about what you eat as it could have a major impact on your condition. Changes such as substituting low-fat products for full-fat ones, cutting the amount of saturated fat in your diet, substituting low-fat dairy foods for high-fat varieties, using monounsaturated oils, and increasing your intake of omega-3 fatty acids can all be beneficial. The Therapeutic Lifestyle Changes (TLC) diet, as outlined below, is a great starting point.

| FOOD GROUP | GOOD CHOICES | POOR CHOICES |
| --- | --- | --- |
| **Bread, pasta, rice, and potatoes (5 servings daily)** | Whole-grain breakfast cereals, crispbreads, oatcakes, wholemeal bread, and muesli bars; brown rice and wholemeal pasta; lentil burgers; reduced-fat hummus | Products high in saturated and trans fats, such as doughnuts, croissants, pastries, pies, and biscuits; white rice and pasta; crisps and snack mixtures; buttered popcorn |
| **Vegetables (2–3 servings daily)** | Steamed vegetables and baked root vegetables (no butter); roast vegetables drizzled with olive oil; raw vegetables with low-fat dips | Vegetables fried or prepared with butter, cheese, or cream sauce; raw vegetables with full-fat dips |
| **Fruits (2–3 servings daily)** | Fresh fruits; canned fruit in own juice; baked fruit served with low-fat crème fraîche or yogurt; low-fat fruit tarts and pies | Fruits served with butter or cream; canned fruit in sugary syrup; fruit tarts and pies with butter-rich pastry |
| **Dairy foods (2–3 servings daily)** | Skimmed and semi-skimmed milk; low-fat yogurt; fat-free frozen yogurt; reduced-fat cheeses; low-fat fromage frais | Whole milk; cream; whole-milk yogurt; ice cream; full-fat hard and soft cheeses; soured cream; cream cheese |
| **Eggs (2 yolks a week)** | Egg whites; egg substitutes; omelettes made from egg whites or egg substitutes | Egg yolks; whole eggs; omelettes made from whole eggs |
| **Fish, poultry, and meat (125g/4oz daily)** | Baked, grilled, or griddled fish; baked, grilled, or griddled skinless poultry; baked, grilled, or griddled lean cuts of meat, such as loin or leg; sausages made with lean meat or soya protein | Fried fish; fried poultry with skin; fatty cuts of meat such as spareribs; sausages; ready-to-eat meats such as salami, pastrami, and corned beef; offal; hot dogs |
| **Fats and oils (1–2 tbsp daily)** | Rapeseed and olive oils; cholesterol-lowering spreads; trans-fat-free tub margarine | Butter; lard; hard margarine; full-fat salad dressings; coconut cream and milk |

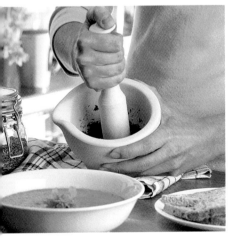

# Linseeds are rich in omega-3

The seeds of flax, linseeds have been valued for their therapeutic properties since ancient times. These nutty-tasting seeds are one of the richest sources of omega-3 fatty acids, and are excellent for regulating blood pressure (*see pp.39–40*). They contain both soluble and insoluble fibre. Soluble fibre helps reduce cholesterol, while insoluble fibre helps eliminate toxins from the bowel.

**Grinding linseeds** Boost your omega-3 intake by crushing linseeds with a pestle and mortar and sprinkling over soups and salads.

It is easy to incorporate linseeds into your diet. When ground, they provide the greatest nutritional benefit since the body cannot digest whole seeds. Crushed or milled seeds can be added to breakfast cereals, yogurt, salads, soups, or smoothies. You can also add linseeds to breads, burgers, and sauces before baking or cooking.

Oil extracted from the seeds also offers omega-3, but does not contain any fibre. It can be used as a salad dressing, but is unsuitable for cooking and must be refrigerated at all times as it is sensitive to light, oxygen, and heat.

# Nutrients that help cardiovascular disease

In addition to limiting your intake of saturated fats, increasing omega-3 fats, and including more fibre in your diet, there are specific changes that you can make in order to help prevent and treat cardiovascular disease.

## CHOOSE SOYA PRODUCTS
Studies have shown that eating 25g (1oz) soya protein every day will lower levels of LDL cholesterol by about five per cent. In the US the Food and Drug Administration has approved a health claim for soya foods that encourages eating soya protein daily as part of a diet low in saturated fat, to reduce the risk of cardiovascular disease.

## REDUCE HOMOCYSTEINE LEVELS
An emerging risk factor for developing cardiovascular disease is a high level of an amino acid called homocysteine in the blood. This can be caused by a genetic defect in the enzymes that break down homocysteine, as well as by a diet low in folate. Vitamins $B_6$ and $B_{12}$ are also needed to break it down in the body, so most doctors prescribe a supplement that contains these three vitamins for anyone with elevated homocysteine levels. If you are at risk of cardiovascular disease, ask your doctor about taking a multivitamin supplement.

## EAT PLANT OILS
Plant sterols and stanols, derived from natural plant oils, have been shown to lower LDL-cholesterol levels in the blood by up to 14 per cent. As a result sterols and stanols have been incorporated into some brands of spreads.

For those with elevated LDL levels the American National Cholesterol Education Program recommends that 2g of plant stanol/sterol (esters) be included daily in a diet low in cholesterol and saturated fat. In the gastrointestinal tract sterols/stanols compete with cholesterol for absorption, so less dietary and biliary cholesterol is absorbed by the body.

Since spreads with added sterol/stanol are the main source of these compounds, it is important to substitute these for other added fats, such as butter, margarine, oil, or cream cheese, so that your total calories will not be increased by adding these to your diet.

## What about alcohol?
The antioxidant properties of red wine may protect your heart by increasing HDL-cholesterol levels and reducing LDL cholesterol from being oxidized and deposited in arteries. However, if you regularly have more than three to four units a day (for men) or two to three units a day (for women), you may increase your risk of developing high blood pressure, elevated triglyceride levels, enlarged heart, and stroke. The best approach is to drink alcohol in moderation.

# Boosting your fibre intake

Since a high-fibre diet has been proved to reduce the risk of heart attack and other cardiovascular diseases, it is vital that you eat lots of fibre-rich foods.

## HIGH-FIBRE FOODS
Eating a diet rich in soluble fibre daily has been shown to reduce levels of LDL cholesterol by about five per cent.

Foods that are high in soluble fibre include pulses, whole grains such as oats and rye, and vegetables, as well as fruits, which are rich in the soluble fibre pectin. They will help decrease harmful LDL-cholesterol levels and reduce your risk of cardiovascular disease.

One meal that is easy to transform into a fibre-rich one is breakfast (*right*). By making simple changes, such as substituting whole-grain cereals and breads for refined varieties and adding fruit, you can increase the amount of soluble fibre that you eat every day.

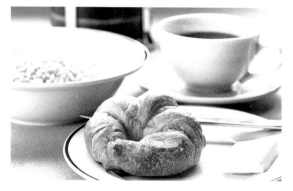

**Low-fibre breakfast**
This breakfast of sweetened, puffed-wheat cereal, coffee, and a croissant provides just 1.5g of fibre, as well as 27g fat and 105mg of cholesterol.

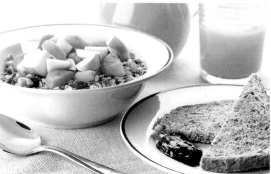

**High-fibre breakfast**
With whole-grain muesli and fruit, wholemeal toast, and orange juice, this breakfast provides 3.0g of fibre, 7.0g fat, and only 4.9mg of cholesterol.

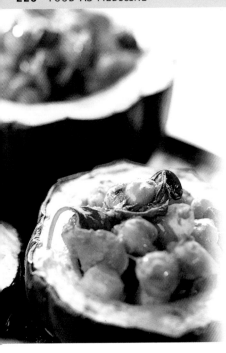

# Dietary advice for high blood pressure

By making some simple changes to your diet you can can help reduce high blood pressure. In addition to the changes outlined here it is also important that you reduce the amount of salt in your diet (*opposite*). Always check with your doctor before implementing changes.

## POTASSIUM AND CALCIUM

The DASH diet recommends increasing your dietary intake of potassium and calcium (*below*). Potassium can be found in all the food groups – fruit and vegetable sources include oranges,

pears, acorn squash, and spinach, as well as potatoes. Dairy products are excellent sources too, as are protein foods such as red meat, poultry, and pulses. Dairy products are, of course, rich in calcium (opt for the lower fat versions), as are green leafy vegetables such as kale and broccoli (*see p.62*).

## ALCOHOL

People who drink large amounts of alcohol are more likely to develop high blood pressure, whereas small amounts of alcohol raise HDL-cholesterol levels and are beneficial for cardiovascular health. Larger amounts of alcohol cause blood vessels to constrict or narrow, forcing the heart to pump harder. Alcohol can thus raise your blood pressure and make your high blood pressure more difficult to manage.

**Potassium-rich acorn squash** Make a tasty vegetarian meal by baking acorn squash halves, then filling them with a spicy mixture of chickpeas and wilted baby leaf spinach in a tomato sauce.

# DASH diet for high blood pressure

The Dietary Approaches to Stop Hypertension (DASH) diet for people with high blood pressure promotes increasing the intake of potassium and calcium in your diet (*above*) by eating plenty of fruits and vegetables and low-fat dairy products. Meat portions are limited, and nuts provide magnesium and additional fibre. Saturated fat intake is limited to less than seven per cent of total calories, and cholesterol to less than 200mg per day. Sugar and sweets can be eaten only sparingly.

## BENEFITS OF THIS DIET

Research shows that people on the DASH diet were able to reduce their diastolic blood pressure (the lower measurement of blood pressure, taken between heartbeats when the heart is relaxed) by up to 5mmHg, regardless of their age, gender, ethnicity, or initial blood pressure levels. For those with high blood pressure that ranged from 140/90 to 159/99mmHg, the DASH diet's effectiveness was similar to that of medication for high blood pressure.

| FOOD GROUP | INTAKE | SERVING SIZES AND SUGGESTIONS |
|---|---|---|
| Breads, pasta, rice, and potatoes | 7–8 daily servings | • 1 slice wholemeal bread<br>• 25g (1oz) cereal<br>• 75g (2½oz) cooked rice or pasta |
| Vegetables | 4–5 daily servings | • 50g (2oz) raw leafy vegetables<br>• 75g (2½oz) cooked vegetables<br>• 180ml (6floz) vegetable juice |
| Fruits | 4–5 daily servings | • 120ml (4floz) fruit juice<br>• 1 medium fruit<br>• 75g (2½oz) fresh, dried, frozen, or canned fruit |
| Reduced- or low-fat dairy foods | 2–3 daily servings | • 225ml (8floz) milk<br>• 225ml (8floz) yogurt<br>• 40g (1½oz) cheese |
| Meats, poultry, and fish | 2 or fewer daily servings | • 100g (3½oz) cooked lean meat, poultry, or fish |
| Fats and oils | 2–3 daily servings | • 1 tsp soft margarine<br>• 1 tbsp reduced-fat mayonnaise<br>• 2 tbsp low-fat salad dressing<br>• 1 tsp vegetable oil |
| Nuts, seeds, and pulses | 4–5 servings per week | • 3 tbsp nuts<br>• 3 tbsp seeds<br>• 3–4 tbsp cooked beans |

# Dietary advice for heart failure

Many people with heart failure tend to lose weight and become undernourished because they follow restrictive diets and may not get enough calories. They need to work with their GP to find a way of reducing their sodium intake and limiting their fluid intake. They should also try to maintain or increase body weight with high-calorie, nutrient-dense foods and food supplements.

## MAINTAIN A HEALTHY WEIGHT

It is important to maintain an adequate calorie intake to prevent weight loss. If you have already lost weight due to loss of appetite, you may need to take in more calories. Having small, frequent, nutrient-dense and high-calorie meals may help you meet your caloric needs. See page 224 for some suggestions for nutrient-dense snacks and meals.

## REDUCE SODIUM INTAKE

People with heart failure retain sodium and fluid, so restricting sodium (salt) in the diet is usually necessary. The level of sodium restriction varies depending on the severity of the condition. Those with long-term heart failure with symptoms such as shortness of breath should aim to reduce their dietary intake of sodium to less than 2000mg per day.

If you suffer from heart failure you must do more than just "stay away from salt". You must check food labels for sodium content, select only foods with less than 400mg per serving, and use herbs and other non-salt seasonings when cooking (*right*).

## LIMIT FLUID INTAKE

People who have heart failure may be advised by their GP to limit fluid intake to six to eight glasses per day, which is about 1.5–2 litres (2½–3½ pints). Fluids may be restricted slightly more than this for patients in hospital.

## TAKE FOOD SUPPLEMENTS

High-protein, high-calorie supplements can help to increase calorie intake in a relatively small volume, and they are especially useful for people who have a poor appetite. The supplements are available in a variety of flavours. Note though that supplements should only be taken on the advice of your doctor or a state-registered dietitian.

## Reducing salt intake

People who suffer from heart failure and those with high blood pressure should follow a low-salt diet. Reducing sodium has been proved to be one of the best ways of lowering high blood pressure.

### Tips for cutting down sodium

Convenience foods, ready meals, and canned foods, as well as eating out frequently, all contribute to a higher sodium intake, so if you are following a low-sodium diet read labels carefully.
• Use fresh or dried herbs and spices, such as cinnamon and cumin, to flavour vegetables.
• Avoid using salt at the table.
• Use soy sauce sparingly: 1 tsp contains about 1200mg of sodium.
• Buy fresh or frozen vegetables or those canned without salt.
• Rinse canned foods, such as beans, to remove excess salt.
• Choose breakfast cereals that are lower in sodium.
• Buy low- or reduced-sodium or no-salt-added versions of foods.

---

# Recipe  Low-sodium spicy chicken kebabs

### INGREDIENTS

**4 skinless chicken fillets**

**black pepper**

**3 lemons**

**1 tbsp grated fresh ginger**

**3 garlic cloves, crushed**

**½ tsp ground cumin**

**1 green chilli**

**Serves 4**

1 Cut each chicken fillet into 2.5cm (1in) cubes. Season with black pepper and the juice of one lemon. Marinate in the refrigerator for 30 minutes.

2 In a small bowl, combine the grated ginger, crushed garlic, ground cumin, and chopped chilli. Rub this into the chicken, then cover and refrigerate for 1 hour

3 Cut the remaining lemons into wedges. Thread the chicken cubes and lemon wedges on to skewers.

4 Barbecue or grill for about 5 minutes on each side until the chicken is browned and cooked through.

If you like, serve the kebabs with cucumber raita.

### Each serving provides

Cal. 160, Total fat 1.6g (Sat. 0.5g, Poly. 0.3g, Mono. 0.8g), Cholesterol 105mg, Protein 36g, Carbohydrate 0.2g, Fibre 0.3g, Sodium 90mg. Good source of – Mins: Ca, K, Mg, P, Se.

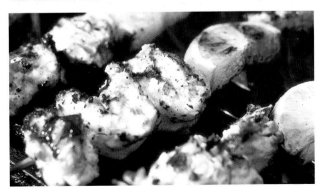

# Respiratory disorders

**If you suffer from a respiratory disease, changing your diet and lifestyle can help.**

The respiratory system – the lungs and airways – together with the cardiovascular system (*see p.214*), is responsible for delivering oxygen from the lungs to every cell in the body and then for removing carbon dioxide and returning it to the lungs to be exhaled.

## How we breathe

With each breath, a fresh supply of oxygen enters the bloodstream. It is the job of the red blood cells to transport the oxygen from the lungs to the tissues. The work of emptying and filling the lungs is done by the respiratory muscles.

The main respiratory muscle is the diaphragm, a layer of muscle situated between the chest and the abdomen. As this contracts and relaxes, air is drawn in and forced out at regular intervals. Other muscles that contribute to respiration are located between the ribs, in the neck, and in the abdomen. Any disease that affects these muscles, the passage from the nose to the lungs, or the bones of the chest wall will interfere with normal respiratory function.

## Respiratory disorders

Chronic obstructive pulmonary disease (COPD) is a result of progressive damage to the lungs, and is due mainly to smoking.

Sleep apnoea is a condition in which breathing is interrupted, usually by the soft tissues of the throat relaxing and blocking the flow of air. It most commonly occurs in overweight people. When the airway is obstructed, breathing becomes laboured and can stop for at least ten seconds, leading to dangerously low levels of oxygen in the blood.

In asthma, there is an intermittent narrowing of the airways, causing shortness of breath and wheezing. If asthma is severe, just trying to breathe can cause exhaustion.

## Dietary and lifestyle changes

Some dietary changes can help relieve these disorders. Since COPD often leads to weight loss, making sure you have a nutrient-dense diet will help. Conversely, if you have sleep apnoea you may be overweight, and losing a little weight may successfully treat the disorder. If you have asthma and know of a particular food that triggers an attack, make sure you avoid that food.

Lifestyle changes are also very important. Giving up smoking and increasing your level of exercise will benefit all respiratory disease. You should consult your doctor, however, before embarking on an exercise programme.

## The respiratory system

This includes the upper airway (the nasal passages to the trachea), the lower airways, and lungs.

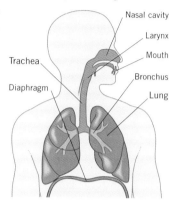

Nasal cavity

Larynx

Mouth

Trachea

Bronchus

Diaphragm

Lung

# Who is most at risk for respiratory disorders?

There are a number of risk factors for the respiratory diseases discussed in this section. The most common of these are outlined below.

**Diet and lifestyle** Excess body fat, especially if it is around the neck, can cause sleep apnoea, which is also more common in people who are overweight, who smoke, and who drink too much alcohol. Chronic obstructive pulmonary disease (COPD) is almost always due to smoking. In addition, smoking can trigger asthma in some people.

**Age** Asthma occurs more commonly in children, while COPD is more common in people over the age of 40.

**Gender** COPD is twice as common in men than women, whereas adult-onset asthma is more common in women.

**Family history** Asthma has been found to run in families.

**Other risk factors** Children with eczema or other allergies are at greater risk of developing asthma. Dust, noxious gases, and other lung irritants can cause COPD and trigger asthma.

## Warning signs

A morning cough and shortness of breath are two early signs of chronic bronchitis and emphysema, which together are known as chronic obstructive pulmonary disease (COPD).

Since smoking cigarettes greatly increases your risk of emphysema, it is important to take the symptoms seriously – you should avoid people who smoke and kick the habit if you smoke. Giving up smoking will produce quite dramatic effects in improving your lung function.

# What are respiratory disorders?

Chronic obstructive pulmonary disease (commonly known as COPD), asthma, and sleep apnoea are three common respiratory disorders that you can avoid or help to treat by making sensible changes to your diet and lifestyle – as summarized in the chart below.

COPD and asthma are disorders of the lungs and the lower airways (bronchioles), whereas sleep apnoea results from obstruction of the upper airway (usually the nasopharynx – the passage that leads from the back of the nasal cavity to the throat).

In general, the changes that you need to make are sensible and include maintaining a healthy nutrient-dense diet, cutting out or limiting the amount of alcohol that you drink, and giving up smoking or avoiding passive smoking.

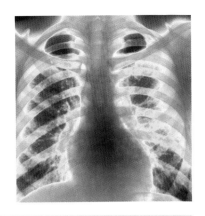

**Chronic bronchitis**  Damage to lung tissue is shown in this X-ray of chronic bronchitis, which is usually caused by smoking.

| DISORDER | WHAT IS IT? | HOW YOU CAN HELP |
|---|---|---|
| **Chronic obstructive pulmonary disease (COPD)** | People with COPD usually have one of two lung conditions – chronic bronchitis or emphysema. In COPD, the airways (bronchi and bronchioles) and tissues of the lungs become damaged over time, causing a shortness of breath. Damage to the lungs caused by COPD is usually irreversible. | • Eat nutrient-dense foods in order to prevent or reverse weight loss and undernutrition, which are both common with this condition<br>• Stop smoking |
| **Sleep apnoea** | Obstructive sleep apnoea is defined as recurrent episodes of apnoea, which is the cessation of breathing during sleep, caused by blockage of the upper airway. | • Lose weight<br>• Avoid alcohol<br>• Stop smoking |
| **Asthma** | Asthma is a form of chronic lung disease caused by inflammation and swelling of the lining of the airways in the lungs. It is associated with exposure to allergens (substances that trigger an allergic reaction). | • Maintain a healthy diet<br>• Avoid foods that trigger attacks<br>• Exercise to improve your stamina<br>• Stop smoking |

# Nutritional advice if you have COPD

Many people with chronic obstructive pulmonary disease (COPD) do not eat enough. Weight loss is very common and can increase breathing difficulties. It is therefore very important that people with COPD eat a balanced diet and take in enough calories to avoid undernutrition.

Recent studies suggest that foods high in antioxidants, such as fruits and vegetables, and omega-3 fatty acids (*see p.90*), such as oily fish, may be helpful in protecting against COPD. Taking a multivitamin supplement will also help you get the right nutrients.

## MAINTAIN ADEQUATE CALORIES
If you are underweight and trying to regain your strength, gradually increase the amount you eat with small, frequent, nutrient-dense meals that are easy to consume (*see p.224*). Other ideas that can help include:
• Eat three small meals each day plus between-meal snacks to get the calories you need. Smaller meals may help you breathe more easily and may be less tiring to eat than large meals.
• Time your main meal for when you have the most energy and feel your best (often in the morning), and rest before and after mealtimes.
• Avoid foods that cause uncomfortable wind or bloating.
• Increase your intake of fibre-rich foods to avoid constipation.

**Fruit salad is a healthy dessert**  Fruit is high in antioxidants, which have been found to help protect against COPD.

• Select soft foods that are easy to chew.
• For easy preparation, choose meals that can be cooked in the microwave, such as healthy ready meals (check the labels for salt and saturated fat levels).
• Make sure you drink enough fluids – at least eight glasses of water or other caffeine-free drinks per day – to keep your body hydrated.

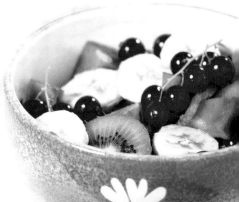

# High-calorie meals to counteract weight loss in COPD

If your condition has led to weight loss and you are trying to gain weight, it does not mean that you should simply eat fatty foods, such as cheese, mayonnaise, and butter, although you can eat them in moderation. High-calorie snacks should be as healthy as possible and packed with nutrients, especially vitamins, minerals, and proteins. Bearing in mind the benefits of whole grains and the need to moderate saturated fat, try:

- Guacamole with raw vegetables or baked tortilla chips
- Tuna, chicken, or salmon and salad on wholemeal bread
- Full-fat cheese, cream cheese, ham and salad, or peanut butter stuffed in pitta bread pockets
- Two-egg omelette with cheese and ham or tomato
- Falafel in pitta bread with salad, red peppers, and hummus
- Whole-grain cereals with whole milk
- Fruits with full-fat yogurt or Greek yogurt
- A glass of whole (full-fat) milk, or a mug of cocoa made with whole milk
- Nuts, such as almonds or brazils, or home-made trail mix

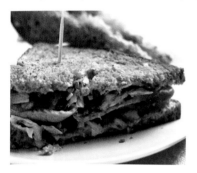

**Ham sandwich** Packed with protein and fibre, this sandwich of ham and salad on wholemeal bread is easy to eat.

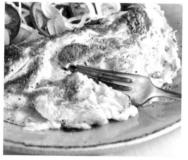

**Omelette** Easy to prepare, an omelette made with two eggs and grated cheese is high in protein and calcium. Serve with a bagel.

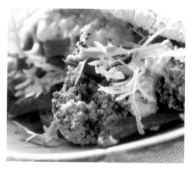

**Falafels in pitta bread** Spicy chickpea croquettes, served in pitta bread with salad, peppers, and hummus, is a nutritious snack.

# Case study   Woman with severe COPD who is losing weight

**Name** Patty

**Age** 53 years

**Problem** Patty was diagnosed with COPD eight years ago. Her symptoms include shortness of breath, which seems to worsen when she is unwell, stressed, cold, in high humidity, or after a large meal. She often feels too tired to prepare food and gets short of breath when she chews and swallows because these affect her breathing. Patty complains of being tired all the time and feeling weak, especially at mealtimes. Within the last year, she has lost 4.5kg (10lb).

**Lifestyle** Patty lives with her husband. They have four children and 14 grandchildren. She retired last year because of her illness. Lately, she has been too tired to go out, and her husband has taken over the food shopping. Patty usually follows a low-salt, low-fat diet at home. She smoked for 30 years but stopped five years ago.

In the morning, Patty eats cereal and a slice of toast. For lunch she has a pot of low-fat yogurt and apple juice, and for dinner a chicken breast, baked potato, and a vegetable. She often has fruit after dinner. Her calorie intake is about 1000 per day. She is 1.57m (5ft 2in) tall and her present weight is 67kg (147lb).

**Advice** Patty's calorie intake of about 1000 calories per day provides only two-thirds of her needs. Because of reduced lung function, she requires more energy to breathe; the normal daily intake of calories required to maintain body weight is not enough to meet the excessive demands of breathing for people with COPD.

Providing enough calories and protein to restore and maintain her weight and keep her respiratory muscles strong is the major goal of nutritional treatment for people with COPD.

Patty's dietitian advised her to rest before mealtimes and to eat foods that are easy to chew, such as soft meats and casseroles. She can get additional calories from high-protein, high-calorie shakes, drinking at least one can per day. Eating small, frequent meals consisting of nutrient-dense foods, such as peanut butter or cheese sandwiches, will help meet her nutritional needs. Using extra spread on her bread, potatoes, and vegetables will also supplement her intake of calories.

Patty should have her main meal at a time of the day when her energy level is highest. She should also limit her intake of fluids during meals, and instead drink fluids between meals.

# Tips for treating sleep apnoea

Obesity contributes to the development of sleep apnoea (see p.223) and a weight loss of as little as 4.5kg (10lb) can dramatically improve symptoms.

## WEIGHT-REDUCTION TIPS
If you need to lose weight because of sleep apnoea, you should consult a state-registered dietitian for nutritional counselling. However, you may find the following suggestions useful as well.
• Stay out of the kitchen after dinner. Eating late at night adds extra calories.
• If you are hungry and have to snack, have fresh fruit or cut-up vegetables ready in the refrigerator. Use low-calorie dressings for dipping.
• If you are tempted by snacks and junk food around the house, don't buy or bring those foods into your house. If you have lots of snack foods for the children, consider them "off limits".
• Be aware of your quantities and portion sizes both at home and when eating out: skip the starter or share one, and have bread without butter. If you want a dessert, you could share it and skip the wine.
• Regular exercise, such as walking, swimming, or cycling, will give you more energy and help you sleep better.
• Alcohol may promote throat closure during sleep and should be avoided.

## OTHER TIPS FOR SLEEP APNOEA
In addition to losing weight, there are important lifestyle factors that can help improve your condition.
• Avoid smoking.
• Do not go to sleep immediately after eating; take a walk instead.
• Treat allergies, colds, or sinus problems. Avoid using antihistamines or tranquillizers.
• Try to sleep exclusively on your side or with the head of the bed elevated.

# Asthma and nutrition

People with asthma generally have the same nutritional needs and food considerations as anyone else, but if you have asthma it is important to make a healthy diet a regular part of your life. Asthma can place additional stress on your body – especially if you take oral corticosteroids, which can deplete your body of vitamins and minerals.

## EAT A HEALTHY DIET
Eat plenty of fruits and vegetables, pulses, wholemeal bread, and whole-grain cereals; moderate amounts of low-fat dairy products, lean meats, fish, and poultry; and small amounts of fats, oils, and sugar. A healthy diet and regular exercise go a long way towards helping improve your well-being. Certain foods and additives, however, have been found to trigger or exacerbate asthma.

## FOODS THAT TRIGGER ASTHMA
Asthmatics are usually affected by at most two or three foods; it is a common misconception that people are sensitive to a wide variety of foods.

The factors that set off and exacerbate asthma symptoms are called "triggers". Identifying and avoiding asthma triggers are essential in preventing flare-ups. The most common trigger foods are milk, yogurt, and other dairy products, eggs, prawns, fish, citrus fruits, soya, and wheat. These foods are more likely to trigger asthma in children than in adults, and fortunately most children outgrow such allergies. Check food labels because additives found in many canned and processed foods, such as tartrazine, sulphur, benzoic acid, and monosodium glutamate, can trigger asthma. If you can identify the specific food or the additive that triggers your asthma, you should simply avoid it.

**Avoiding additives** By feeding your toddler home-made meals, you can be sure that she is getting the best ingredients, without the addition of potentially harmful chemicals.

## Asthma in babies

This illness is sometimes related to allergies, which may be prevented by close attention to your baby's diet. Early exposure to infant cereals has been linked to an increase in asthma triggered by grass pollen. Just breast-feeding for three months may prevent this occurring.

Probiotic foods, such as yogurt with live cultures, can promote the development of bacteria in the gut (see p.48). The bacteria may play a role in assisting the digestion of proteins that cause food allergy.

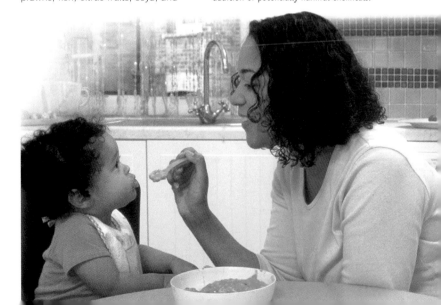

# Digestive disorders

## The digestive tract and associated organs can be affected by many disorders.

The digestive system is made up of the digestive tract, the salivary glands, liver, gall bladder, and pancreas. The digestive tract is essentially a long tube. In total, it is about 7.3m (24ft) long and composed of a series of joined sections made up of the mouth, oesophagus, stomach, small and large intestines, rectum, and anus.

### How it works
The role of the digestive tract is to break down food and transport nutrients throughout the body for energy, growth, and repair. It is also responsible for eliminating waste from the body.

The rhythmic contraction of the muscles lining the oesophagus is called peristalsis. This action moves food into the stomach and prevents any stomach contents from going backwards into the oesophagus

(reflux). To aid in this function there is a ring of muscles at the bottom of the oesophagus called the lower oesophageal sphincter.

Medical problems occur when there is a structural or functional change along the digestive tract or in the associated organs.

### What can go wrong?
Disorders of the digestive system that can in some way be relieved, treated, or prevented by dietary or lifestyle measures are outlined in the chart on the opposite page.

The most common digestive disorders are usually short-term problems and include indigestion, diarrhoea, and constipation. A common cause of indigestion is gastro-oesophageal reflux disease (GORD), in which acidic stomach juices are regurgitated. Peptic ulcers, which affect either the stomach or the duodenum (the first part of the small intestine) may persist or recur.

Some disorders, for example Crohn's disease and ulcerative colitis, cause inflammation of the intestine and affect the absorption

## The digestive system
The digestive system includes the digestive tract (from mouth to anus) and associated organs, such as the liver and gall bladder.

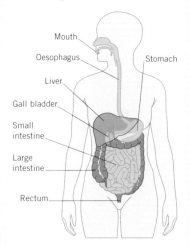

Mouth

Oesophagus

Stomach

Liver

Gall bladder

Small intestine

Large intestine

Rectum

of nutrients. Other disorders, such as lactose intolerance and coeliac disease, are a result of a reaction to a substance that is present in food. The dietary and lifestyle changes you can make to combat these disorders, and treat any side effects, are discussed in detail on the following pages.

## What are the risk factors for digestive disorders?

Some of the known risks for digestive disorders are outlined below. These include diet and lifestyle, age, gender, and family history.

**Diet and lifestyle** A diet that does not include a sufficient amount of fibre may lead to some digestive diseases. For example, diverticular disease is more common in the West, where intake of fibre tends to be low because of the popularity of refined grain products.

Anyone who is overweight or has a high-fat diet is at risk of developing gall stones. Drinking alcohol, smoking cigarettes, and emotional stress may all trigger or aggravate existing stomach ulcers or interfere with their healing.

**Age** As people grow older, the motility of their intestinal tract decreases, and therefore food and waste move through the intestine at a slower rate, which increases the risk of constipation.

Similarly, diverticular disease is more common in people over the age of 50, and over half of the population in the UK over the age of 70 and nearly everyone over 80 has this disorder.

About ten per cent of people in the UK suffer from irritable bowel syndrome (IBS), a condition that is most common in those aged 15–40 years. Similarly, Crohn's disease and ulcerative colitis most commonly first develop in young people aged 15–30 years.

**Gender** Some gastrointestinal diseases, such as peptic ulcers, do occur more commonly in men than in women. But gall stones and IBS are more common in women than in men.

**Family history** Some digestive disorders, such as coeliac disease, are genetic and can run in families. Family members of people who have been diagnosed with a genetic digestive disorder may be offered tests to see if they are at risk of developing the disorder.

Between 15 and 30 per cent of people with Crohn's disease and ulcerative colitis have a family history of these conditions, suggesting that genetics are involved in their development too.

# What are digestive disorders?

Diarrhoea, constipation, and indigestion are common, and there are measures you can take to prevent and treat them. However, diarrhoea may be a symptom of an infection or a long-term problem, such as irritable bowel syndrome (IBS) or an inflammatory bowel disorder such as ulcerative colitis or Crohn's disease. If diarrhoea persists, see your GP.

Gastro-oesophageal reflux (GORD) is a common disorder of the oesophagus and a cause of indigestion. Attacks can be mild, but may leave your oesophagus scarred. Peptic ulcer is commonly due to a bacterium called *Helicobacter pylori*.

Many digestive disorders can be successfully managed by following your doctor's advice and making lifestyle changes. See the table below for tips.

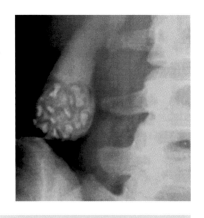

**Gall stones**  A gall bladder full of gall stones is visible in this colour-enhanced X-ray. The stones are in the green area on the left.

| DISORDER | WHAT IS IT? | HOW YOU CAN HELP |
|---|---|---|
| **Indigestion** | Pain or discomfort in the upper abdomen that usually develops after eating | • Avoid foods that irritate the stomach such as spicy foods and citrus fruits<br>• Eat small, low-fat meals and snacks |
| **Constipation** | Infrequent and difficult passage of stools | • Eat plenty of soluble and insoluble fibre<br>• Drink plenty of fluids |
| **Diarrhoea** | Frequent passage of loose, watery stools, often caused by an infection | • Avoid high-fibre foods if short term<br>• Increase soluble fibre if long term<br>• Avoid sorbitol, and drink plenty of fluids |
| **Irritable bowel syndrome (IBS)** | A combination of abdominal pain, bloating, excessive wind, and changes in bowel habits | • Follow a low-fat, high-fibre diet<br>• Avoid caffeinated drinks |
| **Gastro-oesophageal reflux disease (GORD)** | Regurgitation of acidic stomach juices into the oesophagus, causing pain in the chest | • Follow a low-fat, high-fibre diet<br>• Control weight; stop smoking |
| **Peptic ulcer** | Damage to the stomach lining and part of the small intestine (duodenum) | • Eat three meals daily; stop smoking<br>• Limit alcohol, caffeine, and spicy foods |
| **Cholecystitis and gall stones** | Inflammation of the gall bladder, often with stones formed in the gall bladder | • Follow a low-fat, high-fibre diet<br>• Lose weight; exercise regularly |
| **Lactose intolerance** | The inability to digest lactose, the natural sugar present in milk | • Avoid milk and milk products<br>• Opt for low-lactose or lactose-free drinks<br>• Take calcium with vitamin D supplements |
| **Coeliac disease** | Damage to the small intestine caused by a reaction to gluten, resulting in malabsorption | • Exclude gluten from your diet<br>• Read labels and choose gluten-free food |
| **Crohn's disease** | An inflammatory disorder that affects mainly the ileum and the colon of the large intestine | • Follow a diet low in fat, fibre, and lactose<br>• Take a vitamin and mineral supplement |
| **Ulcerative colitis** | Inflammation and ulcers affecting the rectum and the colon (large intestine) | • Eat plenty of insoluble fibre<br>• Take a vitamin and mineral supplement |
| **Diverticular disease** | Small pouches in the colon (diverticulosis) that may become inflamed and painful (diverticulitis) | • Eat plenty of insoluble fibre<br>• Drink plenty of water<br>• If you have abdominal pain, see a doctor |

# Nutrition for digestive disorders

## What you eat and how you eat can have a major impact on digestive problems.

Nutrition plays a big role in many digestive disorders because what you eat has an important effect on your gastrointestinal (GI) tract.

### The role of nutrition

If your GI tract is abnormal in any way, your doctor will suggest specific dietary changes to help alleviate some of your symptoms.

Some of these dietary changes may help correct and prevent the problem. For example, increasing the amount of fibre in your diet and drinking more water will help prevent constipation; and excluding gluten, a specific type of protein, may be required for the rest of your life if you have coeliac disease. Although this may sound difficult, it could save your life and you will

be grateful to be able to enjoy your meals again without suffering from painful symptoms afterwards.

Your doctor may advise you to change your lifestyle. For example, if you have reflux disease you should avoid lying down after eating; and if you have a peptic ulcer you may need to limit foods and drinks containing caffeine.

### Changing your diet

Making the appropriate changes to manage your digestive disorder requires patience and a trial-and-error period. You may find it helps to write down the offending foods that give you wind or cause you to feel bloated. If this continues to happen over and over again, then eliminating these foods may be beneficial to you. But remember, if you eliminate food groups from your diet you may need to take supplements. For example, those who avoid dairy products will need a calcium supplement to prevent osteoporosis from developing.

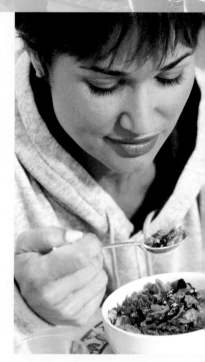

**High-fibre breakfast** To increase your fibre intake and keep your digestive tract active, start your day with a bran or whole-grain cereal, topped with dried or fresh fruit.

A lot has changed over the years with regards to nutrition for digestive disorders and we have provided the most up-to-date advice in this chapter.

## Tips to treat indigestion

The following suggestions can help relieve mild attacks of indigestion – pain or discomfort in the stomach or upper abdomen that usually comes on after eating a meal. The complaint may be accompanied by nausea, belching, and bloating. It is caused by eating or drinking too much or by stress, or may be a symptom of an underlying disorder such as a peptic ulcer (see p.227).

• Avoid foods that may irritate the stomach, such as caffeine, spearmint, peppermint, citrus fruits, spicy foods, high-fat foods, and tomato products.

• Some people find that a cup of herbal tea, such as peppermint, fennel, or camomile, provides relief.

• Eat small, low-fat meals and snacks, such as fruits, pretzels, crispbreads, and low-fat yogurt frequently, and at regular times during the day.

• Always eat slowly and chew your food thoroughly.

• Have drinks between meals, rather than with meals.

• Take a walk after meals, but do not do any strenuous exercise for at least one hour after eating.

• Avoid lying down for at least two hours after eating a meal.

• Try having a warm milk drink before bed, and use extra pillows to raise your head.

• If stress might be a cause of your indigestion, try to include relaxation techniques in your life, such as yoga or meditation.

• If you smoke, you should try to stop, since smoking may worsen the symptoms.

• Try an antacid medication, which can relieve the symptoms of indigestion by neutralizing stomach acid.

• Do not take aspirin or ibuprofen for pain relief since these medications can irritate the stomach.

• If you are overweight, which may worsen symptoms, try to lose weight.

• See your GP if your symptoms become worse or do not improve after two weeks or if your indigestion recurs.

# Treating constipation

A diet that is high in animal fats, such as meat, cheese, and eggs, and refined sugar, but low in fibre from vegetables, fruits, and whole grains is a common cause of constipation.

The infrequent and difficult passage of stools is particularly common in older people. This is because gut motility decreases with age, resulting in food and waste taking longer to pass through the intestine. Stimulant laxatives can make the intestine sensitive to their effects, so you should avoid taking them regularly. It is far more effective to treat constipation through changes to your diet.

In addition, regular exercise will help stimulate intestinal activity and improve the motility of the intestinal tract.

### INCREASE YOUR FIBRE INTAKE

Dietary fibre in food (*see pp.48–49*) traps water and adds bulk to the stool, making it move through the gut more quickly.
• Gradually increase your fibre intake by eating more whole grains, wholemeal bread and pasta, vegetables, fruits, and pulses. Aim to eat five servings of grains and grain products daily.
• Make sure that you eat lots of fresh fruits and vegetables. Include foods with a natural laxative effect, such as prunes or prune juice, apricots, and apples.
• Eat a high-fibre breakfast cereal. Bran cereals are particularly high in fibre and can be livened up with toppings, such as sliced banana, raisins, or strawberries.
• Switch from white bread, pasta, and rice to wholemeal or whole-grain types.
• Avoid eating processed or highly refined foods, which are high in sugar and carbohydrates and low in fibre.

### INCREASE YOUR FLUID INTAKE

If you suffer from constipation, increase your fluid intake. Aim to drink about 2 litres (3½ pints) of water a day. Dry stools are more difficult and painful to pass, but drinks add bulk and fluid to the stool, making it easier to expel. Limit alcohol and caffeine because they can lead to dehydration, creating stools that are hard and more difficult to pass.

### MAGNESIUM AND EXERCISE

Magnesium can help loosen stools, so increase your intake of magnesium-rich foods, such as spinach, almonds, Brazil nuts, raisins, and artichokes (*see p.68*). Alternatively, you can take a magnesium supplement (*see p.271*).

**Eat dried fruit** Soak dried fruits in juice or water for a nutritious fruit salad. Apricots, figs, and raisins are high in soluble fibre, and raisins are also high in magnesium.

## When should I see my doctor?

If you have recently become constipated and the problem has lasted for more than two weeks – even after increasing your intake of fibre and fluids and your level of activity – you should make an appointment to see your GP.

In addition, if you notice blood in your stool, consult your doctor, because bleeding from the intestine can be a symptom of a serious disorder such as colorectal cancer.

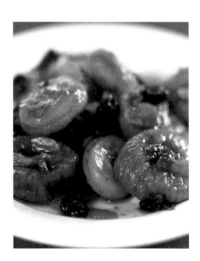

---

## Tips to prevent diarrhoea

Good hygiene and awareness of the sources of food contamination will help you to avoid diarrhoea.
• Wash your hands after using the toilet and changing baby's nappies.
• Frequently wash bathroom and food preparation surfaces.
• When travelling overseas, drink only bottled water, carbonated soft drinks, and drinks made with boiled water such as tea and coffee. Do not drink tap water or have ice that has been made from tap water.
• Avoid meat or fish that is raw or rare, or that is not served hot.
• Peel fruits and vegetables.

# Treating diarrhoea

Diarrhoea – the frequent passage of loose, watery stools – is often caused by infections from contaminated food or water. The following suggestions will help ease your symptoms:
• Replace lost fluid and electrolytes (minerals dissolved in fluids) with water, fruit juices diluted with water, rehydration drinks, or sports drinks. Try to drink at least 500ml (16floz) of fluid every one to two hours to prevent dehydration.
• Avoid very hot or very cold liquids, coffee, alcohol, or caffeinated soft drinks, all of which can irritate the intestine.
• Read product labels and check with your chemist if medications and diet products contain sorbitol or lactulose, both of which can cause diarrhoea; discontinue taking them if possible.
• If you can tolerate food, eat yogurt with live cultures (to replace gut flora) and avoid insoluble fibre (whole grains) until the diarrhoea has resolved.
• Eat bland, non-fatty foods that are easily digested, and avoid milk, red meats, and highly seasoned food.
• If the bout of diarrhoea is a short-term problem, avoid high-fibre foods, such as whole grains and fresh vegetables and fruits, all of which can be difficult for the irritated intestine to digest. If the diarrhoea lasts for more than two weeks, increasing soluble fibre intake may help, but you should see your GP.

# Treating irritable bowel syndrome

Doctors believe that in people with irritable bowel syndrome (IBS) the colon (the major section of the large intestine) is abnormally sensitive to stimuli such as excess wind, stress, high-fat or fibre-rich foods, caffeine, and alcohol. These stimuli can irritate the colon and cause pain, cramps, and diarrhoea. Women with IBS may have more symptoms during menstrual periods, suggesting that reproductive hormones can aggravate the condition. Many people state that the symptoms occur after they eat or when they are under stress.

## IDENTIFY PROBLEM FOODS

A balanced diet can help alleviate IBS symptoms. You may find it helpful to keep a food diary to identify which foods cause the most discomfort and try to eliminate these from your diet. The foods may be different for each person; for example, some people find onions and mushrooms cause wind, bloating, and discomfort, while others find relief from omitting wheat.

## CHOOSE DAIRY PRODUCTS

Even if you find that most dairy products are difficult to tolerate (*see p.232*), do not rule out yogurt. Yogurt may be better tolerated because it contains organisms that supply lactase, the enzyme needed to digest lactose (the sugar in milk). Lactose-free milk is also an option. Since dairy products are an important source of calcium, consider drinks enriched with calcium or take a calcium supplement if your body cannot tolerate dairy products.

## OTHER DIETARY FACTORS

High-fibre foods, such as wholemeal bread, whole-grain cereals, pulses, fruits, and vegetables, help to avoid intestinal cramps and spasms, and constipation – although if you suffer from diarrhoea, a low-fibre diet is better. It is also best to avoid caffeinated drinks such as tea, coffee, and cola, which stimulate the colon. Many find herbal teas, especially peppermint and fennel, soothing. Fruit juice contains a lot of fructose, which

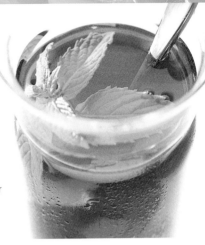

**Peppermint tea** A great alternative to normal tea or coffee, peppermint has anti-spasmodic properties and can ease IBS symptoms by calming the intestinal tract.

can aggravate symptoms of IBS and contribute to diarrhoea. It is best to stick to drinking mineral water to help flush out your system. In addition, smoking can exacerbate the symptoms of IBS, so it is important to quit if you smoke.

---

# Case study Young woman with irritable bowel syndrome (IBS)

**Name** Megan

**Age** 25 years

**Problem** Five years ago, Megan was diagnosed with irritable bowel syndrome (IBS). She complains of crampy abdominal pain, which is relieved by a bowel movement. She often has loose stools or diarrhoea followed by no bowel movements for several days. Her movements are irregular and her symptoms worsen when she is stressed. Her weight is stable and she does not have a fever or bleeding when going to the toilet.

**Lifestyle** Megan is a lawyer and is always busy and often stressed out. Her symptoms occur several times a week and affect her work. She has

two meals a day (pizza or a sandwich for lunch and pasta or take-away for dinner), often on the run. Because of the diarrhoea, she is not sure what to eat, but she drinks apple juice to prevent dehydration. She does not take a multivitamin supplement and does not exercise.

**Advice** Several factors contribute to Megan's IBS. She is stressed at work and would benefit from yoga and exercise. She should eat breakfast – such as wholemeal toast or whole-grain cereal – to encourage more regular bowel movements and to help increase the fibre in her diet.

Megan also experiences cramping and wind from certain foods, the most common being pulses, onions, prunes, and cruciferous vegetables such as cabbage and broccoli. Megan could try to eliminate these foods one

by one to determine any associations. She could also temporarily eliminate dairy products, since an intolerance to lactose (milk sugar) can cause symptoms similar to IBS. She may find, however, that she can tolerate yogurt, which is also high in calcium.

Increasing dietary fibre will help relieve Megan's symptoms, and she should have regular, firmer bowel movements. However, it can be hard to get enough dietary fibre, especially if she eliminates fibre-rich foods that cause wind. She might benefit from taking a fibre supplement, and should talk to her doctor about this.

Megan should make sure she drinks plenty of water with the supplements to reduce the symptoms of excessive wind, which may occur initially. The fructose in the apple juice can also contribute to diarrhoea, so drinking water instead could help.

# Treating gastro-oesophageal reflux disease (GORD)

GORD is a common cause of indigestion that occurs when acidic stomach juices are regurgitated into the oesophagus (the tube from the throat to the stomach). These stomach juices irritate the oesophagus, causing inflammation and pain (heartburn), and this can cause permanent scarring if the condition persists. The main causes of GORD are poor tone in the ring of muscle at the end of the oesophagus (the lower oesophageal sphincter) and increased abdominal pressure due to obesity or pregnancy. It is important to follow a low-fat diet since high-fat meals tend to decrease sphincter pressure, slowing the movement of food to the stomach and exposing the oesophagus to irritants. Other key ways to treat GORD include losing weight if you are overweight and avoiding fatty foods, alcohol, chocolate, and coffee as much as possible.

| AIM | TREATMENT |
|---|---|
| **Decreasing the frequency and amount of regurgitated stomach juices** | • Eat small, frequent meals<br>• Drink fluids between meals rather than with meals<br>• Eat plenty of fibre to avoid constipation, as straining increases abdominal pressure |
| **Decreasing irritation in the oesophagus** | • Avoid or limit foods that may give you symptoms of GORD or aggravate the condition. These vary with different people, but may include fatty foods, citrus fruits, tomato products, spicy foods, and carbonated drinks |
| **Improving clearance of food from the oesophagus** | • Do not recline after eating – sit upright or, even better, take a walk<br>• Avoid eating for two to three hours before bedtime or prior to lying down<br>• Raise the head of your bed |
| **Avoiding scarring the oesophagus** | • Choose soft foods that are easy to swallow, such as low-fat cottage cheese |
| **Losing weight** | • Eat smaller portions, follow a low-fat diet, and exercise regularly |

# Treating and preventing peptic ulcers

The goals of nutritional treatment for peptic ulcers – damage to the stomach lining (stomach ulcer) or the first part of the small intestine (duodenal ulcer) – are to reduce and neutralize stomach acid and to maintain the stomach lining's resistance to the acid. Reducing stomach acid helps alleviate symptoms and allows sores to heal.

There is no specific diet for ulcers – each person must discover which foods cause discomfort and avoid them. You may find the following tips helpful:

• Eat three meals daily, avoid skipping meals, and limit your intake of spicy, fatty, or other foods that cause discomfort.
• Avoid bedtime snacks, since symptoms often occur in the night.
• Limit caffeine intake by reducing your intake of coffee, tea, cola, and chocolate.
• Limit your alcohol intake and avoid drinking on an empty stomach.
• Avoid smoking and passive smoking as smoke may increase the secretion of stomach acid, increase the frequency of duodenal ulcers, and delay healing.

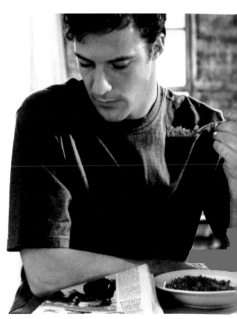

**Make time for regular meals** It is very important not to skip meals, including breakfast, if you suffer from a peptic ulcer.

## Helicobacter pylori infection and peptic ulcers

Peptic ulcers are commonly associated with *Helicobacter pylori* infection. The infection is thought to be spread by unsanitary living conditions. It infects the stomach and releases substances that reduce the effectiveness of the layer of mucus that protects the stomach lining from its own acidic juices. The acidic juices then erode the lining of the stomach or the duodenum, allowing a peptic ulcer to develop. A combination of antibiotics and ulcer-healing drugs will usually clear up the ulcer.

# Preventing and treating gall stones

Gall stones are formed from bile, a cholesterol-rich liquid made by the liver and stored in the gall bladder that aids the digestive process. Gall stones are more common in women, in people over the age of 40, and those who are overweight and eat a high-fat diet. A family history of gall stones is a risk factor.

### LOW-FAT, HIGH-FIBRE DIET
Avoiding fatty foods and increasing your consumption of fibre (see p.49) by eating more high-fibre foods such as bran, soya, guar gum, and pectin, which is found in many fruits and vegetables, can help prevent gall stones and relieve the discomfort caused by existing stones. Regular exercise may also decrease the risk of developing gall stones.

If you are obese, you are at increased risk of developing gall stones. Therefore, following a low-fat diet and increasing your exercise level will not only help you lose weight but also reduce your risk of developing gall stones. However, rapid weight loss can cause the formation of gall stones in some people, so it is important to lose weight gradually.

### GALL BLADDER SURGERY
Surgical removal of the gall bladder is the most effective means of curing gall bladder disease – the effects are immediate. Once the gall bladder has been removed, however, there is no reservoir of bile, and fat absorption may be affected. In this case, following a low-fat diet may be helpful.

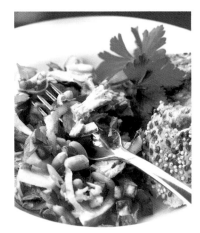

**Healthy high-fibre dish** Tuna and bean salad and some whole-grain bread make a low-fat, high-fibre meal that can help prevent the formation of gall stones.

# Dealing with lactose intolerance

Normally, the enzyme lactase breaks down lactose (a natural sugar found in milk and other dairy products) in the intestine to form the sugars glucose and galactose. These are then easily absorbed through the intestinal wall into the bloodstream.

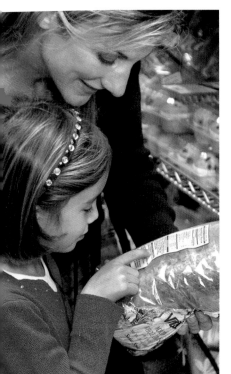

**Checking ingredients** If you or your child has a lactose intolerance, it is important that you check food labels carefully and learn to spot ingredients that contain lactose.

If this enzyme is absent or its levels are low, the unabsorbed lactose ferments, producing painful symptoms such as abdominal bloating and cramping, diarrhoea, and vomiting. The condition usually develops in adolescence or adulthood and is uncommon in babies and young children. No treatment can improve the body's ability to produce lactase, but symptoms can be easily controlled through diet.

### LIMIT OR AVOID LACTOSE
Some people can benefit from just reducing the amount of foods they eat containing lactose, such as milk, yogurt, cheese, cream, and butter, and most are able to tolerate a small amount of lactose without symptoms. However, some people will develop symptoms from just a tiny amount of lactose. For those who cannot tolerate even small amounts of lactose, lactase enzymes are available, which will help them digest foods that contain lactose.

### READ FOOD LABELS
If you are lactose-intolerant, check food labels very carefully for hidden dairy products. There may be small amounts of lactose in breads, cereals, biscuits, margarine, sliced cooked meats, salad dressings, soups, sweets, and many other foods. Lactose-free forms of milk are commonly available.

### SOYA ALTERNATIVES
Try soya milk if you find that you cannot tolerate even lactose-free milk. Soya milk is naturally lactose-free, yet it supplies many of the same nutrients that are in cow's milk. Different brands of soya milk have different tastes, so try a few until you find one that you like.

### WATCH YOUR CALCIUM INTAKE
Dairy products are our prime source of dietary calcium, which is important for maintaining bone health. You should therefore try to include some lactose-free dairy or soya products in your diet every day. Other calcium-rich foods are canned salmon, spinach, and leafy greens (see p.63). If you fall short on calcium, a supplement of 800–1200mg per day is advisable to maintain the recommended daily calcium levels.

# Coping with Crohn's disease and ulcerative colitis

People who have an inflammatory bowel disorder, such as Crohn's disease or ulcerative colitis, cannot absorb nutrients properly and so are at risk of nutrient deficiencies and becoming underweight.

## GETTING ENOUGH NUTRIENTS
If you have an inflammatory bowel disorder, make sure you get enough nutrients. A dietitian can help you in dealing with deficiencies, which can develop because the damaged intestine is not absorbing nutrients effectively. This is very important for children, who are growing and developing.

Symptoms such as nausea, diarrhoea, and recurrent abdominal pain can occur at mealtimes, which often leads to decreased appetite and food intake. In Crohn's disease, inflammation of the intestine can result in overgrowth of bacteria. This, combined with the effects of any previous surgery to remove diseased sections of the bowel, can decrease the absorptive surface area of the intestine and reduce the absorption of essential nutrients. People who have undergone surgery may have problems absorbing fats and this, coupled with frequent bouts of diarrhoea, may also cause deficiencies to develop.

It is crucial to increase the amount of protein you eat as inflammatory bowel disorders can cause excessive intestinal secretion of protein-rich fluids through the inflamed wall of the intestine. Good sources include lean meat, poultry, oily fish, and pulses (*see pp.84–85*).

## PROTECTIVE FOODS
Various foods can help relieve as well as prevent the troublesome symptoms of an inflammatory bowel disorder.
● Complex carbohydrates (*see p.46–47*) from whole grains, vegetables, and fruits are a good source of fibre, which helps the intestine function properly. If the extra fibre causes wind, you can take an over-the-counter product to reduce this.
● Drink lots of fluids, mainly water, but avoid caffeinated drinks. Green tea is thought to be beneficial.
● Eat plenty of foods containing omega-3 fatty acids, such as linseeds, rapeseed oil, soya beans, and oily fish.
● The herb sage may be helpful too.

## FOODS TO AVOID
Certain foods may cause symptoms. Common things to avoid are: alcohol, sugary foods, including sweet fruit such as grapes and pineapple, and caffeine, as they can all cause inflammation; foods containing gluten, which is found in wheat, oats, and barley; milk and dairy products; foods that are common causes of allergic reactions, such as soya, eggs, and peanuts; and vegetables of the brassica family, such as Brussels sprouts, cabbages, and broccoli.

## TAKING SUPPLEMENTS
People who have Crohn's disease or ulcerative colitis are advised to take a multivitamin supplement. Deficiencies of the fat-soluble vitamins (A, D, E, K), vitamin $B_{12}$, and folate are common. A folate supplement is vital for anyone taking sulfasalazine (a drug prescribed for chronic inflammation), which can interfere with folate's absorption. Some patients may need injections of vitamin $B_{12}$. Persistent, watery diarrhoea may require supplementation with the minerals zinc and magnesium.

---

# Recipe  Omega-3-rich trout stuffed with sage

### INGREDIENTS

**2 fresh trout, boned and cleaned**

**bunch of fresh sage**

**2 lemons**

**freshly ground black pepper**

**3 tbsp olive oil**

### Serves 2

1 Preheat the oven to 180°C (350°F, gas 4). Line a baking tray with a large sheet of foil and place the trout on it.

2 Stuff several sprigs of sage into each fish and season with the juice of one lemon and freshly ground black pepper.

3 Cut the remaining lemon into wedges and place around the trout. Drizzle with olive oil.

4 Bring the foil up and over the trout and seal to form a parcel. Bake for 35 minutes or until the fish is cooked.

5 Carefully remove the trout from the foil on to serving plates. Garnish with sprigs of fresh sage. If you like, serve with baby new potatoes and lightly steamed green beans.

### Each serving provides
Cal. 316, Total fat 22g (Sat. 2.0g, Poly. 1.5g, Mono. 12g), Cholesterol 10mg, Protein 29g, Carbohydrate 2.0g, Fibre 0.5g, Sodium 84mg. Good source of – Vits: A; Mins: Ca, K, Mg, P.

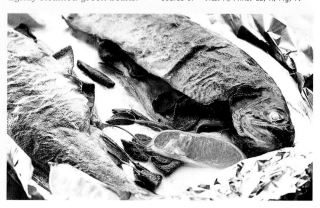

# Diverticular disorders

Diverticulosis is the presence of small pouches (known as diverticuli) in the wall of the colon, which occur when parts of the intestine bulge outwards through weak areas. The increase in pressure in the colon is commonly caused by constipation due to lack of fibre in the diet.

From time to time, one or more of these "pouches" may become inflamed. This condition is known as diverticulitis, and it is possible to treat it with a low-fibre, "soft" diet.

## HIGH FIBRE FOR DIVERTICULOSIS

Diverticulosis is very common among older people and, although it often does not produce specific symptoms, some people may develop cramps, bloating, and irregular bowel movements, with no sign of fever or infection.

Treating and preventing diverticulosis through nutrition often involves just increasing insoluble fibre in the diet; this helps keep stools soft and easy to pass and prevents constipation, and therefore prevents the development of diverticulosis.

Experts recommend an intake of at least 18g of fibre from food every day. Fruits, vegetables, and whole grains are

### HIGH-FIBRE MEAL PLANNER

**Breakfast**
- Muesli with chopped fruit, and wholemeal toast (see p.219)

**Lunch**
- Baked sweet potato with a rocket salad
- Fresh orange
- Glass of semi-skimmed milk

**Dinner**
- Chicken and vegetable stir-fry with brown rice
- Baked apple with vanilla yogurt

**Snacks**
- Six or seven dried apricots
- Low-fat fruit yogurt

### LOW-FIBRE MEAL PLANNER

**Breakfast**
- Puffed rice with semi-skimmed milk and a banana
- Glass of apple juice

**Lunch**
- Omelette with ham, and a bagel
- Stewed apple
- Water or semi-skimmed milk

**Dinner**
- White pasta and tuna bake topped with reduced-fat cheese
- Reduced-fat chocolate mousse

**Snacks**
- Vanilla low-fat yogurt
- Rice cakes with seedless jam

good sources of dietary fibre, and can easily be incorporated into your daily diet (see pp.48–49).

If you suffer from diverticulosis, it is important that you follow a high-fibre diet, and make sure that you also drink plenty of fluids (preferably water) – about 2 litres (3½ pints) a day. It is important that you avoid becoming constipated as hard stools or straining when you go to the toilet will cause more diverticuli (pouches) to form and make your symptoms worse.

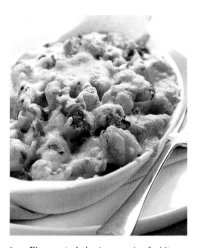

**Low-fibre pasta bake** A casserole of white pasta and tuna topped with grated reduced-fat hard cheese is a great low-fibre option for people suffering from diverticulitis.

## LOW FIBRE FOR DIVERTICULITIS

Diverticulitis is an acute infection or inflammation of the diverticuli that may flare up if stool gets caught in one of the "pouches". Symptoms can include abdominal pain, fever, and nausea. An infection usually lasts for about a week.

When someone with diverticulosis develops diverticulitis, the nutritional advice changes. Rather than following a high-fibre diet, you should instead follow a low-fibre one, which allows the passage of stools through the inflamed, typically narrowed segment of the colon.

In addition, you should eat a soft diet, which means that you should eat things that do not require much chewing, such as soup, mashed potatoes, well-cooked pasta, and bananas. Once the infection has cleared up, patients should go back to their high-fibre diet.

## EATING SEEDS AND NUTS

In the past, doctors recommended that people with diverticulosis should avoid eating nuts and seeds because they could lodge in the diverticula and lead to diverticulitis. There are no known cases of such a blockage, however, and so there is no proven benefit in avoiding seeds and nuts. If you have suffered rectal bleeding, your doctor may still advise you not to eat seeds and nuts, but otherwise you can safely enjoy these foods as part of a high-fibre diet.

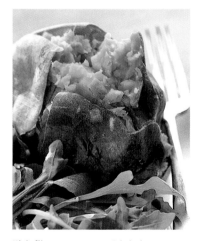

**High-fibre sweet potato** A baked sweet potato served with rocket is a high-fibre dish that is nutritious and easy to prepare, and will help in the treatment of diverticulosis.

# Gluten-free diet for coeliac disease

In coeliac disease, the intestine cannot absorb food properly due to a reaction to gluten, a protein found in wheat, rye, barley, and oats. The only treatment, therefore, is a gluten-free diet, which must be followed for life. A gluten-free diet will improve symptoms within days of starting it, allow existing damage to heal, and prevent further intestinal damage. The table below is a great starting point for anyone embarking on a gluten-free diet. Remember always to check food labels for hidden gluten as it can appear in different forms in places you wouldn't expect to find it, for example in hydrolyzed vegetable protein (HVP).

| FOOD TYPE | FOODS ALLOWED | FOODS NOT ALLOWED |
|---|---|---|
| Breads, pasta, cereal, rice, and grains | Bread or pasta made from corn (maize), rice, soya, potato starch, potato flour, whole-bean flour, tapioca, sago, rice bran, sorghum, and quinoa; cereal containing rice or corn; corn tacos and tortillas | Breads containing wheat, rye, barley, oats, bran, semolina, kamut; pasta made from wheat or wheat starch; couscous; cereals made from wheat, rye, triticale, barley, oats |
| Fruits and vegetables | Fresh, frozen, and canned fruits and vegetables (avoid emulsifiers and stabilizers from unknown sources) | Fruit pie filling, breadcrumbed or creamed vegetables (read labels) |
| Dairy foods | Milk, cream, buttermilk, yogurt, cheese, cream cheese, processed cheese, and cottage cheese | Thickened milkshake (some contain flour); processed cheeses products |
| Protein foods | Fresh meat, fish, and poultry; pulses; nuts and seeds; tofu | Cooked meats, sausages, and canned ham or tuna may contain HVP (check labels) |
| Fats and oils | Butter, margarine, and vegetables oils | Shredded suet; sprays with grain alcohol |
| Alcohol | Wine, potato vodka, rum, tequila, and sake | Beers and ales, grain alcohol, most liqueurs |
| Miscellaneous | Home-made soups; wheat-free soy sauce; non-grain vinegars such as wine or fruit vinegar | Canned soup; stock cubes; most soy sauces; white vinegar made from grains |

# Recipe Gluten-free quinoa-stuffed peppers

### INGREDIENTS

**115g (4oz) quinoa**

**1 onion**

**2 cloves garlic**

**1 courgette**

**85g (3oz) drained canned chickpeas**

**1 lemon**

**4 peppers**

### Serves 4

1 Cook the quinoa according to the directions on the packet. When it is cooked, set it aside, covered, in a warm place for 15 minutes.

2 Preheat the oven to 200°C (400°F, gas 6). Peel and chop the onion; crush the garlic; and dice the courgette. Heat a little oil in a frying pan, add the vegetables, minutes until softened but not browned. Stir in the quinoa, the chickpeas, and 1 tsp of lemon juice, and season with freshly ground black pepper.

3 Cut the tops off the peppers and remove the seeds. Divide the quinoa mixture among the peppers and replace the tops. Place in an ovenproof dish and brush with oil.

4 Bake for about 45 minutes, until the peppers are tender and lightly browned. Serve with a mixed salad.

### Each serving provides:

Calories 219, Total fat 2.5g (Sat. 0.3g, Poly. 1.1g, Mono. 0.6g), Cholesterol 0mg, Protein 8.4g, Carbohydrate 46g, Fibre 4.0g, Sodium 71mg. Good source of – Vits: A, Fol, C; Mins: Ca, K, Mg, P.

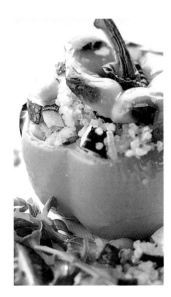

# Disorders of the urinary system

**The urinary system rids your body of waste, so it is crucial that it functions well.**

The urinary system, also known as the urinary tract, consists of a pair of kidneys; the bladder; the ureters, which connect each kidney to the bladder; and the urethra, through which urine leaves the body.

### Role of the kidneys
The main job of the kidneys is to remove waste and excess water from the body in the form of urine, keep a stable balance of salts and other substances in the blood, and produce hormones that stimulate red blood cell production and regulate blood pressure.

Every day, the kidneys filter about 190 litres (about 40 gallons) of blood and then produce about 2 litres (3½ pints) of waste products and water – the amount will vary depending on how much food and drink you have consumed. The waste and water become urine, which is held in the bladder until you go to the toilet. The waste

products in your blood come from the normal breakdown of body tissues and the foods you eat. If your kidneys aren't able to remove these wastes properly, they build up in the blood, which can cause significant medical problems.

### Potential problems
Most kidney diseases affect the filtration capacity of the kidneys, causing them to lose function.

Kidney disorders are broadly classified as acute – the sudden failure of a kidney, which may be fatal – or there may be a gradual reduction in function over months or years, in which case it is chronic.

Although the urinary system is structured in a way that helps ward off infection, infections can occur. They are caused by germs that get into the urethra, which can spread to the kidneys.

## The urinary system

This is different in men and women. The urethra from the male bladder passes through the prostate gland.

The female bladder sits under the uterus. Urination is controlled by the muscles in the neck of the bladder.

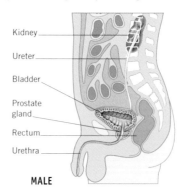

Kidney
Ureter
Bladder
Prostate gland
Rectum
Urethra

**MALE**

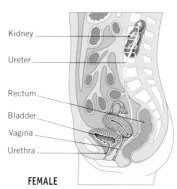

Kidney
Ureter
Rectum
Bladder
Vagina
Urethra

**FEMALE**

# Who is most at risk of developing urinary disorders?

The following are some of the risk factors for disorders of the urinary system discussed in this section:

**Diet and lifestyle** People who live in hot climates and who are susceptible to kidney stones are at increased risk if they do not drink enough fluid to replace that lost through perspiration.

**Gender and age** About 20 per cent of women will contract a urinary tract infection (UTI) at some point in their life. The reasons for this are not fully understood, although it may be because a woman's urethra is short, allowing bacteria quick access to the

bladder. Kidney stones are more common in Caucasians, in men, and in those between the ages of 20 and 40.

**Family history** You are more likely to develop a stone if someone in your family has had a kidney stone. Similarly, anyone who has a kidney stone is at increased risk of having another.

**Other factors** Any abnormality of the urinary tract that obstructs the flow of urine (a kidney stone, for example) sets the stage for a urinary tract infection. An enlarged prostate gland can also slow urine flow, thus increasing the risk of infection. Sexually active women or

those who use a diaphragm for birth control may be more likely to have a UTI. People with diabetes have a higher risk of a UTI because of changes in their immune systems.

People with ulcerative colitis or Crohn's disease, or who have had intestinal bypass surgery for weight loss, are at risk of developing oxalate kidney stones, and these people may be prescribed preventive treatment.

People with diabetes or high blood pressure, or who have suffered repeated kidney infections, are at greatest risk of developing kidney failure.

# Disorders of the urinary system

The table below deals with the major disorders affecting the urinary system, which comprises the kidneys, bladder, and urethra. It keeps the chemistry of the body in balance by removing waste products and excess water.

One of the most common disorders of the urinary system, kidney stones are formed from deposits of calcium, oxalate, uric acid, or citrate. The risk of developing kidney stones is increased by inadequate fluid intake. Kidney failure may be acute (short-term) or chronic (long-term). Chronic failure develops slowly over the years, with symptoms so mild that people may not recognize that they have a kidney disease.

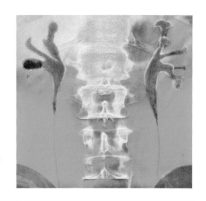

**Kidney stone**  On the left of this X-ray image a reddish brown kidney stone can be seen quite clearly in the right kidney .

| DISORDER | WHAT IS IT? | HOW YOU CAN HELP |
|---|---|---|
| **Urinary tract infection (UTI)** | An infection can occur in any part of the urinary tract when a bacterium, fungus, or virus invades. If the infection reaches the kidneys, it can cause a fever or lower back pain. | • Drink plenty of water and cranberry juice to flush out the system<br>• Do not resist the urge to urinate |
| **Kidney stones** | Stones are one of the most common kidney disorders. A kidney stone is a hard mass that develops from crystals that separate from urine and build up in the kidney. Most stones pass on their own and require no treatment other than pain management. Dietary measures may be effective at reducing the risk of another occurrence. Stones can also form in the bladder from substances in urine. | • Maintaining hydration with plenty of fluids is essential<br>• Maintain your calcium intake and reduce intake of high-oxalate foods<br>• Avoid high-protein diets<br>• Choose complex carbohydrates<br>• Eat more fresh fruit and vegetables |
| **Kidney failure** | Damage to the kidney compromises its ability to filter out and eliminate waste products and water, which build up in the blood, disrupting its chemical balance. | • Control your blood pressure and blood sugar<br>• Eat a low-protein, low-sodium diet |

# Urinary tract infections

Infections can occur if bacteria get into the body via the bloodstream or the urethra. Urinary tract infections (UTIs) are more common in women.

### THE SPREAD OF BACTERIA

Despite containing fluids, salts, and waste products, urine is sterile (free from germs such as bacteria). An infection occurs only when bacteria begin to grow. A woman's urethral opening lies near sources of bacteria from the anus and vagina. Infections often start in the urethra (urethritis). From there, the bacteria can move up into the bladder, causing an infection (cystitis). If the infection is not treated, it can spread to the kidneys, causing pyelonephritis, which is serious and can damage the kidneys.

### TREATING A UTI

There are steps you can take to ease painful symptoms, such as a frequent urge to urinate, a burning feeling when you urinate, and general discomfort.
• Drink plenty of water.
• Drink cranberry juice – it reduces the ability of bacteria to "stick" to the bladder lining and fights off infection.
• Urinate when you feel the need.
• Wipe from front to back.
• Avoid using feminine hygiene sprays.
• Take showers instead of baths.
If symptoms persist, see your doctor, who may prescribe antibiotics.

**Cranberry juice**  Drinking pure cranberry juice can not only treat but can also prevent urinary tract infections.

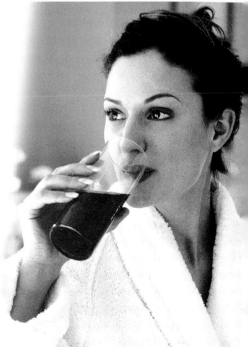

# Dietary treatment for kidney stones

Kidney stones occur when the urine is saturated with waste products that can crystallize into stones or when the chemicals that normally inhibit this crystallization process are absent. The most common type of stone contains calcium with either phosphate or oxalate. Some stones contain uric acid, and these are more common in people with gout (*see p.245*).

The goal of nutritional treatment is to eliminate the diet-related risk factors for stone formation and to prevent the further growth of existing stones.

## THE IMPORTANCE OF FLUIDS
First, and most importantly, a regular intake of plenty of fluids is essential for people with kidney stones. This will dilute the urine, thus reducing the concentration of stone-forming substances in the urine. It is also very important to drink plenty of extra fluid in hot weather and when on holiday in a hot climate. Water is the best choice for maintaining fluid levels.

On the other hand, a moderate intake of alcohol, coffee, and tea may help reduce the risk of stone formation –

due, presumably, to the diuretic effect of the caffeine in these beverages.
• A daily intake of 3–3.5 litres (about 5–6 pints) of fluid is recommended.

## MAINTAIN CALCIUM INTAKE
Most calcium stones are not, in fact, attributable to a diet high in calcium-rich foods. As explained in the box (*right*), it is important to maintain a moderate calcium intake if you suffer from kidney stones. This is because a low intake may promote the formation of calcium oxalate stones.
• A calcium intake of approximately 600–800mg per day is recommended for people with kidney stones.

## CUT OUT HIGH-OXALATE FOODS
A reduction in dietary intake of foods containing high levels of oxalate (*right*) is important for susceptible people, since this is an important factor in the formation of calcium oxalate stones.

Vitamin C supplements should also be avoided by people at risk of kidney stones since this vitamin can break down to oxalate, which is excreted in the kidney (*see p.269*).

## RESTRICT ANIMAL PROTEIN
A high intake of animal protein is acidic and increases the excretion of urinary calcium. In addition, the binding effect of sulphate in dietary protein decreases kidney calcium reabsorption. Therefore, it is recommended that people with kidney stones should limit their intake of animal proteins from meat, fish, poultry, and eggs to 60–70g per day.

## REDUCE SODIUM INTAKE
A high intake of sodium (*see p.221*) increases calcium excretion, which can result in an increase in calcium-containing crystals in the urine. A reduction of high-sodium foods is therefore recommended, with an intake of no more than 2–4g per day.

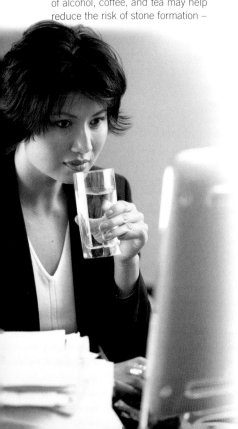

**Drink plenty of water** If you have kidney stones, maintain your fluid intake throughout the day to dilute your urine and reduce the concentration of stone-forming substances.

High-sodium foods include most canned, processed, and packaged foods. Check the labels: any food that has a sodium content greater than 400mg per serving is considered to be high in sodium.

## COMPLEX CARBOHYDRATES
It is also advisable for people with kidney stones to reduce their intake of simple sugars and products made from refined flour (such as white bread, cakes, and biscuits), in favour of whole-grain foods, such as wholemeal bread and pasta and brown rice, which are high in complex carbohydrates (*see pp.46–47*), as well as eating more fruits and vegetables.

## Avoid high-oxalate foods

Although high calcium excretion in the urine is commonly seen in people with calcium stones, kidney stones do not result from a high dietary intake of calcium. On the contrary, a diet that is very low in calcium increases the absorption and subsequent excretion of the chemical oxalate, which promotes the formation of calcium oxalate stones in susceptible people.

The amount of oxalate in the diet, however, is an important factor in the formation of calcium oxalate stones, and people who are prone to this type of kidney stone are advised to cut back on high-oxalate foods in order to help prevent the formation of stones. Foods that are rich in oxalate include:
• Spinach
• Swiss chard
• Spring greens
• Parsley (can be used sparingly)
• Beetroot
• Rhubarb
• Tea
• Chocolate
• Chocolate drinks and cocoa
• Carob powder
• Nuts and nut butters
Strawberries, celery, and instant coffee contain moderate amounts of oxalates, so should be eaten in limited quantities.

# Nutrition in kidney failure

Kidney (or renal) failure occurs when the kidneys cease to function normally. People who have kidney disease will be prescribed special diets by their doctor and dietitian, specifically to reduce their dietary protein, sodium, phosphorus, and potassium intake, depending on the results of weekly blood tests.

Dialysis can be done by filtering the blood through a machine (haemodialysis) or by infusing and removing a saline solution through the abdomen (peritoneal dialysis). People receiving dialysis must also watch their diets with extreme care and may need extra calories to prevent weight loss. The following general dietary points can be made.

## CONTROL PROTEIN INTAKE

Because people with kidney failure have a decreased ability to excrete urea (the product of protein metabolism), it is advisable to control the intake of protein in the diet to help minimize the build-up of these nitrogen-containing wastes in the blood. Recent research suggests that restricting the intake of protein early in the course of kidney failure may slow the progression of the disease and delay the need to initiate dialysis therapy. The generally accepted level of

protein for people with kidney failure is to eat less than 0.6g per 1kg (2¼lb) of body weight per day.

## OBTAIN CALORIES FROM FAT

Since people with kidney failure are at risk of undernutrition, additional dietary fat intake, in the form of mono- and polyunsaturated fats, may be advised as a way of providing adequate calories. However, elevated levels of "bad" LDL cholesterol and total cholesterol are found in 20–70 per cent of people with kidney failure, so regular monitoring of blood lipid levels is important.

## MAINTAIN SODIUM BALANCE

As kidney failure progresses, the ability of the kidneys to excrete sodium declines and dietary intake may have to be limited (*see p.221*). Sodium balance can usually be maintained by limiting sodium intake to 2000–3000mg per day.

## RESTRICT POTASSIUM

A restriction on dietary potassium may be necessary during the later stages of kidney failure, or if certain medications lead to high levels of potassium in the blood. A limit of 2000–3000mg per day may be initiated.

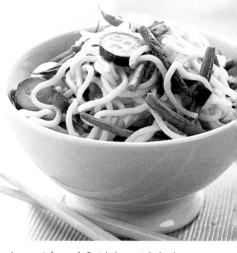

**Low-protein meal** Restricting protein intake may help slow the progression of kidney failure, so low-protein meals, such as noodles with fresh vegetables, are recommended.

## MAINTAIN FLUID BALANCE

Fluid intake in people with kidney failure is determined by the ability of the kidneys to eliminate fluid. As long as the daily urine output essentially equals the daily fluid intake, balance will be maintained. In the later stages of kidney failure, however, fluid intake may need to be restricted in order to prevent fluid retention.

# Maintaining dietary balance

It is usually advisable for people with kidney failure to follow a very specific diet to slow the progression of the condition, alleviate symptoms, and prevent nutrient deficiencies. This will usually be implemented under the supervision of a registered dietitian.

Since many people with chronic kidney failure also have other medical conditions such as high blood pressure, diabetes, and, possibly, high levels of blood cholesterol, the right balance of food is very important; otherwise, the dietary restrictions will cause them to lose weight and become malnourished.

The challenge is to make sure that you get enough calories and the right kind of fat (monounsaturated) so you maintain a healthy weight, as well as

enough vitamins and minerals. Since protein is usually reduced, calories can be added from olive and rapeseed oils and margarine, as well as from small frequent meals and snacks.

## NUTRITIONAL SUPPLEMENTS

Due to dietary restrictions, people with kidney failure need supplements of vitamins $B_1$, $B_2$, $B_6$, C, D, niacin, and folate. Vitamin A, however, may build up as kidney failure progresses and should not be supplemented.

Kidney failure usually leads to anaemia due to decreased production by the kidneys of the hormone erythropoietin, which is needed to make red blood cells. Anaemia can treated with erythropoietin therapy and iron supplementation.

### KIDNEY FAILURE MENU PLANNER

**Breakfast**
- Scrambled egg on a slice of wholemeal toast with margarine
- Slice of melon

**Lunch**
- Low-salt turkey breast and salad on wholemeal bread
- Glass of lemonade

**Dinner**
- Spaghetti with low-salt marinara or tomato sauce
- Green beans
- Baked apple with low-fat yogurt

**Snacks**
- Raw vegetables with low-fat dip

# Bone and joint disorders

## Nutrition plays a vital role in the health of bones and joints.

Bones and joints make up the body's framework, protecting our internal organs and working in conjunction with our muscles to keep us mobile. Good nutrition throughout life is essential for the formation and maintenance of strong bones, while regular exercise is an important factor in maintaining the healthy function of bones and joints.

## Osteoporosis

One of the most common bone diseases, osteoporosis involves a gradual loss of bone tissue, leaving the bones less dense and more prone to fracture. Osteoporosis is a major health problem in the UK, affecting one in three women and

one in 12 men over the age of 50. An estimated three million people in the UK suffer from osteoporosis and this is likely to increase as the population ages.

Adequate calcium intake is crucial for the formation and maintenance of bones (*see p.62*). This mineral must be replaced by dietary means because it is not manufactured by the body. If your dietary intake is inadequate, calcium is lost from the bones, making them weaker.

Vitamin D is also essential for bone health (*see p.57*) because it is needed for calcium absorption, with deficiency contributing to low bone density and disease (*below*). Researchers also believe that isoflavones from soya and other phytoestrogens (*see p.144*) may increase calcium absorption.

## Osteomalacia and rickets

A disease of adults, osteomalacia is characterized by soft bones due to a failure of bone to absorb calcium. The disorder is caused by various factors including too little vitamin D in the diet, insufficient exposure to sunlight, and malabsorption of vitamin D in the intestine due to conditions such as coeliac disease (*see p.235*) or after gastrointestinal surgery. Osteomalacia can lead to pain in the legs, ribs, hips, and muscles, and to easily broken bones and impaired mobility.

In children, the same condition is known as rickets and is usually caused by a vitamin D deficiency. Babies who are breast-fed for more than a year (with no vitamin D supplements) and children deprived of sufficient sunlight are most at risk of developing rickets.

However, the incidence of rickets has almost disappeared in the UK, thanks to better nutrition.

## Fibromyalgia and nutrition

Fibromyalgia is a complex chronic muscle disorder that affects two to five percent of the UK population. The symptoms of fibromyalgia include widespread muscle pain and general stiffness, profound fatigue, and non-refreshing sleep.

While there is little scientific support for dietary treatment, many people turn to nutritional and herbal supplements, including vitamins, magnesium, and amino acids. Studies show that the pain and tenderness of fibromyalgia may be relieved by supplements of magnesium hydroxide and malic acid (a naturally occurring substance in our bodies).

## Key anatomy

Joints occur where bones meet, and enable our bodies to be flexible. The ends of bones are lined with cartilage.

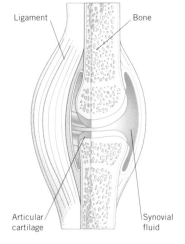

Ligament — Bone

Articular cartilage — Synovial fluid

## Arthritic conditions

There are many different types of arthritis, but in general the term refers to inflammation of one or more joints, accompanied by pain, swelling, and stiffness. Rheumatoid arthritis is the most common form of inflammatory joint disease and affects one to three per cent of adults in the UK. Many tissues in the body may be involved, but the joints are most severely affected.

Osteoarthritis is another common form of arthritis that affects 80 per cent of people over the age of 65. The condition is characterized by a gradual loss of cartilage from the joints and, in some people, joint inflammation. It most commonly affects the joints of the hands, knees, spine, and hips.

Gout is another form of arthritis that usually affects the joint at the base of the big toe. The condition is caused by high levels of uric acid in the bloodstream – which is known as hyperuricaemia – leading to the deposition of uric-acid crystals in the joint. The joint becomes red, swollen, and tender, and the attack may be accompanied by fever.

# Who is most at risk of bone and joint disorders?

Adult bone mass is determined by the amount of bone formed during childhood, with accumulation (known as peak bone mass) complete by age 30–35. Bone mass is influenced by a number of factors: up to 80 per cent is influenced by genetic factors, while about 20–40 per cent is environmental.

**Diet and lifestyle**  A life-long diet low in calcium and vitamin D is one of the major risk factors for many bone disorders. Smoking and heavy alcohol consumption, which are often accompanied by poor nutrition and lack of physical activity, are also associated with low bone density. Gout is often associated with a rich diet and heavy alcohol consumption.

**Age**  Bone and joint disorders are more common among middle-aged and older adults. The onset of rheumatoid arthritis most commonly occurs between ages 40 and 60, and osteoarthritis between ages 60 and 80. Gout most commonly develops between the ages of 40 and 50 in men

and over 60 in women. Asian and Caucasian women over age 65 have a particularly high risk of developing osteoporosis. On the other hand, women of African origin tend to have a higher bone mass than Caucasians and a lower risk of osteoporosis.

**Gender**  Osteoporosis is more common in women since they have less bone mass than men to begin with. Women who have short intervals between pregnancies or several children are at increased risk of this disease. In addition, because the levels of oestrogen – necessary to retain calcium in bones – decrease in women after the menopause, their risk increases at this time. Women have twice the risk of developing rheumatoid arthritis as men, but gout is 20 times more common in men.

**Family history**  Both osteoporosis and gout are conditions in which a family history increases the risk of developing the disease. A history of a maternal hip fracture after age 50 is also considered a risk factor for osteoporosis.

# What are bone and joint disorders?

Disorders that affect the musculoskeletal system are common and range from mild problems such as gout, to more severe problems such as rheumatoid arthritis and osteoarthritis. The most common symptoms are pain and physical disability, which can have a major impact on people's lives. As many as 30 per cent of people in the UK have symptoms related to their bones and

joints, but people rarely die from these conditions. Treatments for bone and joint disorders include medication, surgery, physiotherapy, and nutritional therapy.

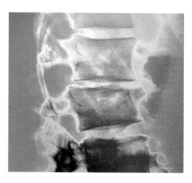

**Osteoporosis**  This coloured X-ray shows how the lower spine is compacted in a person with osteoporosis. The vertebrae (dark blocks) are touching, causing back pain and immobility.

| DISORDER | WHAT IS IT? | HOW YOU CAN HELP |
|---|---|---|
| **Osteoporosis** | Loss of bone density, leaving bones brittle, and prone to fracture. Since it occurs without symptoms, it is often diagnosed only after a bone is fractured in a fall or a vertebra collapses, causing back pain. | • Ensure adequate intake of calcium and vitamin D; stop smoking; exercise regularly |
| **Osteomalacia** | Softening and weakening of bones in adults, due to a failure of bone to absorb the mineral calcium. | • Increase vitamin D intake <br> • 20–30 minutes sunshine daily |
| **Rickets** | Childhood condition causing retarded growth, joint malformation, and swelling and tenderness at bone ends. May lead to bowed legs, spinal curvature, and chest-bone malformations. | • Increase vitamin D and calcium intake <br> • 20–30 minutes sunshine daily |
| **Rheumatoid arthritis (RA)** | Inflammation of synovial membrane, which encloses joints, causing joint stiffness, pain, and swelling; may lead to a loss of movement and deformity of joints. | • Eat a varied diet rich in essential vitamins and minerals <br> • Exercise regularly |
| **Osteoarthritis (OA)** | Degeneration of cartilage covering bone ends, within joints, causing pain, swelling, and stiffness, usually in knees and hips. | • Exercise regularly <br> • Lose weight if overweight |
| **Gout** | Deposits of uric acid crystals within joints, causing sudden pain and inflammation; joint at base of big toe most commonly affected. | • Avoid high purine foods <br> • Restrict alcohol intake |

# Treating osteoporosis

One of the most common bone diseases, osteoporosis involves a gradual loss of bone tissue, leaving the bones less dense and more prone to fracture. An estimated three million people in the UK suffer from osteoporosis. It is possible to slow the progress of the condition by making changes to your diet and lifestyle:

**Take adequate calcium** The body does not manufacture calcium, and it is lost from the body every day. It is therefore important to maintain adequate daily calcium intake (*below*).

**Take adequate vitamin D** This vitamin is needed for normal calcium absorption by the body, as well as playing a role in the uptake of calcium into bone (*see p.57*). Thus it is important that you get sufficient vitamin D from your diet as well as from exposure to the sun.

**Stop smoking** Studies have shown that smokers have poorer bone density than non-smokers. Giving up smoking, even later in life, may help limit bone loss. Research shows that while hormone replacement therapy protects women from bone fractures, this may not be the case in female smokers, as tobacco may have an anti-oestrogenic effect. In addition, smokers tend to drink more alcohol and exercise less.

**Limit alcohol intake** Those who drink alcohol heavily are more prone to bone loss and fractures, mainly because of poor nutrition but also due to their increased risk of falling.

**Exercise regularly** Regular physical activity helps increase bone mass and reduce bone loss. Weight-bearing exercises such as walking, dancing, and weightlifting are best.

## Checking bone density

A DEXA scan is currently the most widely used method of measuring bone-mineral density of the spine and extremities. Scanning takes a few minutes and is a sensitive and accurate test of bone density. The report compares your values with those of a young person and with a person of your age with normal bone density (age-related bone loss is normal). You are at risk of osteoporosis if you take medication that affects your bones (such as steroids); if you have a history of menstrual cycle cessation; if you have inflammatory bowel disease; or if you had an early menopause. In such circumstances, ask your GP about having a baseline bone scan that can be repeated over time.

# Boosting your dietary calcium intake

Calcium is vital for bone formation and keeping bones strong. It is important to boost your calcium intake if you are at risk of developing, or if you already suffer from, osteoporosis.

The recommended daily calcium intake is 350mg for children aged one to three years; 450mg for four- to six-year-olds; 550mg for children aged seven to ten; 1000mg for boys aged 11–18 and 800mg for girls the same age; and at least 700mg for adults. Anyone who has been diagnosed with osteoporosis may need to increase their intake to 1200mg per day.

## CALCIUM-RICH FOODS

The mineral calcium is better absorbed by the body from food rather than in a supplement. Obvious sources of calcium are dairy products such as milk, yogurt, and cheese, but calcium is also found in green vegetables such as spinach and broccoli, canned fish eaten with the bones, tofu, dried apricots, and figs.

Once you know how, it is relatively easy to make meals calcium-rich – see right for an easy lunch transformation to boost calcium intake.

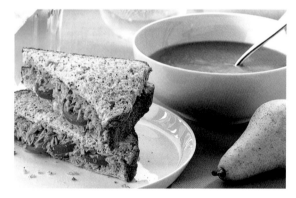

**Low-calcium lunch**
Although healthy in many respects, this lunch of tomato soup, tuna and tomato sandwich on wholemeal bread, fresh pear, and glass of water provides just 94mg of calcium.

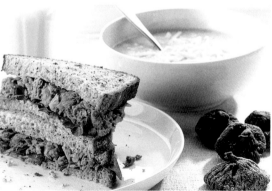

**High-calcium lunch**
A bowl of cream of broccoli soup topped with grated reduced-fat Cheddar, a canned salmon and watercress sandwich, dried figs, and glass of skimmed milk will provide 821mg of calcium.

# Preventing and treating osteomalacia and rickets

Osteomalacia and rickets (the name given to osteomalacia when it occurs in babies and children) are caused by a deficiency of vitamin D in the body (*see p.57*).

### INCREASING VITAMIN D
Deficiency is due to inadequate dietary intake of foods containing vitamin D, or to insufficient sunlight, which is necessary for the conversion of vitamin D in our skin to its active form (a form that the body can use). There are few dietary sources of vitamin D, but many common foods, such as margarine and breakfast cereals, are fortified with the vitamin. Good natural sources of vitamin D include cod liver oil, egg yolks, butter, canned salmon and sardines (eaten with their bones), herring, green leafy vegetables, and tofu.

There is no recommended daily amount (RDA) for vitamin D for individuals who are under the age of 65 years and living a normal lifestyle. For anyone who is confined indoors, and people over the age of 65, the RDA is 10mcg a day.

# Treating rheumatoid arthritis

Depending on the stage of the disease, treatment of rheumatoid arthritis varies but initial treatment is usually aimed at reducing inflammation while minimizing the side effects of such treatment. The presence of other disorders, particularly liver or kidney complaints, also affects the type of treatment. In some cases, treatment may involve surgery.

### INCREASED NUTRIENT INTAKE
People with active rheumatoid arthritis may have a poor dietary intake due to loss of appetite. At the same time, some of the medications that treat rheumatoid arthritis, such as anti-inflammatory drugs, may increase the requirement for certain nutrients and reduce their absorption.

Like osteoarthritis (*see p.245*), weight loss is recommended for overweight and obese people to reduce the stress on inflamed joints. Nutritional guidelines, therefore, focus on eating a varied diet that provides essential nutrients while helping control weight.

- Sufficient intake of vitamin E (*see p.58*) is important for the health of your joints; vitamin E-rich foods include oils, fish, nuts, and seeds.
- You should also choose foods that provide an adequate intake of B vitamins (*see pp.53–56*), vitamin D (*see p.57*), calcium (*see p.62*), iron (*see p.66*), and omega-3 fatty acids (*see p.90*).
- Try to include adequate amounts of antioxidants (*see p.20*) in your diet.

### MAINTAINING BONE DENSITY
Rheumatoid arthritis causes bone loss, which can also lead to osteoporosis (*see p.241*). Bone loss is more likely with an increasing level of disability, resulting from rheumatoid arthritis and the decreasing level of weight-bearing activity. The use of steroid drugs further accelerates bone loss, particularly in post-menopausal women.

Bone loss can be countered by ensuring that you consume adequate amounts of calcium-rich foods and those that provide vitamin D, or by taking supplements.

### EXERCISE AND MOBILITY
Pain and stiffness often cause people with rheumatoid arthritis to stop using their inflamed joints. However, such decrease of activity can lead to loss of joint motion and loss of muscle strength, which leads to decreased joint stability and increased fatigue. Exercise can help prevent and reverse these effects, but programmes should be designed by a physiotherapist and tailored to the severity of your condition, your former activity level, and your body build.

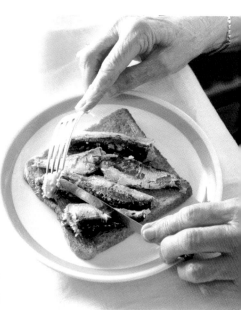

**Sardines are good for rheumatoid arthritis**
Containing high levels of calcium, B vitamins, iron, and omega-3 fatty acids, sardines on toast is a quick, easy, and nutritious snack.

## Omega-3 fatty acids and rheumatoid arthritis

Studies have shown that people with rheumatoid arthritis who were treated with fish-oil supplements for three to four months had a reduction in the number of affected joints.

It is thought that omega-3 fatty acids, which are found in oil-rich fish as well as some plant oils (*see p.90*), might reduce inflammation and help alleviate the troublesome symptoms of rheumatoid arthritis by reducing the number of inflammatory "messenger molecules" made by the body's immune system.

High doses of omega-3 fatty acids should be taken under the supervision of a doctor to prevent side effects or interactions with medications that you may be using to treat rheumatoid arthritis. Eating oil-rich fish, such as tuna, salmon, and mackerel, at least twice a week should be an integral part of your diet if you suffer from rheumatoid arthritis.

# Can diet cure arthritis?

Theories abound that eliminating certain foods, such as tomatoes, potatoes, and peppers, taking specific supplements, or adding honey, vinegar, or herbs to the diet will alleviate arthritis. However, with the exception of gout, which may benefit from a change of diet, there is no conclusive scientific evidence that diet can cure joint disorders.

Tests have shown that diets low in saturated fats, or that include certain omega-3 fatty acids, seem to have a mild anti-inflammatory effect, but there is insufficient evidence that these are useful in the treatment of arthritis. (You should note that cod liver oil is not the best source of these oils and should not be taken in large quantities.)

Neither is there any evidence that fasting and "cleansing" diets, which are sometimes promoted as methods of treating arthritis, have any long-term benefits. On the contrary, these may lead to malnutrition and health problems.

## GLUCOSAMINE SUPPLEMENTS
There is a certain amount of evidence that glucosamine, in a dose of 1500mg per day, may help relieve the pain of osteoarthritis, and studies are now underway to try to determine whether this supplement helps preserve or regenerate damaged cartilage. Since glucosamine may affect the action of insulin in the body and cause digestive upsets and allergic reactions, it should be taken only under medical supervision and avoided entirely if you are pregnant or breast-feeding. The usefulness of other supplements, such as chondroitin S-adenosylmethionine, sulphate, zinc, and copper is still uncertain.

## TIPS FOR ARTHRITIS
If you suspect that a particular food is aggravating your arthritis, try keeping a food diary for a month, writing down everything that you eat and drink, and then see your doctor for advice. If you eliminate a food, be sure to find an alternative source for the nutrients that this food supplies. The best advice is to maintain a healthy lifestyle and to eat a balanced diet, choosing foods low in sugar and fat and including a variety of foods from the five major food groups every day. Other general dietary tips for people with arthritis include:
- Avoid crash dieting or fasting.
- Increase dietary calcium intake.
- Drink plenty of non-alcoholic fluids.
- Keep within a normal weight range.
- If you do drink alcohol, make sure you do so in moderation.

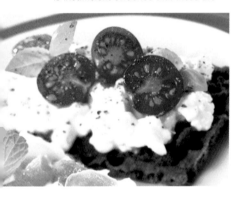

**Soft cheese on crispbread** Maintaining calcium levels is important for arthritis sufferers, but it is a good idea to choose low-fat dairy products to help control weight.

---

# Case study Chef with severe foot pain

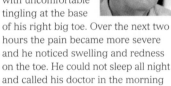

**Name** Michael

**Age** 62 years

**Problem** Michael woke up in the night with uncomfortable tingling at the base of his right big toe. Over the next two hours the pain became more severe and he noticed swelling and redness on the toe. He could not sleep all night and called his doctor in the morning for an emergency appointment.

**Lifestyle** Michael is a chef at a small restaurant. He is on his feet for ten to 12 hours every day and is very upset that this pain in his foot will prevent him from going to work. He has a history of mild high blood pressure, for which his doctor has prescribed a diuretic medication. Michael is moderately overweight and his only exercise is playing a round of golf at the weekend.

Michael's GP diagnosed an acute attack of gout and placed him on anti-inflammatory medication. He is advised to stay off of his foot for five to seven days and then to make a follow-up appointment to discuss how to prevent future attacks of gout. His GP also advised him to reduce his intake of purines (*opposite*).

At his follow-up visit, Michael's doctor explained that gout has been linked to "rich" diets high in meat and wine. Michael's doctor changed his blood pressure medications because diuretics may make gout worse, and explained that he wanted to check his blood levels of uric acid and LDL cholesterol. He explained that gout can be a sign of a serious condition, known as metabolic syndrome, which he may have because he is overweight and has high blood pressure (*see p.214*).

**Advice** By losing weight and limiting his intake of alcohol and foods high in purine, Michael can reduce his risk of another attack. Gout is more common in those who overeat or are overweight. Rapid weight loss can precipitate a gout attack, so a reduced-calorie diet for gradual weight loss is important. Too much alcohol can cause an attack and so should be avoided or limited. Some beers even contain purines. Plenty of water is recommended to ensure dilute urine and prevent the formation of uric-acid kidney stones.

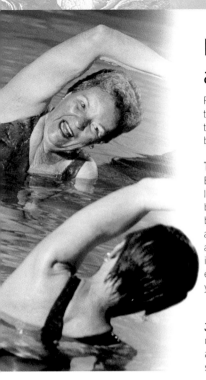

# Benefits of increasing physical activity for osteoarthritis

People who exercise regularly to control their weight and manage their arthritis typically are in less pain and function better than those who are inactive.

## THE BENEFITS OF EXERCISE

Being overweight not only increases the likelihood of developing osteoarthritis, but also worsens the stress on weight-bearing joints, such as the hips, knees, and lower spine, that may already be affected by the condition. Therefore, it is important for you to increase your exercise level to control your weight if you have osteoarthritis.

**Joint-friendly exercise** Exercising in water minimizes stress on any joints affected by arthritis, while helping to maintain flexibility, strengthen muscles, and control weight.

Regular stretching routines and exercises will help increase flexibility and reduce stiffness by keeping your joints moving, whereas strengthening exercises, which should also be performed regularly, will help to maintain or increase muscle strength and increase bone mineral density. Having strong muscles will help keep your joints stable. Cardiovascular exercise can also help with weight loss.

## DIFFERENT TYPES OF EXERCISE

When starting to exercise, build up gradually as your joints may be stiff. Water exercises such as swimming or aqua-aerobics are particularly good for arthritis sufferers as your body weight is supported by the water. In addition, low-impact exercises such as walking or Tai Chi are gentle on the joints, and easy to incorporate into a daily routine.

# Nutritional therapy for gout

A common form of arthritis, gout is a very painful condition, usually affecting the base of the big toe. The condition is due to high levels of uric acid in the blood, leading to the deposition of uric-acid crystals in joint tissue. Treatment is therefore aimed at controlling uric acid in the blood and involves weight loss where appropriate, reduction or elimination of alcohol intake, and possibly the discontinuation of diuretic drugs or other medication.

## PROTEIN AND PURINE FOODS

Because foods with high protein and purine content contribute to high levels of uric acid, eliminating such foods may be beneficial for people who suffer from gout. Beer, in particular, contains high levels of purines in addition to alcohol. Milk, eggs, and cheese are good sources of protein and do not contain high levels of purine, but if you are trying to lose weight, you should choose reduced- or low-fat varieties of dairy products.
● Restrict or avoid alcohol; in particular, you should stop drinking beer.

● Avoid high-purine meats, such as liver, kidneys, sweetbreads, and brains.
● Cut down or avoid meat extracts, such as gravy made from meat drippings.
● Eat no more than 85–115g (3–4oz) of meat at any meal.
● Avoid foods that are high in fat.
● Try to avoid shellfish, fish roe, and oily fish such as anchovies and herring.
● Do not overeat, especially on a regular basis. Control your portion sizes, and share dishes when eating out.
● Take your time when eating.
● Lose weight if necessary, but do it gradually and avoid going on a very low-calorie diet.
● Drink plenty of non-alcoholic fluids.
● Do not take vitamin C supplements.
● Exercise regularly.
● Take your medications if you have high blood pressure or high cholesterol.

**Low-purine protein** Since they are low in purine, eggs are an ideal source of protein for gout sufferers. Here, with leeks and potatoes they make the filling for a filo-topped pie.

# Jargon buster

**Purine** This is a product of protein breakdown that causes a high level of uric acid in the blood. Foods that are high in purine include crab, herrings, anchovies, mackerel, sardines, roe, scallops, game, offal, stock cubes, and meat extracts. Vegetables high in purine include asparagus, cauliflower, spinach, and mushrooms.

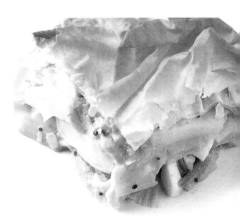

# Diabetes

## Nutrition plays a vital role in the treatment of this chronic illness.

Diabetes is a condition that affects how the body uses carbohydrates for energy (see p.46). It is diagnosed when a random venous plasma glucose concentration is greater than 11.1mmol per litre or a fasting plasma glucose concentration is greater than 7.0mmol per litre.

### Role of insulin
The body's main source of energy comes from carbohydrates, which are turned into glucose in the body. For glucose in the bloodstream to be able to enter into body cells, the hormone insulin, produced by the pancreas, is required.

Sometimes, the body cannot make enough insulin or use the insulin it does make effectively – this is known as insulin resistance –

which causes blood glucose levels to rise. The reasons why insulin resistance develops are becoming more defined. It is now known that genetics, diet, and level of physical activity are all involved.

Insufficient insulin action and the resulting high blood-glucose levels can lead to diabetes. Most of the treatments for diabetes are aimed at restoring and maintaining normal blood-glucose levels.

### How common is diabetes?
One of the most common chronic diseases, diabetes affects 1.4 million people in the UK, which is about three in every 100 people. And it is estimated that one million more have diabetes but don't yet know it.

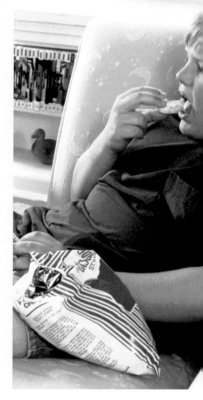

**Control your child's eating** Children who snack on fatty foods such as crisps and have a low level of activity are at risk of becoming overweight and developing diabetes.

## Who is most at risk of diabetes?

By identifying the risk factors for diabetes you can detect it early, and prevent or delay the complications of the disease.
**General risk factors** Whatever your age, if you have any of the risk factors below, ask your GP to measure the levels of glucose in your blood.
• A family history of diabetes. If anyone in your family has type 2 diabetes, you should exercise regularly and maintain a healthy weight in order to minimize your risk of developing the condition.
• A body mass index (BMI) above 25 (see pp.26–27). Overweight people often suffer from insulin resistance, which is associated with type 2 diabetes because the accumulated fat cells interfere with the action of insulin.
• You are a member of a high-risk ethnic group (right).
• You have been diagnosed with gestational diabetes during pregnancy.

• You have high blood pressure.
• You have HDL-cholesterol levels less than 1.0mmol per litre (men) or 1.4mmol per litre (women), and/or a triglyceride level greater than 2.0mmol per litre. This could indicate metabolic syndrome (see p.214), and the risk of type 2 diabetes and cardiovascular disease is high.
• You had borderline elevated glucose levels on previous testing (pre-diabetes).
• You are a woman with polycystic ovary syndrome.
**Age** The risk of diabetes increases with age, and those over the age of 65 have the highest rates. If you have a family history of diabetes, at age 45 you should talk to your GP about having your blood tested for glucose levels – even if the results are normal, the test should be repeated every three years. Children should be screened if:
• They have two or more of these risk

factors: family history of type 2 diabetes, from a high-risk ethnic group (below), signs of insulin resistance (such as grey-brown skin pigmentation round the neck).
• They are overweight with a BMI above the 85th percentile for their age and gender (see p.113).
**Gender** Women with polycystic ovary syndrome are at increased risk. The risk of gestational diabetes (see p.141) is more likely in overweight women and those with a family history of diabetes. Women with a history of delivering a baby weighing more than 4kg (9lb) at birth, or a history of miscarriages or stillbirths, are also at risk. If you are at risk, your GP will measure your blood-glucose levels during pregnancy.
**Ethnicity** In the UK, African-Caribbean and South Asian people are three to five times more likely to develop diabetes than Caucasians.

## Type 1 diabetes

This accounts for one-third of all diagnosed cases of diabetes, and is the form that is more likely to affect children and people under 30 years of age. Type 1 diabetes, also known as insulin-dependent diabetes, results from the insulin-producing cells of the pancreas being destroyed, thus causing insulin deficiency in the body. It can be treated with injections of synthetic insulin.

Without sufficient insulin, people with type 1 diabetes may develop weight loss, excessive thirst and hunger, frequent need to urinate, lack of energy, nausea, vomiting, and dehydration. If it is untreated or poorly controlled type 1 diabetes can also lead to ketoacidosis (*right*).

## Type 2 diabetes

The development of type 2 diabetes, or non-insulin-dependent diabetes, is strongly related to lifestyle factors. Increasing the amount of exercise you do; losing weight if necessary and maintaining a healthy weight; increasing your fibre intake; and cutting your fat intake (particularly saturated fats) have all been shown to delay or prevent the development of type 2 diabetes in susceptible people.

Type 2 diabetes accounts for the majority of all diagnosed cases of diabetes in the UK, and is the type that usually occurs in adults over the age of 40 who are often overweight (this is why it used to be called adult-onset diabetes). It is now also being diagnosed in overweight children.

People with type 2 diabetes do not need insulin injections because the pancreas continues to secrete insulin. Symptoms develop slowly and are not usually obvious. Some people may simply feel tired, but when blood-glucose levels are very high symptoms similar to those related to type 1 diabetes can develop. Eventually about 40 per cent of people who have type 2 diabetes will require insulin to maintain adequate control of their blood-glucose levels.

## Gestational diabetes

This type of diabetes occurs in some women during pregnancy due to an increase in hormones, some of which may have anti-insulin properties. Women who are diagnosed with elevated blood-sugar levels in pregnancy can usually control the problem with diet and exercise, although some may have to take insulin (*see p.141*).

## Jargon buster

**Ketoacidosis** When the body's tissues cannot take up glucose from the blood, fat is broken down for energy instead. The breakdown of fat produces chemicals called ketone bodies, or ketones. When these build up to high levels, a ketoacidosis occurs. The symptoms of ketoacidosis include abdominal pain, rapid deep respiration, fruity breath odour, weakness, fatigue, confusion, stupor, and shock. It can lead to severe dehydration, coma, or even death.

# Managing diabetes

Diabetes is a chronic disease requiring important changes to your lifestyle. These include diet, physical activity, managing the condition on a daily basis, and, for many people, medications.

## DEALING WITH YOUR CONDITION

Taking responsibility for your diabetes will improve your quality of life both in the short and long term. Achieving the best possible control of your blood sugar, cholesterol, and triglyceride levels and blood pressure can prevent or delay any complications while minimizing low-blood-sugar episodes and weight gain.

Many doctors encourage people with diabetes to manage their condition themselves, with the support of their family. Some diabetes specialists, in addition to giving medical care, provide nutrition and physical activity plans. Your specialist can also put you in contact with a state-registered dietitian who can help you with an individual nutrition management plan.

## MONITORING BLOOD SUGAR

People with diabetes can easily and quickly monitor blood-sugar levels with a simple finger stick or blood-glucose meter. By monitoring your blood-sugar levels daily, you can determine what effect your food choices and physical activity have on the levels. These results can help you modify your diet and make adjustments to help you achieve blood-sugar levels as close to normal as is possible. If you have type 1 or type 2 diabetes and are taking insulin, it is best to monitor your blood sugar three or four times a day. If you have type 2 diabetes and are taking oral medications, testing of glucose levels by urinalysis is done several times a week.

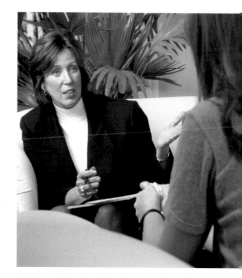

**Meeting with a dietitian** A state-registered dietitian (SRD) will help you manage your diabetes by suggesting menu plans for healthy and nutritious meals.

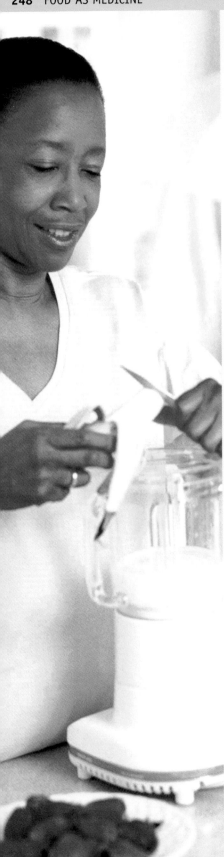

# Nutrition for diabetes

## Use food to maintain control of your blood-sugar levels, and lose weight if necessary.

If you have diabetes, the primary goal of medical nutrition therapy is to keep your blood-sugar levels in the normal range to prevent diabetes-related complications. Diet is therefore the cornerstone of treating your illness. You can manage blood-sugar levels, lower your blood pressure, and avoid hypoglycaemia just by watching what you eat, when you eat, and learning to manage your condition.

### Hyperglycaemia

This term means "high glucose in the blood" and is what all people with diabetes are trying to control. Severe hyperglycaemia can occur if you eat something very high in sugar, or if you have not produced enough insulin. The symptoms are similar to those you may have had before you were diagnosed with diabetes – fatigue, thirst, and excessive urination.

### Treating your condition

Research shows that treating your diabetes through a combination of dietary changes, weight control, and exercise – implemented and supervised by a state-registered dietitian – can have a dramatic effect, and in some cases remove the need for medications that lower high blood-sugar levels.

By managing your diabetes in this way you can effectively lower your levels of haemoglobin A1c. Testing for this type of haemoglobin shows your average blood-sugar levels over the last three months, and regular testing can help you track blood-sugar levels over time.

### Healthy eating

Having diabetes does not mean that you have to follow a strict nutritional regime, nor do you have to eat a carbohydrate-free or sugar-free diet (*see p.250*); it just means that what you eat must be healthy and well balanced.

### Weight control

Being overweight contributes to an increased risk of developing diabetes because the body cannot make enough insulin to keep the levels of blood sugar normal.

If you have a family history of type 2 diabetes and are overweight it is important to lose weight and maintain a healthy weight: even modest amounts of weight loss can improve insulin resistance and help correct high blood-sugar levels.

### Cardiovascular disease

If you have diabetes, you are at increased risk of developing cardiovascular disease (*see pp.214–215*). Reducing saturated fat is one of the most important changes you can make to reduce your risk. If you have high blood pressure, you should limit your total sodium intake (*see p.221*).

## Jargon buster

**Hypoglycaemia** This is when blood sugar levels drop dangerously low. It is caused by too high a dose of insulin, missed meals, or being more active than usual. Symptoms are similar to drunkenness – unsteady movement, slurred speech, nausea, sweating, dizziness, headache, or weakness. Any carbohydrate-rich food will raise blood-sugar levels, including glucose tablets, sugar, juice, regular cola, or a sports drink.

**Make a delicious fruit smoothie** Blend soft fruits, such as bananas and strawberries, with low-fat yogurt to make a healthy drink.

# What to eat

Knowing what you are eating will make it easier to control and maintain your blood-glucose levels. It is especially important for you to control your intake of carbohydrates if you have diabetes (*see p.250*). Eating a high-fibre diet can help lower your blood-glucose levels, reduce your insulin needs, and improve your blood-glucose control.

## MAINTAIN PROTEIN LEVELS

There is no evidence to suggest that your usual intake of protein (15–20 per cent of your total calories) should be changed if you have diabetes. Protein has a small effect on blood-sugar levels, so following a healthy diet should be sufficient for your needs. See page 45 for a list of healthy protein sources.

The long-term effects of diets high in protein and low in carbohydrate are unknown. Initially, blood-sugar levels may improve and you may lose weight, but it is not known whether long-term weight loss is maintained any better

# When to eat

It is important to recognize when you need to eat or drink in order to balance the effect of any medication or insulin on your blood-sugar levels. People with diabetes need to eat at regular intervals throughout the day to maintain blood-sugar levels and ensure they do not drop to a point that may cause hypoglycaemia.

with these diets than with other low-calorie diets. Since they are usually high in saturated fat, the long-term effect of such diets on LDL cholesterol is also an important concern (*see p.38*).

## LIMIT DIETARY FAT

It is important to limit your intake of saturated fats, trans fatty acids, and dietary cholesterol, especially if you have LDL levels greater than 3.0mmol per litre. Fats have a limited effect on blood-sugar levels, but you should cut your total fat intake to reduce calories,

If you only eat one large meal a day you run the risk of causing an imbalance in blood-glucose levels, as your body struggles to turn a large amount of food into energy quickly. It is better to eat regularly, with snacks in between your main meals, although watch that you do not overeat as a result.

especially if you have type 2 diabetes. For more information about fats and their role in your diet, see pages 38–43.

## EAT LOW-FAT DAIRY PRODUCTS

Dairy products are a mix of fat, protein, and carbohydrate, and they do not directly affect your blood-sugar levels. If you have diabetes, make sure that you always choose low- or reduced-fat versions. Also, do remember that your favourite ice cream or milkshake may be high in added sugar, so opt for a low-sugar version.

# Sample day's menu

We have developed a low-fat, low-calorie one-day menu to help guide your food selection and enable you to make better choices. Remember to eat three small meals every day. If you are taking insulin, try to eat at the same time each day, to keep sugar levels balanced. For breakfast, instead of porridge and banana, you could try low-sugar cereal with strawberries. If you would like a small glass of 100 per cent juice, skip the fruit. Snacks are more important if you are on insulin. If you have type 2 diabetes and are not on insulin, then you may not need two snacks every day.

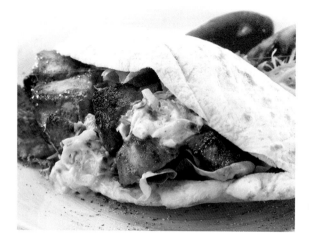

**Pitta pocket**
Grilled chicken breast and salad in pitta bread makes a tasty low-calorie lunch – perfect if you have diabetes. Make sure you use a low-fat dressing.

## DIABETES MEAL PLANNER

**Breakfast**
- ½ medium banana
- Bowl of porridge
- Glass of semi-skimmed milk

**Snack**
- Low-fat sugar-free yogurt
- Unsalted mixed nuts

**Lunch**
- Pitta bread with grilled chicken, salad, and low-fat dressing
- Raw carrots with low-fat dip
- 1 medium apple

**Snack**
- Baked nacho chips
- Salsa

**Dinner**
- Baked salmon steak
- Steamed broccoli and courgettes and boiled or steamed brown rice
- Small pancake with blueberries

# Maintaining carbohydrate levels

It is important to remember that foods containing complex carbohydrates are an important component of a healthy diet and should be included in your daily meal planning, even if you have diabetes. Carbohydrates provide your

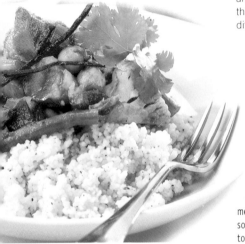

body with fuel and also help to prevent sharp increases or decreases in blood-sugar levels, which is very important for people with diabetes.

There is a great deal of discussion around rating all carbohydrates into low and high categories (see p.47). It is true that different carbohydrates do cause different responses in blood-sugar levels – there is some evidence that low-glycaemic-index (GI) diets have a greater long-term benefit than high-GI diets. For diabetics, the glycaemic index is best used for fine-tuning post-meal responses after first focusing on your total carbohydrate intake (see p.47).

**Vegetables and chickpeas with couscous** This colourful and satisfying meal is low in fat, high in fibre, and a good source of slow-release complex carbohydrate to help keep blood-sugar levels in balance.

## BLOOD SUGAR LEVELS

For those who have type 1 diabetes, the amount of carbohydrate to eat is the key component that affects your blood-sugar levels and the amount of insulin you need to control them. If you are receiving fixed insulin regimens rather than adjusting pre-meal doses, you should keep the amount of carbohydrate at meals consistent.

People with diabetes need to focus on eating low-glycaemic-index carbohydrates, which take longer to break down in the body, thereby reducing the risk of high blood-sugar levels. These include oats, pasta, pulses, apples, tomatoes, and yogurt. By making sound food choices, you will find it easier to control your blood-sugar levels.

You will soon learn the quantity of carbohydrate you can or cannot eat and how to control your insulin requirements. For more information, consult your GP or specialist, a specialized diabetic nurse, or a state-registered dietitian.

# Eating your favourite foods

The first thing that people with diabetes ask is "Can I still eat my favourite foods?" The answer is yes. No foods are banned; just try every day to reach a balance.

## YOU CAN EAT SUGAR

If you have diabetes, it does not mean you have to cut sugar out of your diet completely, but you should limit your intake as much as possible. Sugary foods can cause your blood-sugar levels to rise steeply, especially if you eat them on an empty stomach. If you do want something sweet, have it as part of a meal. If you do choose to eat a food containing sugar, you need to adjust the total amount of carbohydrate you eat accordingly, because both contribute to raised blood sugar (hyperglycaemia).

## ADAPT YOUR FAVOURITE MEALS

You do not need to forget your favourite meals if you have diabetes, you just need to learn how to adapt them. Opt for low- or reduced-fat dairy products, choose

lean cuts of meat or skinless poultry, and grill, steam, poach, or bake food rather than frying or roasting. Also, reduce the sugar content when baking. Use calorie-free sweeteners to cook with as well as sweeten food after cooking.

When eating out, ask what is in a dish, and have any sauces served separately. Most airlines offer a meal option for those with diabetes – check before you travel.

## Calorie-free sweeteners

These compounds have the unique property of providing an intensely sweet flavour in minute amounts. Although some do have an energy value, their calorific content is negligible as they are used in such small quantities. Intense sweeteners are classified as food additives; their use is controlled by the Sweeteners in Food Regulations, which specify the types of food in which they can

## ALCOHOL AND DIABETES

You should always avoid drinking alcohol on an empty stomach since it can cause blood-sugar levels to rise dramatically. If you have type 1 diabetes and choose to drink, always have a snack or a meal with alcohol, and drink sensibly – limit your consumption to three to four units of alcohol per day for men and two to three units per day for women.

be used and the maximum amount that can be used. Acesulfame-K, aspartame, sucralose, and saccharin are the most widely used sweeteners (see p.280). They are added to many processed foods and are available for use at home in tablet, liquid, and sprinkle forms. Most "sugar-free" products contain artificial sweeteners and they can be a valuable asset if you are trying to lose weight.

# Exercise is important

Physical activity has many benefits for people with diabetes. Studies continue to show that exercise lowers after-meal glucose levels by increasing the body's uptake of insulin and helping improve insulin sensitivity. In addition, exercise reduces your risk of cardiovascular disease, for example by reducing high blood pressure. It also helps control weight, increases energy levels, and generally brings about a healthier outlook on life.

Remember that exercise can lower blood-sugar levels, as your muscles use up the glucose in your body for energy.

## DELAY THE ONSET OF DIABETES

For people who have an increased risk of diabetes, regular physical activity has been shown to prevent or delay the onset of the disease. If you are overweight, have a family history of diabetes, have metabolic syndrome, or have any other risk factors, it is time to be more active. Prevention is the key.

## MAKE AN EXERCISE PLAN

Your exercise plan will depend on your age, general health, and level of fitness, so check with your GP before starting. Make sure that you start off gently and do not overexert yourself. Try walking, swimming, and cycling, which can all be carried out at a pace that you find comfortable, and increased as your level of fitness improves.

Wear a visible diabetes ID, carry some carbohydrate with you, and exercise with a friend who knows that you have diabetes in case your blood sugar drops and you become hypoglycaemic.

## ENERGY-BOOSTING SNACKS

You need enough carbohydrate in your system to sustain you during exercise. Good energy-boosting snacks include:
- Low-fat, sugar-free fruit yogurt
- Banana or apple
- Slice of wholemeal toast or a bagel with peanut butter or low-fat spread
- Rice crackers with hummus.

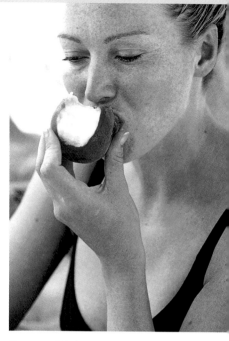

**Have a snack to boost your energy** It is important to regulate your blood-sugar level at all times, so make sure you have a snack before you start exercising to keep you going.

# Case study Sedentary computer engineer with type 2 diabetes

**Name** David

**Age** 45 years

**Problem** David visited his doctor because he has felt tired for the past six months. He is 1.72m (5ft 6in) tall and weighs 98kg (216lb) with a BMI of 33, making him clinically obese. He also has high blood pressure. From blood tests, David was diagnosed with type 2 diabetes. His 49-year-old brother also has this type of diabetes.

**Lifestyle** David is married with two children. He is an engineer and spends most of the day sitting at a computer. He occasionally plays tennis, takes no medication, and has smoked a pack of 20 cigarettes every day for 25 years.

For breakfast, David has a large bagel with cream cheese and orange juice. He has a doughnut and coffee mid-morning. Lunch is usually a meat or cheese sandwich with a packet of crisps and fruit juice. For dinner, he sometimes eats out with clients, or the family will get take-away Chinese or Indian food with large servings of fried rice or breads. David usually drinks two bottles of beer with his evening meal.

**Advice** David's goals are to achieve and maintain normal or near-normal levels of blood glucose and blood pressure to prevent or reduce the complications of diabetes and risk for cardiovascular disease. In order to achieve this, he has to cut down on calories, saturated fat, cholesterol, and salt. Giving up smoking is very important, and exercising more will also be beneficial.

David can take medication for his blood pressure and diabetes, but to help him change his dietary habits and lose weight, he should consult a state-registered dietitian who will be able to help him focus on foods that he can eat. Involving David's wife in these discussions would also be very helpful.

David should choose whole-grain and low-GI carbohydrates. Being made aware of low-calorie, low-fat, and low-salt alternatives to what David has been eating will also help him lose weight and reduce his blood pressure (see pp.220–221). For example, if he still wants Chinese for dinner, he can have a small portion of steamed rice and vegetables with prawns, scallops, or chicken breast, and an extra vegetable dish such as green beans with garlic sauce. Adding more fibre from whole grains, pulses, fruit, and vegetables is advisable.

David should also start an exercise programme during his lunch break and after work, which he could build up to walking for 30 minutes a day at least five days a week.

# Food allergies and intolerances

## Some foods cause adverse reactions in susceptible people.

Food allergies occur when your body reacts to a food by triggering an immune response. Common foods that cause allergies are nuts, eggs, and shellfish (*opposite*). Food intolerances, on the other hand, do not trigger an allergic reaction but cause a response from the digestive system. The best-known example of a food intolerance is lactose (milk sugar)

### Symptoms of an allergy

These range from a tingling in the mouth, eczema, hives, vomiting, abdominal cramps, and diarrhoea to swelling of the tongue and throat, breathing difficulties, and a drop in blood pressure. Symptoms typically appear within minutes to two hours after eating a suspect food.

intolerance (*see p.232*). Up to ten per cent of northern Europeans suffer from lactose intolerance.

### How reactions develop

The first time you eat a potentially allergenic food, you do not usually have symptoms, but your immune system mistakenly prepares to protect you against it. The next time you eat that food you release chemicals that cause symptoms such as eczema or life-threatening anaphylaxis (*see p.254*).

Food allergies usually begin in childhood and may be lifelong. However, some allergies, such as milk allergy, may be outgrown.

People with a food intolerance are not able to digest or process specific foods properly in the body, resulting in bloating, abdominal pain, wind, vomiting, or diarrhoea. The problem usually involves a defect or deficiency in an enzyme necessary to digest some foods. Unlike food allergies, intolerances are usually not dangerous.

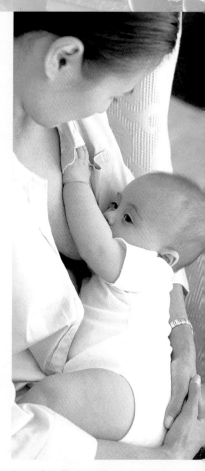

**Preventing allergy problems** Exclusively breast-feeding your baby for at least the first three months can help prevent allergies.

## When do food allergies develop?

Food allergies are common in people who are susceptible to eczema, hay fever (allergic rhinitis), or asthma.

### ALLERGY HISTORY

It is estimated that five to eight per cent of all children may develop a food allergy by the age of two years, although studies suggest that babies with a family history of allergies may be two to four times more likely to develop an allergy or intolerance.

Since infancy is an especially vulnerable time for food allergies to develop, allergy prevention efforts must be started immediately after birth to be effective. Compared to babies fed cow's

or soya milk formula, babies who are exclusively breast-fed for a prolonged period develop less eczema and wheezing in the first year of life.

### ASSESS YOUR CHILD'S RISK

If you answer yes to any of these questions and are pregnant or breast-feeding, talk to your doctor about allergy prevention.
● Do you have a history of allergies (such as a food allergy, allergic eczema, hay fever, asthma, or allergy to furry animals, pollens, dust mites, or mould)?
● Does your spouse have a history of allergies?
● Do your children have any allergies?

## Skin-prick test

In this test for allergy, a drop of a common allergen (a substance that can cause an allergic reaction) is placed on the skin, which is then punctured with a small needle. If the skin reacts to the allergen by producing a weal, or hive, the test result is positive. A positive result should be followed with a diet that eliminates the suspected food and followed later by a food challenge, in which the food is reintroduced to see if symptoms return. Food challenge tests must be medically supervised as they may trigger anaphylaxis (*see p.254*).

# Avoiding foods that trigger allergies

Just eight foods account for 90 per cent of all food allergies. They are eggs, milk, fish, shellfish, soya, gluten, peanuts, and tree nuts (eg walnuts or almonds). It is typically the protein component of a food that is responsible for the allergic response. However, even foods that we do not usually think of as containing protein, such as citrus fruits or potatoes, can actually contain enough protein to cause an allergic reaction.

## TAKE CARE WHEN EATING OUT

It is very important to watch out for trigger foods when eating out. Some types of cuisines frequently serve foods that include peanut protein or oil or may contain gluten or soya products. Ask your waiter to check the ingredients in the dish you are ordering. You must make it clear that if you eat a particular food that you are allergic to, it could have serious implications; it is not just that you do not like something.

When travelling, you should learn how to say the name of any trigger foods, or have the name written down in the language of the country you are visiting.

## HIDDEN INGREDIENTS

If you have a food allergy or a food intolerance it is critical that you learn the different names of the substances that contain the food that affects you and look for them on labels. Dairy products and eggs are often hidden in a wide range of foods, as is gluten, which can be a hidden ingredient in processed meats, cheeses, sauces, gravies, yogurt, and even frozen vegetables. If you are allergic to corn (maize), note that many processed foods contain corn syrup and many products that are labelled with dextrose or fructose or even some food colouring may be made from corn.

The table below outlines foods that commonly contain peanuts, eggs, milk, gluten, or soya as ingredients.

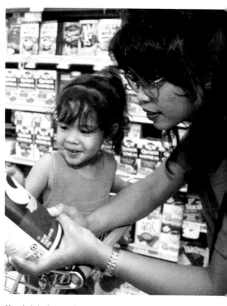

**Check labels carefully** If you or your child has a food allergy or intolerance, check food labels for hidden ingredients, and teach your child to be aware of ingredient labels too.

| FOOD | FOODS AND INGREDIENTS TO AVOID | WHERE FOODS MIGHT BE HIDDEN |
|---|---|---|
| **Peanuts and tree nuts** | • Peanuts are potentially life-threatening for anyone with an allergy to them. Avoid cold-pressured, expelled or extruded groundnut or peanut oil; peanut butter; peanut flavour; and nut butters<br>• Allergies to tree nuts, such as walnuts, pecans, and almonds, are not usually severe, but avoid all nuts | • Breakfast cereals and cereal bars; biscuits, cakes, and pastries; marzipan; nougat; sweets; ice cream<br>• Sauces and salad dressings<br>• African, Chinese, Mexican, Indonesian, Thai, and Vietnamese cuisine |
| **Eggs and egg protein** | • Albumin, ovalbumin, egg lecithin, mayonnaise, meringue or meringue powder, and surimi | • Pasta and noodles; soups<br>• Cakes, pastries, and biscuits; marzipan; nougat<br>• Flu vaccine may contain egg protein |
| **Milk and dairy** | • All forms and types of milk, including goat's milk; all butter products and artificial butter flavourings; buttermilk; casein; all cheeses and curds; whey; custard; yogurt; ghee; all forms and types of cream; sour milk solids; lactoalbumin and lactoalbumin phosphate; lactulose | • Breads, biscuits, cakes, and pastries; processed breakfast cereals; instant potato dishes; soups and sauces; salad dressings and dips; margarine; cooked sliced meats<br>• Mousses; custard-type, instant, and other desserts; protein shakes |
| **Gluten** | • Wheat, spelt, rye, oats, bran, and barley; bread and breadcrumbs; bulgur wheat; couscous; durum; all types of flour; pasta; semolina<br>• Wheat protein may be found in starch, hydrolyzed proteins, and natural and artificial flavourings | • Breads, muffins, cakes, and biscuits; cereals; sliced cooked meats; sausages; sauces; soups; noodles; tomato ketchup; soy sauce<br>• Pancakes; ice cream; chocolate; sweets |
| **Soya** | • Soy sauce; soya beans; soya oil; soya flour; tofu; tempeh; miso; textured vegetable protein (TVP)<br>• Hydrolyzed plant and vegetable proteins | • Baked items; canned tuna in soya oil; cereals; infant formulas; sauces; soups; butter substitutes; peanut butter; frozen pizzas; meat substitutes |

# Preventing food allergies in babies

A food allergy develops when a baby's immune system creates antibodies to a specific food the first time that the food is eaten. The next time the food is eaten, the baby or young child may experience symptoms of a food allergy. Some babies with a family history of allergy may be made allergic to certain food allergens when they are ingested in minute amounts in their mothers' breast milk. Babies at risk for allergy may also become allergic to cow's milk and soya proteins in infant formulas.

### BREAST-FEEDING AND NUTS

Experts recommend that mothers with a family history of food allergy should avoid eating nuts and any products containing nuts while breast-feeding. Apparently peanut protein is secreted into breast milk, which may sensitize a baby who is at risk for developing a food allergy. Page 253 tells you where nuts may be hidden and unexpected ingredients in foods.

### HYPOALLERGENIC FORMULAS

If your child is at high risk for allergies, talk to your GP or health visitor about using hypoallergenic infant formulas to supplement breast-feeding, if necessary, or if you are unable to breast-feed. This can help to reduce your baby's risk of developing a cow's milk allergy and allergic eczema.

### INTRODUCING SOLID FOODS

The introduction of solid foods to a food-allergic or allergy-prone baby should be delayed. Waiting until at least six months to introduce solid foods to a high-risk baby is critical, with dairy products

## Anaphylaxis

This is a severe allergic reaction. The symptoms of anaphylaxis include swelling of the tongue and throat, difficulty breathing, low blood pressure, and loss of consciousness. An injection of an adrenaline medication can reverse the symptoms, but left untreated the condition can result in death.

delayed until he or she is a year old, eggs until two, and peanuts, nuts, and fish until he or she is three years old. While this may seem to be overcautious, it is better to overstate the risk. If you are worried about introducing possibly allergenic foods to your child, it is a good idea to talk to your GP or health visitor or seek advice from a state-registered dietitian or qualified nutritionist.

# Treating food allergies and intolerances

For people with a true food allergy or food intolerance, even a tiny amount of a food that affects you can cause discomfort or, in the case of an allergy, potentially life-threatening anaphylaxis (*above*). Strict avoidance of the food is the only way to prevent symptoms, but avoiding some common foods that cause allergy or intolerance can be difficult, particularly if you often eat ready meals or eat out in restaurants.

### RECOGNIZING PROBLEM FOODS

Since you can be allergic or intolerant to a complete food or to ingredients added during preparation or cooking, it is often difficult to recognize the foods that affect you. Therefore, your own observation is important in helping identify these foods. Keeping a food diary of what you or your child eats every day and any reaction to particular foods is very helpful. Over a period of four to six weeks, you may be able to recognize foods that cause symptoms, such as eczema or abdominal pain. It is then time to start eliminating specific foods from the diet to find the food that is responsible for these symptoms.

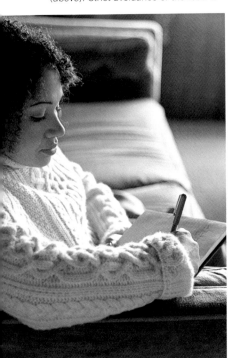

**Keeping a food diary** If you suspect that you have a food allergy or intolerance, keep a food diary to help you identify which foods may be the cause of your symptoms.

### ELIMINATION DIET

Many studies have shown that the best dietary restrictions should start with elimination of foods suspected of causing the allergy or intolerance. Under a doctor's care, try eliminating possibly offending foods to see if there is any improvement in your symptoms.

If you then do a "food challenge", in which suspected foods are reintroduced one at a time, and one or more foods lead to the return of symptoms, the diagnosis is confirmed and you know which food or foods to avoid.

For example, studies in children who are allergic to cow's milk protein have shown that the diagnostic procedure must begin with a diet that eliminates the suspected food component or with a diet containing a limited variety of foods for seven to 14 days or more. When the diagnosis is confirmed, the cow's milk is eliminated from the diet and substituted with a less harmful but nutritionally equivalent food. If more than one food is eliminated, you must make sure that important nutrients are not being left out and that you are getting a balanced diet (*see p.255*).

# Getting a balanced diet

If you have a food allergy or intolerance, and avoid a whole food group, such as milk and dairy products, you may be missing out on key nutrients. This is especially important for those needing extra calories, vitamins, and minerals, such as growing children, pregnant and breast-feeding women, and older adults.

## MILK ALLERGY OR INTOLERANCE

People who are allergic to dairy products or lactose-intolerant may fall short on the minerals calcium (see p.62) and phosphorus (see p.63).

Many foods contain calcium. Good substitute sources for those people who have to avoid milk and dairy products include calcium-enriched soya milk, tofu, calcium-fortified fruit juices, canned salmon eaten with the bones, and leafy greens such as broccoli and spinach. A good intake of vitamin D (from eggs and oily fish as well as from the skin being exposed to sunlight) will facilitate the body's uptake of calcium. Phosphorus is found in meat, poultry, fish, eggs, and whole-grain foods.

## WHEAT ALLERGY

People who avoid eating foods that contain wheat due to an allergy may not get sufficient B vitamins, especially $B_1$, $B_2$, niacin, and folate (see pp.53–56), as well as the minerals potassium (see p.63), magnesium (see p.63), iron (see p.66), and phosphorus (see p.63).

You can get additional folate from orange juice, fruits, leafy greens, and pulses. Meat, poultry, and fish are good sources of iron, niacin, potassium, and phosphorus. Magnesium is found in many fruits, as well as in pulses and leafy green vegetables. Again, taking a multivitamin supplement (see p.267) may help fill some nutritional gaps.

## CHECK FOOD LABELS

If you have a food allergy or intolerance, be sure to avoid the food that affects you by checking packets and labels and being extra careful when eating out in restaurants. You should also check labels to ensure that you are getting a balanced intake of the key nutrients, vitamins, and minerals.

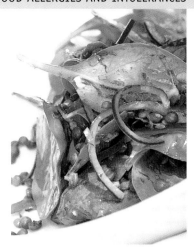

**Leafy greens** Spinach is a good source of nutrients that you may miss if you have to exclude milk or wheat from your diet.

## TALK TO A DIETITIAN

Anyone with multiple food allergies, or those who are allergic to difficult-to-avoid foods such as milk or wheat, may benefit from seeing a state-registered dietitian. He or she can analyze your diet to identify nutritional inadequacies and help you achieve a healthy plan.

# Case study  Active child with food allergies

**Name** Malik

**Age** 10 years

**Problem** At age two and a half, Malik developed eczema and a runny nose. After repeated episodes, his doctor suggested that his mum keep a food and symptom diary. This helped identify eggs and chocolate as potential triggers of his symptoms. A skin-prick test (see p.252) gave positive results for walnuts, chocolate, watermelon, and eggs, but negative for peanuts, soya, citrus, gluten, and dairy. Since then, an elimination diet has kept Malik free of symptoms. As he gets older he will be exposed to more situations where he is at risk. He wants to know what he can and cannot eat.

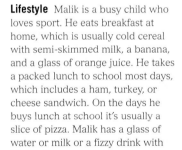

**Lifestyle** Malik is a busy child who loves sport. He eats breakfast at home, which is usually cold cereal with semi-skimmed milk, a banana, and a glass of orange juice. He takes a packed lunch to school most days, which includes a ham, turkey, or cheese sandwich. On the days he buys lunch at school it's usually a slice of pizza. Malik has a glass of water or milk or a fizzy drink with his lunch.

After school, Malik has either football or lacrosse practice for most of the year. He usually eats a snack before practice – some oatcakes with peanut butter or a piece of fruit and a sports drink.

For dinner, he eats whatever is prepared for the family, which may be pasta with tomato sauce, or steak or chicken with green vegetables.

**Advice** Malik has continued to show signs of a food allergy when he has been tested by the doctor and has therefore not yet outgrown it, which happens with many children. Being allergic to chocolate, eggs, and walnuts can be a challenge for a child, as well as his parents. Reading labels for these ingredients is the best bet for preventing exposure to the trigger foods. Home-made cakes and biscuits may also be a problem since they are likely to contain eggs. Now that Malik is more independent, he will need to make some decisions on his own. Because his symptoms are annoying but not dangerous, he can be allowed to make choices and may make some mistakes. He needs to learn to ask questions and to read food labels to avoid the foods that give him symptoms.

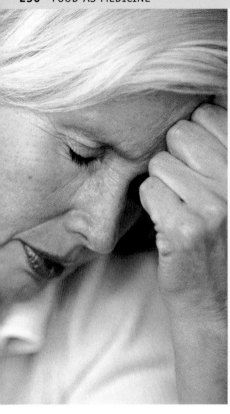

# Migraine headache

## Certain foods can trigger a migraine, while other foods may help prevent it.

Up to one in ten people regularly experience the misery of migraine. A migraine is a type of headache, but not all headaches are migraines; for example, a headache that occurs every day would not normally be described as a migraine. A migraine can occur as often as several times a week, or as seldom as once or

**One-sided pain** The symptoms of a migraine include a severe, throbbing headache that is usually felt on one side of the head, above one eye, or around one temple.

twice a year. The condition can be so debilitating that it completely wipes you out for several days at a time. People usually have their first migraine attack before age 30. Initial attacks rarely occur in those over 40, but they can occur in children as young as three.

### What are the symptoms?
The differences between migraine and other types of headaches are the characteristic symptoms. Up to half of people who suffer from migraines get a warning, known as an aura, that a migraine attack is coming on. The aura is a visual disturbance that occurs before the onset of the headache and can include flashing lights, zigzag lines, and blind spots. Other symptoms of a classic migraine aura include

## Preventing and treating migraines

There are several things you can do to reduce your risk of geting a migraine. Eating regularly, drinking plenty of water or other caffeine-free drinks, and eating magnesium-rich foods can be beneficial.

### EAT AT REGULAR INTERVALS
This is really important if you suffer from migraines or other types of headaches. Low blood sugar, caused by insufficient food, is a well-known trigger, especially when combined with fatigue and/or stress. Skipping meals, having fast-food snacks, and following drastic weight-loss diets can also cause attacks.

### DRINK PLENTY OF WATER
Dehydration is another trigger for headache and migraine. If you don't drink enough during the day, the body takes fluid from the blood and other body tissues. The blood vessels constrict in an effort to conserve body fluids, and this can cause a headache. Drink plenty of water to avoid dehydration, especially when you are exercising or drinking

alcohol – alcohol consumption is a major contributor to dehydration, so drink plenty of water after you drink alcohol.

### BOOST YOUR MAGNESIUM INTAKE
Eating foods rich in magnesium can help treat migraines. Magnesium deficiency may be due to reduced dietary intake, smoking, alcohol consumption, stress, or genetic problems, and can result in blood vessels in the brain constricting, which can cause a migraine. You should aim to boost your daily magnesium intake to the RDA (300mg for men and 270mg for women), to help increase the flow of blood to the brain.

Plant foods such as grains, pulses, and vegetables are rich in magnesium, whereas refined foods have a low content – processed grains, for example, lose up to 80 per cent of their magnesium.

**Add tofu to a vegetable stir-fry** Tofu is high in magnesium, which can help treat a migraine, so add it to your shopping list.

Boost your daily intake by eating bran and wheat cereals for breakfast and by substituting brown rice for white rice at dinner. All nuts and seeds are good sources of magnesium too. Magnesium-rich vegetables include broccoli, spinach, and Swiss chard. Taking a magnesium supplement may also be helpful.

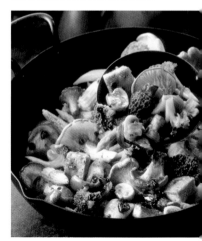

difficulty speaking, confusion, weakness of an arm or leg, or tingling of the face or hands. The symptoms of aura usually occur 10–30 minutes before the onset of the migraine headache.

Migraine headaches, both with or without an aura, are sometimes preceded by a group of symptoms, collectively known as prodrome. These symptoms tend to appear approximately one hour before the headache pain develops, and often include anxiety or mood changes, an altered sense of taste and smell, and either an excess of or a lack of energy.

Symptoms common to all types of migraines include a severe, throbbing headache that is made worse by movement, and usually felt on only one side of the head, over one eye, or around one temple; nausea or vomiting; or discomfort with bright light or loud noises.

Generally, if a headache and/or associated symptoms prevents you from continuing with normal activities, it could be a migraine.

## What causes a migraine?

There appear to be many general triggers of a migraine, including stress, hunger, and dehydration. Many women often experience an attack around the time of menstrual periods, which might be why the condition occurs more commonly in women. In addition, migraine attacks usually run in families.

Migraines are sometimes linked to intolerance to particular foods, including cheese, chocolate, and red wine. Therefore, you may be able to reduce or even eliminate migraine attacks by identifying your particular trigger food and avoiding it in future. Magnesium deficiency may also contribute to a migraine (*opposite below*).

## Trigger foods

Some foods, such as dairy products, hard cheeses, and alcohol, contain amines, which migraine sufferers can find hard to process in the body. The result is that these substances remain in the body longer, and when detected by the nervous system can cause the brain to dilate or the blood vessels in the brain to constrict.

Research suggests that when people who suffer from migraines eat foods containing substances that cause blood vessels in the brain to constrict, this reduces the blood flow to the brain and causes a migraine. People can also have reactions to other foods, such as monosodium glutamate (MSG), chocolate, citrus fruits, caffeine, and certain additives, so keep track of reactions you have.

# Case study  Busy solicitor's clerk suffering from migraines

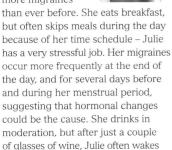

**Name**  Julie

**Age**  30 years

**Problem**  Julie is finding that she is suffering from more migraines than ever before. She eats breakfast, but often skips meals during the day because of her time schedule – Julie has a very stressful job. Her migraines occur more frequently at the end of the day, and for several days before and during her menstrual period, suggesting that hormonal changes could be the cause. She drinks in moderation, but after just a couple of glasses of wine, Julie often wakes up the next day with a severe migraine headache and nausea.

**Lifestyle**  Julie works as a solicitor's clerk and is responsible for running a busy office. She spends quite a lot

of time in front of her computer screen. She rarely takes a lunch hour and keeps herself going with coffee and sugary snacks. She works full-time and takes law classes two nights a week. She does not exercise regularly, although she has a free membership for a health club through work.

On Friday evenings, she unwinds with a couple of glasses of red wine, either at home or out with friends. Sometimes her whole weekend is ruined because of the migraine she suffers as a consequence. She often takes over-the-counter medication for her migraine headache.

**Advice**  Since Julie is complaining about more and more migraines at the end of the day, the easiest and most realistic change that she can accomplish now is to make time to eat lunch. Julie could either plan to take a frozen meal that can be

microwaved quickly in the office kitchen or prepare a sandwich at home. Leftovers from dinner the night before could also be used in her packed lunch. This would give her a break from staring at her computer screen, and would also help to reduce her stress levels. Rather than having coffee and sugary snacks, she could eat fresh fruit and a yogurt.

Although Julie does not drink excessive amounts of alcohol, she may not be drinking enough water with or after she has drunk alcohol. Alcohol can dehydrate the body and this can cause a headache. If drinking more water does not improve her condition, she may want to avoid red wine for a few weeks to see if her weekend migraines are reduced.

To further reduce her stress levels, she could try to exercise at least once a week, maybe after work on the days that she is not taking classes or even during her lunch break.

# Cancer

## The second leading cause of death, cancer is a major concern in the 21st century.

Cancer is a group of diseases characterized by the uncontrolled growth and spread of abnormal cells. Of the many different types of cancer, most form tumours in a specific part of the body, most commonly the skin, breast, lung, large intestine, or prostate gland. The disease may then spread within the body through the blood and lymphatic system (a system of glands that filters out infectious organisms from the body).

Because public knowledge and understanding of the disease has developed and increased over the last few decades, we have been able to implement lifestyle changes, effective screening programmes, and new types of therapies in order to improve the prevention and treatment of cancer.

### Different types of cancer
There are many different types of cancers, and the disease can affect organs (such as the colon, breast, or prostate) as well as tissues (such as the blood or bones). The most common types of cancer in the UK

are skin, lung, breast, prostate, and colorectal. About one in three people in the UK will develop cancer at some point in their life.

### Risk factors
Cancer risk is influenced by both external factors (tobacco smoke, chemicals, radiation, and infectious organisms) and internal factors (genes, mutations, hormones, and immune conditions). Exposure to the most common carcinogens (cancer-causing agents), such as tobacco smoke, ultraviolet light, and other types of radiation, should be avoided when possible.

Your physical state, what you eat, your age, whether you are obese or not, and hereditary factors all influence whether you are more or less likely to get cancer.

### Treating cancer
The treatment for cancer usually depends on the stage the disease has reached. Surgically removing tumours can be successful if the cancer has not yet spread to the lymph nodes or other sites in the body. For certain types of cancers, treatment with chemotherapy and radiation therapy may be used instead of, or in combination with, surgery. New therapies include inactivating damaged genes and boosting the immune system's

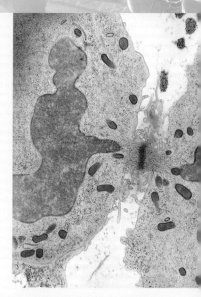

**Cancerous cells multiply very quickly**
In this magnified image, a cancerous cell is dividing to form two cells that contain damaged genetic material.

ability to destroy cancerous cells. However, the most effective way to lower the number of deaths is to prevent cancer from developing by screening to detect it early, eating healthily, and exercising regularly.

### Nutrition and cancer
We deal primarily with three types of cancer in this section – breast, prostate, and colorectal cancer – because nutritional and lifestyle changes can be effective in their prevention and treatment. If you are undergoing chemotherapy or radiation therapy, nutrition can play an essential role in helping you feel better, giving you energy and increasing your sense of well-being (see p.262).

Because some drugs used in chemotherapy can deplete vitamin and mineral levels in the body, your doctor may recommend a supplement. During treatment, however, you should not exceed the recommended daily amounts (RDAs) for vitamins and minerals. This is because high doses of certain micronutrients could interfere with the processing of some chemotherapy drugs.

## Obesity and cancer
Scientific evidence suggests that about one-third of cancer deaths in the UK each year are related to problems associated with poor nutrition and physical inactivity, particularly resulting from obesity.

Calculations from a long-term study of over 900,000 men and women in the United States suggest that deaths from cancer could be attributed to overweight and obesity in 14 per cent of men and 20 per cent

of women. In subjects with a BMI of at least 40, death rates from cancer increased by 52 per cent in men and 62 per cent in women. In both men and women increasing BMI was also associated with higher death rates from cancer of the oesophagus, colon, rectum, liver, gall bladder, pancreas, and kidney.

It is therefore very important that you maintain a healthy weight for your height to reduce your risk.

# Who is most at risk of cancer?

The risk of developing any type of cancer generally increases with age. Older people are more likely to develop the disease, largely because their cells have had more time to accumulate genetic damage, but also because their immune system is not as efficient at finding and destroying abnormal cells. It takes a long while for some tumours to grow large enough to be diagnosed.

## BREAST CANCER
This is the most common cancer in women – nearly one in three of all cancers in women occur in the breast. Most cases of breast cancer develop in women over 50. At age 30, a woman's risk of developing breast cancer is about one in 1900, but by age 50 her chances are one in 50, rising to one in 15 by the age of 70. Women who have a first-degree relative (mother, sister, or daughter) diagnosed with breast cancer are at increased risk of developing the disease, as are women who started their menstrual periods before the age of 12, overweight or obese women, and those who reach the menopause after 55.

Women who have their first pregnancy after the age of 35 and those who have never had a full-term pregnancy also seem to have a higher risk of breast cancer. In addition, evidence shows that long-term use of hormone replacement therapy (HRT) may increase a woman's risk of breast cancer.

## PROSTATE CANCER
The causes of prostate cancer are not well understood. Many studies have shown that certain factors may increase the risk of the disease. Age is the most important risk factor: prostate cancer is not usually found in men under 50, and half of all cases occur in men aged 75 and over. A family history of the disease also raises your risk. About 73 men out of every 1000 get prostate cancer at some point in their lives. So the average risk in the UK is about one in 11 men. This is lifetime risk – your risk at any single point in your life will be much lower than this; the older you are, the greater the risk.

## COLORECTAL CANCER
About 35,000 people are diagnosed with colorectal cancer (cancer in either the colon or rectum) each year in the UK. Excluding non-melanoma skin cancer, this makes colorectal cancer the second most common cancer affecting women and the third most common cancer in men. There appears to be a genetic component to the risk for developing colorectal cancer, but the relationship is complex. About 25 per cent of people with colorectal cancer have a family history of the cancer. It is rare in people under the age of 40, and usually occurs in people who are aged 60 and over.

# Ways to reduce your risk

If you have a family history of cancer, it is important that you adapt your lifestyle to decrease your risk of getting cancer.

## YOUR WEIGHT AND EXERCISE
Even a small weight gain can increase your risk, so maintain a stable weight right for your height. If you are currently overweight, exercise and reduce your caloric intake. Regular exercise is linked with a reduced risk of prostate, breast, and colorectal cancer.

## SMOKING
If you smoke, it is very important to give up. A recent study of 3000 smokers aged 40 and over showed that female smokers are twice as likely as male smokers to develop lung cancer. The risk of lung cancer also increases with age and how much you smoke.

## ALCOHOL
It is important to limit or avoid alcohol – many studies have shown that alcohol consumption increases the risk of some cancers, such as breast and colon cancer. People who drink alcohol should limit their daily intake to no more than three to four units for men and no more than two to three units for women.

## LIMIT FREE-RADICAL DAMAGE
Smoking, not washing fruits and vegetables (to remove harmful nitrates and fertilizers), and other environmental poisons can promote the production of free radicals in the body (see p.58). Free radicals can cause ageing, cancer, and cardiovascular disease, so adapt your lifestyle accordingly.

## BREAST-FEED YOUR BABY
Recent studies have found that for every year that a woman breast-feeds, her risk of breast cancer goes down by just over four per cent, on top of the seven per cent reduction for each child she has. This may be because breast-feeding triggers a hormonal change in a woman's body that can make her cells more resistant to becoming cancerous.

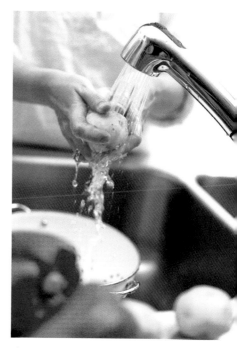

**Always wash fruit and vegetables** This will help reduce the risk of eating nitrates and fertilizers, which can promote free radicals.

# Nutritional guidelines for preventing cancer

By eating a healthy, balanced diet emphasizing fruits, vegetables, whole grains, and pulses, and maintaining a healthy weight, as many as one-third of all cancer deaths could be prevented. You should therefore try to include a least one of our "super" cancer-fighting foods in your diet each day (*below*). In addition, you should exercise regularly and limit your consumption of alcohol.

## FIVE A DAY

Vegetables and fruits contain many vitamins, minerals, fibre, and hundreds of beneficial phytochemicals (*see p.59*), some of which have been proved to prevent and fight cancer. For example, some phytochemicals protect DNA (the substance that makes up our genes) from damage and promote DNA repair, which helps explain how these foods reduce the risk. The World Cancer Research Fund has estimated that approximately 20 per cent of all cancers could be prevented by eating five or more servings of fruit and vegetables every day. So it is well worth increasing your intake if necessary.

## CUT DOWN ON FATTY FOODS

Diets high in saturated fats are also high in calories and contribute to obesity, which is associated with an increased risk of many cancers, so make sure you eat a low-fat diet. Limit the amount of red meat you eat, especially any that is high in fat, and opt for poultry breast, fish, and shellfish instead.

## EAT A HIGH FIBRE DIET

Fibre can help eliminate cancer-related toxins and, like antioxidants, helps the body eradicate free radicals. In addition to fruits and vegetables, eating plenty of whole grains will boost your intake of dietary fibre. Whole grains are also a good source of several of the B vitamins and compounds called lignans – which are also found in linseeds – that may have a protective role against breast, prostate, and colorectal cancers.

## LOSE WEIGHT

By losing excess weight, you can make a big difference in reducing your risk for developing cancer. An increase in body weight of as little as five per cent in pre-

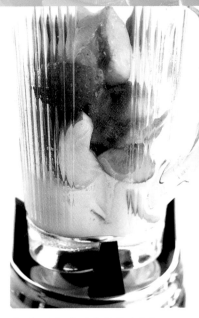

**Blend or juice fresh fruit** Fresh fruit contains essential vitamins, minerals, and phytochemcials that help prevent cancer.

menopausal women has been shown to significantly increase the risk of breast cancer after the menopause, so you should lose a little weight if necessary. Once you have reached your target weight, work hard to maintain it.

# "Super" cancer-fighting foods

No single food can protect you against cancer, but the right combination of foods can really help boost your immune system in the fight against cancer.

**Cruciferous vegetables** Broccoli, cabbage, cauliflower, and Brussels sprouts all contain substances that increase the antioxidant defences of cells to fight cancer, and switch on enzymes that detoxify carcinogens.

**Orange vegetables and fruits** Carrots, pumpkins, and mangoes all contain antioxidants in the carotenoid family, including beta-carotene, which helps cells defend themselves against the changes that can lead to cancer.

**Tomatoes** These are rich in lycopene, a potent antioxidant that may protect against prostate cancer. Lycopene levels are higher in cooked tomatoes.

**Pulses** These contain substances called saponins, which are thought to prevent cancer cells from multiplying.

**Berries** Strawberries and raspberries contain ellagic acid, a type of phenolic acid that reduces the damage to cells caused by smoke and air pollution.

**Whole grains** Wheat, rice, oats, and barley, and the foods made from them, are high in fibre and other nutrients, and can reduce your risk of cancer.

**Nuts and seeds** These are rich in essential fatty acids and phenolic acids, which can help combat prostate cancer. Brazil nuts are also an especially good source of the mineral selenium, which studies suggest can help protect against prostate cancer.

**Linseeds** Phytochemicals called lignans, which can help combat cancer,

are found in linseeds; this is possibly due to their high fibre content.

**Green and black tea** Both of these teas contain numerous active ingredients, including polyphenols, which may protect against stomach cancer, and flavonoids, which may protect against viral infections.

## Antioxidants

These chemicals are mainly found in fruits and vegetables and have been shown to reduce the amount of free radicals in the body. They can neutralize free radicals and help repair their damage to body cells. A combination of antioxidants is most beneficial as they all have different protective roles.

# Nutritional concerns and cancer

If you are suffering from cancer, there are likely to be times when you feel very weak, your energy levels are down, and you cannot face eating. This may be due to the cancer itself or the treatment you are receiving (*see p.262*).

## MALABSORPTION
This may happen if your body is unable to properly absorb nutrients in the normal way. Malabsorption can lead to weight loss because the body does not get the nutrients it requires. Many disorders can cause malabsorption, and it can be treated. The most common symptoms include diarrhoea, dehydration, fatigue, and weight loss. To avoid malnutrition, discuss your diet with your doctor or a state-registered dietitian.

## FEELING FULL
The feeling of being full after just a small amount of food is quite common. However, this will quickly lead to weight loss if you do not get enough calories to

sustain you. You must make sure you do not become malnourished, so try to eat little but often. Choose small snacks that are packed with vital nutrients, vitamins, and minerals to boost your calorie intake, give you energy, and prevent weight loss (*right*).

## LOSS OF APPETITE
As with feeling full after a small meal, loss of appetite is a common side effect among people with cancer. You may start to lose interest in food, or your appetite may decrease due to pain, nausea, or vomiting (*see p.262*), or because you are anxious or depressed about having cancer. Remember that for your body to be strong enough to fight against your condition you need energy. Even if you do not feel like eating, prepare something small that has an appetizing aroma to stimulate your appetite, such as home-made chicken noodle soup (*below*) or a high-protein snack (*see p.224 and right for ideas*).

## Snacks when you are ill with cancer

If you are receiving chemotherapy or radiation treatment, your energy levels may be low and foods may take on unpleasant tastes. For example, meats such as beef and pork may not appeal to you; substituting chicken or veal may be helpful because they have a milder flavour. The following high-protein, calorie-dense foods are good choices for meals or snacks to help you maintain your weight and keep your energy levels up:
- Cereal with fruit and whole milk
- Fruit yogurt with muesli
- Instant porridge with raisins
- Soup with a bread roll
- Cream cheese on an English muffin or crumpet
- Soft flour tortilla (wrap) filled with melted cheese
- Mixed nuts and crackers

# Recipe Nutrient-dense chicken noodle soup

### INGREDIENTS

**400g (14oz) chicken breast**

**1 small onion**

**1 stick celery**

**1 clove garlic**

**Handful of fresh, flat-leaf parsley**

**1 litre (1¾ pints) chicken stock**

**½ tsp dried thyme**

**85g (3oz) egg noodles**

### Serves 4

1 Remove the skin and bone from the chicken breast and cut into fine strips. Peel and finely dice the onion; dice the celery; and crush the garlic clove. Chop the parsley, reserving a few leaves for garnish.

2 Place the stock in a large saucepan and bring to the boil. Add the chicken breast, onion, celery, garlic, chopped parsley, and thyme.

3 Return the soup to the boil, then reduce the heat, cover, and simmer for 30 minutes, or until the chicken breast is tender.

4 Add the egg noodles to the soup. Bring back to the boil,

then reduce the heat, cover again, and simmer for a further 10 minutes, or until the noodles are cooked.

5 Season the soup to taste with freshly ground black pepper. Serve hot, topped with grated Parmesan cheese and

a garnish of a few leaves of flat-leaf parsley.

**Each serving provides**
Calories 200, Total fat 3.0g (Sat. 0.7g, Poly. 0.5g, Mono. 0.3g), Cholesterol 40mg, Protein 27g, Carbohydrate 16g, Fibre 1.0g, Sodium 600mg. Good source of – Vits: Fol; Mins: Ca, K, P, Se.

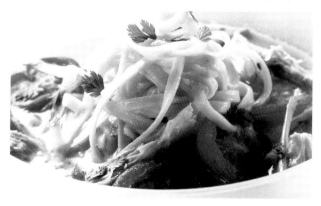

# Dealing with the effects of chemotherapy and radiation

Although you may not feel much like eating due to the side effects of your treatment, you can adapt your eating to ensure you still get important nutrients.

### SIDE EFFECTS OF TREATMENT
Chemotherapy drugs can damage both healthy and cancerous cells. The cells lining the entire gastrointestinal tract may be particularly affected, interfering with your ability to absorb food. You may experience changes in the way food tastes and smells or you may lose your appetite. The following are common side effects associated with these treatments.

### LOSS OF APPETITE
To improve your appetite, try to eat by the clock. Make breakfast and lunch your main meals, since you may find that you have more energy at these times. If possible, have someone help you prepare meals. Try to avoid having treatment on an empty stomach, which might aggravate symptoms such as nausea, vomiting, and diarrhoea. Eat small, frequent meals and choose high-calorie snacks, such as smoothies, milk shakes, supplement drinks, desserts, avocados, nuts, and sandwiches.

### NAUSEA
This is a common complaint among people undergoing cancer treatment. If you have nausea, try frequent small meals or snacks such as crackers and toast, and foods that are easy to digest, such as porridge, noodles, and boiled potatoes. Choose low-fat protein sources and avoid fried, greasy, and rich foods. Cold foods may be better tolerated, particularly if the smell of food makes you feel sick. Rest, sitting up, after eating, and sip apple juice or ginger or peppermint teas through the day.

### VOMITING
Do not eat or drink anything until you have stopped vomiting. When you feel better, try sipping small amounts of water, apple or cranberry juice, ginger ale, sports drinks, broths, and tea. Once these liquids are tolerated, move on to bland foods such as mashed potatoes, rice, and yogurt. Bananas, apricots, and juice can be added when you feel better.

### DIARRHOEA AND CONSTIPATION
When chemotherapy affects intestinal cells, it can cause diarrhoea. Tips for treating diarrhoea are on page 229.

Constipation can be caused by some anti-cancer drugs, pain relievers, and other medications. Tips for treating constipation are on page 229.

### CHEWING AND SWALLOWING
Mouth sores are a common side effect of chemotherapy. To make foods easier to chew, cut them into bite-sized pieces or mince them. Choose soft foods and add gravy, sauces, or butter to foods to make them easier to swallow. Avoid highly seasoned, spicy, tart, or acidic foods because they will aggravate the sores. In addition, you should add liquid nutritional supplements to your diet to ensure that it is balanced.

### KIDNEY AND BLADDER
Some anti-cancer drugs can irritate the bladder or cause temporary or permanent damage to the bladder or kidneys. To treat irritation, drink plenty of fluids, such as water and diluted fruit juice, and choose liquid or soft foods, such as broth, soup, soft fruits, and fruit sorbet, to assure good urine flow and help prevent infection. Cranberry juice, in particular, may reduce your chances of getting a bladder infection.

## Weight gain
This can result from medication given during cancer treatment, and is more common during the treatment of breast and prostate cancers. Weight gain may also result from overeating due to the stress of having cancer.

To avoid excessive weight gain, choose lean cuts of red meat, chicken and turkey breast, and fish; opt for low-fat dairy products; eat more vegetables and fruits; avoid high-fat, high-calorie snacks such as crisps, sweets, biscuits, and ice cream; and make sure you exercise regularly. See pages 156–209 for more hints and tips.

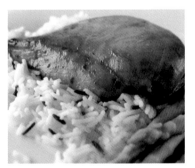

**Dealing with nausea or difficulty swallowing** A bowl of vegetable soup is easy to prepare and a good way to boost your nutrient intake if you do not feel like eating much.

**Loss of appetite** Quick and easy to make, this grilled chicken and rice dish can be big or small. This dish contains a good low-fat protein, and rice is easy to digest.

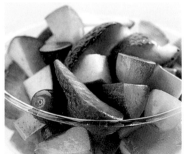

**Difficulty chewing** Cut food into small pieces, and choose soft fruit, such as berries. To make other fruits easier to eat, you can soften them by stewing or poaching.

# Diets and cancer

Some people feel the need to go on a radical diet when diagnosed with cancer. But the body needs nutrients, so a diet can be counter-productive.

## FAD DIETS

In the past, fad diets, such as eating only grapes or eating just raw food, totally eliminating dairy foods, and other radical approaches, have all been tried. In fact, eating raw food is not a good idea – people having radiation therapy are especially susceptible to infection and therefore may be advised to follow a germ-free (neutropenic) diet (below).

## MACROBIOTIC DIET

This vegetarian diet (see p.101) has long been promoted as an alternative cancer therapy, and has been proved to reduce rates of progression of prostate cancer and reduce the risk of colon cancer by 25 per cent. However, the diet lacks certain vitamins and minerals, and supplements are often required.

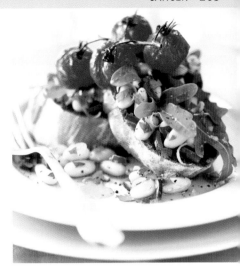

**Crostini with protein-rich cannellini beans**
If you follow a macrobiotic diet, which is vegetarian, make sure that you get enough protein – for example from pulses.

# Germ-free (neutropenic) diet

People who receive chemotherapy often have a suppressed immune system and are therefore more likely to develop infections. Such infections can be caused by bacteria found in foods. Do not keep perishable foods such as milk, yogurt, and sandwiches at room temperature for more than two hours. Hot food should be kept hot (above 74°C/165°F), and cold food must be kept cold (under 4°C/40°F). If necessary, buy a thermometer for your refrigerator, to keep a consistent temperature of 1–4°C (34–40°F). Proper food handling and food preparation are discussed in the next chapter (see pp.284–293). The table below shows high-risk foods that are likely to promote an infection and low-risk alternatives.

| FOOD GROUP | HIGH-RISK FOODS | LOW-RISK ALTERNATIVES |
|---|---|---|
| **Vegetables and fruits** | Raw fresh fruits and vegetables, including those from salad bars; unpasteurized fruit and vegetable juices; dried fruits; raw nuts | Well-washed and peeled fresh fruit; canned and frozen fruit (except berries); cooked, peeled or washed fresh vegetables; cooked frozen and canned vegetables |
| **Meat, poultry, and fish** | Raw or rare-cooked meat, poultry, or fish; processed meats and cooked meats from the deli counter, such as salami and ham; cold smoked salmon; raw or lightly cooked eggs | Well-cooked or canned meat, poultry, and fish; ready-packaged salami, ham, etc; canned tuna; well-cooked eggs (they should be boiled for ten minutes) |
| **Bread, rice, pasta, and potatoes** | Raw grain products; bought baked items such as breads, cakes, doughnuts, and muffins | Cooked pasta, rice, and grains; frozen breads, bagels, waffles, and bought biscuits; crisps, popcorn, pretzels, and snack crackers |
| **Dairy foods** | Unpasteurized or raw milk, cheese, yogurt, and other milk products; naturally-aged mouldy cheeses (such as Stilton, blue, and gorgonzola); soft cheeses (such as brie and camembert) | All pasteurized milk products (including yogurt); individually wrapped ice cream bars or frozen yogurt; vacuum-packed hard cheese |
| **Drinks** | Fresh apple juice; home-made lemonade; mineral or spring water; freshly ground coffee | Pasteurized apple juice; canned, bottled, and powdered drinks; tap water; instant coffee |
| **Miscellaneous** | Raw honey; herbal and non-traditional nutritional supplements; leftover food | Pasteurized honey, jam, and syrups; commercial liquid and powdered nutritional supplements; frozen ready meals |

# Vitamin and mineral deficiencies

## Make sure you get enough of the right vitamins and minerals.

A varied diet should provide you with all the vitamins and minerals you need and in their necessary amounts. The people most at risk of vitamin and mineral deficiencies are those who – for one reason or another – exclude certain foods or food groups from their diet.

For example, vegetarians and vegans may not get enough vitamin $B_{12}$, which occurs naturally only in foods of animal origin; and people who avoid milk and dairy products may miss out on sufficient amounts of calcium or phosphorus.

In addition, at different stages of life you may need extra vitamins; for example, extra folate is needed during pregnancy.

However, isolated vitamin and mineral deficiencies are rarely seen, and the symptoms listed below provide an indication that you may not be getting adequate amounts of many nutrients. The chart lists potential symptoms of deficiencies and indicates which particular nutrients may be deficient.

### Do I need a supplement?

If you have any of the symptoms in the chart, see your GP, who may suggest that you have a blood test. Only take a supplement on the advice of your doctor.

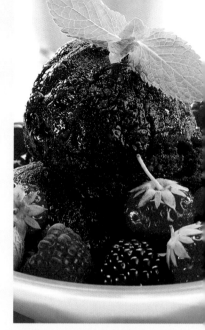

**Fruit sorbet with fresh berries** Packed with essential vitamins, fruits can be presented in a number of ways, such as this refreshing mixed fruit sorbet with fresh fruits.

## Increase vitamin and mineral intake through your diet

This chart lists common signs and symptoms of vitamin or mineral deficiencies, together with suggestions of which particular nutrients may be deficient in your diet. However, it is rare to see an isolated vitamin deficiency, and the symptoms listed here may indicate that you are lacking in many nutrients. People who do not eat a wide variety of different foods are most likely be at risk of deficiencies. See page 296 for a key to the abbreviations used for vitamins and minerals in the chart.

| BODY REGION | SIGNS AND SYMPTOMS | POSSIBLE VITAMIN / MINERAL DEFICIENCY |
|---|---|---|
| **General** | • Lack of energy | • Vitamins $B_1$, $B_6$, $B_{12}$, Fol, Nia |
| | • Weight loss | • Vitamins $B_1$, Nia |
| | • Poor appetite, or loss of appetite | • Vitamins $B_1$, Biotin, Fol, Nia / Minerals Fe, Mg, Zn |
| | • Fatigue | • Vitamins $B_6$, C, D / Mineral Fe |
| **Skin** | • Easily bruised skin | • Vitamins C, Vit K |
| | • Small red or purple spots on skin | • Vitamin C |
| | • Poor wound healing | • Vitamins A, C, E / Mineral Zn |
| | • Scaly, dry, flaky skin, eczema, or dermatitis; rash | • Vitamins A, $B_2$, $B_6$, $B_{12}$, Biotin, Fol, Nia / Mineral Zn |
| | • Pale skin (pallor) | • Vitamins A, $B_2$, $B_{12}$ / Mineral Fe |
| **Hair and fingernails** | • Hair loss | • Vitamins Biotin, D / Mineral Zn |
| | • Poor hair condition | • Vitamins $B_{12}$, Biotin |
| | • Dull or oily hair | • Vitamin $B_2$ |
| | • Spoon-shaped (concave), brittle, and split fingernails | • Vitamin $B_2$ / Mineral Fe |

| BODY REGION | SIGN AND SYMPTOMS | POSSIBLE VITAMIN / MINERAL DEFICIENCY |
|---|---|---|
| **Mouth** | • Dry, cracked lips; inflamed mouth | • Vitamins $B_2$, $B_6$, Fol, Nia |
| | • Cracking at angles of mouth | • Vitamins $B_2$, $B_6$, Fol, Nia / Mineral Fe |
| | • Sore or bleeding gums | • Vitamins $B_2$, C, Vit K |
| | • Sore and inflamed tongue | • Vitamins $B_2$, $B_6$, $B_{12}$, Fol, Nia |
| | • Dental cavities | • Mineral F |
| | • Delayed tooth eruption in babies | • Vitamins C, D |
| | • Poor tooth enamel formation | • Vitamin D / Minerals Ca, F, P |
| | • Peridontal disease | • Vitamin C |
| | • Decline in sense of taste | • Vitamin A / Mineral Zn |
| **Abdomen and gastrointestinal tract** | • Diarrhoea | • Vitamins $B_6$, $B_{12}$, Fol, Nia / Minerals Mg, Zn |
| | • Nausea and/or vomiting | • Mineral Mg |
| | • Abdominal pain | • Vitamin Nia |
| | • Blood in stool | • Mineral Fe |
| | • Poor motility of the intestine | • Minerals K, P |
| | • Constipation | • Mineral Mg |
| **Respiratory system** | • Frequent colds | • Vitamin C |
| | • Shortness of breath on exertion | • Vitamin C |
| **Eyes** | • Blurred vision; blood-shot, itchy, watery eyes; sensitivity to bright light | • Vitamin $B_2$ |
| | • Poor night vision; dry eyes | • Vitamin A |
| **Cardiovascular system** | • Rapid heart beat | • Vitamin $B_1$ / Mineral Mg |
| | • Irregular heart rhythm (arrhythmia) | • Minerals Ca, K, Mg |
| | • Electrocardiogram abnormalities | • Vitamin K |
| | • Congestive heart failure | • Vitamin $B_1$ |
| **Blood** | • Microcytic (small-cell) anaemia | • Mineral Fe |
| | • Macrocyctic (large-cell) anaemia | • Vitamins $B_6$, $B_{12}$, Fol |
| | • Prolonged blood-clotting time | • Vitamin K |
| | • Haemolytic anaemia in babies | • Vitamin E |
| | • Haemorrhage in babies | • Vitamin K |
| | • Heavy menstrual periods or blood loss | • Mineral Fe |
| **Bones, muscles, and joints** | • Aching or weak bones | • Vitamins C, D / Minerals Ca, P |
| | • Muscle cramps | • Vitamin $B_6$ / Minerals Ca, K, Mg, Na |
| | • Sore, tender, or aching muscles | • Vitamins $B_1$, $B_{12}$, Biotin |
| | • Joint pain | • Vitamins C, D / Mineral Ca |
| | • Muscle weakness | • Vitamins $B_6$, C, D / Minerals K, Mg, P, Se |
| | • Swollen legs (fluid retention) | • Vitamin $B_1$ |
| | • Growth retardation | • Vitamin D / Mineral Zn |
| | • Softening of bones | • Vitamin D / Minerals Ca, P |
| | • Abnormally curved spine | • Vitamin D / Mineral Ca |
| **Nervous system** | • Spasms and twitching | • Vitamin D / Minerals Ca, Mg |
| | • Headaches | • Vitamin Nia / Mineral Mg |
| | • Tingling hands and feet | • Vitamins $B_1$, $B_6$, $B_{12}$ / Mineral Ca |
| | • Irritability | • Vitamins $B_1$, $B_6$, $B_{12}$, Nia / Mineral Zn |
| | • Lack of concentration | • Vitamin Nia / Minerals Fe, Mg |
| | • Anxiety | • Vitamins $B_{12}$, Fol, Nia |
| | • Depression | • Vitamins $B_6$, Fol, Nia, C / Mineral Zn |
| | • Insomnia; sleeplessness | • Vitamins $B_6$, Nia |

# Dietary supplements

## Vitamin and mineral supplements can improve your health.

Evidence continues to grow that certain vitamin and mineral supplements can improve your health and possibly even prevent cardiovascular disease, cancer, and the bone disease osteoporosis.

According to recent surveys, one in three people in the UK take a dietary supplement. A survey by the Pharmaceutical Association of Great Britain found that in 2000, £305.3 million was spent on vitamin and mineral supplements. In this section, we review the most popular vitamin and mineral supplements and tell you who may benefit from taking them and any precautions to be noted.

**Supplements for health** In the last decade, public interest in the benefits of vitamin and mineral supplements has rocketed.

## Safety of supplements
The Department of Health (DOH), Food Standards Agency (FSA), and the EC all have to approve the safety and health claims made about dietary supplements by their manufacturer before they can be marketed. Unlike medications, which are rigorously tested and their manufacturing processes monitored, the DOH, FSA, and EC do not examine the purity of supplements or determine their medical effectiveness. However, they can prevent the sale of a supplement if they have proof that it is unsafe for consumption.

Manufacturers are allowed to make general health claims about their products as long as they do not contain reference to preventing or curing a specific disease.

## Safe intake
The Department of Health sets Dietary Reference Values (DRVs) for Food Energy and Nutrients in the UK. Within these guidelines it lists reference nutrient intakes (RNIs), which are more commonly known as recommended daily amounts (RDAs), for vitamins and minerals. RDAs vary from country to country. Those in the UK tend to be modest compared with other countries and with the RDAs for the EC. Where there is insufficient information on the physiological requirements for an RDA to be suggested, a safe intake (SI) is recommended instead.

## Buyer beware
Supplements may be in the form of capsules, tablets, gel caps, liquids, or powders. However, even though they may look like medicine, they are classified under the category of food, and it is important for companies to label their products accordingly. Unfortunately, this confusion gives rise to a situation in which the buyer is at risk of purchasing supplements that have absolutely no benefit or that may be harmful.

## Chelated minerals
Minerals in supplements are often bound – or chelated – to another substance in order to improve their absorption and use by the body. Chelated minerals are also better tolerated and may be less harmful to the body than pure forms.

Substances to which a mineral can be chelated include amino acids, gluconates, citrates, and picolinates. If you read the labels on supplements, you will see different forms of minerals. For example, zinc as zinc picolinate, magnesium as magnesium oxide, iron as ferrous fumarate, and calcium as calcium carbonate.

Manufacturers of supplements choose a certain form of a mineral, depending on digestive factors and how well the intestine tolerates it.

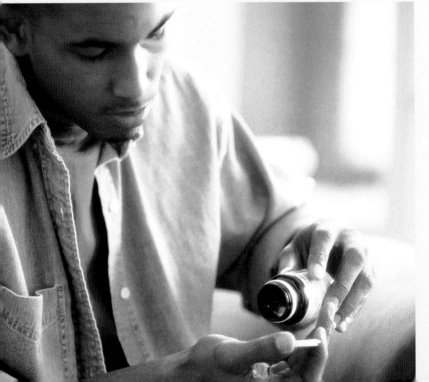

# Can you benefit from supplements?

A general multivitamin may provide some nutritional "insurance" against missing specific nutrients due to lack of variety in your diet or to make sure you get enough nutrients when you need extra, such as during pregnancy.

However, nutritionists are still trying to demonstrate a specific benefit for supplements with regard to prevention and treatment of chronic diseases. The use of vitamins and minerals in this way is different from correcting "classic" vitamin deficiencies, which fortunately are rare in the UK.

### NO PROVEN BENEFITS

The efficacy of vitamin E for treating and preventing cardiovascular disease has been studied for over 30 years, and tested in people with or at risk for the disease. However, it has not been shown to be effective, and recent trials have shown that it may even have a negative impact on cardiovascular health.

Chromium is needed by the body to process the hormone insulin and control levels of glucose in the blood, but supplements do not seem to help people with or at risk of developing diabetes. Beta-carotene is effective at blocking steps in cancer development when tested on cells in the laboratory, but when given to people at high risk of cancer it appears to have no effect.

### GET PROFESSIONAL ADVICE

People who want to supplement their diet with any form of nutrient should consult a properly qualified health-care professional such as a state-registered dietitian. He or she can provide advice on which supplements you should or should not take if you have a pre-existing disorder or are taking certain medications.

A general multivitamin and mineral supplement may be helpful as long as the contents are at the recommended daily amount (RDA) levels (*see p.35*). Data is lacking to support the benefits of taking isolated supplements of single nutrients or combinations, such as the antioxidant vitamins C and E, carotenes, and selenium. The charts on pages 268–271 show who would benefit from taking specific supplements. In fact, the body actually absorbs vitamins in food more easily than from supplements.

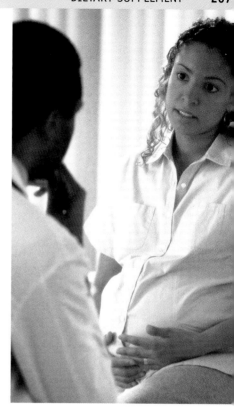

**Taking a supplement** You may need to take a vitamin or mineral supplement for various reasons, including pregnancy or illness.

---

# Can you take too much?

Harmful effects of vitamins and minerals usually result from taking too much, misusing supplements, or dosage errors. If you are taking large doses of vitamins or minerals, your doctor should be closely monitoring you. The fat-soluble vitamins – vitamins A, D, E, and K – are stored

## Jargon buster

### Upper safe level (USL)
This indicates the maximum safe amount of a nutrient to eat or take as a supplement without risk of side effects from poisoning. It is often divided into limits for long-term and short-term use. In the charts on the following pages, the upper safe level (USL) for long-term use is given for the supplements.

in the liver, and if they are taken in excess may build up to harmful levels more quickly compared to the water-soluble vitamins – the B vitamins and vitamin C (*see pp.268–271*).

If you do take a supplement, select a sensible one with the levels of nutrients recognized as safe and avoid going over the upper safe level (*left*).

### VITAMINS
Some vitamins can be harmful if taken in excess. Too much vitamin A can lead to headaches, blurred vision, cracked lips, and dry and rough skin. An excess of vitamin D can cause a poor appetite, nausea, and vomiting, plus deposits of calcium in body tissues. Large doses of the B-complex vitamins can produce symptoms ranging from itching, flushing, nausea, lightheadedness, and tingling

sensations in the fingers, to progressive loss of balance and sensation in the legs. Excessive doses of vitamin C can cause diarrhoea and have also been reported to predispose those people susceptible to oxalate kidney stones (*see p.237*). Symptoms usually disappear when the offending vitamin is withdrawn.

### MINERALS
In children, excessive intake of iron is dangerous and too much fluoride turns the teeth brown. People being treated for ulcers may develop milk–alkali syndrome, due to excessive intake of calcium from medication, causing muscle pain and weakness. Excessive intake of vitamin D can cause overabsorption of calcium, and excessive zinc may suppress the immune system and interfere with the absorption of copper.

# Vitamin and mineral supplements

This chart outlines who would benefit from taking a vitamin or mineral supplement and any relevant warnings. You are more likely to need a supplement if you are pregnant or breast-feeding; have had a recent severe injury or surgery; have a serious infection; are anaemic; if you drink alcohol and/or smoke; or eat a restrictive or unusual diet. In general, it is best to first consult your GP or a dietitian before taking supplements, especially if you are taking any medication.

The amount of a vitamin and mineral supplement that the body absorbs depends on its needs. For example, women and growing children have a greater need for calcium and iron than adult males and therefore absorb more. How much the body absorbs depends on the chemical form of the vitamin or mineral and the acidity or alkalinity where absorption occurs in the digestive tract. For example, the acidic environment of the stomach increases the solubility of calcium and iron in food, resulting in increased absorption. In contrast, people suffering from achlorhydria, who have a reduced production of acid in the stomach, or those who take antacid medication, may be at risk of poorer absorption of calcium and iron.

| SUPPLEMENT | WHO MIGHT BENEFIT FROM A SUPPLEMENT? | WARNINGS |
|---|---|---|
| **Vitamin A** (*see p.52*) USL for long-term use: 2300mcg per day | • People with skin problems such as acne and psoriasis <br> • Those with infections such as measles or peritonitis, which is inflammation of the membrane lining the abdominal cavity (taken together with antibiotics) <br> • People with osteoarthritis (*see p.241*) <br> • Those with poor night vision | • Avoid if you are taking any vitamin A-derived medications for skin problems, if you are taking oral contraceptives, or if you are pregnant. <br> • High doses can cause flaking, itching skin, blurred vision, and headache. <br> • Toxic levels can lead to enlarged spleen and liver and joint pain. |
| **Vitamin B$_1$** (*see p.53*) USL for long-term use: 100mg per day | • People with a weakened immune system <br> • Regular alcohol drinkers or smokers | • No known problems. |
| **Vitamin B$_2$** (*see p.53*) USL for long-term use: 200mg per day | • Vegetarians (*see pp.100–101*) <br> • Athletes (*see pp.146–149*) <br> • Those who suffer regularly from migraine headaches (*see pp.256–257*) <br> • People with skin problems such as acne, eczema, and ulcers <br> • Those with carpal tunnel syndrome (tingling and pain in hand and forearm) | • High doses may upset the stomach. |
| **Niacin** (*see p.53*) USL for long-term use: 150mg per day | • People with high blood cholesterol | • Niacin is prescribed at high doses for treating high blood-cholesterol levels. <br> • It is best to take niacin with meals to reduce the likelihood of stomach upset. <br> • Avoid if you have liver problems or a peptic ulcer. <br> • You should check first with your doctor before taking niacin if you have diabetes, gout, gall bladder disease, internal bleeding from weakened arteries, ulcers, low blood pressure, or the eye disorder glaucoma. <br> • Doses of 50mg per day can cause flushing, itching, headaches, cramps, and nausea. <br> • Very high doses taken over a long period of time can cause liver damage, high levels of glucose in the blood, and irregular heart rhythm (arrhythmia). |

| SUPPLEMENT | WHO MIGHT BENEFIT FROM A SUPPLEMENT? | WARNINGS |
|---|---|---|
| **Vitamin B$_6$** (*see p.54*) USL for long-term use: 100mg per day | • People who have a poor diet, such as heavy alcohol users, or older people, who may have difficulties absorbing vitamin B$_6$ from food <br> • Those sensitive to monosodium glutamate <br> • Women taking oral contraceptives <br> • People using the asthma medication theophylline or the tuberculosis medication isoniazide <br> • Those with high blood levels of homocysteine (*see p.219*) – taken with vitamins B$_{12}$ and folate | • More than 100mg per day can cause numbness and tingling in fingers and toes. <br> • Very high doses taken over a long period of time can cause liver damage and nerve damage. Fortunately, nerve damage is reversible, and diminishes when you discontinue the vitamin. <br> • Check first with your doctor if you have intestinal problems, liver disease, an overactive thyroid gland, or sickle-cell disease, or if you are recovering from illness, injury, or surgery. <br> • Supplements of this vitamin may lead to kidney stones. |
| **Vitamin B$_{12}$** (*see p.55*) USL for long-term use: 3000mcg per day | • Vegetarians and vegans (*see pp.100–101*) <br> • Those with problems absorbing it from food <br> • People with anaemia (*see p.55*) <br> • Those who have had portions of their intestines removed or bypassed <br> • Those with high blood levels of homocysteine (*see p.219*) – taken with vitamins B$_6$ and folate | • No known problems. |
| **Folate** (*see p.56*) USL for long-term use: 400mcg per day | • Pregnant women (*see pp.138–141*) <br> • Those with problems absorbing folate from food <br> • People with liver disease or on kidney dialysis (*see p.237*) <br> • Those with high blood levels of homocysteine (*see p.219*) – taken with vitamins B$_6$ and B$_{12}$ | • Can mask a vitamin B$_{12}$ deficiency. <br> • Consult your doctor if you have anaemia. <br> • High doses may cause bright yellow urine, fever, shortness of breath, rash, diarrhoea, nausea, loss of appetite, flatulence, and a swollen abdomen, and interfere with the effectiveness of medications for epilepsy. |
| **Vitamin C** (*see p.56*) USL for long-term use: 2000mg per day | • Regular drinkers or smokers <br> • People with severe burns, fractures, pneumonia, rheumatic fever (in which there is inflammation of the joints and a high body temperature), or tuberculosis <br> • Those preparing for surgery | • High doses may interfere with absorption of copper and selenium. <br> • Consult your doctor if you have kidney problems, kidney stones, gout, sickle-cell disease, or iron-storage disease. <br> • High doses can cause nausea and vomiting, flatulence, diarrhoea, abdominal cramps, and headache. |
| **Vitamin D** (*see p.57*) USL for long-term use: 10mcg per day | • Those who do not get enough sunlight <br> • People who cannot absorb fats from the intestine, such as those with cystic fibrosis <br> • Those with a family history of osteoporosis (*see p.241*) <br> • People over the age of 65, who make less vitamin D in their bodies when skin is exposed to sunlight | • Consult your doctor if you have epilepsy, cardiovascular disease, persistent diarrhoea, kidney, liver, or pancreas disease, intestinal problems, or the immune disorder sarcoidosis, or if you are planning to become pregnant. <br> • High doses can cause nausea and vomiting, diarrhoea or constipation, headache, extreme fatigue, lack of appetite, weight loss, frequent urination, irregular heart rhythm (arrhythmia), and weak bones and muscles. <br> • High doses taken over a long period of time can lead to kidney stones and irreversible hardening of tissues. <br> • In babies and children, too much vitamin D can lead to retarded growth, rounding of the skull, and learning difficulties. |

| SUPPLEMENT | WHO MIGHT BENEFIT FROM A SUPPLEMENT? | WARNINGS |
| --- | --- | --- |
| **Vitamin E** (*see p.58*) USL for long-term use: 800mg per day | • Pregnant women who smoke, as it can protect their babies from possible harm caused by the mothers' exposure to cigarette smoke <br>• People at risk of Alzheimer's disease | • High doses may cause dizziness, fatigue, headache, abdominal pain, diarrhoea, flu-like symptoms, nausea, and blurred vision; and decrease libido. <br>• Avoid for two weeks before and after surgery. <br>• Consult your doctor if you are taking blood-thinning (anticoagulant) medications or have anaemia, bleeding or problems with blood-clotting, cystic fibrosis, liver disease, or intestinal problems. <br>• High doses can interfere with the absorption of vitamin A and with niacin's ability to lower high levels of blood cholesterol. <br>• High doses may also increase the tendency to bleed and impair the function of white blood cells. |
| **Vitamin K** (*see p.58*) USL for long-term use: not established | • Babies, given as an injection at birth to prevent bleeding <br>• Women during and after the menopause, to decrease bone loss <br>• People with liver disease, jaundice, or problems absorbing nutrients, or with long-term use of aspirin or antibiotic medications | • Vitamin K reverses the effects of blood-thinning (anticoagulant) drugs (*see p.153*). <br>• High doses may cause allergic reactions and brain damage in babies. |
| **Calcium** (*see p.62*) USL for long-term use: 1500mg per day | • Pregnant (*see p.140*) and breast-feeding women (*see p.142*) <br>• People at risk of osteoporosis (*see p.241*) <br>• Those wanting to lose weight (*see p.62*) <br>• People with diabetes (*see pp.246–247*) | • Calcium supplements are available in various forms, so consult your doctor for advice. <br>• Do not take calcium and iron supplements together since calcium limits iron absorption. Calcium may also limit the absorption of the mineral zinc. <br>• Consult your doctor if you want to take more than 5000mg per day or if you suffer from sarcoidosis, kidney disease, long-term constipation, colitis, diarrhoea, stomach or intestinal bleeding, or heart problems. <br>• Calcium supplements may cause flatulence, constipation, headache, confusion, muscle or bone pain, and nausea and vomiting, and affect heart rhythm. <br>• Very high doses taken over a long period of time may lead to kidney stones. |
| **Fluoride** (*see p.65*) USL for long-term use: not established | • People who do not have fluoride added to their public drinking water (*see p.66*) <br>• Some breast-fed babies, who do not get enough fluoride in breast milk (*see p.109*) <br>• People with the bone disorder osteoporosis (*see p.241*) | • Various forms are available, so consult your doctor for advice on the best one for you. <br>• Do not swallow fluoridated tooth products. <br>• Children under the age of six should use only a pea-sized amount of fluoridated toothpaste and be supervised by an adult when brushing. <br>• 20–40mg per day can interfere with how the body uses calcium. <br>• 40–70mg per day can cause heartburn and pains in the extremities. |

| SUPPLEMENT | WHO MIGHT BENEFIT FROM A SUPPLEMENT? | WARNINGS |
|---|---|---|
| **Iron**<br>(*see p.66*)<br>USL for long-term use: 15mg per day | • People with a low dietary intake of iron, such as vegetarians and vegans<br>• Those with problems absorbing iron, with kidney disease, or who have lost a lot of blood, such as after an injury<br>• People with iron-deficiency anaemia<br>• Pregnant and breast-feeding women<br>• Women who have heavy menstrual periods | • Take only under the supervision of your doctor or a state-registered dietitian.<br>• Take vitamin C with iron supplements to aid absorption of the iron.<br>• People with haemochromatosis store too much iron and should avoid iron supplements.<br>• Prolonged high doses of iron supplements can cause bronzed skin, damage to the liver and pancreas, and diabetes. |
| **Magnesium**<br>(*see p.63*)<br>USL for long-term use: 300mg per day | • Athletes and those with muscle cramps<br>• Pregnant women at risk of premature labour<br>• People with high blood pressure or other cardiovascular diseases (*see pp.214–215*), or irregular heart rhythm (arrhythmia)<br>• Those with asthma or frequent migraines<br>• People with diabetes, to increase the production of the hormone insulin<br>• Those with chronic constipation<br>• People with excessive urinary loss of magnesium, very low blood levels of magnesium, long-term problems absorbing nutrients, severe diarrhoea, or long-term vomiting | • Check with your doctor before taking magnesium supplements.<br>• High doses may cause diarrhoea and nausea, muscle weakness, dizziness, lethargy, confusion, and difficulty breathing. |
| **Zinc**<br>(*see p.67*)<br>USL for long-term use: 15mg per day | • People with poor taste and smell<br>• Those with a weakened immune system<br>• People with a cold, influenza, or a sore throat | • Do not take with either calcium or iron supplements as these interfere with zinc absorption.<br>• Avoid if you have a peptic ulcer.<br>• Doses of over 15mg per day may weaken the immune system.<br>• Side effects include diarrhoea, heartburn, nausea, vomiting, and abdominal pain.<br>• High doses taken over a long period of time can lower levels of HDL cholesterol, which is protective, and cause copper deficiency, producing brittle nails.<br>• If you are taking antibiotics, take zinc supplements at least 2 hours afterwards. |
| **Multivitamin and mineral**<br>No more than manufacturer recommends | • Pregnant (*see p.142*) or breast-feeding women (*see p.142*)<br>• Those who are recovering from surgery or severe injury<br>• People who have infections, such as HIV<br>• Those who are anaemic or have a low red blood cell count (haemoglobin) (*see p.55*)<br>• Regular drinkers and smokers<br>• People who avoid entire food groups, such as dairy products if lactose-intolerant<br>• Those who are following a low-calorie diet or have irregular eating habits and skip meals<br>• Older people or anyone with a condition that affects their ability to absorb nutrients<br>• Women taking oral contraceptives | • Those taking other supplements listed above may get too much of some nutrients.<br>• Those taking anti-seizure or blood-thinning (anticoagulant) medications as listed above. |

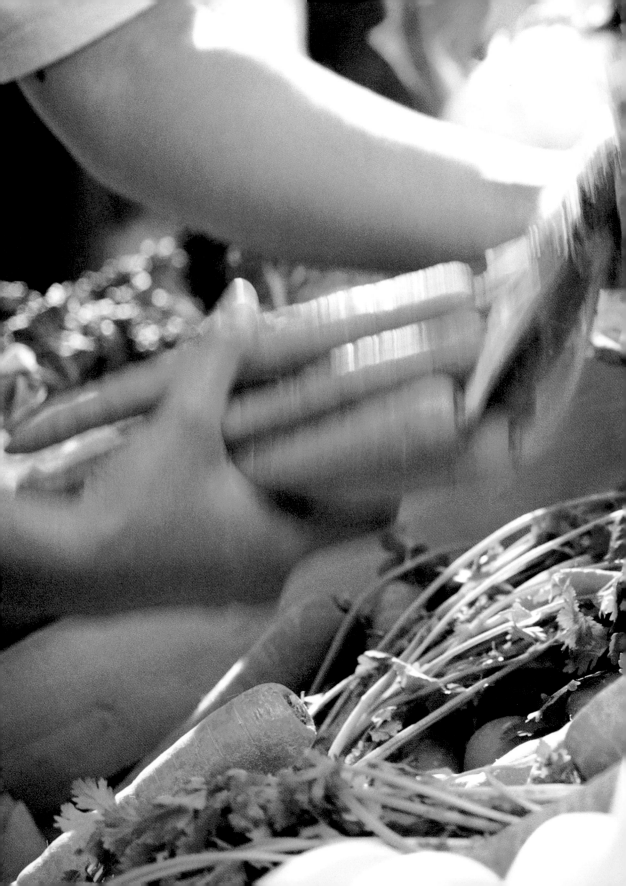

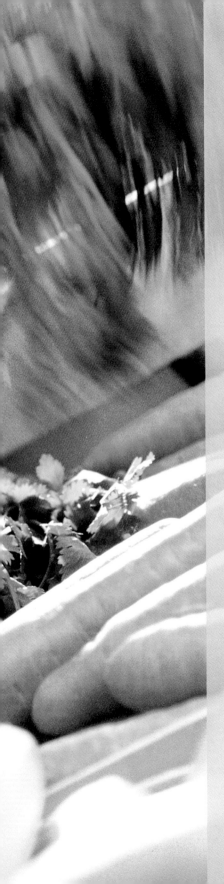

# The food you buy

In this chapter, we explain nutritional theories and provide practical advice on how to make the best and healthiest choices when you go food shopping, hints on comparing products, and tips on storing, preparing, and cooking the food when you get it home.

# Nutrition and modern food production

**Modern technology allows year-round availability of a vast array of foods.**

From fridges and freezers to cans, jars, and bottles that enable us to keep food on our shelves for weeks or longer, the British kitchen is now packed with appliances and products that have revolutionized

our way of eating. These products of modern technology save us a lot of time and energy, enabling us to assemble healthy meals whenever we want them, instead of having to make daily shopping trips for fresh produce. Food producers can now supply us year round with food of uniform size, shape, colour, and quality.

## Impact on nutrition

The mass availability of food, at affordable prices, is made possible only by highly sophisticated food-production methods, some of which are now being questioned because of their impact on nutrition and health. For example, public concern

**Mass food production** Supermarket shelves stacked with cans, jars, bottles, and frozen and chilled products, as well as fresh produce, offer a year-round choice of affordable foods.

## Is fresh food best?

There is no doubt that fresh food is best from a nutritional point of view: newly dug potatoes or freshly picked peas, taken straight from the garden to the kitchen, have more nutrients than either canned or frozen alternatives – not to mention being incomparably better in taste and texture. Not everyone has the luxury of growing and eating their own produce, however, and "fresh" produce on supermarket shelves may have been picked and kept in cold storage for a considerable time. Then, the distinction between "fresh" and canned or frozen becomes less clear-cut.

### FRESH, FROZEN, OR CANNED?

Here are some guidelines to help you decide on the most nutritious food choices for your family.
• When buying fruits and vegetables, choose locally grown produce whenever possible, as this is likely to be almost as fresh as home-grown varieties.
• In supermarkets, if no locally grown produce is available, buy fruits and

vegetables in season, as they are least likely to have been in lengthy storage.
• Frozen fruits and vegetables are as nutritious as fresh varieties, if they were frozen immediately after picking.
• When choosing pre-packaged foods, check the contents on the food label. It may include a long list of undesirable ingredients including additives, sugar, sodium, and oil (see pp.278–280).
• Choose fresh meat, preferably low-fat varieties such as poultry breast and lean beef, instead of processed meats such as sausages and burgers, which are likely to contain high levels of saturated fat, salt, and additives.
• Buy freshly baked wholemeal bread rather than sliced, packaged varieties, which often contain additives that give them a prolonged shelf life.

**Choosing fresh foods** While freshly picked fruits and vegetables are highest in nutritional content, remember that supermarket stock may have been in storage for several months.

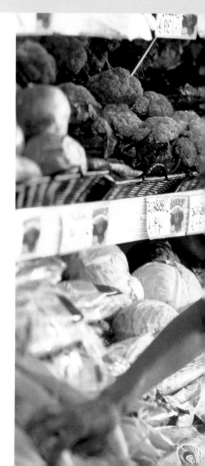

about the use of pesticides and herbicides, and the knowledge that meat and poultry can be infected with harmful bacteria, such as salmonella and *E. coli*, has led to a growing demand for organic foods produced by ecologically sensitive methods.

Some research has shown that organic crops contain significantly higher levels of nutrients than crops grown conventionally. However, it is worth bearing in mind that organic vegetables and fruits may spoil faster as they are not treated with preservatives. In addition, organic produce tends to cost considerably more than food produced by conventional means. This is because the production of organic foods necessitates more expensive farming practices, with tighter regulations and lower crop yields. However, as demand for organic foods increases, they should become less expensive, which will make them a more viable option for a greater number of consumers.

## Food and health claims

In addition to meeting the demand for an affordable variety of year-round products, the food industry now caters to a growing interest in nutrition and health, with consumer demand for foods that are lower in fat, salt, sugar, and cholesterol. More recently, products claiming additional health benefits, such as cholesterol-lowering margarines, have been launched.

In conclusion, while we may take for granted the convenience, abundance, and huge variety of affordable food that is available today, we must remain alert to the health implications of what we eat and strive to make the best choices from what is available.

## Genetically modified food

Modern developments in genetics have been applied to agricultural crops, which can be modifed by transferring specific inherited traits from one species to another. This technique, known as genetic modification (GM), has been used to increase crop yields and improve pest resistance. Other benefits may also be possible in the future, such as improving crops' nutritional value and disease resistance and allowing them to survive flood, drought, or frost.

There is considerable concern, however, that GM crops may pose threats to human health and to the environment, such as allergic responses to substances in foods, inadvertent toxicity to wildlife, and herbicide tolerance. Therefore, the debate continues.

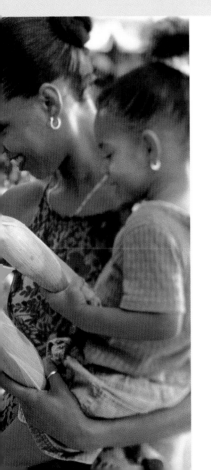

## Tips on choosing organic foods

Before a product can be marketed as organic, strict conditions set by European legislation must be fulfilled. Organic fruit, vegetables, and grains must be grown on land that has been farmed organically for at least two years, and only fertilizers and pesticides that are approved for organic production can be used. Organic meat, poultry, eggs, and dairy products must come from animals that are given veterinary drugs only to treat disease and not for growth promotion.

• Organic fruits and vegetables are not treated with preservatives; therefore, you should always choose the freshest produce available. Ask your greengrocer on which day new produce is delivered, so you can buy it the day it arrives. Choose locally grown produce whenever possible. Select fruits and vegetables with care, avoiding those with blemishes or insect holes.

• Read labels carefully: organic products are not necessarily "healthy" in every respect as they can be high in fat, sugar, or calories.
• Do not confuse foods labelled "natural" with organic products; only foods bearing the organic logo have met defined standards.
• It is not always possible to make products entirely from organic ingredients because all those needed may not be available in organic form. Therefore, manufacturers of organic foods are permitted to use specific non-organic ingredients provided that ingredients which are organic make up at least 95 per cent of the food. If the product contains 70–95 per cent organic ingredients, the organic description can only be mentioned in the ingredients list, and a clear statement must be given on the front label of the food packet showing the total percentage of ingredients that are organic.

# How food is preserved

## Various techniques are used to preserve the quality of food for long-term storage.

Since ancient times, food has been preserved by techniques such as curing, smoking, storing in salt or brine, and freezing: methods that ensure supplies will not run out when adverse conditions limit the availability of fresh products.

The commercial food producers of today use a variety of methods to prolong the life of their products, including canning, pasteurization, and irradiation, in addition to more traditional methods.

Preserving food not only helps maintain plenty of choices for the consumer throughout the year, but also saves time and energy, since fewer shopping trips are needed to stock up on the ingredients for daily meals.

### Preservation methods
Freezing, which is one of the most common methods of preserving food, protects the flavour, colour, moisture content, and nutritive value of food. Frozen vegetables, in particular, are often of excellent quality, since they are processed and packaged very quickly after harvesting, with the result that few of the nutrients are lost.

Canned foods are an excellent standby as they have a long shelf-life. Fruits, vegetables, soups, sauces, and basic meals are all available in this form, providing the basis for a quick meal at any time. All such products carry a food label listing ingredients and a detailed nutritional analysis of the contents (*opposite*).

To make milk and milk products safe for consumption, they usually undergo pasteurization, a process involving heating to a temperature high enough to eliminate bacteria. This process also extends the shelf-life of the product without affecting taste or nutritional value. A variety of other preservation methods are used with milk products, including evaporation, condensation, and UHT (*see p.82*).

One of the oldest forms of food preservation, smoking involves exposing foods such as fish, meat, or poultry to the smoke of burning aromatic woods. The process also imparts extra flavour to the food. Traditionally, fish and meats were salted before being smoked, giving a particularly strong taste.

### Good and bad additives
A quick look at the food label on commercially produced food products reveals lengthy lists of substances that are added to the basic food ingredients to prolong the shelf-life of the contents and improve its colour and taste. These substances are discussed on the following pages (*see pp.278–280*).

**Well-stocked shelves** Mass food production methods ensure a plentiful year-round supply of food, preserved by a variety of methods from canning to freezing.

## Food irradiation

A relatively recent addition to the range of preservation techniques, irradiation involves the use of electromagnetic waves to eradicate the microorganisms that cause food spoilage and deterioration. Scientists believe it to be a useful, controlled, and predictable process that does not change the important characteristics – appearance and texture – of most products. Foods that have been irradiated must be labelled as "irradiated" or "treated with ionising radiation".

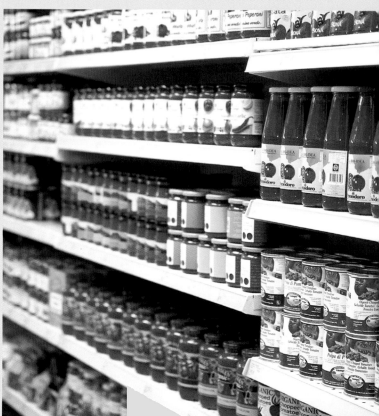

# What do food labels mean?

Food labels can tell us a lot about the nutrient content of food. At present nutrition labelling is voluntary, unless a manufacturer makes a claim about the product on the packet or in an advert, such as that it is low in fat or high in vitamin C. However, at least 75 per cent of all pre-packaged products provide some nutrition information on the label. And there are laws and guidelines that prevent manufacturers from making misleading claims about their products.

A European Directive has set a standard format for nutrition labelling, which is used in the UK. This makes it easy to compare similar products and to make a choice. When looking at labels, always compare the figures per 100g or 100ml rather than per portion or serving because portion sizes can vary.

Vitamins and minerals can be listed on the label if the product contains at least 15 per cent of the recommended daily amount (RDA) for that nutrient. The RDAs used on food labels are those set by the EC, which differ slightly from UK recommendations (*see pp.35 and 266*).

## INGREDIENTS LISTING

If there is more than one ingredient in a product, the label must list all of the ingredients, including all additives and preservatives, which are often identified by their E (European) numbers (*see pp.278–279*). The ingredients are listed in descending order according to weight.

If the list of ingredients includes hydrogenated or partially hydrogenated oil, then trans fatty acids (*see p.38*) will be present in the food.

## Date marks

The use-by date appears on labels of food that is highly perishable; do not eat the food after this date, even if it looks and smells fine. The best-before date, used on foods that can be kept longer, is the date up to which a food can be expected to be at its best, if it is properly stored. Dates such as "display until!" or "sell by" are for shops, not shoppers.

### ADDITIONAL INFORMATION

Food labels must also give the following:
- The name of the food or a description
- The weight of the food
- How long the food can be kept – the use-by or best-before date (*above*)
- How to store the food
- How to prepare and cook it.

**Typical or average values** This is important, since the nutritional information that follows is given per 100g or 100ml of the food (and sometimes also per average portion or serving), not for the entire contents of the container. These values can help you determine if the food is a good or poor source of certain nutrients.

**Energy** The amount of total energy provided by 100g or 100ml of the food is shown, both in kcals (kilocalories) and in kilojoules (kj). A kcal is equal to 4.2kj.

**Carbohydrate** The weight of carbohydrate provided by 100g or 100ml of the food is shown in grams. This may be followed by a similar analysis showing how much of the total carbohydrate content is from sugars. It will not distinguish between added sugar and naturally occurring sugars.

**Sodium** The total amount of sodium in 100g or 100ml of the product is listed in grams. A gram of sodium is equal to 2.5g of salt.

**Additional information** A label may show if the food is suitable for people with dietary restrictions or for those who have food allergies or intolerances.

### NUTRITION INFORMATION

| Typical values per | 100g | Portion |
|---|---|---|
| **Energy** | 1741kJ | 1219kJ |
|  | 414kcal | 290kcal |
| **Protein** | 3.5g | 2.5g |
| **Carbohydrate** | 65.8g | 46.1g |
| of which sugars | 49.1g | 14.4g |
| **Fat** | 15.2g | 10.6g |
| of which saturates | 3.6g | 2.5g |
| **Fibre** | 2.3g | 1.6g |
| **Sodium** | 0.1g | 0.1g |

Based on 8 portions per cake

**INGREDIENTS:**
Raisins, glacé cherries, wheatflour, egg, partially hydrogenated vegetable oil, pecan nuts, sugar, glucose syrup, honey, flavourings, emulsifiers (E471, E435), spices, salt, preservative (E202), gelling agent (E440), acidity regulator (E330), colours (E127, E133, E102, E129)

- **THIS PRODUCT CONTAINS NUTS**
- **SUITABLE FOR VEGETARIANS**

**Portion size and portions per container** Pay attention to this because it's common to eat more than one portion.

**Protein** The total amount of protein provided by 100g or 100ml of the food is shown in grams. The protein content is shown even if there is very little or none.

**Fat** The amount of fat provided by 100g or 100ml of the food is shown. This may be followed by a similar analysis showing how much of the total fat content is saturated, which is the type of fat known to raise blood cholesterol levels and be a risk factor for heart disease.

**Fibre** The total amount of fibre provided by 100g or 100ml of the food is shown in grams. A food is considered to be a source of fibre if it contains 3.0g or more; if it contains 6.0g or more it is considered to be a good source of fibre.

**Nutrition Information** This is found on the label of most pre-packaged foods. It includes information on calorie content and the amounts of various nutrients contained in the product.

# Why are additives needed?

Food additives are substances that are added to processed foods in order to improve their flavour, appearance, or texture, maintain freshness, increase shelf life, and enhance their nutritional value. Additives may be extracted from natural sources or synthesized in the laboratory to be chemically the same as the natural materials (known as "nature identical"), or they may be synthetic compounds that do not occur in nature. Within the EU, additives may be listed on food labels either by name or their E (European) number.

Food manufacturers use at least 3000 different additives, ranging from familiar substances such as sugar and salt to chemicals or preservatives such as citric acid. European legislation regulates the use of additives in various categories. For example, additives can include colouring agents to make foods look more attractive; sweeteners, natural and synthetic flavours, and flavour

enhancers to make foods taste better; and thickeners, emulsifiers, and stabilizers to give texture to foods.

Additives can also protect foods from adverse conditions, such as variations in temperature and damage during the distribution process. Preservatives slow the spoilage of foods and help protect consumers from food-borne illnesses. They also help retain a food's natural colour and freshness and keep oils and fats from turning rancid during storage and transportation. Acids, which help in the release of the gas carbon dioxide from yeast, may also have preservative effects in certain foods.

### FORTIFIED AND ENRICHED FOODS

Many common foods, such as breakfast cereals and breads, are also fortified with vitamins and minerals that might otherwise be lacking in the diet, or they are enriched with nutrients that were lost in the refining process (see p.50).

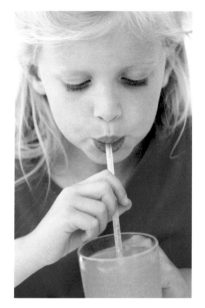

**Growing needs** Some brands of orange juice are fortified with calcium (see p.62), a mineral that is particularly important for growing children, to build strong bones.

## Case study  Young boy with a soya allergy

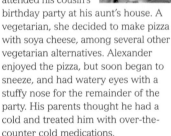

**Name** Alexander

**Age** Five years

**Problem** This past winter, Alexander attended his cousin's birthday party at his aunt's house. A vegetarian, she decided to make pizza with soya cheese, among several other vegetarian alternatives. Alexander enjoyed the pizza, but soon began to sneeze, and had watery eyes with a stuffy nose for the remainder of the party. His parents thought he had a cold and treated him with over-the-counter cold medications.

Now it is summer and Alexander still has symptoms of what seems to be a persistent cold. He has developed an itchy rash that prompted a visit to the doctor. Their GP discovered that soon after the birthday party Alexander's parents had decided to incorporate some of his aunt's healthy

eating ideas into their own diet. Since Alexander liked the pizza, they tried other soya products, such as soya nuggets and sausages, in addition to pizza made with soya cheese. The GP referred Alexander to an allergy specialist, who did a skin-prick test that came back positive only for soya. The test was negative for milk, eggs, chocolate, and peanuts, which are other common food allergens.

**Lifestyle** Alexander is a typical five-year-old with a lot of energy. He attends school five days a week, from 9am to 3.30pm. His mother prepares a packed lunch for him to take along, and he enjoys staying at school with his friends to eat his lunch. He eats breakfast and dinner at home, and usually has a snack when he gets home from school. His weekends are filled with playing in the garden with his sister, riding his bicycle, and going to the playground.

**Advice** Since Alexander is allergic to the proteins found in soya, his parents must make sure he does not consume it in any form. They will need to read labels for soya and other ingredients that may contain soya. These include hydrolyzed vegetable or plant protein, vegetable broth, gums, and starches. Soya lecithin, which is made from fatty substances in soya beans, can usually be eaten by people allergic to soya.

Alexander's parents should maintain their healthy eating, but without soya products. The nuggets can be prepared with chicken breast and then sautéed in a little olive or rapeseed oil. They can buy reduced-fat sausages and pizza with reduced-fat mozzarella. When they eat out, they must be careful of hidden sources of soya, such as salad dressings, mayonnaise, soya cheese, and certain sauces, such as soy and teriyaki sauces. They should include more grains, vegetables, and fruits as Alexander gets older.

# Understanding food additives

The following are some of the additives or groups of additives that have been approved by the European Union for inclusion in foods.

**Agar (E406)** Vegetable gum used as a stabilizer or thickener.

**Alginates (E400–404)** Seaweed product used as a thickener.

**Ammonium chloride** Chemical used to help yeast grow in bread.

**Annatto (E160b)** Used to colour yogurt, margarine, and smoked fish.

**Anti-caking agents** Used to absorb moisture and prevent caking or lumping in powdered products.

**Antioxidants (E300–321)** Protect food from oxidation or breakdown on exposure to air.

**Baking powder** Mix of bicarbonate of soda and an acid such as cream of tartar, used to raise cakes.

**Calcium chloride** Chemical that helps bread rise. It is also used to keep fruits and vegetables firm during cooking.

**Calcium propionate (E282)** Used to prevent mould from growing in cheese and baked items.

**Calcium sulphate (E516)** Used to boost calcium content in bread and keep tomato products and canned vegetables firm.

**Caramel (E150)** Colouring agent made from toasted sugar.

**Carob (locust bean) gum (E410)** Thickener used to improve texture and to blend ingredients together.

**Carrageenan (Irish moss, E407)** Seaweed product used in ice cream to stabilize the size of ice crystals.

**Cellulose (E460)** Plant additive used to improve texture and to retain moisture in sweets and jams.

**Citric acid (E330)** Chemical derived from citrus fruits that is used to maintain food colour, increase tartness, and prevent foods from becoming rancid.

**Dextrin** A starch, commonly used as a thickener in gravies, sauces, and baking mixes.

**Emulsifiers** Substances that help prevent the separation of ingredients that would not normally mix, such as oil and water. Used in salad dressings and mayonnaise where they prevent oil separating from vinegar.

**Guar gum (E412)** Plant substance used as a thickening agent in sauces, milk products, and baking mixes.

**Humectants** Help maintain moisture in foods by absorbing water from the air. They may be listed as glycerol, propylene glycol, and sorbitol.

**Hydrolyzed vegetable protein** Derived from soya beans, wheat, or corn and used as a flavour enhancer.

**Lecithin (E322)** Typically derived from eggs and soya beans and used to keep foods from separating. Also prevents loss of flavour and rancidity.

**Modified food starch (E1414)** Substance made from grains, potatoes, or tapioca that keeps ingredients from separating and prevents lumps in powdered foods.

**MSG (E612)** Monosodium glutamate (MSG) is used as a flavour enhancer in a variety of foods.

**Pectin (E440)** Fruit-derived additive used in jams and soft sweets as a thickener, to prevent separation of ingredients and give a gel-like texture.

**Phosphoric acid (E338)** Used to make food acidic and to give texture to soft drinks.

**Polysorbates** Blending agents used to keep oil and water from separating.

**Potassium sorbate (E202)** Used in cheese, margarine, and wine to stop microbes causing food spoilage.

**Raising agents** Products such as yeast and baking powder that cause cakes and batters to increase in volume during cooking.

**Sequestrants** Chemicals that prevent discoloration or rancidity in food.

**Silicon dioxide** Used to keep salt from clumping or foaming.

**Sodium aluminium phosphate** Used in cheese processing to help congealing. Also used to keep processed fruits and vegetables firm.

**Sodium benzoate (E211)** Prevents microbes spoiling processed foods.

**Sodium erythorbate (E316)** Keeps flavour and colour in cured meats.

**Sodium sulphate (E515)** Used as an acidity regulator.

**Sodium stearoyl-2-lactylate (E481)** Helps bread dough bake evenly and prevents spoilage. Prevents the separation of oil and water in salad dressings and non-dairy creamers.

**Sulphur dioxide (E220)** Used to prevent discoloration in dried fruits and inhibit bacterial growth in wine.

**Tartrazine (E102)** A coal-tar derivative used to colour foods.

**Xanthan gum (E415)** Used as a thickener, emulsifier, and stabilizer in dairy products, puddings and desserts, and dressings.

# Sugar and calorie-free sweeteners

In addition to adding sweetness, sugar's distinctive properties enable it to play an important role in food preservation. For example, sugar (otherwise known as sucrose) absorbs and retains water very easily and is therefore included in breads and muffins to help keep them moist and tender. Sugar also helps to prevent the growth of bacteria in jams and preserves, and to retain the bright colours of canned fruits when they are packed in a sugar solution. Sugar, however, is also a source of "empty calories" (*see p.129*) and, as such, contributes to a number of health risks, including overweight and tooth decay.

A diet rich in sugar can also blunt your appetite for more nutritious foods, such as those containing complex carbohydrates, vitamins, and minerals. Therefore, try to limit your intake of sugary foods.

## SWEETENERS

A variety of sweeteners – calorie-free sweeteners and sugar alcohols (polyols) – are used by food manufacturers in their products. These are many times sweeter than sugar and much less is needed, with a corresponding decrease in the calorie content. The following are among the most commonly used sweeteners.

**Acesulfame-K (E950)** This is 200 times sweeter than sugar, yet contains only four calories per teaspoon. It is safe and, since it is not absorbed by the body, is ideal for people with diabetes.

**Aspartame (E951)** This synthetic sugar is 200 times sweeter than sugar, yet contains less than four calories per teaspoon. It is not suitable for baking or cooking. A review in 2002 by the European Commission's Scientific Committee on Food (SCF) confirmed the safety of this sweetener for adults and children. However, aspartame is potentially life-threatening for people who have the inherited condition phenylketonuria (PKU), in which the body cannot process the amino acid phenylalanine. Products containing aspartame are marked with a warning.

**Saccharin (E954)** This was the first substitute sweetener and remains one of the most popular. It is 300 times sweeter than sugar and is suitable for baking and cooking. Studies confirm it is safe and poses no danger to humans.

**Sucralose** This is 600 times sweeter than regular sugar, and is the most versatile sweetener. It is available in granular form that can be used to replace sugar in drinks and recipes.

**Sorbitol (E420)** Used as a sweetener and to protect against moisture loss in food products, sorbitol is 60 per cent as sweet as sugar, with one-third fewer calories. It provides a cool, pleasant taste and withstands high temperatures.

**Mannitol (E421)** This sweetener is also used in food products as a stabilizer, bulking agent, and humectant. It is more than 70 per cent as sweet as sugar and has a cool, sweet taste.

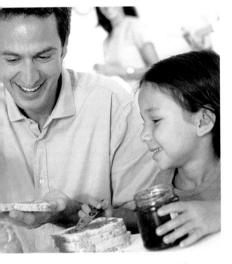

**Limit sugar intake** Children often like sweet things, but it is important to offer them reduced-sugar foods, such as low-sugar jam.

---

# Claims about fat

Increasing public awareness of the links between certain components of food, such as fat and sodium, and health have led manufacturers to market products with those concerns in mind. However, it is not always obvious what is meant by the various claims that are made.

The most confusing area of food labelling is with products that claim to be low- or reduced-fat. For example, a vegetable oil labelled "94 per cent saturated-fat-free" may be mistakenly perceived as 94 per cent fat-free and therefore much lower in calories than it actually is. If you take a second look at the nutritional information on the back of the bottle, you will see that 100 per cent of the calories come from fat.

# Understanding nutritional claims on food labels

Food labelling regulations produce standard definitions for nutritional claims on food labels. Many of these relate to fat content per serving size. However, claims are also made about sodium, fibre, and calorie content. Here are some definitions:

**Reduced fat** The product must contain at least 25 per cent less fat than a comparable product.

**Low fat** The product must contain less than 3.0g of fat per serving.

**Fat-free** The product must contain less than 0.15g of fat per serving.

**Low saturated fat** The product must contain less than 1.0g of saturated fat per serving.

**Reduced sodium** The product must contain 25 per cent less sodium than a standard equivalent.

**Low sodium** The product must contain less than 40mg of sodium per serving.

**High fibre** The product must contain at least 6.0g fibre per serving.

**Source of fibre** The product must contain at least 3.0g fibre per serving.

# Smart shopping

## Healthy eating starts with the choices you make when shopping.

With so much choice available, it is easier than ever to eat well. This section will help you to develop some strategies to cope with the temptations that assail you each time you walk through the door of the supermarket, and to maintain control over what you buy. We give you strategies for supermarket shopping, tips for what to choose from each food group, and advice on making healthier choices.

### Maintaining control
One of the best ways of ensuring that your kitchen is stocked only with healthy foods and that you are always in a position to prepare a nutritious meal or snack for yourself and your family is to plan all the week's menus in advance. Compile your shopping list on this basis. Then, when you get to the supermarket, you will be less likely to be tempted by clever marketing promotions to buy items that were not on your list and you did not intend to purchase.

### Making healthy choices
Shopping involves making choices – not just about which foods to buy, but between different brands and varieties. Health and nutrition should be the guiding factor in making choices – look at the list of ingredients, read the nutrition information, consider what you know about nutrition and health, and choose appropriately. In this section, we help you do this.

### Shopping on a budget
If you shop on a limited budget, it does not have to mean forfeiting nutritional quality, but it may mean adjusting your shopping habits.
- Compare prices and sizes to make the best value purchases.
- Don't buy ready meals and prepared vegetables: it is healthier and cheaper to do it yourself.
- Remember you do not need meat every day: there are cheaper sources of protein (see pp.84–85).
- Keep money-off coupons and use them when you go shopping.
- Take advantage of special offers.
- Choose fruits and vegetables in season, when they cost much less than they do out of season.

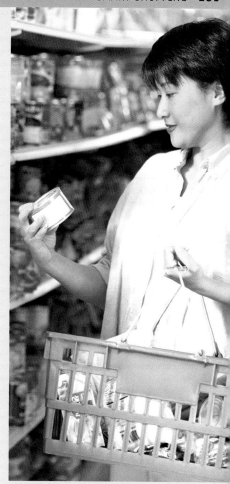

**Check your choices** Before putting anything in your basket, check that it has not passed its use-by or best before date, and that you are happy with its nutritional contents.

# Supermarket strategies

There are always tantalizing sights and smells and unmissable offers to distract you in supermarkets. Here are some strategies to help you achieve your goal.

**Plan your shopping** Advance meal-planning is an effective way to manage your eating habits. Before you go out shopping, make a list and stick to it.

**Eat before you go** Shop after a meal, when you are less likely to find yourself buying biscuits and pastries.

**Start with fresh fruits and vegetables** These are the most nutritious foods you can buy, supplying a variety of valuable nutrients, so load up on fruits and vegetables when you enter the shop.

**Shop the perimeter** Most supermarkets display fruits, vegetables, bread, dairy products, meat, poultry, and fish around their perimeter. Since you want to buy mainly from those groups, shop the perimeter first and then go down only those aisles that contain other items that are on your shopping list.

**Avoid impulse buys** Supermarkets are designed to take advantage of impulse buyers. To avoid these distractions, stick to your menu-based shopping list.

**Read food labels** When comparing products, take time to read food labels, since this will help you make informed decisions. Pay special attention to calories, and total and saturated fat content. Compare figures per 100g or 100ml rather than per serving or portion as serving sizes vary.

**Use a delivery service** Shopping on the Internet offers a great way of avoiding supermarket temptations, and such services are now widely available at low delivery charges. This is an ideal way to prevent unhealthy impulse buys.

# Making choices from the food groups

When shopping, aim for a wide variety of foods from all the major foods groups (*see pp.70–71*).

**Breads, rice, and pasta** Choose wholegrain or wholemeal varieties, which are naturally low in fat and high in dietary fibre, B vitamins, and minerals.

• Pasta is available in hundreds of forms. Although traditionally made from refined grain, wholemeal versions that boost fibre intake are your best choices.

• Brown rice is best as it has not had its nutritious bran coating removed.

• The healthiest breads are wholemeal, Granary, and fibre-enriched white.

**Vegetables** Buy firm, brightly coloured, blemish-free vegetables. Discard any damaged specimens – bruises and nicks attract mould, which can lead to spoilage of an entire bagful.

• Leaves or greens should be crisp and free of wilting.

• Buy only what you can use within a few days, since long storage times diminish nutrient levels and flavour.

• Some frozen vegetables such as sweetcorn, peas, and spinach, which are processed quickly after picking, offer more nutrients than their fresh counterparts that have been on the greengrocer's shelves too long.

• Canned vegetables are a very useful standby: look for those packed without added salt or sugar.

## Healthy treats

Totally avoiding junk foods can be counter-productive, leading to over-indulgence when the perceived deprivation becomes too great to bear. Instead, include a few "treats" in your weekly shopping, so you do not feel deprived. For example:

• Sorbet
• Angel cake
• Ginger nuts
• Wafer biscuits
• Cereal bars
• Baked tortilla chips
• Plain popcorn
• Pretzels
• Nuts (unsalted or dry-roasted)
• Frozen yogurt

**Fruits** For the best flavour and price, buy fruits in season. Some fruits, such as bananas and pears, should be bought before they are completely ripe, so that they do not spoil quickly.

• Choose fruits with a good colour and smooth skin, and avoid any that have blemishes or insect holes.

• Bear in mind that dried fruits are a concentrated source of dietary fibre, but higher in calories than fresh fruit.

**Dairy foods** Wherever possible, choose low- or reduced-fat dairy products.

• Compared to whole or full-fat milk at 3.9 per cent fat, skimmed milk contains 0.1–0.3 per cent fat and semi-skimmed milk 1.8 per cent fat

• Cheese is milk in concentrated form, so it has far more fat than milk, and the fat is highly saturated. So choose lower fat cheeses such as cottage cheese, fromage frais, and ricotta, or reduced-fat varieties of other cheeses.

• Full-fat yogurt contains three per cent fat, whereas low-fat yogurt has less than one per cent.

**Eggs** Available in many different sizes and types. Check use-by or best-before dates and always open the box to check for broken or cracked eggs.

**Poultry** Select poultry that looks moist and supple: the younger the bird, the more tender. Avoid poultry with signs of drying, discoloration, blemishes, or bruising. Check the packaging is intact.

• The leanest choice is white meat from the breast of chicken or turkey.

• Although skinless dark meat (legs and thighs) is also lean, it has almost twice the fat calories of breast.

**Fish and shellfish** You should always buy the freshest seafood possible: scales, skin, or shell should be moist, bright, and lustrous, with no dry spots or discoloration. Eyes should be bright, clear, and bulging, and the flesh should be firm and bounce back when lightly pressed. All seafood should have a clean smell.

• If you are buying fillets or steaks, they should not have brown edges.

• Frozen fish should be completely frozen rather than partially thawed, should be odourless, and should show no discoloration.

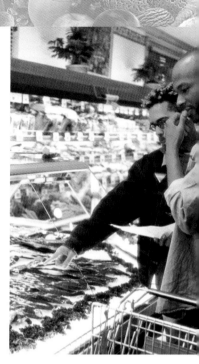

**Fresh fish** For the best nutritional value and flavour, buy the freshest fish possible, and cook it on the day you buy it. Look for fish with a fresh odour, firm flesh, and bright eyes.

**Meat** Choose well-trimmed lean cuts of meat and avoid those that are heavily marbled with fat.

• Look for meat that has a good healthy colour and that is fresh and moist.

• Check labels on minced meat for fat content and opt for the leanest. Or buy lean meat and mince it yourself in a food processor or mincer.

• When choosing meats from the deli counter, the best are turkey breast, lean ham, and roast beef. Processed meats such as salami, pastrami, and chorizo sausage are high in fat.

• On packaged meats, check the use-by or best-before date.

**Pulses** Look for dried beans, peas, and lentils of a bright colour and uniform size, clear of defects such as cracked seed coats, foreign matter, or pinholes made by insects. Buying in bulk is the cheapest option; however, to ensure freshness buy from a source with a rapid turnover. For convenience, you can use canned beans and lentils. Before using, drain and rinse them to reduce the salt content. This is also thought to minimize flatulence.

# Buying healthier alternatives

Shopping is often a routine activity, when purchases are made by habit rather than by considered choice. If you are serious about improving your health and well-being, then you must also change your approach to buying food. You are what you eat – and what you eat is what you buy – so your choices in the supermarket are vitally important for you and your family. To help you make better choices and save thousands of calories, check out the list below.

| FOOD TYPE | HIGH-CALORIE CHOICE | LOWER-CALORIE CHOICE |
|---|---|---|
| **Breads, rice, pasta, and grains** | • Sweetened breakfast cereal<br>• Ciabatta bread<br>• Chocolate or fruit muffin<br>• Croissant<br>• Chocolate or carrot cake<br>• Chocolate chip cookies<br>• Flapjack | • Whole-grain cereal, muesli, or porridge<br>• Wholemeal bread<br>• Plain muffin<br>• Bagel or baguette<br>• Angel cake with berries<br>• Fig bars or digestive biscuits<br>• Low-fat cereal bar |
| **Dairy foods** | • Channel Island milk<br>• Half cream<br>• Full-fat yogurt<br>• Full-fat cheese<br>• Soured cream<br>• Butter<br>• Double or whipping cream<br>• Cream cheese dip<br>• Creamy salad dressing | • Skimmed or semi-skimmed milk<br>• Whole (full-fat) milk or plain yogurt<br>• Low-fat, low-sugar or sugar-free yogurt<br>• Reduced-fat cheese<br>• Low-fat plain yogurt or fromage frais<br>• Margarine or olive oil<br>• Greek yogurt<br>• Salsa<br>• Vinaigrette dressing |
| **Meat, poultry, and fish** | • Beef on the bone<br>• Pork spareribs<br>• Streaky bacon<br>• Dark chicken or turkey meat<br>• Breadcrumbed chicken fillet<br>• Breadcrumbed fish fillet | • Lean boneless beef<br>• Pork fillet<br>• Lean back bacon or Parma ham<br>• Chicken or turkey breast<br>• Grilled chicken fillet<br>• Grilled fish steaks and fillets and shellfish |
| **Deli counter** | • Salami<br>• Corned beef or pastrami<br>• Full-fat cheese<br>• Potato salad or coleslaw<br>• Pâté | • Roast turkey or baked ham<br>• Lean roast beef or turkey breast<br>• Reduced-fat cheese<br>• Roast peppers or carrot and raisin salad<br>• Reduced-fat or vegetable pâté |
| **Frozen** | • Pizza topped with salami or meat<br>• Croissants or brioche<br>• Vegetables with butter or cheese sauce<br>• Beef burger<br>• Breadcrumbed chicken nuggets<br>• Ice cream<br>• Regular ready meal | • Pizza topped with vegetables<br>• Bagels<br>• Vegetables without sauce<br>• Vegetable burger<br>• Chicken fillet<br>• Frozen yogurt or sorbet<br>• Low-fat ready meal |
| **Canned food** | • Tuna in oil or brine<br>• Fruit in heavy syrup<br>• Vegetables with salt and/or sugar<br>• Creamy pasta sauce<br>• Regular baked beans | • Tuna in water<br>• Fruit in fruit juice<br>• Vegetables without salt and/or sugar<br>• Tomato pasta sauce<br>• Low-sugar, low-salt baked beans |
| **Snacks** | • Fried potato crisps<br>• Tortilla chips | • Baked low-fat potato crisps<br>• Breadsticks or pretzels |

# How to store food

## Food storage is easy and convenient with modern appliances.

Having bought the freshest and healthiest food, you must handle it carefully and store it correctly when you get it home in order to maintain the quality and taste.

### Fridges and freezers

Indispensable for storing fresh food, the fridge is the modern-day equivalent of the larder. Invest in the most capacious fridge that you can fit in your kitchen as over-crowding the fridge will reduce its efficiency and may also shorten its life. Check that the fridge temperature remains at a constant 5°C (40°F) or lower.

Freezing is a convenient way of storing food for longer periods while avoiding loss of nutrients and taste. The length of freezer storage time varies according to the type of food (see p.287). Be sure your freezer temperature is -18°C (0°F) or below. To help you keep a check on the contents of your freezer, label everything with the date of its freezing and, if necessary, add a brief description of the contents of the packet.

### Keep them in the dark

Grains can be stored for up to a year in a cool, dark cupboard, as can canned vegetables, fruits, fish, and soups, and bottles of sauces, vinegar, and oil. Be sure to check the contents of your cupboards on a regular basis and discard any out-of-date products. Potatoes should also be kept in the dark, to prevent them from sprouting.

**Well-stocked storecupboard** Keep pasta, grains, and pulses in a cool, dark place; once opened transfer to jars with close-fitting lids.

## Fridge storage tips

To ensure that your food does not become contaminated while it is stored in the fridge, bear these points in mind. (Note that the coldest part of the fridge is against the back wall.)

• Allow warm food or drinks to cool down before placing them in the fridge.

• Wrap or cover food to be stored.

• Place wrapped uncooked meat, poultry, fish, and shellfish on a tray on the bottom shelf.

• Place dairy products, pastries, cooked food, and ready meals on the upper shelves.

• Keep all fruits and vegetables (except potatoes) in the drawers at the bottom of the fridge.

• Store bottles and cartons upright in the door compartments.

• Once a month, clean the inside of your fridge with tepid water that has a mild antibacterial washing up liquid added. After cleaning, rinse the fridge interior thoroughly.

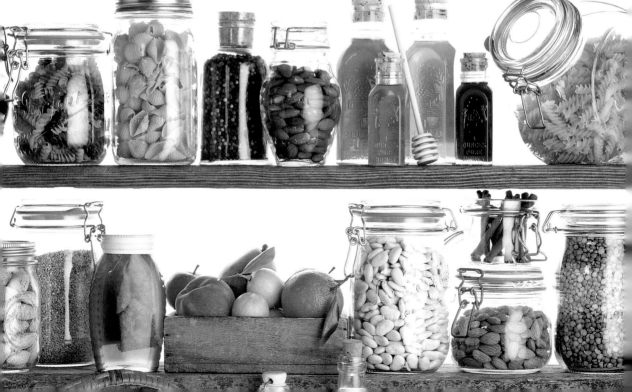

# How to store the food you buy

Having chosen your purchases carefully, and brought them home safely, it is important to store foods correctly, so that they remain fresh and maintain their flavour and nutritional value. Different types of foods have to be stored in different ways – some require refrigeration, while others keep best in a cool, dark place. Others can be frozen and then thawed as required (*see p.287*). Keep an eye on best-before or use-by dates and make sure that you discard out-of-date foods.

| FOOD TYPE | STORAGE HINTS |
|---|---|
| **Grains and cereals** | Store whole grains and cereals at room temperature in a dark place. After opening, tightly reseal the original packaging or transfer the contents to containers with tightly fitting lids. Whole grains should be used within a year of purchase; alternatively, freeze for up to a year. |
| **Pasta and noodles** | Dried pasta and noodles are stored in the same way as grains. Keep fresh varieties in the refrigerator and use within two days, or freeze for up to two months. |
| **Bread** | Keep bread in a sealed bag or container, at room temperature for two to four days, in the fridge for seven to 14 days, or in the freezer for six months. |
| **Vegetables** | Before storing vegetables, check and discard any that are damaged or blemished. Keep potatoes and other root vegetables in a cool, dark place; store all other vegetables and salad leaves in the fridge. Store frozen vegetables in the freezer for up to 12 months. |
| **Fruit** | Discard any damaged or blemished fruits to prevent further spoilage. Make sure that all produce is dry, and do not wash before storing. Canned fruits, once opened and transferred to a glass or plastic container, can be stored in the fridge for one week. Many fruits are also suitable for freezing (*see p.287*). Keep unopened packets of dried fruit in the fridge or storecupboard for six months; once opened, keep in the fridge for one month. |
| **Dairy foods** | Refrigerate dairy products immediately after purchase, with the exception of items such as long-life milk in cartons. Store fresh milk in the fridge for five days. Hard cheeses, once opened, can be kept in the fridge for three to four weeks. Keep all cheese tightly packaged in moisture-proof wrap. Soft cheeses can be refrigerated for one to two weeks; grated Parmesan will keep for at least one month in the fridge or three months in the freezer. |
| **Fish and shellfish** | Store in the coldest part of the fridge, wrapped in a polythene bag or moisture-proof paper, and use within two days of purchase. Alternatively, wrap tightly in air- and moisture-proof wrapping and store in the freezer for up to six months. Cook shellfish as soon as possible after purchase; once cooked it can be stored in the fridge for three to four days, or in the freezer for up to three months. |
| **Poultry** | Use fresh poultry within two days of purchase. Store, loosely wrapped, in the coldest part of the fridge. Alternatively, wrap in an airtight freezer bags and store in the freezer for up to eight months. Never leave poultry at room temperature as this encourages the growth of bacteria. |
| **Meat** | Keep meat, in its original packaging, in the coldest part of the fridge. Use joints, steaks, and chops within three to four days, and minced meat within two days of purchase. Before freezing meat, wrap in an airtight freezer bag in addition to its original packaging and label with date of purchase. |
| **Eggs** | Store fresh eggs, in their box (large end up), in the fridge for up to one month. Do not store eggs near strong-smelling foods as they easily absorb unwanted flavours. Freeze egg whites for up to six months. Egg yolks can be frozen only if mixed first with a pinch of salt or $1\frac{1}{2}$ tsp sugar per four yolks. Thaw frozen egg yolks and whites overnight in the fridge before use. |
| **Pulses** | Store dried peas, beans, and lentils for up to one year in tightly covered containers, in a dry, cool place. Do not mix pulses bought at different times, since older ones are drier and will take longer to cook. Pick over pulses before use and discard stones, fibres, and misshapen or discoloured beans. |

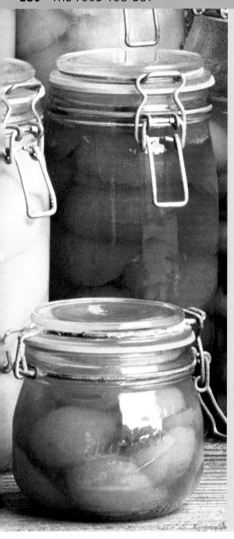

# Preserving food at home

Freezing and home preserving enable you to store fresh foods for extended use.

Whether you grow your own fruits and vegetables, or want to take advantage of buying them in bulk, preserving is an effective way of storing food for future use. It can also be a great time-saver if you prepare batches of food and freeze them until required – or even freeze whole meals for times when you are too busy to cook.

## Traditional and modern

In the past, before home freezers became widely available, various preservation techniques were employed. These methods included drying, salting, smoking, pickling, and bottling. While the use of such methods has become less common due to the year-round availability of supermarket foods, they provide a satisfying and healthy way of preserving home-grown produce.

Traditionally, freezing involved packing food in ice, but modern freezers have streamlined the process with carefully regulated temperatures. How long you can keep food in your freezer depends on how cold the temperature is, because you want to ensure the food maintains its quality.

## Keeping control

Whichever method you choose, preserving allows you to provide a constant supply of nutritious home-made food for your family, rather than relying on ready meals and other convenience foods that are likely to contain more salt, sugar, and other additives.

**Home preserves** There is something deeply satisfying about stocking your larder with jars of home-made jam, pickles, and chutneys, and your own bottled fruits and vegetables.

## Preserving your own produce

If you have a garden or allotment and grow your own fruits and vegetables, you may find yourself at certain times of the year with more than you can possibly eat. Preserving by traditional techniques such as making jams and pickles means that you can enjoy your harvest all year round.

### PRESERVING FRUITS

Unlike shop-bought varieties, fruits preserved at home as jam, jelly, or marmalade, or in a chutney or sweet pickle, will be free of additives and contain only the best of ingredients. For the best results, try these tips.
- Use only freshly picked, just ripe fruits for jam and jelly as these are highest in the setting agent pectin.
- Prepare fruit by washing and, if necessary, removing the peel, pith, any damaged flesh, stalks, and stones.
- Wash jars with hot soapy water, rinse with hot water, and dry well. Warm the jars in the oven before filling.

- Seal the jars tightly to make sure germs do not get in; if you use jars with self-sealing lids, use new rubber seals each time to ensure a close fit.

### PICKLING VEGETABLES

Choose firm young vegetables. For specific information, follow your favourite recipe. The following tips will help you.
- Cauliflower florets, shredded cabbage, cucumbers, beetroot, and gherkins are ideal for pickling.
- Wash and drain selected vegetables and prepare for pickling by dry-salting or packing in brine: this draws moisture from the vegetables, making them more receptive to the pickling vinegar. Remove the vegetables from the brine, rinse well, and then pack in the prepared jars.
- Add whole spices such as allspice, black peppercorns, cloves, mustard seeds, and coriander seeds.
- Fill the jars with vinegar, then seal them tightly.

# Tips for freezing

The easiest, most effective technique for preserving the flavour, colour, moisture content, and nutritive value of food is freezing. For the best results, wrap the food first in special freezer paper and then in a sealed freezer bag or container. This helps prevent freezer burn, which occurs when frost forms on the outside of the food and can alter the taste and quality.

• Cool all foods and liquids completely before placing in the freezer container or bag. Depositing warm foods in the freezer raises the temperature and may thaw neighbouring foods.

• Pack food in quantities that will be used for a single serving, so you need to thaw only the amount that you require.

• When placing food to be frozen in freezer bags, exclude all air before sealing tightly with a wire tie.

• Ensure that lids on rigid freezer containers are properly sealed to prevent spillages.

• Before freezing, label each packet with the name of the product, any added ingredients, and the date.

• Avoid overloading your freezer with unfrozen food as this slows the freezing rate: some freezers offer a fast freeze mode that ensures rapid freezing.

• While food is freezing, leave space between the packages so that air can circulate; once it is is frozen, you can store the packages close together.

• To save space in the freezer, freeze liquids in shallow, rectangular trays; transfer the frozen slabs to freezer bags that can then be stacked up.

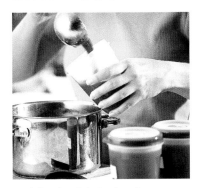

**Batch freezing**  Make batches of soup, stew, or baby's meals when you have time, and freeze in individual-size portions for later use.

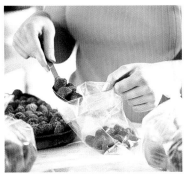

**Seasonal fruits**  Most fruits freeze well. Soft fruits such as raspberries should be open frozen, then transferred to bags or containers.

## Thawing frozen food

Apart from vegetables, most of which can be cooked from frozen by adding them straight to boiling water, frozen foods should be thawed before cooking. This can be done in the fridge, at room temperature, or in a microwave oven. Which method you choose depends mainly on how soon you want to cook the food. Thawing times at room temperature are given below; thawing in the fridge will take longer.

# Which foods can be frozen?

Most foods, including bread, pizza bases, fruits, vegetables, meat, poultry, fish, and ready-made soups and stews, are suitable for freezing.

In general, any vegetable that is eaten steamed or boiled can be frozen, while those that are eaten raw, such as spring onions, lettuce, and radishes, are not suitable. In order to retain the vitamin content and colour of vegetables, it is advisable to blanch them first, before freezing. This involves immersing the prepared vegetables in boiling water for a few minutes.

Eggs cannot be frozen in their shells, but the yolk and white can be frozen separately or stirred together and frozen in plastic containers or ice-cube trays.

| FOOD | FREEZER STORAGE | THAWING TIME |
| --- | --- | --- |
| Bread | 6 months | 2–3 hours |
| Pizza | 2–3 months | 2–4 hours |
| Broccoli | 9–12 months | Cook from frozen |
| Carrots | 12 months | Cook from frozen |
| Corn-on-the-cob | 12 months | 3–4 hours |
| Plums | 10–12 months | 5–10 hours |
| Raspberries | 10–12 months | 3–7 hours |
| Beef | 6–12 months | 10–12 hours |
| Chicken (1–1.35kg/2–3lb) | 8 months | 10–12 hours |
| Fish fillets | 2–3 months | 6–8 hours |
| Ricotta cheese | 1 month | 3–4 hours |
| Soup | 3–6 months | Reheat from frozen |

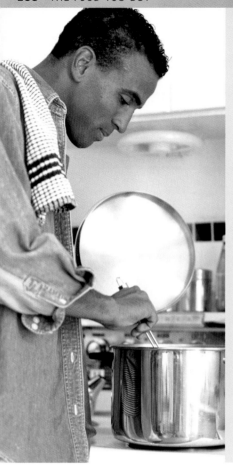

# Food preparation and cooking

## Make the most of nutritious ingredients by adopting healthy cooking methods.

Cooking food in a healthy way does not take extra time, effort, or special equipment. A few simple adjustments to your usual cooking methods may be all you need to improve the nutritional quality of the food you cook. It won't lose flavour. In fact, in many cases it will taste even better.

Reducing the amount of saturated fat in your diet is one of the most important changes that you can

make to benefit your health (*see pp.42–43*). This means choosing ingredients carefully, removing all visible fat, adding as little extra fat as possible while cooking, and discarding any excess. The cooking techniques listed opposite are all healthy and retain the nutritional content of food as well as enhance natural flavours and textures.

Reducing added salt is another dietary change that will benefit your health, especially if you have a tendency for high blood pressure (*see p.221*). This requires a gradual reduction in the amount of salt you add to your food and becoming accustomed instead to healthier flavourings, such as seasonings, herbs, and spices.

On the following pages we give you a few ideas to help you find healthier ways of preparing and cooking food at home.

**Home cooking** Preparing meals at home allows you to choose the best ingredients and to use the healthiest cooking methods.

## Experiment with seasoning

Healthy food need not taste bland or uninteresting. It does, however, require an adjustment in your sense of taste if you are used to seasoning everything you eat with salt and enjoy the flavour that fat gives to meat, poultry, breads, and pastries. You can experiment with herbs and spices, or try marinating foods in citrus juices before cooking.

### HEALTHY SEASONING

By trying out different ways of flavouring food you will soon begin to appreciate the lighter, fresher flavours of herbs, spices, and other seasonings.
• For the best flavour, dry roast and grind your own spices.
• Use fresh or dried herbs.
• Lemon or lime juice squeezed over food during and after cooking imparts a fresh, tangy taste; grated lemon zest can also be added during cooking.

• A dash of vinegar – balsamic, red or white wine, herb, or fruit – added towards the end of the cooking time adds a zesty flavour.
• Sprinkle some toasted nuts or seeds over a dish for a crunchy topping.
• Garnish a dish with roast peppers for a sweet, smoky taste.

### BENEFITS OF MARINATING

In addition to flavouring poultry, meat, fish, and vegetables, marinating also helps to tenderize meat. And studies have shown that marinating foods prior to cooking them on a barbecue reduces the harmful hydrocarbons that are produced by this cooking method.

To make a simple marinade, use any combination of citrus juice and fresh herbs. Pour the mixture over the raw ingredients, cover, and marinate in the fridge for a few hours before cooking.

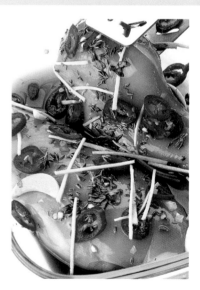

**Adding flavour** Marinades are a good way to add lots of healthy flavouring. Here fresh red chillies, garlic, fresh ginger, and coriander give a lift to chicken breasts.

# Healthy cooking methods

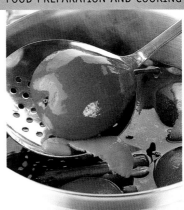

All cooking destroys nutrients to some extent, but some methods are better than others in both this respect and in minimizing other unhealthy factors, such as fat and salt content.
- Non-stick pans and tins are a healthy investment, since they reduce the need for added fat during cooking.
- A light spray of vegetable oil should be enough to avoid food sticking to the pan.
- Sauté vegetables and meat in wine, water, or stock instead of using butter.
- Remove fat from soups, stews, sauces, and gravies by chilling after cooking and skimming fat off the surface.
- Substitute healthy oils such as olive or rapeseed for butter or dripping.

**Poaching**  This is a healthy, low-fat method for cooking fruits, fish, eggs, or meat in a suitably flavoured liquid.

| METHOD | HOW IT WORKS |
|---|---|
| **Barbecuing** | This quick method of cooking fish and shellfish, meat, poultry, vegetables, and even fruit infuses the food with a smoky flavour. The food is cooked on a rack above hot coals, and little or no fat is needed depending on what is being barbecued. Marinating will enhance flavour (*opposite below*). Griddling on a ridged grill pan is similar to barbecuing but doesn't give a smoky flavour to the food. |
| **Braising** | Braising cooks food in a small amount of liquid in an open or covered pan, either on top of the cooker or in the oven. There is no need for any fat to be added, since the cooking liquid keeps the food moist. The juices from the food add flavour to the cooking liquid, which may be reduced by rapid boiling to provide an intensely flavourful, nutrient-rich sauce of thickened consistency. |
| **Grilling** | Ideal for thin cuts of poultry, meat, and fish, grilling cooks food quickly. If the food is cooked on a rack fat can drip into the pan beneath and be discarded. If the food is very lean, it may be necessary to brush it first with a little oil to prevent it from sticking to the rack and drying out during cooking. |
| **Microwaving** | Microwave ovens cook food by emitting high-frequency radio waves that cause food molecules to vibrate. This creates friction, which heats and cooks food very quickly. No added fat and very little liquid is required, so microwaving is a healthy cooking method that retains nutrients well. It is particularly suitable for vegetables, which retain all their colour, taste, and texture. |
| **Poaching** | In this low-fat method, fruit, fish, eggs, and meat are gently simmered in water, stock, tomato or fruit juices, or wine until tender. Food can be poached in a saucepan, or it can be cooked in a baking dish in the oven. |
| **Roasting** | For healthy roasting of large joints of meat or whole poultry, place the food on a rack in a roasting tin. The rack allows the fat to drain into the tin and be discarded. Use a meat thermometer to ensure that meat and poultry are thoroughly cooked (*see p.292*). |
| **Sautéing** | This involves cooking food quickly in a sauté pan or frying pan over direct heat. Use a good quality non-stick pan to minimize the need for added oil. If necessary, use just a light spray of oil to prevent the food from sticking to the bottom of the pan. Sautéing is a healthy alternative to shallow frying, which uses more fat. |
| **Steaming** | Ideal for cooking fish, poultry, and vegetables, this quick cooking method retains nutrients and does not require any added fat. Place a steamer basket or rack with the food to be cooked over a pan of boiling water, cover, and cook over a low heat. Some steamers incorporate several separate baskets so that a variety of foods can be steamed at the same time. |
| **Stir-frying** | This is a fast and healthy method of cooking, particularly if you use a non-stick wok. Cut ingredients into similarly sized small pieces and use just a small amount of oil or cooking spray to prevent them from sticking to the wok. Fry quickly over a high heat, constantly moving the food around. |

# Storecupboard basics to stock

Keep your storecupboard (and freezer) well stocked with basic ingredients in cans, jars, and packets that can form the foundation of a healthy diet. If you choose wisely, these basic items can be transformed into healthy meals, either alone or with the addition of other fresh products. For example, if you have wholemeal pasta and brown rice – rather than regular pasta and white rice – then you are already halfway to nutritious meals.

Copy our healthy shopping list (*right*), amending it to fit your food preferences, and stick it to the fridge door. Get your family to add to it, then take it with you to the supermarket every week.

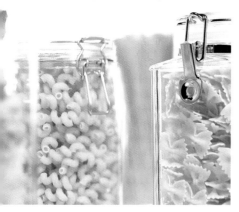

**Satisfying pasta** Pasta is cheap, filling, and quick to prepare. Wholemeal pasta is an excellent source of B vitamins and folate.

## Healthy shopping list

Stock up on these healthy basics so that you can prepare a nutritious meal at any time.

### Cans, jars, and cartons
- Apple sauce (no added sugar)
- Beans
- Fruit in fruit juice
- Fruit juice (no added sugar)
- Lentils
- Low-salt chicken broth
- Low-salt soy sauce
- Low-salt vegetable juice
- Peeled whole or chopped tomatoes
- Salsa
- Sardines in olive oil
- Sweetcorn (sugar- and salt-free)
- Tomato passata
- Tomato pasta sauce
- Tomato purée
- Tuna in water
- UHT (long-life) skimmed milk
- Vegetable juice

### Frozen foods
- Chicken and turkey breasts
- Low-fat ready meals
- Low-fat frozen yogurt
- Mini wholemeal bagels
- Part-baked bread and rolls
- Pizza bases
- Prawns
- Salmon steaks
- Sorbet
- Summer berries
- Vegetable or bean burgers
- Vegetables (no added salt)

### Grains and cereals
- Brown rice
- Bulgur wheat
- Couscous
- Muesli
- Porridge oats
- Whole-grain cereal
- Wholemeal pasta

### Desserts
- Digestive biscuits
- Fromage frais
- Fruit jelly
- Gingernuts
- Low-fat fruit yogurt

### Snacks
- Baked potato crisps
- Baked tortilla chips
- Dried fruit
- Fig bars
- Plain popcorn
- Pretzels
- Rice cakes
- Unsalted nuts (almonds, walnuts)
- Wholemeal crackers

### Oils and spreads
- Low-sugar preserves
- Margarine
- Non-stick vegetable oil spray
- Olive oil
- Peanut butter
- Rapeseed oil

### Drinks
- Bottled water and herb teas

# Tips on safe microwave cooking

The speed and convenience of microwave cooking has ensured the popularity of these appliances, which can be used for thawing, reheating, and cooking. However, it is important to be aware of the potential hazards of this form of cooking in order to avoid health risks. Microwaves do not enter the oven uniformly and cold spots can occur in food being cooked, allowing bacteria to survive and possibly leading to food poisoning.
- To minimize uneven cooking, stir the food once or twice during microwaving, arrange foods uniformly, and turn large items over halfway through cooking.
- Remove plastic wraps and foam trays from shop-bought

frozen food before thawing as these might melt and allow chemicals to be absorbed by the food.
- Frozen meat and poultry may begin to cook during thawing in the microwave and should be cooked immediately after.
- Never use any metal or foil utensils or wraps in the microwave oven; this includes recycled or coloured kitchen towel and newspapers, which may contain metal.
- If microwaves are used to heat baby food, always stir well to ensure even cooking and no hot spots.
- Use a meat thermometer or probe (*see p.292*) to check that food has reached a safe temperature. Check in several places when cooking large pieces of meat.

# Fast, home-cooked healthy food

If you have followed our suggestions on storecupboard basics (*opposite*), you will be in a position to create quick, nutritious meals for yourself and your family at short notice and at any time. Here are some suggestions:

**Pasta**  Serve with a ready-made fat-free sauce – or make your own sauce and freeze in serving-size portions until required. If there is any leftover pasta, use it in a salad, adding chopped raw vegetables and a little low-fat dressing.

**Rice**  Brown rice can form the basis of a satisfying meal. For a spicy pilaf, add chopped cooked vegetables, shredded chicken breast, or tofu, and season with cumin, coriander, and ginger.

**Pizza**  Top a ready-made pizza base with chopped tomatoes, mushrooms, onions, and peppers, finishing with grated reduced-fat cheese.

**Omelette**  An omelette takes just a few minutes to prepare and cook, but can make a satisfying light meal. Add lightly steamed vegetables to the eggs before cooking. For a low-fat cheese omelette, you can blend ricotta or cottage cheese in a food processor until smooth, then mix with the eggs before cooking.

**Grilled chicken or salmon**  Rub ground spices or dried herbs over a chicken breast or a salmon fillet or steak, then grill until cooked through; serve with steamed vegetables and rice.

**Stir-fry**  Buy a prepared stir-fry mixture of carrots, broccoli, onions, mushrooms, and beansprouts, and stir-fry it with cubes of tofu, peeled prawns, or strips of skinless chicken breast to make a satisfying dish. Season the dish with a little low-salt soy sauce.

**Jacket baked potato**  Split open a baked potato and top it with a ready-made salsa, vegetarian chilli, grated reduced-fat cheese, or low-fat hummus.

**Vegetable couscous**  This nutritious type of pasta is quick and simple to prepare. While the couscous is being soaked in boiling water, stir-fry cubes of tofu and some sliced vegetables, then add a little vegetable stock. Top the couscous with the vegetable and tofu mixture (*below*).

**Vegetarian burgers**  For a quick and nutritious meal, grill a vegetable burger and serve in toasted ciabatta with sliced tomato, salsa, and a green salad.

**Cottage cheese dip**  For a simple dip to serve with vegetable crudités, or as a quick pasta sauce or salad dressing, purée plain cottage cheese in a food processor, then add garlic powder and dill, basil, or Italian seasoning to taste.

**Griddled vegetables**  Brush vegetables with a little olive oil and cook on a hot ridged grill pan for 3–5 minutes on each side. Serve as a starter with ciabatta or French bread, as a side dish with meat or poultry, or spooned over rice or pasta as a satisfying meal. Vegetables that are ideal for griddling include sliced onion, sliced aubergine, halved mushrooms, quartered peppers, asparagus tips, long slices of courgette, sweet potato rounds, and cherry tomatoes.

# Recipe  Quick vegetable couscous

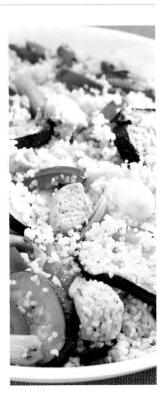

| INGREDIENTS |
| --- |
| 1 stock cube |
| 115g (4oz) couscous |
| 2 courgettes |
| 2.5cm (1in) piece of fresh ginger |
| 6 spring onions |
| 2 red peppers |
| 350g (12oz) firm tofu |
| 2 garlic cloves |

Serves 4

1 Dissolve the stock cube in 350ml (12floz) boiling water.

2 Place the couscous in a medium-sized bowl. Pour over the boiling stock and stir well. Leave until the couscous has absorbed all the liquid.

3 Slice the courgettes into rounds. Peel and grate the fresh ginger; slice the spring onions; core, seed, and slice the peppers; cut the tofu into cubes; and peel and crush the garlic.

4 Spray a wok with a little oil and place over a medium heat. Add the courgettes to the wok and stir-fry for 5 minutes.

5 Add the tofu and the rest of the vegetables to the wok. Stir-fry for a further 5 minutes.

6 Remove the vegetables and tofu from the wok and stir gently into the couscous, taking care not to break up the vegetables. Serve immediately.

**Variation**  You can replace the tofu with cubes of chicken breast; flavour with ground cumin and coriander; and garnish with flaked almonds.

**Each serving provides**
Calories 171, Total fat 4.5g (Sat. 0.6g, Poly. 2.0g, Mono. 1.0g), Cholesterol trace, Protein 11g, Carbohydrate 22g, Fibre 2.0g, Sodium 189mg. Good source of – Vits: A, Fol, C, K; Mins: Ca, K, Mg, P.

# Food hygiene

## Prevent food-borne illnesses by adopting safe food practices.

According to a 2002 survey by the Food Standards Agency, as many as 5.5 million people in the UK could have experienced food poisoning in the previous year. Bacteria such as *E.coli*, *Listeria*, and salmonella can cause life-threatening illnesses, especially in vulnerable people.

Food contamination may occur during the storage, handling, or cooking of food, at home and in shops and restaurants, and it is important that you bear this issue in mind whenever you are dealing with food. For example, when you are shopping, always check the condition of food packages and reject those that are damaged in any way, such as dented cans and torn plastic wrapping. Keep frozen and chilled foods cold on the way home, and put them in your fridge or freezer as soon as possible.

### Keeping food separate
Because cooked foods can become contaminated through contact with raw foods, make sure that you keep them separate in your basket or trolley at the supermarket, pack them separately, and keep them apart in the fridge. You should always use separate cutting boards for preparing raw and cooked foods, and wash utensils and surfaces thoroughly after use.

### Cook thoroughly
Most food-borne illnesses occur after eating raw or inadequately cooked meat, poultry, or fish, since animals sometimes carry bacteria that are killed only by thorough cooking. Traditionally, advice was to cook meat for a specified time per weight and poultry until the juices run clear; however, the most accurate way to ensure that any bacteria is destroyed is to use a meat thermometer. Safe cooked temperatures vary for different kinds of meat (*below*).

### Safe refrigeration
Refrigerated foods should be kept at temperatures below 5°C (40°F). Make a point of regularly checking the temperature in your

## Using a food thermometer

To ensure that food is cooked to a high enough temperature to destroy bacteria, it is recommended that you use a thermometer to check the internal temperature. There are two types of food thermometers: one is inserted into a joint of meat or whole poultry at the start of cooking and left in throughout; the other is inserted towards the end of the suggested cooking time for an instant reading. Always insert the thermometer into a meaty part, avoiding bone. The instant-read thermometers can also be used to check whether egg dishes are thoroughly cooked. There are also thermometers for microwave cooking.

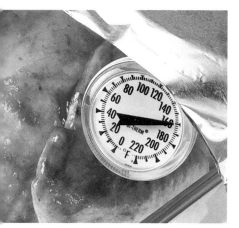

**Is it done?** The best way to check whether meat and poultry have been cooked long enough to destroy bacteria is to use a food thermometer. Some, like the one shown, are left in the food throughout cooking; others are inserted towards the end.

| FOOD | TEMPERATURE |
|---|---|
| **Minced beef, pork, veal, and lamb** | • 71°C (160°F) |
| **Joints and cuts of beef, veal, and lamb** | • Medium-rare 63°C (145°F)<br>• Medium 71°C (160°F)<br>• Well-done 77°C (170°F) |
| **Poultry** | • Whole birds 82°C (180°F)<br>• Breasts, legs, thighs, and wings 77°C (170°F)<br>• Minced 74°C (165°F) |
| **Pork** | • Medium 71°C (160°F)<br>• Well-done 77°C (170°F) |
| **Gammon and ham** | • Uncooked 71°C (160°F)<br>• Precooked 60°C (140°F) |
| **Fish** | • 63°C (145°F) |
| **Egg dishes** | • 71°C (160°F) |
| **Casseroles, stews, combination dishes, leftovers, and stuffings** | • 74°C (165°F) |

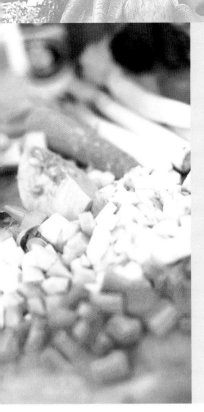

fridge, and ensure that you adjust the setting as you fill and empty the shelves. You can keep a special thermometer in the fridge to help you monitor the temperature.

## Keep food hygiene in mind

Plastic cutting boards should be washed thoroughly every day and replaced regularly. Wooden boards and kitchen sponges can be microwaved to kill bacteria. Wash dishes or utensils in very hot water. Disinfect work surfaces daily.

By taking sensible precautions, you will protect yourself and your family from the health dangers posed by food-borne illnesses.

**Cutting board hygiene** To prevent cross-contamination, use separate boards for raw and cooked food. Keep them scrupulously clean and replace them regularly.

## Kitchen hygiene

Scrupulous cleanliness is essential in the handling of food to prevent the risk of food-borne illnesses.
● Wash your hands every time you handle, prepare, or cook food. Use warm, soapy water and wash your hands front and back, up to the wrists, between your fingers, and under fingernails and rings.
● Dry your hands thoroughly using disposable kitchen towels or hand-dryers. Do not use fabric towels, which can harbour bacteria.
● Wash your hands after using the telephone or toilet, blowing your nose or sneezing, touching your pet, or changing nappies.
● Keep your fingernails clean and trimmed, and cover any cuts or abrasions on your hands with a waterproof dressing.

# Keeping food safe at picnics

Ensuring that cold food remains cold and hot food stays hot are major safety concerns when planning a picnic. This will affect not just the food you choose to take, but also how you pack it and store it before you sit down to eat.

Hot food that has been allowed to cool in a picnic basket provides an ideal environment for bacteria to grow, so take hot food with you only if you can keep it piping hot until you are ready to eat it. The best way is to keep it in a vacuum flask. Similarly, cold food that is allowed to warm and become tepid becomes potentially hazardous to consume.
● Pack salads and cooked meats with ice packs in a cooler box or bag, and keep food in the cooler until required.
● Discard any uneaten food that has been left out in the sun.
● Keep the cooler inside the car rather than putting it in the boot.
● Your body needs plenty of water in the summer months, especially when it is very hot, so take a cooler box filled with bottles of water and juice boxes to keep you refreshed.

## FOOD IDEAS FOR PICNICS

Here are some tips on what to take on your picnic, bearing in mind both food safety and nutritional factors.
● Pack chilled, refreshing salads, such as shredded carrot and raisin or tomato and onion drizzled with olive oil.
● Pasta, rice, and couscous salads are perfect for picnics. Try different kinds of pasta, adding canned tuna chunks, vegetables, olives, and low-fat dressing.
● Pack a selection of sliced meats, such as turkey, ham, or lean roast beef, and crunchy bread and rolls.
● Snack on pretzels rather than crisps.
● Chilled fruit makes a refreshing snack. Pack soft fruits such as grapes, cherries, and slices of Galia or honeydew melon in re-sealable polythene bags.
● Take a portable, disposable barbecue and a selection of vegetables, including corn on the cob and skewered peppers, red onions, courgettes, and aubergine.
● If you plan to barbecue meat or fish, store them in a cooler bag with ice packs until required, then cook them until piping hot and cooked thoroughly.

## Food safety while travelling

When travelling in regions where the water supply and food hygiene are less than ideal, take sensible precautions to avoid becoming ill.
● Give your body time to adjust by moderating your intake of unfamiliar foods.
● Eat in busy restaurants where there is a rapid turnover of food.
● Make sure that food is piping hot and cooked thoroughly before you sit down to eat it.
● Drink only pasteurized or boiled milk, dairy products, and juice.
● Wash raw fruits and vegetables in bottled water if you have any doubts about the local water.
● Avoid salads (including fruit salads) in areas where they might have been washed in unsafe water.
● If the local tap water is unsafe to drink, boil it, use sterilizing tablets, or drink only bottled water; check that bottle seals are unbroken.

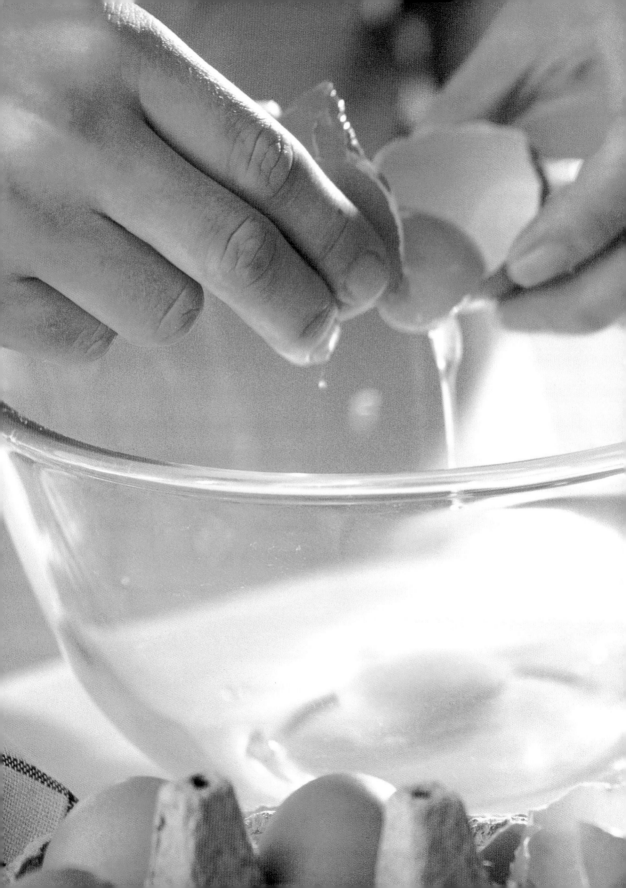

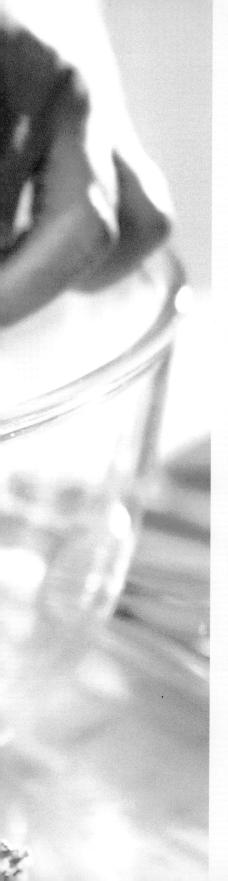

# Food analysis

Knowing which nutrients are contained in the food you eat helps you make healthy choices within a balanced diet. In this chapter, we offer you a reference that provides you with the nutritional breakdown (fat, protein, carbohydrate, fibre, and vitamin and mineral content) of almost 500 different foods.

# What is in the food you eat?

## Understanding what food contains is the key to healthy eating.

A basic knowledge of what is in the food you eat and how many calories it provides is vital to ensure that you eat a balanced diet. This chapter is an important resource that you can use as a reference guide now and in the future. We have also used the information in this chapter as the basis for all the charts and menus that we have given throughout the book.

## Macronutrients

Knowing which foods are high in protein or carbohydrate is the best way to get enough of these key macronutrients. Understanding which foods to avoid because of high saturated fat content and which to choose for unsaturated fats or fibre will help you plan a diet that optimizes health and reduces your risk of disease.

## Micronutrients

In these tables, we also list many of the vitamins and minerals that are found in the foods we eat. We have included this information so you can compare different foods as sources of specific nutrients.

Including a variety of foods that provide vitamins and minerals in your diet is the sensible way to ensure optimum health. Scientific studies have shown that the more of these essential nutrients you have in your diet, the healthier you are likely to be. While many people take a multivitamin to make sure they get all of the nutrients they need each day, the best way to obtain vitamins and minerals is from the foods you eat.

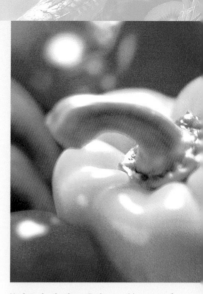

**Variety is the key** Eating a wide range of healthy foods – including fresh vegetables and fruits – every day is the best way to get the nutrients your body needs to stay healthy.

# Understanding the charts

On the following pages, we detail the calorie, fat, protein, carbohydrate, and fibre content of almost 500 foods, as well as the vitamins and minerals they supply. Information is either given per 100g/100ml or, where appropriate, per serving. You will find some figures are missing, mainly for types of fats and fibre. This is because information is not currently available.

Foods are listed in categories that, for the most part, follow the basic groups covered in the book (*see Elements of a Healthy Diet, pp.68–103*).Unless otherwise stated, foods are raw or uncooked.

**Carbohydrate foods** We have divided these into the following categories in the food analysis charts: Grains; Cereals, breakfast; Pasta and noodles; Breads; and Potatoes.

**Vegetables** Fresh, canned, frozen, and dried are included.

**Fruits** Fresh, canned, frozen, and dried are included.

**Dairy foods** Various fat contents are included for comparison.

**Protein foods** These have been subdivided into Eggs; Meat and poultry; Meat products; Fish and shellfish; Pulses and soya products; and Nuts and seeds.

**Fluids and foods to eat sparingly** The remaining items in the charts are grouped as Fats, oils, spreads, and syrups; Drinks; Frozen and chilled desserts; Cakes and biscuits; Pastries and puddings; and Snacks.

# Abbreviations used in the book

In the following charts, and throughout the book, the names of vitamins and minerals have been abbreviated. Those that may not appear obvious are explained below.

**Vitamins**
**Fol** Folate or folic acid
**Nia** Niacin
**Pant** Pantothenic acid
**Vit K** Vitamin K

**Minerals**
Macrominerals (*see p.60*):
**Ca** Calcium
**K** Potassium
**Mg** Magnesium

**Na** Sodium
**P** Phosphorus
**S** Sulphur
Microminerals (*see p.60*):
**Cr** Chromium
**Cu** Copper
**F** Fluoride
**Fe** Iron
**I** Iodine
**Se** Selenium
**Zn** Zinc

**Other abbreviations and symbols used in the book**
**cal** calories
**g** gram
**kcal** kilocalories
**mcg** microgram

**mg** milligram
**tr** trace of a nutrient
**-** no information available for nutrient at present

| | Cal (kcal) | Total fat (g) | Sat. fat (g) | Mono. fat (g) | Poly. fat (g) | Protein (g) | Carb. (g) | Fibre (g) | Useful source Vitamins/Minerals |
|---|---|---|---|---|---|---|---|---|---|
| **GRAINS** | | | | | | | | | |
| **Barley, pearl** 100g (3½oz) | 360 | 1.7 | 0.2 | 0 | 0 | 7.9 | 83.6 | 0.5 | Nia / Cu, Fe |
| **Barley, pearl, cooked** 100g (3½oz) | 120 | 0.6 | 0.1 | 0 | 0 | 2.7 | 27 | - | Cu |
| **Buckwheat groats** 100g (3½oz) | 364 | 1.5 | 0.2 | 0.3 | 0.3 | 8.1 | 84 | 2.1 | $B_1$, $B_2$, Nia / Ca, Fe, K, Mg, P, Zn |
| **Bulgur wheat** 100g (3½oz) | 353 | 1.7 | 0.1 | tr | tr | 9.7 | 76.3 | tr | $B_1$, Nia / Fe, Zn |
| **Couscous** 100g (3½oz) | 227 | 1.0 | tr | tr | tr | 5.7 | 51 | tr | $B_1$, Nia |
| **Quinoa** 100g (3½oz) | 309 | 5.0 | 0.5 | 1.3 | 2.0 | 13.8 | 57 | tr | $B_1$, $B_2$, Fol, Nia, Pant / Fe, K, Mg, P, Zn |
| **Rice, brown, long-grain** 100g (3½oz) | 357 | 2.8 | 0.7 | 0.7 | 1.0 | 6.7 | 81.3 | 1.9 | $B_1$, Nia / Mg, P, Zn |
| **Rice, brown, long-grain, cooked** 100g (3½oz) | 141 | 1.1 | 0.3 | 0.3 | 0.4 | 2.6 | 32 | 0.8 | $B_1$, Nia / Mg, P, Zn |
| **Rice, white, long-grain** 100g (3½oz) | 383 | 3.6 | 0.9 | 0.9 | 1.3 | 7.3 | 85 | 0.4 | $B_1$, Nia / Fe |
| **Rice, white, long-grain, cooked** 100g (3½oz) | 138 | 1.3 | 0.3 | 0.3 | 0.5 | 2.6 | 31 | 0.1 | $B_1$, Nia / Fe |
| **Semolina** 100g (3½oz) | 350 | 1.8 | 0.2 | 0.2 | 0.1 | 10.7 | 77.5 | 2.1 | P |
| **CEREALS, BREAKFAST** | | | | | | | | | |
| **All bran** 100g (3½oz) | 270 | 3.5 | 0.7 | 0.5 | 0.5 | 13 | 48 | 24.5 | A, B vitamins, C / K, Mg, P, Zn |
| **Bran flakes** 100g (3½oz) | 330 | 1.9 | 0.3 | 0.3 | 1.5 | 10.2 | 71.2 | 13 | A, most B vitamins / Fe, K, Mg, P, Zn |
| **Cornflakes** 100g (3½oz) | 376 | 0.7 | 0.2 | 0.2 | 0.4 | 7.9 | 89.6 | 0.9 | A, $B_1$, $B_2$, $B_6$, Fol, Nia, C / Fe, Zn |
| **Crunchy oat cereal** 100g (3½oz) | 453 | 20 | - | - | - | 8.0 | 59.3 | 6.6 | $B_1$, $B_2$, Nia |
| **Fruit and fibre** 100g (3½oz) | 353 | 15 | 2.5 | 1.0 | 0.7 | 9.0 | 72.5 | 7.0 | $B_1$, $B_2$, $B_6$, $B_{12}$, Fol, Nia / Fe, Zn |
| **Grapenuts** 100g (3½oz) | 346 | 0.5 | tr | tr | tr | 10.5 | 79.9 | 0.2 | $B_1$, $B_2$, $B_6$, $B_{12}$, Nia / Fe, Zn |

| | Cal (kcal) | Total fat (g) | Sat. fat (g) | Mono. fat (g) | Poly. fat (g) | Protein (g) | Carb. (g) | Fibre (g) | Useful source Vitamins/Minerals |
|---|---|---|---|---|---|---|---|---|---|
| **Muesli (no added sugar)** 100g (3½oz) | 366 | 7.8 | 1.5 | 3.5 | 2.4 | 10.5 | 67.1 | 7.6 | $B_1$, $B_2$, Nia / Fe |
| **Muesli, Swiss style** 100g (3½oz) | 363 | 6.7 | 0.8 | 2.8 | 1.6 | 9.8 | 72 | 6.4 | $B_1$, $B_2$, Nia / Fe |
| **Porridge oats** 100g (3½oz) | 401 | 8.7 | - | - | - | 12.4 | 72.8 | 6.8 | $B_1$, $B_2$, Nia / Ca, Fe |
| **Porridge, cooked with whole milk** 200g (7oz) | 226 | 10 | 5.6 | 2.9 | 1.2 | 10 | 25 | 2.0 | $B_1$, $B_2$, $B_{12}$ / Ca, Mg, P, Zn |
| **Puffed rice** 100g (3½oz) | 380 | 3.0 | - | - | - | 8.0 | 80 | 9.0 | $B_1$, $B_2$, Nia / Fe |
| **Puffed wheat** 100g (3½oz) | 321 | 1.3 | 0.2 | 0.2 | 0.6 | 14.2 | 67.3 | 5.6 | $B_1$, $B_2$, Nia / Fe |
| **Shredded wheat** 1 biscuit | 73 | 0.5 | 0.1 | 0.1 | 0.2 | 2.5 | 15.8 | 2.2 | $B_1$, Nia / Fe, K, P, Zn |
| **Weetabix** 1 biscuit | 70 | 0.4 | 0.1 | 0.1 | 0.4 | 2.2 | 15 | 1.9 | $B_1$, $B_2$, Fol, Nia / Fe, P |
| **PASTA AND NOODLES** | | | | | | | | | |
| **Egg noodles, Chinese** 100g (3½oz) | 391 | 8.2 | 2.3 | 3.5 | 0.9 | 12.1 | 71.7 | 2.9 | $B_1$, $B_2$, Nia / Cu, Zn |
| **Egg noodles, Chinese, cooked** 100g (3½oz) | 62 | 0.5 | 0.1 | 0.2 | 0.1 | 2.2 | 13 | 0.6 | $B_1$, $B_2$, Nia / Cu, Zn |
| **Macaroni** 100g (3½oz) | 348 | 1.8 | 0.3 | 0.1 | 0.8 | 12 | 75.8 | 3.1 | $B_1$, $B_2$, Nia / Fe |
| **Macaroni, cooked** 100g (3½oz) | 86 | 0.5 | 0.1 | tr | 0.2 | 3.0 | 18.5 | 0.9 | $B_1$, $B_2$, Nia / Fe |
| **Rice noodles** 100g (3½oz) | 360 | 0.1 | 0 | 0 | 0 | 4.9 | 81.5 | tr | P |
| **Rice noodles, cooked** 100g (3½oz) | 60 | 0.2 | 0.1 | 0 | 0 | 2.0 | 13 | 0.7 | P |
| **Spaghetti** 100g (3½oz) | 342 | 1.8 | 0.2 | 0.2 | 0.8 | 12 | 74 | 2.9 | $B_1$, $B_2$, Nia / Fe |
| **Spaghetti, cooked** 100g (3½oz) | 104 | 0.7 | 0.1 | 0.1 | 0.3 | 3.6 | 22.2 | 1.2 | $B_1$ / Cu, Mg, P |
| **Spaghetti, wholemeal** 100g (3½oz) | 324 | 2.5 | 0.4 | 0.3 | 1.1 | 13.4 | 66.2 | 8.4 | $B_1$, Nia / Mg, Zn |
| **Spaghetti, wholemeal, cooked** 100g (3½oz) | 113 | 1.0 | 0.1 | 0.1 | 0.4 | 5.0 | 23 | 3.5 | $B_1$ / Cu, Mg, P |

|  | Cal (kcal) | Total fat (g) | Sat. fat (g) | Mono. fat (g) | Poly. fat (g) | Protein (g) | Carb. (g) | Fibre (g) | Useful source Vitamins/Minerals |
|---|---|---|---|---|---|---|---|---|---|
| **BREADS** | | | | | | | | | |
| **Bagel, oat bran** 1 bagel | 181 | 0.9 | 0.1 | 0.2 | 0.3 | 7.6 | 37.8 | 1.3 | $B_1$, $B_2$, Nia / Fe, Zn |
| **Bagel, plain** 1 bagel | 195 | 1.1 | 0.2 | 0.1 | 0.5 | 7.5 | 37.9 | 0.7 | $B_1$, $B_2$, $B_6$, Fol, Nia / Fe, Zn |
| **English muffin** 1 muffin (60g) | 134 | 1.0 | 0.2 | 0.3 | 0.4 | 6.0 | 26.2 | 1.1 | $B_1$, $B_2$, Nia / Fe |
| **French bread** 1 thin slice (40g) | 105 | 0.8 | 0.1 | 0.1 | 0.3 | 3.6 | 22.4 | 1.0 | $B_1$, Nia |
| **Granary bread** 1 slice (38g) | 90 | 0.9 | 0.3 | 0.2 | 0.3 | 3.6 | 18 | 1.3 | $B_1$, $B_6$, Fol / Ca, P |
| **Irish soda bread** 1 slice (50g) | 129 | 1.3 | 0.5 | 0.4 | 0.1 | 3.9 | 27.3 | 1.1 | $B_1$ / Ca, P |
| **Malt bread** 1 slice (35g) | 103 | 0.8 | 0.2 | 0.3 | 0.4 | 2.7 | 22.7 | 0.9 | $B_1$, $B_2$ |
| **Matzo** 1 matzo (25g) | 96 | 0.5 | 0.1 | 0.1 | 0.2 | 2.6 | 21.6 | 0.8 | |
| **Naan bread** 1 bread (160g) | 456 | 11.7 | 1.6 | 4.9 | 3.8 | 12.5 | 80.3 | 3.2 | $B_1$, Fol / Ca, Cu, Fe, Mg, P, Zn |
| **Pitta bread, white** 1 small bread (75g) | 191 | 1.0 | 0.1 | 0.1 | 0.3 | 6.8 | 41.3 | 1.8 | $B_1$, Nia / Ca, Fe, P |
| **Pizza base, home-made** 1/8 of 23cm (9in) base | 121 | 8.0 | 2.0 | 3.5 | 2.1 | 1.5 | 10.9 | 0.4 | $B_1$, Nia / P |
| **Roll, hamburger** 1 roll | 123 | 2.2 | 0.5 | 1.1 | 0.4 | 3.7 | 21.6 | 1.2 | $B_1$ / Cu, P, Se |
| **Roll, hotdog** 1 roll | 110 | 2.0 | 0 | 0 | 0 | 4.0 | 21 | 1.0 | $B_1$ / Cu, P, Se |
| **Roll, oat bran** 1 roll | 78 | 1.5 | 0.2 | 0.5 | 0.5 | 3.1 | 13.3 | 1.4 | $B_1$ / Cu, P, Se |
| **Roll, rye** 1 roll | 81 | 1.0 | 0.2 | 0.4 | 0.2 | 2.9 | 15.1 | 1.4 | $B_1$ / P |
| **Roll, white** 1 roll | 85 | 2.1 | 0.5 | 1.1 | 0.3 | 2.4 | 14.3 | 0.9 | $B_1$ / Cu, Se |
| **Roll, wholemeal** 1 roll | 75 | 1.3 | 0.2 | 0.3 | 0.6 | 2.5 | 14.5 | 2.1 | $B_1$, $B_6$, Fol / Cu, Fe, Mg, P, Zn |
| **Rye bread** 1 slice (25g) | 55 | 0.4 | 0.1 | 0.1 | 0.1 | 2.1 | 11.4 | 1.1 | $B_1$ / P |

| | Cal (kcal) | Total fat (g) | Sat. fat (g) | Mono. fat (g) | Poly. fat (g) | Protein (g) | Carb. (g) | Fibre (g) | Useful source Vitamins/Minerals |
|---|---|---|---|---|---|---|---|---|---|
| **Rye crispbread** 1 crispbread (10g) | 31 | 0.1 | 0 | 0 | 0.1 | 0.9 | 7.1 | 1.2 | $B_1$ |
| **Scone, cheese** 1 scone (50g) | 182 | 8.9 | - | - | - | 5.0 | 21.6 | 0.8 | P |
| **Scone, fruit** 1 scone (50g) | 158 | 6.7 | 1.2 | 2.0 | 0.8 | 3.3 | 28.1 | 1.0 | $B_1$ / P |
| **Scone, plain** 1 scone (50g) | 182 | 7.4 | 1.8 | 2.2 | 2.9 | 3.6 | 26.9 | 0.9 | $B_1$ / P |
| **Scone, wholemeal, fruit** 1 scone (50g) | 162 | 6.4 | 1.8 | 2.2 | 2.9 | 4.0 | 23.6 | 2.5 | $B_6$ / P |
| **Scone, wholemeal, plain** 1 scone (50g) | 164 | 7.3 | 1.8 | 2.2 | 2.9 | 4.4 | 21.5 | 2.6 | $B_6$ / P |
| **Tortilla, flour (wrap)** 1 tortilla (60g) | 157 | 0.6 | 0.1 | 0.2 | 0.1 | 4.3 | 35.8 | 1.4 | |
| **Wheatgerm bread** 1 slice (38g) | 76 | 1.9 | - | - | - | 7.0 | 32.3 | 2.5 | $B_1$ / P, Zn |
| **White bread** 1 slice (38g) | 89 | 0.7 | 0.2 | - | - | 3.2 | 18.7 | 0.6 | Se |
| **White bread, fibre-enriched** 1 slice (38g) | 87 | 0.6 | 0.2 | 0.2 | 0.1 | 2.9 | 18.8 | 1.2 | Se |
| **Whole-grain bread** 1 slice | 65 | 1.0 | 0.2 | 0.4 | 0.2 | 2.6 | 12.1 | 1.7 | $B_1$, Nia / Mg, P, Se |
| **Wholemeal bread** 1 slice (38g) | 82 | 1.1 | 0.2 | 0.2 | 0.3 | 3.6 | 16 | 1.9 | $B_1$, Nia / Mg, P, Se |

## POTATOES

| | Cal (kcal) | Total fat (g) | Sat. fat (g) | Mono. fat (g) | Poly. fat (g) | Protein (g) | Carb. (g) | Fibre (g) | Useful source Vitamins/Minerals |
|---|---|---|---|---|---|---|---|---|---|
| **Potato, baked** 1 small potato (100g) | 136 | 0.2 | 0.1 | 0 | 0.1 | 3.9 | 31 | 2.7 | $B_1$, $B_6$, C / P, K |
| **Potato, boiled, peeled** 100g (3½oz) | 72 | 0.1 | 0 | 0 | 0.1 | 1.8 | 17 | 1.2 | $B_1$, $B_6$, C / K |
| **Potato, mashed with butter** 100g (3½oz) | 104 | 4.4 | 2.8 | 1.0 | 0.2 | 1.8 | 15.5 | 1.1 | $B_1$, $B_6$, C / K |

## VEGETABLES

| | Cal (kcal) | Total fat (g) | Sat. fat (g) | Mono. fat (g) | Poly. fat (g) | Protein (g) | Carb. (g) | Fibre (g) | Useful source Vitamins/Minerals |
|---|---|---|---|---|---|---|---|---|---|
| **Alfalfa sprouts** 100g (3½oz) | 2 | tr | 0 | 0 | 0.1 | 0 | 0 | 0 | C |
| **Artichoke (globe), boiled** 1 medium | 150 | 0.5 | 0.1 | 0 | 0.2 | 10.4 | 33.5 | 7.0 | A, $B_1$, $B_2$, Nia, Pant, C / Fe, K, Mg, P, Zn |

| | Cal (kcal) | Total fat (g) | Sat. fat (g) | Mono. fat (g) | Poly. fat (g) | Protein (g) | Carb. (g) | Fibre (g) | Useful source Vitamins/Minerals |
|---|---|---|---|---|---|---|---|---|---|
| **Asparagus, cooked** 80g (3oz) | 21 | 0.6 | 0.1 | 0.2 | 0.2 | 2.7 | 1.1 | 1.0 | Fol, C |
| **Aubergine** 100g (3½oz) | 15 | 0.4 | 0.1 | tr | 0.2 | 0.9 | 2.2 | 2.0 | $B_6$ |
| **Aubergine, fried in corn oil** 80g (3oz) | 302 | 32 | 4.0 | 8.0 | 18.5 | 1.2 | 2.8 | 2.3 | $B_6$ |
| **Avocado** 1 medium (145g) | 276 | 28 | 5.0 | 17 | 3.0 | 2.0 | 2.0 | 4.0 | $B_1$, $B_6$, C, E / Cu, Mg, P |
| **Bamboo shoots, boiled** 100g (3½oz) | 11 | 0.2 | 0.1 | tr | 0.1 | 1.5 | 0.7 | 1.7 | C |
| **Bean sprouts** 100g (3½oz) | 31 | 0.5 | 0.1 | 0.1 | 0.2 | 2.9 | 4.0 | 1.5 | C |
| **Beetroot, boiled** 1 small beetroot (35g) | 16 | 0.1 | 0 | 0 | 0.1 | 0 | 3.0 | 0.5 | Fol |
| **Beetroot, pickled** 35g (1¼oz) | 10 | 0.1 | 0 | 0 | 0.1 | 0 | 2.0 | 0.3 | Fol |
| **Broccoli** 100g (3½oz) | 33 | 0.9 | 0.2 | 0.1 | 0.5 | 4.4 | 1.8 | 2.6 | A, $B_6$, Fol, C, Vit K |
| **Broccoli, boiled** 80g (3oz) | 24 | 0.7 | 0.2 | 0.1 | 0.3 | 2.6 | 0.9 | 2.0 | A, $B_6$, Fol, C, Vit K |
| **Brussels sprouts, boiled** 80g (3oz) | 28 | 1.0 | 0.2 | 0.1 | 0.6 | 2.8 | 2.0 | 3.4 | A, Fol, C, Vit K |
| **Cabbage, green** 100g (3½oz) | 26 | 0.4 | 0.1 | tr | 0.3 | 1.7 | 4.1 | 2.4 | $B_6$, Fol, C, Vit K / S |
| **Cabbage, green, boiled** 80g (3oz) | 11 | 0.2 | tr | tr | 0.1 | 0.8 | 1.8 | 1.2 | Fol, C / S |
| **Cabbage, red** 100g (3½oz) | 21 | 0.3 | tr | tr | 0.2 | 1.1 | 3.7 | 2.5 | A, Fol, C / S |
| **Cabbage, red, boiled** 80g (3oz) | 12 | 0.2 | tr | tr | 0.2 | 0.6 | 1.8 | 1.6 | A, Fol, C / S |
| **Cabbage, savoy** 100g (3½oz) | 27 | 0.5 | 0.1 | tr | 0.3 | 2.1 | 3.9 | 3.1 | $B_1$, Fol, C / S |
| **Cabbage, savoy, boiled** 80g (3oz) | 14 | 0.4 | 0.1 | tr | 0.2 | 0.9 | 1.8 | 1.6 | A, $B_1$, Fol, C / S |
| **Carrots** 100g (3½oz) | 35 | 0.3 | 0.1 | tr | 0.2 | 0.6 | 7.9 | 2.4 | A, $B_1$, $B_6$, C, Vit K |
| **Carrots, boiled** 80g (3oz) | 19 | 0.3 | 0.1 | tr | 0.2 | 0.5 | 3.9 | 2.0 | A |

| | Cal (kcal) | Total fat (g) | Sat. fat (g) | Mono. fat (g) | Poly. fat (g) | Protein (g) | Carb. (g) | Fibre (g) | Useful source Vits / Mins |
|---|---|---|---|---|---|---|---|---|---|
| **Cassava** 100g (3½oz) | 142 | 0.2 | 0.1 | 0.1 | tr | 0.6 | 36.8 | 1.6 | C |
| **Cauliflower** 100g (3½oz) | 34 | 0.9 | 0.2 | 0.1 | 0.5 | 3.6 | 3.0 | 1.8 | $B_1$, $B_6$, C, Vit K / K |
| **Cauliflower, boiled** 80g (3oz) | 22 | 0.7 | 0.2 | 0.1 | 0.4 | 2.3 | 1.7 | 1.3 | $B_6$, C |
| **Celeriac** 100g (3½oz) | 18 | 0.4 | tr | tr | tr | 1.2 | 2.3 | 3.7 | $B_1$, $B_6$, Fol, C, Vit K / K, P |
| **Celeriac, boiled** 80g (3oz) | 12 | 0.4 | tr | tr | tr | 0.7 | 1.5 | 2.6 | $B_1$, Fol, C / K |
| **Celery** 1 stalk (30g) | 2.0 | 0.1 | tr | tr | tr | 0.1 | 0.3 | 0.3 | |
| **Chicory** 100g (3½oz) | 11 | 0.6 | 0.2 | tr | 0.3 | 0.5 | 2.8 | 0.9 | $B_1$, Pant, C |
| **Chinese cabbage** 100g (3½oz) | 12 | 0.2 | tr | tr | 0.1 | 1.0 | 1.4 | 1.4 | C |
| **Courgette** 100g (3½oz) | 18 | 0.4 | 0.1 | tr | 0.2 | 1.8 | 1.8 | 0.9 | $B_6$, Fol, C / K |
| **Courgette, boiled** 80g (3oz) | 15 | 0.3 | 0.1 | 0 | 0.2 | 1.6 | 1.6 | 1.0 | Fol, C |
| **Cucumber** 100g (3½oz) | 10 | 0.1 | tr | tr | tr | 0.7 | 1.5 | 0.6 | |
| **Endive** 100g (3½oz) | 13 | 0.2 | 0.1 | tr | 0.1 | 1.8 | 1.0 | 2.0 | $B_1$, C |
| **Fennel (bulb)** 100g (3½oz) | 13 | 0.2 | 0.1 | tr | 0.1 | 1.8 | 1.0 | 2.0 | Fol, C / K |
| **French beans, boiled** 80g (3oz) | 18 | 0.4 | 0.1 | tr | 0.2 | 1.4 | 2.3 | 1.9 | A, Fol, C |
| **Garlic** 3 cloves (10g) | 9 | 0.1 | tr | tr | tr | 0.7 | 1.5 | 0.4 | |
| **Jerusalem artichoke, boiled** 80g (3oz) | 33 | 0.1 | tr | tr | tr | 1.3 | 8.5 | 2.8 | K |
| **Kale** 100g (3½oz) | 33 | 1.6 | 0.2 | 0.1 | 0.9 | 3.4 | 1.4 | 3.0 | A, C / S |
| **Leeks** 100g (3½oz) | 22 | 0.5 | 0.1 | tr | 0.3 | 1.6 | 2.9 | 2.2 | $B_1$, $B_6$, Fol, C |
| **Lettuce, cos** 100g (3½oz) | 16 | 0.6 | 0.1 | tr | tr | 1.0 | 1.7 | 1.2 | A, $B_1$, Fol, C |

| | Cal (kcal) | Total fat (g) | Sat. fat (g) | Mono. fat (g) | Poly. fat (g) | Protein (g) | Carb. (g) | Fibre (g) | Useful source Vits / Mins |
|---|---|---|---|---|---|---|---|---|---|
| **Lettuce, iceberg** 100g (3½oz) | 13 | 0.3 | tr | tr | tr | 0.7 | 1.9 | 0.6 | C |
| **Mushrooms** 100g (3½oz) | 13 | 0.5 | 0.1 | tr | 0.3 | 1.8 | 0.4 | 1.1 | $B_1$, $B_2$, $B_6$, Fol, Nia, Pant / Cu, Fe, K, P |
| **Mushrooms, dried** 10g (⅓oz) | 28 | 0.2 | tr | tr | tr | 1.0 | 6.0 | tr | |
| **Mushrooms, fried in butter** 100g (3½oz) | 157 | 16.2 | 10.7 | 3.9 | 0.5 | 2.4 | 0.3 | 1.5 | $B_1$, $B_6$, Nia / Cu, K, P |
| **Mushrooms, shiitake, cooked** 100g (3½oz) | 55 | 0.2 | 0.1 | 0.1 | tr | 1.6 | 12.3 | tr | $B_2$ |
| **Mustard and cress** 1 level tbsp | 1.0 | 0 | 0 | 0 | 0 | 0.1 | tr | tr | |
| **Okra** 100g (3½oz) | 31 | 1.0 | 0.3 | 0.1 | 0.3 | 2.8 | 3.0 | 4.0 | A, $B_1$, $B_2$, $B_6$, Fol, C / Ca, Cu, K, Mg |
| **Okra, boiled** 80g (3oz) | 22 | 0.7 | 0.2 | 0.1 | 0.2 | 2.0 | 2.2 | 2.9 | $B_6$, Fol, C |
| **Olives, black** 1 medium | 5.0 | 0.4 | 0.1 | 0.3 | 0 | 0 | 0.3 | 0.1 | |
| **Onion** 100g (3½oz) | 36 | 0.2 | tr | tr | 0.1 | 1.2 | 7.9 | 1.4 | C |
| **Onion, fried in corn oil** 80g (3oz) | 164 | 11 | 1.4 | 2.8 | 6.5 | 2.3 | 14 | 3.0 | |
| **Pak choi** 100g (3½oz) | 25 | 0.8 | 0.1 | 0.1 | 0.5 | 2.8 | 1.6 | 2.1 | A, $B_1$, Fol, C |
| **Parsley** 100g (3½oz) | 34 | 1.3 | tr | tr | tr | 3.0 | 2.7 | 5.0 | A, C |
| **Parsnip** 100g (3½oz) | 64 | 1.1 | 0.2 | 0.5 | 0.2 | 1.8 | 12.5 | 4.6 | $B_1$, $B_6$, Fol, C / K, P |
| **Parsnip, boiled** 80g (3oz) | 66 | 1.2 | 0.2 | 0.5 | 0.2 | 1.6 | 12.9 | 4.7 | Fol, C / P |
| **Peas, frozen, boiled** 80g (3oz) | 55 | 0.7 | 0.2 | 0.1 | 0.4 | 4.8 | 7.8 | 4.1 | $B_1$, Fol, C / P |
| **Pepper, red** 100g (3½oz) | 32 | 0.4 | 0.1 | tr | 0.2 | 1.0 | 6.4 | 1.6 | A, $B_6$, C |
| **Pumpkin, boiled** 80g (3oz) | 10 | 0.2 | 0.1 | 0 | 0 | 0.5 | 1.7 | 0.9 | A, $B_1$, C |
| **Radicchio** 30g (1oz) | 5.0 | 0.1 | 0 | 0 | 0 | 0.3 | 0.9 | 0.2 | C |

| | Cal (kcal) | Total fat (g) | Sat. fat (g) | Mono. fat (g) | Poly. fat (g) | Protein (g) | Carb. (g) | Fibre (g) | Useful source Vitamins/Minerals |
|---|---|---|---|---|---|---|---|---|---|
| **Radish, red** 1 radish (8g) | 1.0 | 0 | 0 | 0 | 0 | 0.1 | 0.2 | 0.1 | C |
| **Radish, white (mooli)** 100g (3½oz) | 15 | 0.1 | tr | tr | tr | 0.8 | 2.9 | tr | C |
| **Rocket** 30g (1oz) | 4.0 | 0.1 | tr | tr | tr | 0.2 | 0.5 | 0.3 | C |
| **Runner beans** 100g (3½oz) | 22 | 0.4 | 0.1 | tr | 0.2 | 1.6 | 3.2 | 2.0 | A, Fol, C |
| **Runner beans, boiled** 80g (3oz) | 14 | 0.4 | 0.1 | tr | 0.2 | 1.0 | 1.8 | 1.5 | A, Fol, C |
| **Salsify** 100g (3½oz) | 27 | 0.3 | tr | tr | tr | 1.3 | 10.5 | 3.2 | $B_2$, Fol |
| **Seaweed, nori (dried)** 28g (1oz) | 38 | 0.4 | 0.1 | 0 | 0.2 | 8.6 | 0 | 12.4 | $B_{12}$ / Cu, Fe, I, P |
| **Seaweed, wakame** 100g (3½oz) | 71 | 2.4 | 0.3 | 0.1 | 1.5 | 12 | tr | 47 | $B_{12}$ / I |
| **Shallots** 100g (3½oz) | 20 | 0.2 | 0 | 0 | 0.1 | 1.5 | 3.3 | 1.4 | $B_6$, C |
| **Spinach** 100g (3½oz) | 25 | 0.8 | 0.1 | 0.1 | 0.5 | 2.8 | 1.6 | 2.1 | A, $B_6$, Fol, C, Vit K / Ca, Fe, K, Mg |
| **Spinach, boiled** 80g (3oz) | 17 | 0.6 | 0.1 | 0.1 | 0.4 | 2.5 | 0.4 | 1.7 | A, $B_6$, Fol, C, Vit K / Ca, Fe, K, Mg |
| **Spring onion** 1 onion (10g) | 2.0 | 0.1 | tr | tr | 0 | 0.2 | 0.3 | 0.1 | |
| **Squash, acorn** 100g (3½oz) | 40 | 0.1 | tr | 0 | 0.1 | 0.8 | 9.0 | 2.3 | A, $B_1$, $B_6$, Fol, C / K, P |
| **Squash, butternut** 100g (3½oz) | 36 | 0.1 | tr | 0 | 0 | 1.1 | 8.3 | 1.6 | A, $B_1$, $B_6$, Fol, C / K, P |
| **Swede** 100g (3½oz) | 24 | 0.3 | tr | tr | 0.2 | 0.7 | 5.0 | 1.9 | $B_1$, $B_6$, Fol, C |
| **Swede, boiled** 80g (3oz) | 9.0 | 0.1 | 0 | 0 | 0 | 0.2 | 1.8 | 0.6 | $B_1$, C |
| **Sweetcorn, boiled** 1 corn-on-the-cob | 135 | 2.5 | 0.3 | 0.8 | 1.0 | 5.1 | 24.8 | 2.3 | $B_1$, $B_6$, Fol, Nia, C / Mg, P |
| **Sweetcorn, canned** 100g (3½oz) | 66 | 0.8 | 0.1 | 0.2 | 0.4 | 2.1 | 15.2 | 1.6 | $B_6$, Fol / P |
| **Sweetcorn, kernels** 100g (3½oz) | 93 | 1.8 | 0.2 | 0.5 | 0.7 | 3.4 | 17 | 1.5 | $B_1$, $B_6$, Fol, Nia, C / Mg, P |

| | Cal (kcal) | Total fat (g) | Sat. fat (g) | Mono. fat (g) | Poly. fat (g) | Protein (g) | Carb. (g) | Fibre (g) | Useful source Vitamins/Minerals |
|---|---|---|---|---|---|---|---|---|---|
| **Sweetcorn, baby, canned** 100g (3½oz) | 23 | 0.4 | tr | tr | tr | 2.9 | 2.0 | 1.5 | $B_6$, Fol |
| **Sweet potato** 100g (3½oz) | 87 | 0.3 | 0 | 0 | 0.1 | 1.2 | 21.3 | 2.4 | A, $B_1$, $B_6$, C, E / K |
| **Sweet potato, baked** 100g (3½oz) | 115 | 0.4 | 0.2 | 0 | 0.1 | 1.6 | 27.9 | 3.3 | A, $B_1$, $B_6$, C, E / Cu, P |
| **Tomato** 1 tomato (85g) | 14 | 0.3 | 0.1 | 0.1 | 0.2 | 0.6 | 2.6 | 0.8 | A, $B_6$, C |
| **Tomato, canned** 100g (3½oz) | 16 | 0.1 | tr | tr | tr | 1.0 | 3.0 | 0.7 | $B_6$, C |
| **Tomato, sun-dried, in oil** 100g (3½oz) | 495 | 51 | 6.7 | 15 | 27 | 3.3 | 5.0 | tr | A / Cu, Fe, Zn |
| **Turnip** 100g (3½oz) | 23 | 0.3 | tr | tr | 0.2 | 0.9 | 4.7 | 2.4 | $B_6$, C / S |
| **Turnip, boiled** 80g (3oz) | 10 | 0 | 0 | 0 | 0.1 | 2.2 | 0.2 | tr | C |
| **Water chestnuts, canned** 100g (3½oz) | 31 | 0 | 0 | 0 | 0 | 0.9 | 7.4 | tr | |
| **Watercress** 100g (3½oz) | 22 | 1.0 | 0.3 | 0.1 | 0.4 | 3.0 | 0.4 | 1.5 | A, $B_1$, $B_6$, C / Ca, Fe |

## FRUITS

| | Cal (kcal) | Total fat (g) | Sat. fat (g) | Mono. fat (g) | Poly. fat (g) | Protein (g) | Carb. (g) | Fibre (g) | Useful source Vitamins/Minerals |
|---|---|---|---|---|---|---|---|---|---|
| **Apple, with skin** 1 medium (100g) | 47 | 0.1 | 0 | 0 | 0 | 0.4 | 11.8 | 1.8 | C |
| **Apple sauce, unsweetened** 100g (3½oz) | 64 | 0.1 | 0 | 0 | 0 | 0.2 | 16.7 | 1.1 | C |
| **Apricot** 1 medium (40g) | 12 | 0 | 0 | 0 | 0 | 0.4 | 2.9 | 0.7 | A |
| **Apricots, canned in juice** 100g (3½oz) | 34 | 0.1 | 0 | 0 | 0 | 0.5 | 8.4 | 0.9 | A |
| **Apricots, dried** 100g (3½oz) | 158 | 0.6 | tr | tr | tr | 4.0 | 36 | 6.0 | A, $B_2$, $B_6$, Nia / Ca, Cu, Fe, K, Mg |
| **Banana** 1 medium (100g) | 95 | 0.3 | 0.1 | 0 | 0.1 | 1.2 | 23 | 1.1 | $B_6$, C / K, Mg |
| **Blackberries** 100g (3½oz) | 25 | 0.2 | tr | 0 | 0.1 | 0.9 | 5.1 | 3.1 | Fol, C |
| **Blueberries** 100g (3½oz) | 55 | 0.4 | tr | tr | 0 | 0.5 | 12 | 2.5 | C, E |

| | Cal (kcal) | Total fat (g) | Sat. fat (g) | Mono. fat (g) | Poly. fat (g) | Protein (g) | Carb. (g) | Fibre (g) | Useful source Vitamins/Minerals |
|---|---|---|---|---|---|---|---|---|---|
| Cantaloupe melon 100g (3½oz) | 56 | 0.4 | 0.1 | 0 | 0.2 | 1.4 | 13.4 | 1.3 | A, B₆, C |
| Cherries 100g (3½oz) | 48 | 0.1 | tr | 0 | 0 | 0.9 | 11.5 | 0.9 | A, C |
| Cherries, canned in syrup 100g (3½oz) | 71 | 0 | 0 | 0 | 0 | 0.5 | 18.5 | 0.6 | A, C |
| Cranberries 100g (3½oz) | 15 | 0.1 | 0 | 0 | 0.1 | 0.4 | 3.0 | 3.0 | B₆, C |
| Currants, black 80g (3oz) | 28 | 0 | 0 | 0 | 0 | 0.9 | 6.6 | 3.6 | C |
| Currants, red and white 100g (3½oz) | 21 | 0 | 0 | 0 | 0 | 1.1 | 4.4 | 3.0 | C |
| Dates, dried 100g (3½oz) | 270 | 0.2 | 0.1 | 0.1 | 0 | 3.3 | 68 | 4.0 | B₆, Nia / Cu, K, Mg |
| Figs 100g (3½oz) | 43 | 0.3 | 0.1 | 0.1 | 0.1 | 1.3 | 9.6 | 1.6 | B₆ |
| Figs, dried 100g (3½oz) | 227 | 1.6 | 0.1 | tr | tr | 3.6 | 53 | 7.5 | B₆ / Ca, Cu, Fe, K, Mg, P, Zn |
| Fruit cocktail, canned in juice 100g (3½oz) | 29 | 0 | 0 | 0 | 0 | 0.4 | 7.0 | 1.0 | C |
| Gooseberries, dessert 100g (3½oz) | 40 | 0.3 | 0.1 | 0.1 | 0.1 | 0.7 | 9.0 | 2.4 | C |
| Grapefruit, pink and red ½ medium (80g) | 24 | 0.1 | 0 | 0 | 0 | 0.6 | 5.4 | 1.0 | Fol, C |
| Grapes 100g (3½oz) | 60 | 0.1 | 0.1 | 0 | 0.1 | 0.4 | 15.8 | 0.7 | B₆, Vit K / Cr, Cu |
| Guava 1 medium | 46 | 0.5 | 0.2 | 0 | 0.2 | 0.7 | 10.7 | 3.0 | C |
| Honeydew melon 100g (3½oz) | 28 | 0.1 | 0 | 0 | 0.1 | 0.6 | 6.6 | 0.6 | |
| Kiwi fruit 1 medium (60g) | 25 | 0.2 | 0 | 0 | 0 | 0.6 | 5.5 | 1.0 | B₆, C |
| Kumquat 1 medium | 12 | 0 | 0 | 0 | 0 | 0.2 | 3.1 | 0.5 | C |
| Lemon 1 medium | 17 | 0.2 | 0 | 0 | 0.1 | 0.6 | 5.4 | 1.0 | C |
| Lime 1 medium | 20 | 0.1 | 0 | 0 | 0 | 0.5 | 7.1 | 1.5 | C |

| | Cal (kcal) | Total fat (g) | Sat. fat (g) | Mono. fat (g) | Poly. fat (g) | Protein (g) | Carb. (g) | Fibre (g) | Useful source Vitamins/Minerals |
|---|---|---|---|---|---|---|---|---|---|
| **Loganberries** 100g (3½oz) | 17 | 0 | 0 | 0 | 0 | 1.1 | 3.4 | 2.5 | C |
| **Lychees** 100g (3½oz) | 58 | 0.1 | tr | tr | tr | 0.9 | 14.3 | 0.7 | C |
| **Lychees, canned in syrup** 100g (3½oz) | 68 | 0 | 0 | 0 | 0 | 0.4 | 17.7 | 0.5 | C |
| **Mandarins, canned in juice** 100g (3½oz) | 32 | 0 | 0 | 0 | 0 | 0.7 | 7.7 | 0.3 | C |
| **Mandarins, canned in syrup** 100g (3½oz) | 52 | 0 | 0 | 0 | 0 | 0.5 | 13 | 0.2 | C |
| **Mango** 1 medium (150g) | 86 | 0.3 | 0.1 | 0 | 0 | 1.1 | 21 | 3.9 | A, $B_6$, C / Cu |
| **Mango, canned in syrup** 100g (3½oz) | 77 | 0 | 0 | 0 | 0 | 0.3 | 20 | 0.7 | A, C / Cu |
| **Nectarine** 1 medium (100g) | 36 | 0.1 | 0 | 0 | 0 | 1.2 | 8.0 | 1.1 | A, C |
| **Orange** 1 medium (160g) | 60 | 0.1 | 0 | 0 | 0 | 1.8 | 13.6 | 2.7 | $B_1$, Fol, C / Ca, K |
| **Papaya** 150g (5oz) | 41 | 0.1 | 0 | 0 | 0 | 1.4 | 8.3 | 2.3 | A, C / K, Mg |
| **Passion fruit (granadilla)** 1 medium (15g) | 5.0 | 0.1 | 0 | 0 | 0.1 | 0.4 | 0.9 | 0.5 | |
| **Peach** 1 medium (110g) | 37 | 0.1 | 0 | 0 | 0 | 1.1 | 8.4 | 1.7 | A, C |
| **Peach, canned in juice** 100g (3½oz) | 39 | 0 | 0 | 0 | 0 | 0.6 | 9.7 | 0.8 | A, C |
| **Pear** 1 medium (150g) | 60 | 0.1 | 0 | 0.1 | 0 | 0.5 | 15 | 3.3 | C |
| **Pear, canned in juice** 100g (3½oz) | 33 | 0 | 0 | 0 | 0 | 0.3 | 8.5 | 1.4 | C |
| **Pineapple** 100g (3½oz) | 52 | 0 | 0 | 0 | 0 | 0.4 | 13 | 0.5 | $B_6$, C |
| **Pineapple, canned in juice** 100g (3½oz) | 47 | 0 | 0 | 0 | 0 | 0.3 | 12 | 0.5 | C |
| **Pineapple, canned in syrup** 100g (3½oz) | 64 | 0 | 0 | 0 | 0 | 0.5 | 16.5 | 0.7 | C |
| **Plantain** 100g (3½oz) | 117 | 0.3 | 0.1 | 0 | 0.1 | 0.1 | 29 | 1.3 | A, $B_6$, Fol, C / K, Mg |

| | Cal (kcal) | Total fat (g) | Sat. fat (g) | Mono. fat (g) | Poly. fat (g) | Protein (g) | Carb. (g) | Fibre (g) | Useful source Vitamins/Minerals |
|---|---|---|---|---|---|---|---|---|---|
| **Plum** 1 medium (60g) | 22 | 0.1 | 0 | 0 | 0 | 0.4 | 5.3 | 1.0 | |
| **Pomegranate** 1 medium (150g) | 77 | 0.3 | 0.1 | 0.1 | 0.1 | 2.0 | 17.7 | 5.0 | $B_6$, C / Cu, K |
| **Prunes** 100g (3½oz) | 141 | 0.4 | 0 | tr | tr | 2.5 | 34 | 6.0 | A, $B_2$, $B_6$, Nia / Cu, K, Mg, P |
| **Quince** 100g (3½oz) | 26 | 0.1 | 0 | 0 | 0 | 0.3 | 6.3 | tr | C |
| **Raisins, seedless** 100g (3½oz) | 272 | 0.5 | 0.1 | 0 | 0.1 | 2.1 | 69 | 2.0 | $B_1$, $B_6$ / Cu, Fe, K, Mg, P, Se |
| **Raspberries** 100g (3½oz) | 25 | 0.3 | 0.1 | 0.1 | 0.1 | 1.4 | 4.6 | 2.5 | $B_6$, Fol, C |
| **Raspberries, canned in syrup** 100g (3½oz) | 88 | 0.1 | 0 | 0 | 0.1 | 0.6 | 22.5 | 1.4 | C |
| **Raspberries, frozen** 100g (3½oz) | 25 | 0.3 | 0.1 | 0 | 0.1 | 1.4 | 4.6 | 2.5 | $B_6$, Fol, C |
| **Rhubarb** 100g (3½oz) | 7.0 | 0.1 | 0 | 0 | 0.1 | 0.8 | 0.8 | 1.4 | C / Ca |
| **Rhubarb, stewed without sugar** 100g (3½oz) | 7.0 | 0.1 | 0 | 0 | 0 | 0.9 | 0.7 | 1.3 | Ca |
| **Satsuma** 1 small (50g) | 18 | 0.1 | tr | 0 | 0 | 0.5 | 4.3 | 0.7 | C |
| **Strawberries** 100g (3½oz) | 27 | 0.1 | 0 | 0 | 0 | 0.8 | 6.0 | 1.1 | C |
| **Tangerine** 1 medium (70g) | 25 | 0.1 | 0 | 0 | 0 | 0.6 | 5.6 | 0.9 | A, C |
| **Watermelon** 100g (3½oz) | 31 | 0.3 | 0.1 | 0.1 | 0.1 | 0.5 | 7.0 | 0.1 | A, $B_6$, C |
| **DAIRY FOODS** | | | | | | | | | |
| **Brie** 28g (1oz) | 96 | 7.8 | 5.1 | 1.9 | 0.2 | 5.9 | 0.1 | 0 | A, $B_2$, $B_{12}$ / Ca, P |
| **Buttermilk** 100ml (3½floz) | 37 | 0.5 | 0.3 | 0.1 | 0.1 | 3.4 | 5.0 | 0 | $B_2$ / Ca, P |
| **Camembert** 28g (1oz) | 81 | 6.9 | 4.3 | 2.0 | 0.2 | 5.6 | 0.1 | 0 | A, $B_2$, $B_{12}$ / Ca, P |
| **Cheddar cheese** 28g (1oz) | 114 | 9.4 | 6.0 | 2.7 | 0.3 | 7.1 | 0.4 | 0 | A, $B_2$, $B_{12}$ / Ca, P |

| | Cal (kcal) | Total fat (g) | Sat. fat (g) | Mono. fat (g) | Poly. fat (g) | Protein (g) | Carb. (g) | Fibre (g) | Useful source Vitamins/Minerals |
|---|---|---|---|---|---|---|---|---|---|
| **Cheddar cheese, half-fat** 28g (1oz) | 76 | 4.4 | 2.8 | 1.3 | 0.1 | 9.2 | 0.2 | 0 | A, $B_2$, $B_{12}$ / Ca, P |
| **Cheshire cheese** 28g (1oz) | 106 | 8.7 | 5.5 | 2.5 | 0.2 | 6.6 | tr | 0 | A, $B_2$, $B_{12}$ / Ca, P |
| **Cheshire cheese, half-fat** 28g (1oz) | 75 | 4.3 | 2.7 | 1.3 | 0.1 | 9.2 | tr | 0 | A, $B_2$, $B_{12}$ / Ca, P |
| **Cottage cheese, plain** 28g (1oz) | 28 | 1.1 | 0.6 | 0.3 | 0 | 3.5 | 0.9 | 0 | $B_{12}$ |
| **Cottage cheese, plain** 100g (3½oz) | 101 | 3.9 | 2.3 | 1.2 | 0.1 | 12.6 | 3.1 | 0 | $B_{12}$ |
| **Cottage cheese, reduced-fat** 28g (1oz) | 22 | 0.4 | 0.3 | 0.1 | 0 | 3.7 | 0.9 | 0 | $B_{12}$ |
| **Cottage cheese, reduced-fat** 100g (3½oz) | 79 | 1.5 | 1.0 | 0.4 | 0 | 13.3 | 3.3 | 0 | $B_{12}$ |
| **Cream, double** 100ml (3½floz) | 496 | 54 | 33 | 13.8 | 1.9 | 1.6 | 1.7 | 0 | $B_{12}$ |
| **Cream, single** 100ml (3½floz) | 193 | 19 | 12.2 | 5.0 | 0.6 | 3.3 | 2.2 | 0 | $B_{12}$ |
| **Cream cheese** 28g (1oz) | 123 | 13.3 | 8.3 | 3.8 | 0.4 | 0.9 | 0 | 0 | $B_{12}$ |
| **Cream cheese, reduced-fat** 28g (1oz) | 50 | 3.7 | 2.8 | 0.5 | 0.5 | 0.2 | 0.9 | 0 | $B_{12}$ |
| **Crème fraîche** 100g (3½oz) | 378 | 40 | 27 | 8.6 | 1.1 | 2.2 | 2.4 | 0 | $B_2$ |
| **Crème fraîche, half-fat** 100g (3½oz) | 162 | 15 | 10.2 | 3.2 | 0.4 | 2.7 | 4.4 | 0 | $B_2$ |
| **Danish blue cheese** 28g (1oz) | 96 | 8.1 | 5.4 | 2.1 | 0.3 | 5.7 | 0 | 0 | A, $B_2$, $B_{12}$ / Ca, P |
| **Edam cheese** 28g (1oz) | 95 | 6.9 | 4.4 | 1.5 | 0.1 | 7.5 | 0 | 0 | A, $B_2$, / Ca, P |
| **Emmenthal cheese** 28g (1oz) | 107 | 8.3 | 5.0 | 2.4 | 0.3 | 8.0 | 0 | 0 | A, $B_2$, $B_{12}$ / Ca, P, Zn |
| **Evaporated milk, light** 100ml (3½floz) | 107 | 4.1 | 2.5 | 1.1 | 0.1 | 7.8 | 10.3 | 0 | $B_2$ |
| **Evaporated milk, whole milk** 100ml (3½floz) | 151 | 9.4 | 5.9 | 2.7 | 0.3 | 8.4 | 8.5 | 0 | $B_2$ |
| **Feta cheese** 28g (1oz) | 70 | 5.7 | 3.8 | 1.1 | 0.2 | 4.4 | 0.4 | 0 | A, $B_2$, $B_{12}$ / Ca, P |

| | Cal (kcal) | Total fat (g) | Sat. fat (g) | Mono. fat (g) | Poly. fat (g) | Protein (g) | Carb. (g) | Fibre (g) | Useful source Vitamins/Minerals |
|---|---|---|---|---|---|---|---|---|---|
| Fontina cheese 28g (1oz) | 110 | 8.8 | 5.4 | 2.5 | 0.5 | 7.3 | 0.4 | 0 | A, $B_2$, $B_{12}$ / Ca, P |
| Fromage frais, fruit 100g (3½oz) | 124 | 5.6 | 3.5 | 1.6 | 0.2 | 5.3 | 13.9 | 0 | $B_1$, $B_2$, $B_{12}$ / Ca, P |
| Fromage frais, plain 100g (3½oz) | 113 | 8.0 | 5.5 | 1.8 | 0.2 | 6.1 | 4.4 | 0 | $B_1$, $B_2$, $B_{12}$ / Ca, P |
| Fromage frais, virtually fat-free, fruit 100g (3½oz) | 50 | 0.2 | 0.1 | 0.1 | 0 | 6.8 | 5.6 | 0.4 | $B_2$, $B_{12}$ / P |
| Fromage frais, virtually fat-free, plain 100g (3½oz) | 49 | 0.1 | 0.1 | 0 | 0 | 7.7 | 4.6 | 0 | $B_2$, $B_{12}$ / P |
| Goat's cheese, hard 28g (1oz) | 90 | 7.2 | 5.0 | 1.7 | 0.3 | 5.9 | 0.3 | 0 | A, $B_2$, $B_{12}$ / Ca, P |
| Goat's milk 100ml (3½floz) | 62 | 3.7 | 2.4 | 0.9 | 0.2 | 3.0 | 4.4 | 0 | A, $B_2$, $B_{12}$ / Ca, P |
| Gouda cheese 28g (1oz) | 106 | 8.6 | 5.7 | 2.1 | 0.3 | 7.1 | 0 | 0 | A, $B_{12}$ / Ca, P, Zn |
| Gruyère cheese 28g (1oz) | 117 | 9.2 | 5.4 | 2.8 | 0.5 | 8.5 | tr | 0 | A, $B_{12}$ / Ca, P, Zn |
| Lancashire cheese 28g (1oz) | 104 | 8.7 | 5.5 | 2.5 | 0 | 6.5 | 0 | 0 | $B_{12}$ / Ca, P |
| Limburger cheese 28g (1oz) | 93 | 7.7 | 4.7 | 2.4 | 0.1 | 5.7 | 0.1 | 0 | A, $B_2$, $B_{12}$ / Ca |
| Milk, Channel Island 100ml (3½floz) | 78 | 5.1 | 3.3 | 1.3 | 0.1 | 3.6 | 4.8 | 0 | $B_2$, $B_{12}$ / Ca, P |
| Milk, semi-skimmed 100ml (3½floz) | 46 | 1.7 | 1.1 | 0.4 | 0 | 3.4 | 4.7 | 0 | $B_2$, $B_{12}$ / Ca, P |
| Milk, skimmed 100ml (3½floz) | 32 | 0.3 | 0.1 | 0.1 | 0 | 3.4 | 4.4 | 0 | $B_2$, $B_{12}$ / Ca, P |
| Milk, whole/full-fat 100ml (3½floz) | 66 | 3.9 | 2.5 | 1.0 | 0.1 | 3.3 | 4.5 | 0 | $B_2$, $B_{12}$ / Ca, P |
| Monterey Jack cheese 28g (1oz) | 106 | 8.6 | 5.4 | 2.5 | 0.3 | 6.9 | 0.2 | 0 | A, $B_2$, $B_{12}$ / Ca, P |
| Mozzarella cheese 28g (1oz) | 80 | 6.1 | 3.7 | 1.9 | 0.2 | 5.5 | 0.6 | 0 | A, $B_2$, $B_{12}$ / Ca, P |
| Mozzarella cheese, reduced-fat 28g (1oz) | 72 | 4.5 | 2.9 | 1.3 | 0.1 | 6.9 | 0.8 | 0 | A, $B_2$, $B_{12}$ / Ca, P |
| Muenster cheese 28g (1oz) | 104 | 8.5 | 5.4 | 2.5 | 0.2 | 6.6 | 0.3 | 0 | A, $B_2$, $B_{12}$ / Ca, P |

| | Cal (kcal) | Cal (kcal) | Total fat (g) | Sat. fat (g) | Mono. fat (g) | Poly. fat (g) | Protein (g) | Carb. (g) | Fibre (g) | Useful source Vitamins/Minerals |
|---|---|---|---|---|---|---|---|---|---|---|
| **Neufchatel cheese** 28g (1oz) | 74 | 6.6 | 4.2 | 1.9 | 0.2 | | 2.8 | 0.8 | 0 | A, $B_2$, $B_{12}$ / Ca, P |
| **Parmesan cheese** 28g (1oz) | 111 | 7.3 | 4.7 | 2.1 | 0.2 | | 10.1 | 0.9 | 0 | $B_2$, $B_{12}$ / Ca, P |
| **Pecorino cheese** 28g (1oz) | 110 | 7.6 | 4.9 | 2.2 | 0.2 | | 9.0 | 1.0 | 0 | $B_2$, $B_{12}$ / Ca, P |
| **Port du Salut cheese** 28g (1oz) | 100 | 8.0 | 4.7 | 2.6 | 0.2 | | 6.7 | 0.2 | 0 | A, $B_2$, $B_{12}$ / Ca |
| **Provolone cheese** 28g (1oz) | 100 | 7.5 | 4.8 | 2.1 | 0.2 | | 7.3 | 0.6 | 0 | A, $B_2$, $B_{12}$ / Ca, P |
| **Red Leicester cheese** 28g (1oz) | 112 | 9.4 | 5.9 | 2.7 | 0.3 | | 6.8 | 0 | 0 | A, $B_2$, $B_{12}$ / Ca, P |
| **Ricotta cheese** 28g (1oz) | 40 | 3.0 | 1.9 | 0.8 | 0.1 | | 2.6 | 0.6 | 0 | A, $B_2$, $B_{12}$ / Ca, P |
| **Roquefort cheese** 28g (1oz) | 105 | 8.7 | 5.5 | 2.4 | 0.4 | | 6.1 | 0.6 | 0 | A, $B_2$, $B_{12}$ / Ca, P |
| **Stilton cheese** 28g (1oz) | 115 | 9.5 | 6.4 | 2.6 | 0.3 | | 6.6 | 0 | 0 | A, $B_2$, $B_{12}$ / Ca, P |
| **Tilsit cheese** 28g (1oz) | 96 | 7.4 | 4.8 | 2.0 | 0.2 | | 6.9 | 0.5 | 0 | A, $B_2$, $B_{12}$ / Ca, P |
| **Wensleydale cheese** 28g (1oz) | 106 | 8.8 | 5.5 | 2.3 | 0.3 | | 6.5 | 0 | 0 | $B_{12}$ / P, Zn |
| **Yogurt, Greek, plain** 100g (3½oz) | 92 | 6.0 | 4.2 | 1.6 | 0.2 | | 4.8 | 5.0 | 0 | $B_2$, $B_{12}$ / Ca, P |
| **Yogurt, low-fat, fruit** 100g (3½oz) | 78 | 1.1 | 0.8 | 0.3 | 0 | | 4.2 | 13.7 | 0 | $B_2$, $B_{12}$ / Ca, P |
| **Yogurt, low-fat, plain** 100g (3½oz) | 56 | 1.0 | 0.7 | 0.2 | 0 | | 4.8 | 7.4 | 0 | $B_2$, $B_{12}$ / Ca, P |
| **Yogurt, whole-milk, fruit** 100g (3½oz) | 109 | 3.0 | 2.0 | 0.7 | 0.1 | | 4.0 | 17.7 | tr | $B_2$, $B_{12}$ / Ca, P |
| **Yogurt, whole-milk, plain** 100g (3½oz) | 79 | 3.0 | 1.7 | 0.9 | 0.2 | | 5.7 | 7.8 | 0 | $B_2$, $B_{12}$ / Ca, P |

**EGGS**

| | Cal (kcal) | Cal (kcal) | Total fat (g) | Sat. fat (g) | Mono. fat (g) | Poly. fat (g) | Protein (g) | Carb. (g) | Fibre (g) | Useful source Vitamins/Minerals |
|---|---|---|---|---|---|---|---|---|---|---|
| **Egg, duck** 1 egg (75g) | 122 | 8.8 | 2.2 | 3.7 | 1.5 | | 10.7 | tr | 0 | A, $B_1$, $B_{12}$ / Fe, P, Zn |
| **Egg, hen's** 1 medium (65g) | 98 | 7.0 | 2.0 | 2.9 | 1.1 | | 8.1 | 0 | 0 | A, $B_2$, $B_6$, $B_{12}$ / P, Zn |

| | Cal (kcal) | Total fat (g) | Sat. fat (g) | Mono. fat (g) | Poly. fat (g) | Protein (g) | Carb. (g) | Fibre (g) | Useful source Vitamins/Minerals |
|---|---|---|---|---|---|---|---|---|---|
| **Egg, hen's, white** white of 1 large egg | 17 | 0 | 0 | 0 | 0 | 3.5 | tr | 0 | $B_2$ |
| **Egg, hen's, yolk** yolk of 1 large egg | 61 | 5.2 | 1.6 | 2.4 | 0.6 | 2.8 | tr | 0 | A, $B_2$, $B_6$, $B_{12}$ / P, Zn |
| **Egg, quail** 1 egg | 14 | 1.0 | 0.3 | 0.4 | 0.1 | 1.2 | 0 | 0 | $B_2$ / P |
| **MEAT AND POULTRY** | | | | | | | | | |
| **Beef brisket, lean, braised** 100g (3½oz) | 218 | 10.1 | 3.6 | 4.7 | 0.3 | 29.8 | 0 | 0 | $B_2$, $B_6$, $B_{12}$, Nia / Fe, P, Zn |
| **Beef fillet, lean, grilled** 100g (3½oz) | 188 | 8.0 | 3.6 | 3.2 | 0.5 | 29.0 | 0 | 0 | $B_1$, $B_2$, $B_6$, $B_{12}$, Nia / Fe, P, Se, Zn |
| **Beef mince, lean, grilled** 100g (3½oz) | 244 | 14.3 | 5.5 | 5.7 | 0.5 | 27.0 | 0 | 0 | $B_2$, $B_6$, $B_{12}$, Nia / Fe, P, Zn |
| **Beef sirloin, lean, grilled** 100g (3½oz) | 166 | 6.7 | 3.0 | 2.9 | 0.2 | 26.0 | 0 | 0 | $B_1$, $B_2$, $B_6$, $B_{12}$, Nia / Fe, P, Zn |
| **Boar, wild, roast** 100g (3½oz) | 160 | 4.4 | 1.3 | 1.7 | 0.6 | 28.3 | 0 | 0 | $B_1$, $B_2$, Nia / K, Fe, Zn |
| **Chicken, dark meat no skin, roast** 100g (3½oz) | 205 | 9.7 | 2.7 | 3.6 | 2.3 | 27.4 | 0 | 0 | $B_2$, $B_6$, $B_{12}$, Nia / P, Se, Zn |
| **Chicken, white meat no skin, roast** 100g (3½oz) | 173 | 4.5 | 1.3 | 1.5 | 1.0 | 30.9 | 0 | 0 | $B_2$, $B_6$, Nia / P, Se, Zn |
| **Chicken, white meat with skin, roast** 100g (3½oz) | 222 | 10.8 | 3.0 | 4.3 | 2.3 | 29 | 0 | 0 | $B_2$, $B_6$, Nia / P, Zn |
| **Duck, no skin, roast** 100g (3½oz) | 201 | 11.2 | 4.2 | 3.7 | 1.4 | 23.5 | 0 | 0 | $B_1$, $B_2$, $B_6$, $B_{12}$, Nia / Cu, Fe, P, Se, Zn |
| **Goose, no skin, roast** 100g (3½oz) | 238 | 12.7 | 4.6 | 4.3 | 1.5 | 29 | 0 | 0 | $B_2$, $B_6$, $B_{12}$, Nia / Fe, P, Zn |
| **Guinea fowl, no skin** 100g (3½oz) | 110 | 2.5 | 0.6 | 0.7 | 0.6 | 20.6 | 0 | 0 | $B_2$, $B_6$, $B_{12}$, Nia / P, Zn |
| **Kidney, lamb's, braised** 100g (3½oz) | 137 | 3.6 | 1.2 | 0.8 | 0.7 | 23.6 | 1.0 | 0 | A, $B_2$, $B_6$, $B_{12}$ / Cu, Fe, P, Zn |
| **Lamb leg, lean, roast** 100g (3½oz) | 258 | 16.5 | 6.9 | 7.0 | 1.2 | 25.6 | 0.0 | 0 | $B_2$, $B_6$, $B_{12}$, Nia / Fe, P, Zn |
| **Lamb loin, roast** 100g (3½oz) | 202 | 9.8 | 3.7 | 4.0 | 0.9 | 26.6 | 0 | 0 | $B_2$, $B_6$, $B_{12}$, Nia / Fe, P, Zn |
| **Lamb neck fillet** 100g (3½oz) | 203 | 13.9 | 6.4 | 5.3 | 0.7 | 19.4 | 0 | 0 | $B_1$, $B_2$, $B_6$, $B_{12}$, Nia / P, Zn |

| | Cal (kcal) | Total fat (g) | Sat. fat (g) | Mono. fat (g) | Poly. fat (g) | Protein (g) | Carb. (g) | Fibre (g) | Useful source Vitamins/Minerals |
|---|---|---|---|---|---|---|---|---|---|
| **Lamb shoulder, lean, roast** 100g (3½oz) | 204 | 10.8 | 4.1 | 4.4 | 0.9 | 24.9 | 0 | 0 | $B_2$, $B_6$, $B_{12}$, Nia / Fe, P, Zn |
| **Liver, calf's, braised** 100g (3½oz) | 161 | 4.9 | 1.9 | 0.7 | 1.1 | 24.4 | 3.4 | 0 | A, B vitamins, C / Cu, Fe, P, Zn |
| **Liver, chicken, braised** 100g (3½oz) | 157 | 5.5 | 1.8 | 1.3 | 0.9 | 24.4 | 0.9 | 0 | A, B vitamins, C / Cu, Fe, P, Zn |
| **Liver, lamb's, braised** 100g (3½oz) | 220 | 8.8 | 3.4 | 1.8 | 1.3 | 30.6 | 2.5 | 0 | A, B vitamins, C / Cu, Fe, P, Zn |
| **Pheasant, no skin** 100g (3½oz) | 133 | 3.6 | 1.2 | 1.2 | 0.6 | 20.6 | 0 | 0 | A, $B_2$, $B_6$, $B_{12}$, Nia / Fe, P, Zn |
| **Pigeon, no skin** 100g (3½oz) | 142 | 7.5 | 2.0 | 2.7 | 1.6 | 17.5 | 0 | 0 | $B_1$, $B_2$, $B_6$, $B_{12}$, Nia / Fe, P, Zn |
| **Pork fillet (tenderloin)** 100g (3½oz) | 122 | 4.0 | 1.4 | 1.6 | 0.7 | 21.4 | 0 | 0 | $B_1$, $B_2$, $B_6$, $B_{12}$, Nia / P, Se, Zn |
| **Pork leg, lean, roast** 100g (3½oz) | 211 | 9.4 | 3.3 | 4.5 | 0.8 | 29.4 | 0 | 0 | $B_1$, $B_2$, $B_6$, $B_{12}$, Nia / K, P, Zn |
| **Pork fillet, lean, grilled** 100g (3½oz) | 170 | 4.0 | 1.5 | 1.4 | 0.8 | 33.0 | 0 | 0 | $B_1$, $B_2$, $B_6$, $B_{12}$, Nia / K, P, Zn |
| **Quail, no skin** 100g (3½oz) | 134 | 4.5 | 1.3 | 1.3 | 1.2 | 21.8 | 0 | 0 | $B_1$, $B_2$, $B_6$ / Fe, P, Zn |
| **Rabbit, stewed** 100g (3½oz) | 114 | 3.5 | 1.7 | 0.7 | 0.6 | 29.1 | 0 | 0 | $B_1$, $B_2$, $B_6$, $B_{12}$, Nia / P, Zn |
| **Turkey, dark meat no skin, roast** 100g (3½oz) | 187 | 7.2 | 2.4 | 1.6 | 2.2 | 28.6 | 0 | 0 | $B_2$, $B_6$, $B_{12}$, Nia / P, Zn |
| **Turkey, white meat no skin, roast** 100g (3½oz) | 157 | 3.2 | 1.0 | 0.6 | 0.9 | 29.9 | 0 | 0 | $B_2$, $B_6$, $B_{12}$, Nia / P, Zn |
| **Venison, roast** 100g (3½oz) | 165 | 2.5 | tr | tr | tr | 35 | 0 | 0 | $B_1$, $B_2$, $B_6$, $B_{12}$, Nia / Cu, Fe, P, Zn |
| **MEAT PRODUCTS** | | | | | | | | | |
| **Bacon, lean back, grilled** 2 rashers (50g) | 144 | 10.8 | 4.0 | 4.5 | 1.4 | 11.6 | 0 | 0 | $B_1$, $B_6$, $B_{12}$, Nia / P, Zn |
| **Bacon, streaky, grilled** 3 rashers (60g) | 202 | 16.1 | 5.9 | 6.9 | 2.2 | 14.3 | 0 | 0 | $B_1$, $B_6$, $B_{12}$, Nia / P, Zn |
| **Corned beef** 28g (1oz) | 43 | 1.7 | 0.7 | 0.8 | 0.1 | 6.4 | 0 | 0 | $B_{12}$ / Zn |
| **Frankfurter, beef** 1 sausage (50g) | 135 | 12 | 4.0 | 5.0 | 1.5 | 6.4 | 0.5 | 0 | $B_1$, $B_{12}$ / P |

| | Cal (kcal) | Total fat (g) | Sat. fat (g) | Mono. fat (g) | Poly. fat (g) | Protein (g) | Carb. (g) | Fibre (g) | Useful source Vitamins/Minerals |
|---|---|---|---|---|---|---|---|---|---|
| **Gammon, boiled** 28g (1oz) | 47 | 1.5 | 0.6 | 0.7 | 0.1 | 8.2 | 0 | 0 | $B_1$, $B_6$ / Zn |
| **Ham, lean** 28g (1oz) | 30 | 1.4 | 0.5 | 0.7 | 0.1 | 5.4 | 0.3 | 0 | $B_1$, $B_6$, $B_{12}$, Nia / P |
| **Ham, lean, canned** 28g (1oz) | 34 | 1.4 | 0.5 | 0.6 | 0.2 | 5.2 | 0 | 0 | $B_1$ |
| **Pepperoni** 1 slice (10g) | 30 | 2.6 | 1.0 | 1.3 | 0.3 | 1.3 | 0.2 | 0 | |
| **Salami, beef** 1 slice (10g) | 60 | 4.8 | 2.1 | 2.2 | 0.2 | 3.5 | 0.6 | 0 | |
| **Salami, pork** 1 slice (10g) | 41 | 3.4 | 1.2 | 1.6 | 0.4 | 2.3 | 0.2 | 0 | |
| **Sausage, Italian pork, cooked** 1 sausage | 216 | 17.2 | 6.1 | 8.0 | 2.2 | 13.4 | 1.0 | 0 | $B_1$, $B_2$, Nia / Zn |
| **Sausage, Polish** 28g (1oz) | 92 | 8.1 | 2.9 | 3.8 | 0.9 | 4.0 | 0.5 | 0 | $B_1$, $B_{12}$, Nia |
| **Sausage, pork, cooked** 1 sausage (50g) | 48 | 4.1 | 1.4 | 1.8 | 0.5 | 2.6 | 0.1 | 0 | $B_{12}$ / P |
| **FISH AND SHELLFISH** | | | | | | | | | |
| **Abalone, fried** 80g (3oz) | 161 | 5.8 | 1.4 | 2.3 | 1.4 | 16.7 | 9.4 | 0 | $B_1$, $B_2$, $B_{12}$, Nia / P, K |
| **Anchovies, canned in olive oil** 5 anchovies | 29 | 1.5 | 0.4 | 0.8 | 0.5 | 5.8 | 0 | 0 | $B_{12}$ |
| **Bass, cooked** 80g (3oz) | 105 | 2.5 | 0.6 | 0.7 | 0.9 | 19.3 | 0 | 0 | $B_{12}$ / P |
| **Bream, sea** 100g (3½oz) | 96 | 2.9 | - | - | - | 17.5 | 0 | 0 | $B_6$, $B_{12}$, Nia / P |
| **Carp, cooked** 80g (3oz) | 138 | 6.1 | 1.2 | 2.5 | 1.6 | 19.4 | 0 | 0 | $B_1$, $B_6$, $B_{12}$, Nia / P, Zn |
| **Catfish, cooked** 80g (3oz) | 129 | 6.8 | 1.5 | 3.5 | 1.2 | 15.9 | 0 | 0 | $B_1$, $B_{12}$, Nia, Pant / P, K |
| **Caviar** 128g (4oz) | 26 | 1.5 | 0.2 | 0.3 | 0.5 | 3.1 | 0 | 0 | |
| **Clams, canned in brine, drained** 100g (3½oz) | 65 | 0.5 | 0.2 | 0.1 | 0.1 | 13.6 | 0 | 0 | Nia / Cu, Fe, P, Zn |
| **Cockles, cooked** 100g (3½oz) | 53 | 0.6 | 0.2 | 0.1 | 0.2 | 12 | 0 | 0 | $B_{12}$ / Fe, I, P, Se |

| | Cal (kcal) | Total fat (g) | Sat. fat (g) | Mono. fat (g) | Poly. fat (g) | Protein (g) | Carb. (g) | Fibre (g) | Useful source Vitamins/Minerals |
|---|---|---|---|---|---|---|---|---|---|
| **Cod, poached** 80g (3oz) | 89 | 0.7 | 0.1 | 0.1 | 0.2 | 19.4 | 0 | 0 | $B_6$, $B_{12}$, Nia / I, Se |
| **Coley** 100g (3½oz) | 82 | 1.0 | 0.1 | 0.3 | 0.3 | 18.3 | 0 | 0 | I, P, Se |
| **Crab meat, cooked** 100g (3½oz) | 128 | 5.5 | 0.7 | 1.5 | 1.6 | 19.5 | 0 | 0 | $B_2$, $B_6$ / Cu, Mg, P, Se, Zn |
| **Crab sticks** 100g (3½oz) | 68 | 0.4 | 0.1 | 0.1 | 0.1 | 10 | 6.6 | 0 | $B_{12}$ / Zn |
| **Crayfish, cooked** 80g (3oz) | 75 | 1.0 | 0.2 | 0.2 | 0.3 | 14.3 | 0 | 0 | $B_{12}$, Nia / Cu, P, S, Se, Zn |
| **Flounder, cooked** 80g (3oz) | 100 | 1.3 | 0.3 | 0.2 | 0.5 | 20.5 | 0 | 0 | $B_1$, $B_2$, $B_6$, $B_{12}$, Nia / P, S, Se |
| **Grouper, cooked** 80g (3oz) | 100 | 1.1 | 0.3 | 0.2 | 0.3 | 21.1 | 0 | 0 | A, Pant / K, S |
| **Haddock, cooked** 80g (3oz) | 95 | 0.8 | 0.1 | 0.1 | 0.3 | 20.6 | 0 | 0 | $B_6$, $B_{12}$, Nia / I, K, P, S |
| **Hake** 100g (3½oz) | 92 | 2.2 | 0.3 | 0.6 | 0.5 | 18 | 0 | 0 | P |
| **Halibut, cooked** 80g (3oz) | 119 | 2.5 | 0.4 | 0.8 | 0.8 | 22.7 | 0 | 0 | A, $B_6$, $B_{12}$, Nia / I, K, P, S |
| **Herring, cooked** 80g (3oz) | 173 | 9.9 | 2.2 | 4.1 | 2.3 | 19.6 | 0 | 0 | $B_6$, $B_{12}$, Nia / K, P, S, Zn |
| **Herring, pickled** 28g (1oz) | 59 | 3.1 | 0.4 | 0.3 | 0.8 | 4.7 | 2.8 | 0 | $B_6$ |
| **John dory** 100g (3½oz) | 89 | 1.4 | 0.3 | 0.2 | 0.5 | 19 | 0 | 0 | $B_6$ / P |
| **Kipper** 100g (3½oz) | 111 | 6.2 | 1.0 | 3.3 | 1.3 | 13.8 | 0 | 0 | $B_6$, $B_{12}$, Nia / P |
| **Lobster, cooked** 80g (3oz) | 83 | 0.5 | 0.1 | 0.1 | 0.1 | 17.4 | 1.1 | 0 | $B_{12}$ / Cu, P, S, Se, Zn |
| **Mackerel, cooked** 80g (3oz) | 223 | 15.1 | 3.6 | 6.0 | 3.7 | 20.3 | 0 | 0 | A, $B_1$, $B_2$, $B_6$, $B_{12}$, Nia / I, P, S, Se |
| **Mackerel, smoked** 100g (3½oz) | 354 | 31 | 6.0 | 15 | 6.0 | 19 | 0 | 0 | A, $B_1$, $B_2$, $B_6$, $B_{12}$, Nia / I, P, Se, Zn |
| **Monkfish, cooked** 80g (3oz) | 82 | 1.7 | 0.1 | 0.1 | 0.2 | 15.8 | 0 | 0 | P, S |
| **Mullet, cooked** 80g (3oz) | 128 | 4.1 | 1.2 | 1.2 | 0.8 | 21.1 | 0 | 0 | $B_6$, $B_{12}$, Nia / K, P, Mg, S, Se |

| | Cal (kcal) | Total fat (g) | Sat. fat (g) | Mono. fat (g) | Poly. fat (g) | Protein (g) | Carb. (g) | Fibre (g) | Useful source Vitamins/Minerals |
|---|---|---|---|---|---|---|---|---|---|
| **Mussels, cooked, no shell** 80g (3oz) | 88 | 2.3 | 0.4 | 0.3 | 0.8 | 14.2 | 3.0 | 0 | A, $B_1$, $B_2$, $B_{12}$ / Fe, I, K, P, Se, Zn |
| **Mussels, cooked, in shell** 100g (3½oz) | 28 | 0.7 | 0.1 | 0.1 | 0.3 | 4.5 | 0.9 | 0 | $B_{12}$ / I, Se |
| **Octopus, cooked** 80g (3oz) | 71 | 1.1 | 0.3 | 0.2 | 0.4 | 15 | 0 | 0 | A, $B_6$, $B_{12}$, Nia / Cu, P, S, Se, Zn |
| **Oysters, cooked, no shell** 80g (3oz) | 55 | 1.1 | 0.2 | 0.2 | 0.3 | 9.2 | 2.3 | 0 | A, $B_{12}$, Nia / Cu, Fe, P, S, Se, Zn |
| **Perch, cooked** 80g (3oz) | 100 | 1.0 | 0.2 | 0.2 | 0.4 | 21.1 | 0 | 0 | $B_{12}$, Nia / K, P, S, Zn |
| **Pilchards, canned in tomato sauce** 1 pichard (55g) | 79 | 4.5 | 0.9 | 1.2 | 1.9 | 9.0 | 0.6 | 0 | $B_2$, $B_6$, $B_{12}$, Nia / Ca, P |
| **Pike, cooked** 80g (3oz) | 96 | 0.7 | 0.1 | 0.2 | 0.2 | 21.0 | 0 | 0 | $B_{12}$, Nia / K, P, S |
| **Plaice** 100g (3½oz) | 79 | 1.4 | 0.2 | 0.4 | 0.3 | 16.7 | 0 | 0 | $B_1$, $B_2$, $B_6$, $B_{12}$, Nia / I, P, Se |
| **Prawns, cooked** 80g (3oz) | 85 | 0.8 | 0.2 | 0.2 | 0.2 | 19.6 | 0 | 0 | $B_{12}$, Nia / Cu, Mg, P, S, Se, Zn |
| **Roe, cod's, hard** 28g (1oz) | 7.0 | 0.1 | 0 | 0 | 0.1 | 1.5 | 0.5 | 0 | $B_1$, $B_{12}$, Nia / P |
| **Roe, herring, soft** 28g (1oz) | 25 | 0.7 | 0.1 | 0.2 | 0.2 | 4.7 | 0 | 0 | $B_{12}$ / P |
| **Salmon, grilled** 80g (3oz) | 175 | 10.5 | 2.1 | 3.8 | 3.8 | 18.8 | 0 | 0 | $B_1$, $B_2$, $B_6$, $B_{12}$, Fol, Nia / K, P, S, Se |
| **Salmon, pink, boneless, canned** 80g (3oz) | 130 | 5.6 | 1.1 | 2.0 | 1.6 | 20 | 0 | 0 | $B_2$, $B_6$, $B_{12}$, Nia / I, P, Se |
| **Salmon, red, with bones, canned** 80g (3oz) | 130 | 5.6 | 1.1 | 2.3 | 1.4 | 20 | 0 | 0 | $B_2$, $B_6$, $B_{12}$, Nia / Ca, Mg, P, Se |
| **Salmon, smoked** 80g (3oz) | 121 | 3.8 | 0.7 | 1.5 | 1.1 | 21 | 0 | 0 | $B_6$, $B_{12}$, Nia / P, Se |
| **Sardines, canned in oil** 2 sardines (50g) | 110 | 7.0 | 1.5 | 2.4 | 2.5 | 11.7 | 0 | 0 | $B_2$, $B_6$, $B_{12}$, Nia / Ca, P, S, Se |
| **Sardines, canned in tomato sauce** 2 sardines (50g) | 81 | 5.0 | 1.4 | 1.5 | 1.6 | 8.5 | 0.7 | 0 | $B_2$, $B_{12}$, Nia / Ca, Fe, P, Zn |
| **Sardines, fresh** 1 sardine (25g) | 41 | 2.3 | 0.7 | 0.6 | 0.7 | 5.0 | 0 | 0 | $B_6$, $B_{12}$ / P |
| **Scallops** 100g (3½oz) | 118 | 1.4 | 0.4 | 0.1 | 0.4 | 23 | 3.4 | 0 | $B_{12}$ / P, Se |

| | Cal (kcal) | Total fat (g) | Sat. fat (g) | Mono. fat (g) | Poly. fat (g) | Protein (g) | Carb. (g) | Fibre (g) | Useful source Vitamins/Minerals |
|---|---|---|---|---|---|---|---|---|---|
| **Sea bass, cooked** 80g (3oz) | 105 | 2.2 | 0.6 | 0.5 | 0.8 | 20.1 | 0 | 0 | A, $B_{12}$ / Ca, Fe, P |
| **Shark** 80g (3oz) | 111 | 3.8 | 0.8 | 1.5 | 1.0 | 17.8 | 0 | 0 | $B_1^*$, $B_2$, $B_6$, $B_{12}$, Nia |
| **Skate, grilled** 100g (3½oz) | 79 | 0.5 | 0.1 | 0.1 | 0.2 | 19 | 0 | 0 | $B_1$, $B_2$, $B_6$, $B_{12}$, Nia / I, P |
| **Snapper, red, cooked** 80g (3oz) | 109 | 1.5 | 0.3 | 0.3 | 0.5 | 22.4 | 0 | 0 | $B_6$, $B_{12}$, Nia / I, P, S, Se |
| **Sole, Dover** 80g (3oz) | 76 | 1.5 | 0.3 | 0.2 | 0.5 | 15.4 | 0 | 0 | Nia / Mg, P, S, Se |
| **Squid** 80g (3oz) | 69 | 1.2 | 0.3 | 0.1 | 0.4 | 13.3 | 1.0 | 0 | $B_2$, $B_6$, $B_{12}$, Nia / Cu, I, P, Se, Zn |
| **Swordfish, grilled** 80g (3oz) | 118 | 4.4 | 1.0 | 1.8 | 1.2 | 19.5 | 0 | 0 | $B_1$, $B_2$, $B_6$, $B_{12}$, Nia / P, Se |
| **Trout, cooked** 80g (3oz) | 115 | 3.8 | 0.8 | 1.4 | 1.3 | 20 | 0 | 0 | A, $B_1$, $B_6$, $B_{12}$, Nia / P, Se |
| **Tuna, canned in oil, drained** 80g (3oz) | 161 | 7.7 | 1.3 | 2.0 | 4.1 | 23 | 0 | 0 | $B_6$, $B_{12}$, Nia / Cu, P, Se, Zn |
| **Tuna, canned in water, drained** 80g (3oz) | 84 | 0.5 | 0.2 | 0.1 | 0.2 | 20 | 0 | 0 | $B_6$, $B_{12}$, Nia / P, Se |
| **Tuna steak, fresh** 80g (3oz) | 116 | 3.9 | 1.0 | 1.0 | 1.4 | 20.1 | 0 | 0 | A, $B_6$, $B_{12}$, Nia / Cu, I, P, Se |
| **Turbot, grilled** 80g (3oz) | 104 | 3.2 | 0.8 | 0.7 | 0.6 | 19.3 | 0 | 0 | $B_6$ / Mg, P |
| **Whelks, boiled** 80g (3oz) | 76 | 1.0 | 0.2 | 0.2 | 0.3 | 16 | 0 | 0 | $B_{12}$ / Cu, Fe, Mg, P, Zn |
| **Whitebait, floured and fried** 100g (3½oz) | 525 | 47.5 | - | - | - | 19.5 | 5.3 | 0.2 | Ca, Fe, Mg, P |
| **Whiting, cooked** 80g (3oz) | 78 | 0.8 | 0.1 | 0.3 | 0.2 | 18 | 0 | 0 | $B_2$, $B_6$ / I, P, Se |

## PULSES AND SOYA PRODUCTS

| | Cal (kcal) | Total fat (g) | Sat. fat (g) | Mono. fat (g) | Poly. fat (g) | Protein (g) | Carb. (g) | Fibre (g) | Useful source Vitamins/Minerals |
|---|---|---|---|---|---|---|---|---|---|
| **Aduki beans, boiled** 100g (3½oz) | 123 | 0.2 | 0.1 | tr | tr | 9.3 | 22.5 | 5.5 | $B_1$ / Cu, Fe, K, Mg, P, S, Zn |
| **Baked beans, canned** 100g (3½oz) | 81 | 0.6 | 0.1 | 0.1 | 0.3 | 4.8 | 15.1 | 3.5 | $B_1$, $B_6$, Fol / Mg, P, S |
| **Baked beans, reduced sugar, canned** 100g (3½oz) | 74 | 0.6 | 0.1 | 0.1 | 0.3 | 5.4 | 12.8 | 3.8 | $B_1$, $B_6$, Fol / Mg, P |

| | Cal (kcal) | Total fat (g) | Sat. fat (g) | Mono. fat (g) | Poly. fat (g) | Protein (g) | Carb. (g) | Fibre (g) | Useful source Vitamins/Minerals |
|---|---|---|---|---|---|---|---|---|---|
| **Black-eyed beans, dried** 100g (3½oz) | 311 | 1.6 | 0.5 | 0.1 | 0.7 | 23.5 | 54 | 8.2 | $B_1$, $B_6$, Fol / Cu, Fe, Mg, P, Zn |
| **Black-eyed beans, boiled** 100g (3½oz) | 116 | 0.7 | 0.2 | 0.1 | 0.3 | 8.8 | 19.9 | 3.5 | $B_1$, $B_6$, Fol / P, S, Zn |
| **Broad beans, boiled** 100g (3½oz) | 48 | 0.8 | 0.1 | 0.1 | 0.3 | 5.1 | 5.6 | 5.4 | $B_6$, Fol, Nia, C / Cu, Fe, Mg, P, Zn |
| **Broad beans, canned** 100g (3½oz) | 87 | 0.7 | 0.1 | 0.1 | 0.4 | 8.3 | 12.7 | 5.2 | $B_6$, Fol, Nia / Fe, Mg, P, S, Zn |
| **Butter beans, dried** 100g (3½oz) | 290 | 1.7 | 0.4 | 0.1 | 0.8 | 19.1 | 53 | 16 | Cu, P |
| **Butter beans, boiled** 100g (3½oz) | 103 | 0.6 | 0.1 | 0 | 0.3 | 7.0 | 18 | 5.0 | Cu, P |
| **Chickpeas, canned** 100g (3½oz) | 115 | 2.9 | 0.3 | 0.7 | 1.3 | 7.2 | 16.1 | 4.1 | Fe, P, S, Zn |
| **Chickpeas, dried** 100g (3½oz) | 320 | 5.4 | 0.5 | 1.1 | 2.7 | 21.3 | 49.6 | 10.7 | Fe, P, Zn |
| **Chickpeas, hummus** 100g (3½oz) | 187 | 12.6 | - | - | - | 7.6 | 11.6 | 2.4 | Fe, P, Zn |
| **Haricot beans, dried** 100g (3½oz) | 286 | 1.6 | 0.3 | 0.4 | 0.5 | 21.4 | 49.7 | 17 | $B_1$, $B_6$ / Fe, Mg, P, Zn |
| **Haricot beans, boiled** 100g (3½oz) | 95 | 0.5 | 0.1 | 0.1 | 0.1 | 6.6 | 17.2 | 6.1 | $B_1$, $B_6$ / Fe, Mg, P, Zn |
| **Kidney beans, canned** 100g (3½oz) | 100 | 0.6 | 0.1 | 0.1 | 0.3 | 6.9 | 17.8 | 6.2 | $B_1$, $B_6$ / Fe, P, S, Zn |
| **Kidney beans, dried** 100g (3½oz) | 266 | 1.4 | 0.2 | 0.1 | 0.8 | 22.1 | 44.1 | 15.7 | $B_1$, $B_6$ / Fe, Mg, P, Zn |
| **Lentils, green/brown, dried** 100g (3½oz) | 297 | 1.9 | 0.2 | 0.3 | 0.8 | 24 | 48.8 | 8.9 | $B_1$, $B_6$ / Cu, Fe, Mg, P, Se, Zn |
| **Lentils, green/brown, boiled** 100g (3½oz) | 105 | 0.7 | 0.1 | 0.1 | 0.3 | 8.8 | 16.9 | 3.8 | $B_1$, $B_6$ / Cu, Fe, Mg, P, Se, Zn |
| **Lentils, red, dried** 100g (3½oz) | 318 | 1.3 | 0.2 | 0.2 | 0.5 | 23.8 | 56 | 4.9 | $B_1$, $B_6$, Fol / Cu, Fe, P, Zn |
| **Lentils, red, boiled** 100g (3½oz) | 100 | 0.4 | tr | 0.1 | 0.2 | 7.6 | 17 | 1.9 | $B_1$, $B_6$, Fol / Cu, Fe, P, Zn |
| **Miso** 100ml (3½floz) | 203 | 6.2 | 1.2 | 1.9 | 4.7 | 13.3 | 23.5 | tr | $B_2$, $B_6$, $B_{12}$, Fol / Cu, Fe, Mg, P, S, Zn |
| **Pinto beans, boiled** 100g (3½oz) | 137 | 0.7 | 0.1 | tr | 0.4 | 8.9 | 23 | 12 | $B_1$, $B_6$, Fol / Cu, Fe, K, Mg, P, S, Zn |

| | Cal (kcal) | Total fat (g) | Sat. fat (g) | Mono. fat (g) | Poly. fat (g) | Protein (g) | Carb. (g) | Fibre (g) | Useful source Vitamins/Minerals |
|---|---|---|---|---|---|---|---|---|---|
| **Soya beans, boiled** 100g (3½oz) | 141 | 7.3 | 0.9 | 1.4 | 3.5 | 14 | 5.1 | 6.1 | $B_1$, $B_6$, Fol / Ca, Cu, Fe, K, Mg, P, Zn |
| **Soya milk, sweetened** 100ml (3½floz) | 43 | 2.4 | 0.4 | 0.5 | 1.4 | 3.1 | 2.5 | 0.2 | P |
| **Soya milk, unsweetened** 100ml (3½floz) | 26 | 1.6 | 0.2 | 0.3 | 1.1 | 2.4 | 0.5 | 0.2 | P |
| **Tofu, firm** 100g (3½oz) | 73 | 4.2 | 0.5 | 0.8 | 2.0 | 8.1 | 0.7 | tr | Ca, Cu, P |

**NUTS AND SEEDS**

| | Cal (kcal) | Total fat (g) | Sat. fat (g) | Mono. fat (g) | Poly. fat (g) | Protein (g) | Carb. (g) | Fibre (g) | Useful source Vitamins/Minerals |
|---|---|---|---|---|---|---|---|---|---|
| **Almonds** 100g (3½oz) | 612 | 56 | 4.4 | 38.2 | 10.5 | 21.1 | 6.9 | 7.4 | B vitamins, E / Ca, Cu, Fe, K, Mg, P, S, Zn |
| **Almond milk** 100ml (3½floz) | 51 | 2.3 | 0.6 | 1.3 | 0.4 | 1.0 | 6.6 | 0.3 | |
| **Brazil nuts** 100g (3½oz) | 682 | 68 | 16.4 | 25.8 | 23 | 14.1 | 3.1 | 4.3 | $B_1$, $B_6$ / Ca, Cu, K, Mg, P, S, Se, Zn |
| **Cashew nuts** 100g (3½oz) | 611 | 50.9 | 10.1 | 29.4 | 9.1 | 20.5 | 18.8 | 3.2 | $B_1$, $B_6$ / Cu, Fe, K, Mg, P, S, Se, Zn |
| **Chestnuts, boiled** 100g (3½oz) | 170 | 2.7 | 0.5 | 1.0 | 1.1 | 2.0 | 36.6 | 4.1 | $B_6$ |
| **Coconut, creamed block** 100g (3½oz) | 669 | 68.8 | 59 | 3.9 | 1.6 | 6.0 | 7.0 | tr | Cu |
| **Coconut, desiccated** 100g (3½oz) | 604 | 62 | 53 | 3.5 | 1.5 | 5.6 | 6.4 | 13.7 | Cu |
| **Coconut, fresh (flesh)** 100g (3½oz) | 351 | 36 | 31 | 2.0 | 0.8 | 3.2 | 3.7 | 7.3 | Cu |
| **Hazelnuts** 100g (3½oz) | 650 | 63 | 4.7 | 50 | 5.9 | 14 | 6.0 | 5.0 | $B_1$, $B_6$ / Cu, K, Mg, P, S, Zn |
| **Macadamia nuts** 100g (3½oz) | 784 | 77.6 | 11.2 | 61 | 1.6 | 7.9 | 4.8 | 5.3 | $B_1$, $B_6$ / Cu, P |
| **Peanuts** 100g (3½oz) | 563 | 46 | 8.7 | 22 | 13 | 25.6 | 12.5 | 6.2 | $B_1$, $B_6$, Fol, Nia / Cu, Mg, P, S, Zn |
| **Peanut butter, crunchy** 100g (3½oz) | 606 | 51.8 | 12.8 | 19.9 | 16.8 | 22 | 13 | 5.4 | $B_6$, Fol, Nia / Cu, Mg, P, S, Zn |
| **Pecan nuts** 100g (3½oz) | 689 | 70.1 | 5.7 | 42.5 | 18.7 | 9.2 | 5.8 | 4.7 | $B_1$ / Cu, Mg, P, S, Zn |
| **Pine nuts** 100g (3½oz) | 688 | 68.6 | 4.6 | 19.9 | 41.1 | 14 | 4.0 | 1.9 | $B_1$ / Cu, Mg, P, S, Zn |

| | Cal (kcal) | Total fat (g) | Sat. fat (g) | Mono. fat (g) | Poly. fat (g) | Protein (g) | Carb. (g) | Fibre (g) | Useful source Vitamins/Minerals |
|---|---|---|---|---|---|---|---|---|---|
| **Pistachio nuts** 100g (3½oz) | 601 | 55 | 7.4 | 27.6 | 17.9 | 17.9 | 8.2 | 6.1 | $B_1$ / Cu, Mg, P, Zn |
| **Pumpkin seeds** 100g (3½oz) | 569 | 45 | 7.0 | 11 | 18.3 | 24.4 | 15.2 | 5.3 | Cu, Fe, Mg, P, S, Zn |
| **Sesame seeds** 100g (3½oz) | 598 | 58 | 8.3 | 21.7 | 25.5 | 18.2 | 0.9 | 7.9 | $B_1$, $B_6$ / Ca, Cu, Fe, Mg, P, S, Zn |
| **Sunflower seeds** 100g (3½oz) | 581 | 47 | 4.5 | 9.8 | 31 | 19.8 | 18.6 | 6.0 | $B_1$ / Cu, Fe, Mg, P, S, Se, Zn |
| **Walnuts** 100g (3½oz) | 688 | 68.5 | 5.6 | 12.4 | 47.5 | 14.7 | 3.3 | 3.5 | $B_6$ / Cu, Mg, P |

## FATS, OILS, SPREADS, AND SYRUPS

| | Cal (kcal) | Total fat (g) | Sat. fat (g) | Mono. fat (g) | Poly. fat (g) | Protein (g) | Carb. (g) | Fibre (g) | Useful source Vitamins/Minerals |
|---|---|---|---|---|---|---|---|---|---|
| **Black treacle** 1 tbsp | 39 | 0 | 0 | 0 | 0 | 0.2 | 10.1 | 0 | Fe |
| **Butter** 1 tbsp (15g/½oz) | 112 | 12 | 7.8 | 3.1 | 0.4 | 0.1 | 0 | 0 | A |
| **Cod liver oil** 1 tbsp | 99 | 11 | 2.3 | 4.9 | 3.4 | 0 | 0 | 0 | A, D |
| **Corn oil** 1 tbsp | 99 | 11 | 1.6 | 3.3 | 5.2 | 0 | 0 | 0 | E |
| **Golden syrup** 1 tbsp | 45 | 0 | 0 | 0 | 0 | 0 | 11.9 | 0 | |
| **Groundnut oil** 1 tbsp | 99 | 11 | 2.2 | 4.9 | 3.4 | 0 | 0 | 0 | E |
| **Honey** 1 tbsp | 69 | 0 | 0 | 0 | 0 | 0 | 18.3 | 0 | |
| **Jam, stone fruit** 1 tbsp | 39 | 0 | 0 | 0 | 0 | 0.1 | 10.4 | 0.2 | |
| **Jam, with edible seeds** 1 tbsp | 39 | 0 | 0 | 0 | 0 | 0.1 | 10.4 | 0.3 | |
| **Lard** 1 tbsp | 134 | 14.9 | 6.0 | 6.5 | 1.5 | 0 | 0 | 0 | |
| **Maple syrup** 1 tbsp | 39 | 0 | 0 | 0 | 0 | 0 | 10.1 | 0 | |
| **Margarine, hard** 1 tbsp | 111 | 12.4 | 4.0 | 5.6 | 2.1 | 0 | 0 | 0 | |
| **Margarine, soft polyunsaturated** 1 tbsp | 112 | 12.4 | 2.5 | 4.0 | 5.0 | 0 | 0 | 0 | D, E |

| | Cal (kcal) | Total fat (g) | Sat. fat (g) | Mono. fat (g) | Poly. fat (g) | Protein (g) | Carb. (g) | Fibre (g) | Useful source Vitamins/Minerals |
|---|---|---|---|---|---|---|---|---|---|
| **Marmalade, orange** 1 tbsp | 39 | 0 | 0 | 0 | 0 | 0.1 | 10.4 | tr | |
| **Mayonnaise** 1 tbsp | 109 | 11.9 | 1.7 | 8.2 | 1.3 | 0.2 | 0.1 | 0 | |
| **Mayonnaise, reduced-fat** 1 tbsp | 43 | 4.2 | 0.6 | 1.0 | 2.4 | 0.1 | 1.2 | 0 | |
| **Molasses** 1 tbsp | 40 | 0 | 0 | 0 | 0 | 0 | 10.3 | 0 | B_6 |
| **Olive oil** 1 tbsp | 99 | 11 | 1.6 | 8.0 | 0.9 | 0 | 0 | 0 | E |
| **Rapeseed oil** 1 tbsp | 99 | 11 | 0.7 | 6.5 | 3.2 | 0 | 0 | 0 | E |
| **Safflower oil** 1 tbsp | 99 | 11 | 1.1 | 1.3 | 8.1 | 0 | 0 | 0 | E |
| **Sesame oil** 1 tbsp | 99 | 11 | 1.6 | 4.1 | 4.8 | 0 | 0 | 0 | |
| **Soya bean oil** 1 tbsp | 99 | 11 | 1.7 | 2.3 | 6.5 | 0 | 0 | 0 | |
| **Sunflower oil** 1 tbsp | 99 | 11 | 1.3 | 2.3 | 7.0 | 0 | 0 | 0 | E |
| **Vegetable oil spray** 1 spray | 2.0 | 0.2 | 0 | 0.1 | 0.1 | 0 | 0 | 0 | |
| **Walnut oil** 1 tbsp | 99 | 11 | 1.0 | 1.8 | 7.7 | 0 | 0 | 0 | |

**DRINKS**

| | Cal (kcal) | Total fat (g) | Sat. fat (g) | Mono. fat (g) | Poly. fat (g) | Protein (g) | Carb. (g) | Fibre (g) | Useful source Vitamins/Minerals |
|---|---|---|---|---|---|---|---|---|---|
| **Apple juice** 100ml (3½floz) | 38 | 0.1 | tr | 0 | 0.1 | 0.1 | 9.9 | tr | C |
| **Beer, bitter** 287ml (½ pint) | 86 | tr | 0 | 0 | 0 | 0.9 | 6.3 | tr | B_6 |
| **Beer, lager** 287ml (½ pint) | 83 | 0 | 0 | 0 | 0 | 0.9 | tr | tr | B_2, B_6, Fol, Nia / P |
| **Carrot juice** 100ml (3½floz) | 24 | 0.1 | 0 | 0 | 0.1 | 0.5 | 5.7 | tr | A, B_6, C |
| **Champagne** 1 small glass (125ml) | 95 | 0 | 0 | 0 | 0 | 0.4 | 1.8 | 0 | |
| **Coffee, black** 180ml (6floz) | 0 | 0 | 0 | 0 | 0 | 0 | 0 | 0 | |

| | Cal (kcal) | Total fat (g) | Sat. fat (g) | Mono. fat (g) | Poly. fat (g) | Protein (g) | Carb. (g) | Fibre (g) | Useful source Vitamins/Minerals |
|---|---|---|---|---|---|---|---|---|---|
| **Cola** 1 can (330ml) | 135 | 0 | 0 | 0 | 0 | 0 | 36 | 0 | |
| **Cola, diet** 1 can (330ml) | 0 | 0 | 0 | 0 | 0 | 0 | 0 | 0 | |
| **Cranberry juice** 100ml (3½floz) | 61 | 0 | 0 | 0 | 0 | 0 | 14.4 | tr | C |
| **Fruit squash, made up with water** 100ml (3½floz) | 19 | 0 | 0 | 0 | 0 | 0 | 5.0 | 0 | |
| **Ginger ale, dry** 100ml (3½floz) | 15 | 0 | 0 | 0 | 0 | 0 | 3.9 | 0 | |
| **Grape juice** 100ml (3½floz) | 46 | 0.1 | 0 | 0 | 0 | 0.3 | 11.7 | 0 | C |
| **Grapefruit juice** 100ml (3½floz) | 33 | 0.1 | 0 | 0 | 0.1 | 0.4 | 8.3 | tr | C |
| **Mango juice** 100ml (3½floz) | 39 | 0.2 | 0 | 0.1 | 0.1 | 0.1 | 10 | tr | A, C |
| **Orange juice** 100ml (3½floz) | 36 | 0.1 | 0 | 0.1 | 0 | 0.5 | 8.8 | 0.1 | $B_6$, Fol, C |
| **Pineapple juice** 100ml (3½floz) | 41 | 0.1 | 0 | 0 | 0 | 0.3 | 10.5 | tr | C |
| **Scotch whisky** 1 measure (25ml) | 56 | 0 | 0 | 0 | 0 | 0 | 0 | 0 | |
| **Tea, black** 180ml (6floz) | 0 | 0 | 0 | 0 | 0 | 0 | 0 | 0 | |
| **Tea, green** 180ml (6floz) | 0 | 0 | 0 | 0 | 0 | 0 | 0 | 0 | |
| **Tea, herb** 180ml (6floz) | 0 | 0 | 0 | 0 | 0 | 0 | 0 | 0 | |
| **Tomato juice** 100ml (3½floz) | 14 | 0.1 | 0 | 0 | 0 | 0.8 | 3.0 | 0.6 | A, $B_6$, C |
| **Tonic water** 100ml (3½floz) | 33 | 0 | 0 | 0 | 0 | 0 | 8.8 | 0 | |
| **Vodka** 1 measure (25ml) | 56 | 0 | 0 | 0 | 0 | 0 | 0 | 0 | |
| **Water, bottled** 240ml (8floz) | 0 | 0 | 0 | 0 | 0 | 0 | 0 | 0 | |
| **Water, tap** 240ml (8floz) | 0 | 0 | 0 | 0 | 0 | 0 | 0 | 0 | |

| | Cal (kcal) | Total fat (g) | Sat. fat (g) | Mono. fat (g) | Poly. fat (g) | Protein (g) | Carb. (g) | Fibre (g) | Useful source Vitamins/Minerals |
|---|---|---|---|---|---|---|---|---|---|
| **Wine, red** 1 small glass (125ml) | 85 | 0 | 0 | 0 | 0 | 0.1 | 0.3 | 0 | |
| **Wine, rosé** 1 small glass (125ml) | 89 | 0 | 0 | 0 | 0 | 0.1 | 3.1 | 0 | |
| **Wine, white, medium** 1 small glass (125ml) | 93 | 0 | 0 | 0 | 0 | 0.1 | 3.8 | 0 | |

**FROZEN AND CHILLED DESSERTS**

| | Cal (kcal) | Total fat (g) | Sat. fat (g) | Mono. fat (g) | Poly. fat (g) | Protein (g) | Carb. (g) | Fibre (g) | Useful source Vitamins/Minerals |
|---|---|---|---|---|---|---|---|---|---|
| **Ice cream, chocolate** 100g (3½oz) | 180 | 8.0 | 6.1 | 2.0 | 0.3 | 3.5 | 25 | 0 | $B_2$ |
| **Ice cream, strawberry** 100g (3½oz) | 179 | 8.0 | 5.2 | 2.0 | 0.3 | 3.5 | 24.7 | 0 | $B_2$ |
| **Ice cream, vanilla** 100g (3½oz) | 177 | 8.6 | 6.1 | 2.8 | 0.3 | 3.6 | 19.8 | 0 | $B_2$ |
| **Jelly, made up with water** 200g (7oz) | 122 | 0 | 0 | 0 | 0 | 2.4 | 30.2 | 0 | |
| **Sorbet, lemon** 100g (3½oz) | 97 | 0.3 | 0 | 0 | 0 | 0.2 | 24.8 | 0 | |

**CAKES AND BISCUITS**

| | Cal (kcal) | Total fat (g) | Sat. fat (g) | Mono. fat (g) | Poly. fat (g) | Protein (g) | Carb. (g) | Fibre (g) | Useful source Vitamins/Minerals |
|---|---|---|---|---|---|---|---|---|---|
| **Brownie, chocolate** 100g (3½oz) | 341 | 11.4 | - | - | - | 5.5 | 67.5 | 1.5 | |
| **Carrot cake, iced** 100g (3½oz) | 359 | 22.7 | 5.5 | 5.3 | 10.7 | 4.3 | 37 | 1.0 | |
| **Cereal bar, chewy** 100g (3½oz) | 419 | 16.4 | 5.0 | 8.7 | 1.8 | 7.3 | 64.7 | 3.2 | $B_1$, $B_2$, $B_6$ / Mg, P |
| **Cereal bar, crunchy** 100g (3½oz) | 468 | 22.2 | 4.5 | 11.3 | 5.4 | 10.4 | 60.5 | 4.8 | $B_1$, $B_2$, $B_6$ / Mg, P |
| **Cheesecake** 100g (3½oz) | 426 | 35.5 | 18.8 | 11.4 | 2.8 | 3.7 | 24.6 | 0.4 | |
| **Chocolate cake, with butter icing** 100g (3½oz) | 481 | 29 | - | - | - | 5.7 | 50.9 | tr | |
| **Chocolate chip cookie** 1 cookie (25g) | 119 | 5.7 | 2.7 | 2.2 | 0.6 | 1.5 | 16 | 0.5 | |
| **Digestive biscuit, chocolate** 1 biscuit (17g) | 84 | 4.1 | 2.1 | 1.5 | 0.3 | 1.2 | 11.3 | 0.4 | |
| **Digestive biscuit, plain** 1 biscuit (13g) | 60 | 2.5 | 1.2 | 1.1 | 0.3 | 0.8 | 8.9 | 0.3 | |

| | Cal (kcal) | Total fat (g) | Sat. fat (g) | Mono. fat (g) | Poly. fat (g) | Protein (g) | Carb. (g) | Fibre (g) | Useful source Vitamins/Minerals |
|---|---|---|---|---|---|---|---|---|---|
| **Flapjack** 100g (3½oz) | 493 | 27 | 5.0 | 7.6 | 10.3 | 4.5 | 62.4 | 2.6 | $B_1$ / Fe, Mg, P, Zn |
| **Fortune cookie** 1 cookie | 30 | 0.2 | 0.1 | 0.1 | 0 | 0.3 | 6.7 | 0.1 | |
| **Fruit cake, home-made** 100g (3½oz) | 322 | 12.5 | - | - | - | 4.9 | 50.7 | 1.7 | |
| **Fruit cake, home-made, iced** 100g (3½oz) | 350 | 9.8 | 1.8 | 3.6 | 3.8 | 3.6 | 65 | 1.3 | |
| **Gingerbread** 100g (3½oz) | 379 | 12.6 | - | - | - | 5.7 | 64.7 | 1.2 | |
| **Ginger nut biscuit** 1 biscuit (10g) | 44 | 1.3 | 0.6 | 0.5 | 0.1 | 0.6 | 7.9 | 0.1 | |
| **Meringue (no cream)** 100g (3½oz) | 381 | 0 | 0 | 0 | 0 | 5.3 | 96 | 0 | |
| **Muffin, chocolate chip** 100g (3½oz) | 385 | 18.2 | 10.7 | 5.2 | 0.9 | 6.3 | 52.3 | 1.6 | |
| **Pancake, sweet** 1 small pancake (60g) | 181 | 9.8 | 4.2 | 3.9 | 1.0 | 3.6 | 20.9 | 0.5 | |
| **Pancake, unsweetened** 1 small pancake (60g) | 153 | 9.3 | 2.7 | 2.9 | 3.1 | 3.8 | 14.3 | 0.5 | |
| **Scotch pancake** 1 pancake (31g) | 84 | 3.0 | 0.2 | 1.1 | 0.7 | 1.7 | 13 | 0.5 | |
| **Shortbread** 1 biscuit (13g) | 66 | 3.6 | 2.4 | 0.9 | 0.2 | 0.8 | 8.2 | 0.2 | |
| **Sponge cake** 100g (3½oz) | 467 | 27 | 5.8 | 8.9 | 10.9 | 6.3 | 52 | 0.9 | |
| **Waffle** 1 waffle (50g) | 167 | 8.3 | - | - | - | 4.3 | 19.8 | 0.3 | |

## PASTRIES AND PUDDINGS

| | Cal (kcal) | Total fat (g) | Sat. fat (g) | Mono. fat (g) | Poly. fat (g) | Protein (g) | Carb. (g) | Fibre (g) | Useful source Vitamins/Minerals |
|---|---|---|---|---|---|---|---|---|---|
| **Apple pie, double crust** 100g (3½oz) | 266 | 13.3 | - | - | - | 2.9 | 35.8 | 1.7 | |
| **Crème caramel** 100g (3½oz) | 104 | 1.5 | 0.9 | 0.5 | 0.1 | 3.0 | 21 | 0 | $B_2$, $B_{12}$ / I |
| **Croissant** 1 medium (60g) | 224 | 15.6 | 5.9 | 2.8 | 1.0 | 5.0 | 26.1 | 1.0 | |
| **Custard tart** 100g (3½oz) | 280 | 16.7 | - | - | - | 5.7 | 28.5 | 0.9 | P |

| | Cal (kcal) | Total fat (g) | Sat. fat (g) | Mono. fat (g) | Poly. fat (g) | Protein (g) | Carb. (g) | Fibre (g) | Useful source Vitamins/Minerals |
|---|---|---|---|---|---|---|---|---|---|
| **Danish pastry, fruit** 1 pastry (110g) | 378 | 15.5 | 9.4 | 2.2 | 2.1 | 6.4 | 56 | 1.8 | |
| **Doughnut, jam** 1 doughnut (75g) | 252 | 10.8 | 3.2 | 4.0 | 2.7 | 4.3 | 36 | tr | |
| **Doughnut, ring** 1 doughnut (60g) | 242 | 13.4 | 3.5 | 5.6 | 3.6 | 3.7 | 28 | tr | |
| **Eclair, chocolate, cream-filled** 1 eclair (50g) | 187 | 11.9 | - | - | - | 2.0 | 18.9 | 0.3 | |
| **Lemon meringue pie** 100g (3½oz) | 251 | 8.5 | 3.1 | 3.5 | 1.5 | 2.9 | 43 | 0.7 | |
| **Mince pie** 1 pie (55g) | 239 | 11.7 | - | - | - | 2.3 | 33 | 1.0 | |
| **Rice pudding, home-made** 100g (3½oz) | 85 | 1.3 | 0.8 | 0.3 | 0.1 | 3.3 | 16 | 0.1 | $B_2$ / Ca |
| **Rice pudding, low-fat** 100g (3½oz) | 71 | 0.8 | 0.5 | 0.2 | 0.1 | 3.5 | 13.4 | 0.1 | $B_2$ / Ca |
| **SNACKS** | | | | | | | | | |
| **Cream cracker** 1 cracker (17g) | 29 | 0.9 | 0.4 | 0.4 | 0.1 | 0.7 | 4.8 | 0.2 | |
| **Popcorn, plain** 100g (3½oz) | 108 | 1.0 | - | - | - | 2.0 | 22 | 2.0 | |
| **Potato crisps** 28g (1oz) | 148 | 9.6 | 3.9 | 3.8 | 1.4 | 1.6 | 15 | 1.3 | |
| **Potato crisps, reduced-fat** 28g (1oz) | 128 | 6.0 | 2.6 | 2.4 | 0.7 | 1.8 | 17.8 | 1.7 | |
| **Pretzels** 28g (1oz) | 108 | 1.0 | 0.2 | 0.4 | 0.3 | 2.6 | 22.5 | 0.9 | |
| **Rice cake, unsalted** 1 cake (10g) | 34 | 0.3 | 0.1 | 0.1 | 0.1 | 0.9 | 7.3 | 0.3 | |
| **Rice and corn snacks** 100g (3½oz) | 410 | 8.0 | 1.2 | - | - | 6.5 | 77 | 1.0 | |
| **Tortilla chips** 28g (1oz) | 129 | 6.3 | 1.1 | 3.0 | 1.9 | 2.0 | 16.8 | 1.8 | |
| **Trail mix** 28g (1oz) | 121 | 8.3 | 1.6 | 3.6 | 2.7 | 3.9 | 10.4 | 1.2 | |
| **Wholemeal cracker** 1 cracker (7g) | 29 | 0.8 | 0.2 | 0.2 | 0.3 | 0.7 | 5.0 | 0.3 | |

# Useful addresses

The following organizations and associations provide an additional source of information about the topics covered in this book. They are presented in two broad categories: the first lists organizations dealing with nutritional and fitness-related issues; the second lists organizations that offer information and advice on specific medical conditions.

## Information on nutrition and fitness

**American College of Nutrition**
Online: www.am-coll-nutr.org

**American Dietetic Association**
Online: www.eatright.org

**Association for the Study of Obesity (ORIC)**
Online: www.aso.org.uk

**British Dietetic Association**
Online: www.bda.uk.com
5th Floor, Charles House
148/9 Great Charles Street,
Queensway
Birmingham B3 3HT
Tel: 0121 200 8080

**British Nutrition Foundation**
Online: www.nutrition.org.uk
High Holborn House
52-54 High Holborn
London WC1V 6RQ
Tel: 020 7404 6504

**Centers for Disease Control and Prevention (US)**
Online: www.cdc.gov/nccdphp/dnpa/nutrition.htm

**Centre for Pregnancy Nutrition**
Online: www. shef.ac.uk/pregnancy_nutrition
University of Sheffield
Tel: 0845 130 3646

**Children's Nutrition Research Center (US)**
Online: www.bcm.tmc.edu/cnrc

**Council for Responsible Nutrition (US)**
Online: www.crnusa.org

**European Food Information Council (EUFIC)**
Online: www.eufic.org/gb/home/home.htm
19, rue Guimard
1040 Brussels, Belgium

**Food and Drink Association**
6 Catherine Street
London WC2B 5JJ
Tel: 020 7836 2460

**Food and Drug Administration Center for Food Safety and Applied Nutrition (US)**
Online: vm.cfsan.fda.gov

**Food Standards Agency (FSA)**
Online: www.food.gov.uk
Aviation House, 125 Kingsway
London WC2B 6NH
Tel: 020 7276 8000

**Health Development Agency (HDA)**
Online: www.hda-online.org.uk
Holborn Gate
330 High Holborn
London WC1V 7BA
Tel: 020 7430 0850

**Infant and Dietetic Food Association**
Online: www.idfa.org.uk
6 Catherine Street
London WC2B 5JJ
Tel: 020 7836 2460

**Irish Nutrition and Dietetic Institute**
Online: www.indi.ie
Ashgrove House, Kill Avenue
Dun Laoghaire, Co. Dublin

**NHS-direct**
Online: www.nhsdirect.nhs.uk
Tel: 0845 4647

**National Institutes of Health Office of Dietary Supplements (US)**
Online: ods.od.nih.gov/index.aspx

**National Obesity Forum**
Online: www.nationalobesityforum.org.uk

**National Women's Health Network (US)**
Online: www.womenshealthnetwork.org

**North American Association for the Study of Obesity**
Online: www.naaso.org

**Nutrition Society**
Online: www.nutritionsociety.org
10 Cambridge Court
210 Shepherds Bush Road
London W6 7NJ
Tel: 020 7602 0288

**Soil Association**
Online: www.soilassociation.org
Bristol House
40-56 Victoria Street
Bristol BS1 6BY
Tel: 0117 314 5000

**Vegetarian Society of the United Kingdom**
Online: www.vegsoc.org
Parkdale, Dunham Road
Altrincham, Cheshire WA14 4QG
Tel: 0161 925 2000

**Weight Concern**
Online:: www.weightconcern.com
Brook House, 2-16 Torrington Place
London WC1E 7HN
Tel: 020 7679 6636

## Information on disorders

### ARTHRITIS
**Arthritis Care**
Online: www.arthritiscare.org.uk
18 Stephenson Way
London NW1 2HD
Tel: 020 7380 6500

## CANCER

**Breast Cancer Care**
Online: www.breastcancercare.org.uk
Kiln House
210 New Kings Road,
London SW6 4NZ
Tel: 020 7384 2984

**CancerBACUP**
Online: www.cancerbacup.org.uk
3 Bath Place
Rivington Street
London EC2A 3JR
Tel: 020 7696 9003
Helpline: 0808 800 1234

**Prostate Cancer Charity**
Online: www.prostate-cancer.org.uk
3 Angel Walk
London W6 9HX
Tel: 020 8222 7622
Helpline: 0845 300 8383

**World Cancer Research Fund**
Online: www.wcrf-uk.org
19 Harley Street
London W1G 9QJ
Tel: 020 7343 4200

## CARDIOVASCULAR DISEASES

**British Heart Foundation**
Online: www. bhf.org.uk
14 Fitzhardinge Street
London W1H 6DH
Tel: 020 7935 0185
Heartline: 08450 708 070

**Irish Heart Foundation**
Online: www.irishheart.ie
4 Clyde Road
Ballsbridge, Dublin 4
Tel: 01 668 5001

## DIABETES

**Diabetes UK**
Online: www.diabetes.org.uk
10 Parkway
London NW1 7AA
Tel: 020 7424 1000
Careline: 0845 120 2960

**Diabetes Federation of Ireland**
Online: www.diabetes.ie
76 Lower Gardiner Street
Dublin 1
Tel: 01 836 3022
Helpline: 1850 909 909

## DIGESTIVE DISORDERS

**Coeliac Society UK**
Online: www.coeliac.co.uk
PO Box 220
High Wycombe
Buckinghamshire HP11 2HY
Tel: 01494 437 278
Helpline: 0870 444 8804

**Irritable Bowel Syndrome Network**
Online: www.ibsnetwork.org.uk
Northern General Hospital
Sheffield S5 7AU
Tel: 0114 261 1531
Helpline: 01543 492 192

**National Association for Colitis and Crohn's Disease (NACC)**
Online: www.nacc.org.uk/
4 Beaumont House
Sutton Road
St Albans
Hertfordshire AL1 5HH
Tel: 0845 130 2233

## EATING DISORDERS

**Eating Disorders Association**
Online: www.edauk.com
103 Prince of Wales Road
Norwich NR1 1DW
Youth line: 0845 634 7650
Adult helpline: 0845 634 1414

## FOOD ALLERGIES

**Allergy UK**
Online: www.allergyuk.org
3 White Oak Square
London Road
Swanley
Kent BR8 7AG
Tel: 01322 619 898

**Anaphylaxis Campaign**
Online: www.anaphylaxis.org.uk
PO Box 275
Farnborough
Hampshire GU14 6SX
Tel: 01252 373 793
Helpline: 01252 542 029

**Hyperactive Children's Support Group**
Online: www.hacsg.org.uk
71 Whyke Lane
Chichester
West Sussex PO19 7PD
Tel: 01243 551 313

## KIDNEY DISEASES

**British Kidney Patient Association**
Online: www.Britishkidney-pa.co.uk
Bordon, Hampshire GU35 9JZ
Tel: 01420 472 021/2

## MENOPAUSE

**Menopause Amarant Trust**
Online: www.amarantmenopausetrust.org.uk
Amarant Clinic, 80 Lambeth Road
London SE1 7PW
Helpline: 01293 413 000

**Menopause Exchange**
PO Box 205
Bushey, Hertfordshire WD23 1ZS
Tel: 020 8420 7245

## MIGRAINE

**Migraine Action Association**
Online: www.migraine.org.uk
Oakley Hay Lodge Business Park,
Great Folds Road
Great Oackley
Northamptonshire NN18 9AS
Tel: 01536 461 333

**Migraine Trust**
Online: www.migrainetrust.org
2nd floor, 55–56 Russell Square
London WC1B 4HP
Tel: 020 7436 1336

## OSTEOPOROSIS

**National Osteoporosis Society**
Online: www.nos.org.uk
Camerton, Bath BA2 0PJ
Tel: 01761 471771
Helpline: 0845 4500 230

## RESPIRATORY AND SLEEP DISORDERS

**British Snoring and Sleep Apnoea Association**
Online: www.britishsnoring.co.uk
52 Albert Road North
Reigate, Surrey RH2 9EL
Tel: 01737 245 638

**Asthma UK**
Online: www.asthma.org.uk
Providence House
Providence Place
London N1 0NT
Tel: 020 7226 2260
Advice line: 08457 010 203

# Index

# Picture credits

The publisher would like to thank the following for their kind permission to reproduce their photographs:

(Abbreviations key: t = top, b = bottom, r = right, l = left, c = centre, a = above)

**12-13: Getty Images:** Stewart Cohen (t); **13: Corbis:** John Henley (b); **14: Camera Press:** Richard Stonehouse (tl); **15: Getty Images:** Arthur Tilley; **17: Getty Images:** Jonelle Weaver (br); **18: Corbis:** Darama (tl); **19: Corbis:** Nancy A. Santullo; **20: Zefa Picture Library:** creasource; **22: Getty Images:** Paul Avis (b); **23: Getty Images:** Photodisc; **24: Getty Images:** Ebby May; **25: Getty Images:** Barry Yee (bl); **27: Corbis:** LWA-Dann Tardif; **28-29: Masterfile UK:** Kathleen Finlay (t); **29: Alamy Images:** Imagestate (cl); **30: Retna Pictures Ltd:** Andrew Carruth; **31: Corbis; 34: Getty Images:** Photodisc Blue (br), Mel Yates (tl); **40: Robert Harding Picture Library; 50: Alamy Images:** The Anthony Blake Photo Library; **61: Alamy Images:** Jeff Singer (cl); **70: Getty Images:** Harald Sund; **72: Getty Images:** Gerard Loucel; **79: Getty Images:** Yellow Dog Productions; **83: Rex Features:** Woman's Own; **95: Rex Features** (tr); **Getty Images:** Rita Maas (bc); **96: Getty Images:** Photodisc/Ryan McVay (br), Antony Nagelmann (tr); **102: Getty Images:** Romilly Lockyer (bl); **107: Corbis:** Ariel Skelley; **109: Corbis:** Norbert Schaefer; **110: Getty Images:** Photodisc Collection; **111: Mother & Baby Picture Library:** Ruth Jenkinson; **112: Getty Images:** Paul Thomas; **116: Getty Images:** Bruce Ayers; **117: Corbis:** Rick Gomez; **119: Corbis:** Jose Luis Pelaez, Inc.; **126: Getty Images:** Duncan Smith; **128-29: Corbis:** Charles Gupton; **132: Alamy Images:** David Young-Wolff; **137: Corbis:** David Raymer; **138: Retna Pictures Ltd:** John Powell; **139: Food Features; 141: Getty Images:** Mark Williams; **142: Rex Features:** PHN (br); **Getty Images:** Photodisc (tl); **143: Alamy Images:** Jackson Smith; **144-45: Getty Images:** David Madison; **146: Corbis:** Steve Thornton; **147: Corbis:** Tim McGuire; **148: Empics Ltd; 149: Corbis:** Ed Bock; **150: Alamy Images:** Dennis Hallinan; **151: Photolibrary.com:** IPS Photo Index; **153: Corbis:** Ariel Skelley; **154: Getty Images:** Marc Romanelli; **155: Alamy Images:** Elvele Images (cl); **Anthony Blake Photo Library:** Joy Skipper; **158: Corbis:** Rob & Sas; **159: Corbis:** David Woods; **160: Science Photo Library:** BSIP, Chassenet; **161: Alamy Images:** ImageState/Pictor International (cbl); **Getty Images:** Photodisc (tr); **162: Getty Images:** David Sacks; **198: Science Photo Library:** BSIP Laurent/Pat H.Amer; **199: Getty Images:** Jurgen Reisch; **200: Getty Images:** Yellow Dog Productions; **202: Masterfile UK:** Kevin Dodge (tr); **203: Corbis:** Tom & Dee McCarthy (br); **204: Corbis:** Ken Kaminesky; **205: Alamy Images:** BananaStock (tr); **Getty Images:** Edward Holub (b); **206: Getty Images:** Sean Murphy; **207: Getty Images:** V.C.L.; **208: Alamy Images:** Photofusion Picture Library; **209: Corbis:** George Disario; **212: Alamy Images:** Studio M; **215: Science Photo Library:** Eye of Science; **216: Corbis:** Norbert Schaefer; **217: Alamy Images:** Mick Broughton; **223: Powerstock:** Fichtl (b); **Science Photo Library:** CNRI (t); **224: Alamy Images:** Rex Argent (cl); **Anthony Blake Photo Library:** Amanda Heywood (ca), Roger Stowell (cl), Steve Lee (cra); **225: Bubbles:** Lucy Tizard; **227: Science Photo Library:** Gca; **228: Masterfile UK:** Rick Gomez; **229: Anthony Blake Photo Library:** Georgia Glynn Smith; **230: Alamy Images:** Jackson Smith (b); **231: Getty Images:** Paddy Eckersley; **232: Alamy Images:** David Young-Wolff (b); **237: Science Photo Library:** CNRI (t); Getty Images: Victoria Blackie (b); **238: Masterfile UK:** Kathleen Finlay; **241: Science Photo Library:** Zephyr; **243: Science Photo Library:** Sheila Terry; **244: Alamy Images:** Butch Martin (b); **Anthony Blake Photo Library:** Eaglemoss Consumer Publications (c); **245: Anthony Blake Photo Library:** Sian Irvine (b); **Getty Images:** Zigy Kaluzny (t); **246: Getty Images:** Donna Day; **247: Getty Images:** Photodisc Green/David Buffington; **248: Corbis:** Michael Keller; **251: Alamy Images:** Jackson Smith (b); **252: Getty Images:** Caren Alpert; **253: Alamy Images:** Myrleen Cate; **254: Getty Images:** Photodisc Red/Ryan McVay; **255: Alamy Images:** Imagestate/Pictor (bl); **256: Anthony Blake Photo Library:** Martin Brigdale (b); Getty Images: Laurence Monneret (t); **257: Alamy Images:** Jackson Smith; **258: Science Photo Library; 259: Masterfile UK:** John Lee; **262: Anthony Blake Photo Library:** Joff Lee (bl), Tim Hill (bc); **263: Anthony Blake Photo Library:** Iain Bagwell; **266: Corbis:** Jose Luis Pelaez, Inc.; **267: Corbis:** Jose Luis Pelaez, Inc.; **274-75: Getty Images:** PBJ Pictures; **278: Alamy Images:** Butch Martin (cbl); **Getty Images:** Philippe Gelot (tr); **280: Alamy Images:** BananaStock (cla); **281: Getty Images:** Michael Krasowitz (tr); **282: Getty Images:** Photodisc Green (tr); **284: Getty Images:** Photodisc/K; Ovregaard/Cole Group; **286: Corbis:** Michael Boys (tl); **288: Getty Images:** Alan Becker (tl); **290: Alamy Images:** BananaStock; **293: Rex Features:** OPL (tl).

Every effort has been made to trace the copyright holders. Dorling Kindersley apologizes for any unintentional omissions and would be pleased, if any such case should arise, to add an appropriate acknowledgment in future editions. All other images © Dorling Kindersley

For further information see **www.dkimages.com**

# Authors' acknowledgments

We would like to thank our science editors, Gabriella Maldonado and Jamie Spencer, for their much appreciated assistance in all aspects of *Nutrition for Life*. Gabriella completed the majority of research for the book and developed the majority of tables and charts, and the vitamin and mineral directory, as well as the nutrient and recipe analysis information. Jamie Spencer has been very helpful at editing much of the clinical information we use to teach medical students and doctors into easy to understand text for consumers. We have learned a lot from her and very much appreciated the opportunity to work together.

We would also like to thank DK, our publisher, for recognizing the importance of nutrition to health and the prevention of so many chronic diseases. We thank the entire team for their brilliant editing and production job on *Nutrition for Life*. Jemima Dunne, Senior Managing Editor, provided the leadership needed to direct this immense project and always managed to know what the book needed. She deserves a great deal of credit for her vision and experience, which will help to make the book a success, both in North America and the United Kingdom for many years to come.

Irene Lyford and Liz Coghill, Senior Editors, for being so diligent about everything and including us in all the decisions about the text, photographs, headings, and charts. We are grateful for your writing, editing, and computer expertise and the ability to manage all the information that was sent back and forth via email, without ever losing anything. Sara Kimmins, Project Art Editor, and Marianne Markham, Managing Art Editor, also deserve many thanks for designing the book and directing all photography and selecting visual images.

We would also like to thank Isabel De Cordova, designer, Iona Hoyle, design assistant, Julian Dams, DTP Designer, Wendy Penn, Production Controller, and Sarah Coltman, Production Manager, for making this book a reality. We would not have been able to publish *Nutrition for Life* without you. Thank you!

Finally, we would like to thank our medical students at the University of Pennsylvania School of Medicine for research and writing numerous sections of *Nutrition for Life*. These are Jeremy Brauer, Caitlin Carr, Rex Parker, and Kristen Vierregger. They will surely make great doctors and their patients will benefit from their knowledge and continued interest in nutrition.

### Dedication From Lisa Hark, PhD, RD

To my children, Jamie Erica (10) and Brett Daniel (6), for their never-ending love for their mommy. They are glad that the book is finally finished and look forward to seeing me on television, which they have been asking me about for the past two years.

To my parents, Diane and Jerry, for their incredible support and constant stream of love and attention that they have given me over the years and especially while writing this book. They have been excellent role models by eating healthily and exercising every day for most of their adult life.

To my brothers and their families, David, Cinde, and Nicholas; Richard, Pam, Alexandra, Mitchell, and Samantha; and Jeffrey, Stacy, Rachel, Louis, and Joel, for their love and support for ever and always and for sharing in my excitement for the completion of the book.

To my mentor and friend, Dr Gail Morrison, Professor of Medicine and Vice Dean for Education at the University of Pennsylvania School of Medicine, for helping me reach my full potential during the past 15 years at Penn and for giving me the time and encouragement to complete this huge project.

To Dr Darwin Deen, my Medical Editor and friend, for being so committed to the science of nutrition and always looking for the evidence to support what we have written in this book. I could not have done the book without you, and I thank you for everything!

### Dedication from Darwin Deen, MD, MS

I would like to dedicate *Nutrition for Life* to my family, the crucible for all my ideas. To my mom, Ruth, who taught me that eating well was the path to health. To my dad, Darwin Sr, who stimulated my interest in nutrition. To my brother Anthony and my sister Irene who have always been my best audience, and to my children, Benjamin (17) and Jesse (14), who have challenged everything I ever learned about nutrition.

To my patients, whose demand for a single, easy-to-read, practical, and accurate nutrition book motivated me to write this book. My patients have always stimulated me to learn more so that I can take better care of them. They have always tolerated my exhortations to eat better and exercise more with patience and forbearance. For all of you who have asked your doctor for one comprehensive book about nutrition, we hope that *Nutrition for Life* will go beyond your expectations.

# Publisher's acknowledgments

**Dorling Kindersley would like to thank** Ian O'Leary for new photography; Beth Heald for buying and preparing food; Francis Wong for additional design assistance; Gemma Casajuana Filella and Karen Constanti for DTP assistance; Salima Hirani and Kathryn Wilkinson for editorial assistance; Anna Bedewell for picture research; Romaine Werblow – Picture Library; Babita Bholah, Liz Coghill, Laura Forrester, Martin Gough, Marek Gwiazda, Beth Heald, Iona Hoyle, Crispin Lord, and Francis Wong for modelling; Hilary Bird for the index; and Mary Lindsay and Teresa Pritlove for proofreading.

**Growth charts** are based on information and charts supplied by the Child Growth Foundation, which are subject to copyright. Originals can be purchased from Harlow Printing, Maxwell street, South Shields NE33 4PU.